Percutaneous Image-Guided Biopsy

Kamran Ahrar • Sanjay Gupta

Editors

Percutaneous Image-Guided Biopsy

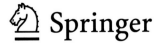

Editors
Kamran Ahrar, MD, FSIR
Department of Interventional Radiology
Department of Thoracic
and Cardiovascular Surgery
The University of Texas MD Anderson Cancer Center
Houston, TX
USA

Sanjay Gupta, MD, DNB
Department of Interventional Radiology
Department of Diagnostic Radiology
The University of Texas MD Anderson Cancer Center
Houston, TX
USA

Medical Illustrator
David L. Bier
The University of Texas MD Anderson Cancer Center

ISBN 978-1-4614-8216-1   ISBN 978-1-4614-8217-8   (eBook)
DOI 10.1007/978-1-4614-8217-8
Springer New York Heidelberg Dordrecht London

Printed on acid-free paper

Springer is part of Springer Science+Business Media (www.springer.com)

Preface

Percutaneous needle biopsy has largely replaced more invasive surgical methods of tissue sampling. The first image-guided biopsies were performed with fluoroscopic guidance; however, the true era of percutaneous image-guided biopsy was ushered in with the advancement of ultrasound, computed tomography, and magnetic resonance imaging technologies. Imaging guidance allows for precise targeting of lesions, resulting in high accuracy and low complication rates.

Traditionally, biopsies were performed to evaluate newly discovered masses or mass-like lesions in order to establish an initial diagnosis of cancer or infection. Biopsies today, in addition to performing a diagnostic function, are commonly obtained for detecting recurrence of metastatic disease and for monitoring response to therapy. Furthermore, in the era of molecular targeted therapy and personalized cancer medicine, accurate subtyping of tumors has necessitated the procurement of larger and more frequent biopsy samples. In the future, image-guided biopsy will likely play an even larger role in drug discovery, assessment of biomarker targets, and evaluation of disease susceptibility. In light of the growing number of indications for targeted tissue acquisition, it will likely become necessary for nearly all practicing radiologists to take part in this important endeavor at some point in their professional career.

Percutaneous Image-Guided Biopsy is a textbook and atlas that offers valuable information to every reader. This well-illustrated book was designed to be a practical, easy-to-use learning and state-of-the-art reference tool. Those in radiology training programs or those with limited previous experience in performing image-guided biopsies may read the entire book from cover to cover. Others may read a particular chapter in preparation for a specific upcoming procedure. Even for experienced radiologists, the book can serve as a quick reference to highlight various approaches to specific anatomic sites, list potential complications, and outline management strategies. Nearly all chapters provide detailed review of relevant anatomy with illustrations and an ample number of clinical cases to demonstrate the salient points of each section.

We hope that the readers will find this book informative and useful. We wish to express our sincere appreciation to all of the authors for sharing their time, knowledge, and skills in producing this volume, which ultimately attempts to enable every radiologist to perform image-guided biopsies safely and effectively.

Houston, TX, USA   Kamran Ahrar, MD, FSIR
Houston, TX, USA   Sanjay Gupta, MD, DNB

Contents

Contributors

Fereidoun Abtin, MD Department of Radiological Sciences, Ronald Reagan UCLA Medical Center, Los Angeles, CA, USA

Judy U. Ahrar, MD Department of Interventional Radiology, The University of Texas MD Anderson Cancer Center, Houston, TX, USA

Kamran Ahrar, MD, FSIR Department of Interventional Radiology, Department of Thoracic and Cardiovascular Surgery, The University of Texas MD Anderson Cancer Center, Houston, TX, USA

Rony Avritscher, MD Department of Interventional Radiology, Division of Diagnostic Imaging, The University of Texas MD Anderson Cancer Center, Houston, TX, USA

John A. Carrino, MD, MPH Radiology and Orthopaedic Surgery, Musculoskeletal Radiology, The Russell H. Morgan Department of Radiology and Radiological Science, The Johns Hopkins University, Baltimore, MD, USA

Debra A. Gervais, MD Division of Abdominal Imaging and Intervention, Department of Radiology, Massachusetts General Hospital, Boston, MA, USA

Sanjay Gupta, MD, DNB Department of Interventional Radiology, Department of Diagnostic Radiology, The University of Texas MD Anderson Cancer Center, Houston, TX, USA

Antonio Gutierrez, MD Department of Radiological Sciences, David Geffen School of Medicine at UCLA Medical Center, Ronald Reagan UCLA Medical Center, Los Angeles, CA, USA

Sanaz Javadi, MD Department of Radiology, Baylor College of Medicine, Houston, TX, USA

A. Kyle Jones, PhD Department of Imaging Physics, The University of Texas MD Anderson Cancer Center, Houston, TX, USA

Savitri Krishnamurthy, MD Department of Pathology, The University of Texas MD Anderson Cancer Center, Houston, TX, USA

David C. Madoff, MD Division of Interventional Radiology, Department of Radiology, New York-Presbyterian Hospital/Weill Cornell Medical Center, New York, NY, USA

David R. Marker, MD The Russell H. Morgan Department of Radiology and Radiological Science, The Johns Hopkins Hospital, Baltimore, MD, USA

Stephen E. McRae, MD Department of Interventional Radiology, The University of Texas MD Anderson Cancer Center, Houston, TX, USA

Department of Diagnostic Radiology, Division of Diagnostic Imaging, The University of Texas MD Anderson Cancer Center, Houston, TX, USA

Bruno C. Odisio, MD Department of Interventional Radiology, Division of Diagnostic Imaging, The University of Texas MD Anderson Cancer Center, Houston, TX, USA

Efe Ozkan, MD Department of Radiology, The Ohio State University, Columbus, OH, USA

Sendasaperumal Navakoti Sendos, MD Department of Radiology, Memorial Hermann Hospital, Houston, TX, USA

Colette M. Shaw, MD Division of Interventional Radiology, Thomas Jefferson University Hospital, Philadelphia, PA, USA

R. Jason Stafford, PhD Department of Imaging Physics, The University of Texas MD Anderson Cancer Center, Houston, TX, USA

Robert D. Suh, MD Department of Radiological Sciences, David Geffen School of Medicine at UCLA Medical Center, Los Angeles, CA, USA

Thoracic Imaging and Intervention, Department of Radiology, Ronald Reagan UCLA Medical Center, Los Angeles, CA, USA

Alda Lui Tam, MD, MBA, FRCPC Department of Interventional Radiology, Department of Diagnostic Radiology, The University of Texas MD Anderson Cancer Center, Houston, TX, USA

Ashraf Thabet, MD Division of Abdominal Imaging and Intervention, Department of Radiology, Massachusetts General Hospital, Boston, MA, USA

Aradhana M. Venkatesan, MD Department of Radiology and Imaging Sciences and Center for Interventional Oncology, NIH Clinical Center, Bethesda, MD, USA

Bradford J. Wood, MD Department of Radiology and Imaging Sciences, Center for Interventional Oncology, Interventional Radiology, NIH Clinical Center, Bethesda, MD, USA

Biopsy Devices and Techniques

Kamran Ahrar and Sanaz Javadi

Background

With the development and refinement of various cross-sectional imaging technologies such as ultrasonography, computed tomography (CT), and magnetic resonance imaging (MRI), masses and tumors are easily identified in virtually any part of the human body. In some cases, a single imaging study or a combination of two or more cross-sectional imaging studies can establish a firm diagnosis and obviate the need for biopsy. For example, simple cysts in the liver or kidney can be adequately characterized by imaging studies [1, 2]. Similarly, tumors of the kidney that contain macroscopic fat are characterized as benign angiomyolipomas on imaging studies [3, 4]. Most liver hemangiomas demonstrate a characteristic enhancement pattern on CT or MRI [5, 6]; thus, a biopsy is not necessary to proceed with the appropriate treatment of these patients.

On the other hand, cross-sectional imaging features of most masses and tumors are nonspecific and may represent either benign or malignant processes. To complement the anatomic characterization of tumors by CT, MRI, or ultrasonography, functional imaging studies such as positron emission tomography have been developed [7]. Currently available radionuclide agents can detect metabolic activity within a mass, which may be the result of benign inflammation or of a malignant process [8, 9]; however, a firm diagnosis of malignancy within a mass cannot be established solely on nonspecific metabolic activity.

Percutaneous image-guided biopsy is often necessary to confirm a diagnosis of malignancy. Without the firm diagnosis of a specific malignancy, a treatment plan cannot be established. Percutaneous image-guided biopsy is also important to characterize locoregional spread, lymph node involvement, and distant metastases [10]. With the emergence of targeted therapeutics aimed at specific molecular defects, the demand for biopsy procedures and tissue sampling has dramatically increased in the past few years [11]. For cancer patients who are undergoing treatment, a repeat biopsy may be necessary to evaluate response to therapy, to characterize residual disease, or to confirm recurrent cancer. In addition to sampling tumors, percutaneous image-guided biopsy of specific organs can help determine the cause of organ dysfunction or failure. For example, in patients who have cirrhosis of the liver, liver failure, graft-versus-host disease, acute renal failure, or renal dysfunction in a transplanted kidney, percutaneous image-guided biopsy is an integral part of the diagnostic workup [12–16].

Over the years, various techniques have been developed to obtain appropriate percutaneous biopsy samples from different parts of the body to establish a definitive pathological diagnosis. Similarly, various needles and devices have been designed, manufactured, and marketed for specific applications. A familiarity with specific devices, including their strengths and weaknesses for particular applications, and an understanding of biopsy techniques will help ensure safe and successful sampling of the targeted organ or tumor.

K. Ahrar, MD, FSIR (✉)
Department of Interventional Radiology, Department of Thoracic and Cardiovascular Surgery, The University of Texas MD Anderson Cancer Center, 1515 Holcombe Boulevard, Unit 1471, Houston, TX 77030, USA
e-mail: kahrar@mdanderson.org

S. Javadi, MD
Department of Radiology, Baylor College of Medicine, One Baylor Plaza, Unit 360, Houston, TX 77030, USA
e-mail: sjavadi@bcm.edu

Devices

Percutaneous Biopsy Needles

Biopsy needles can be divided into two broad categories based on their sampling mechanisms: aspiration needles and cutting needles [17]. Aspiration needles are designed

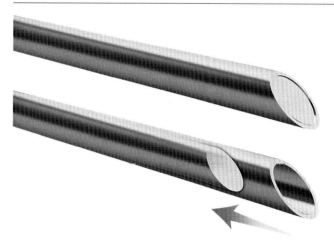

Fig. 1.1 Chiba aspiration biopsy needle. A thin-walled cannula with a beveled tip angled 25° is fitted with a matching stylet

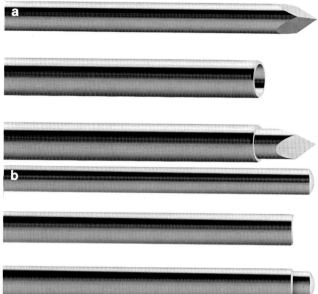

Fig. 1.2 The Hawkins and TruGuide aspiration needles are fitted with a sharp trocar tip (**a**) as well as a blunt-tipped (**b**) stylet. The stylet is shown on *top* of each figure, the cannula is shown in the *middle*, and the appearance of the stylet fitted in the cannula is depicted at the *bottom* of each figure

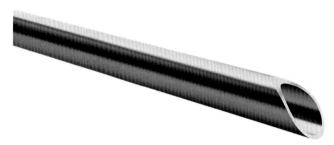

Fig. 1.3 Menghini-type needle has a sharp, beveled convex tip with a 45° angle. When moved forward into the tumor, it cuts out a cylinder of tissue

to obtain samples for cytologic assessment. These needles are generally small in caliber (20–25 gauge) and dissect rather than sever the tissue to obtain individual cells rather than pieces of the tissue [18]. The Chiba needle (Cook, Bloomington, IN), one of the most commonly used aspiration biopsy needles, consists of a thin-walled cannula with a beveled tip angled 25° and a matching stylet (Fig. 1.1) [19]. Spinal needles (Cook) are also commonly used for fine-needle aspiration (FNA) biopsies. In comparison with Chiba needles, spinal needles have a smaller inner lumen and a thicker wall. As such, they are easier to guide if a single-needle technique is used (see the following discussion). Small-caliber aspiration needles cause minimal tissue disruption; therefore, traversing bowel, stomach, liver, or other structures is believed to be well tolerated [20–27]. Within the range of FNA biopsy needles, better samples and increased yield have been reported using 20-gauge needles rather than smaller needles without a significant increase in complication rates [17]. The angle of the beveled tip is another important factor, as a more acute, smaller angle (e.g., the 25° Chiba needle) yields a better specimen than does a less acute, larger angle (e.g., the 90° Green needle or 45° Turner needle) [28].

The Hawkins (Cook) and TruGuide aspiration needles (Bard Biopsy System, Tempe, AZ) are equipped with a sharp trocar tip and a blunt-tipped stylet (Fig. 1.2) [29, 30]. These needles are particularly useful for getting past loops of small bowel and for reaching mesenteric nodes and masses. The blunt-tipped stylet may also prevent puncture of intervening vascular structures [30]. The sharp trocar stylet is used to get through the subcutaneous tissues and peritoneal wall. Once the cannula reaches the peritoneal fat, the blunt-tipped stylet is used to gently advance the needle. A gentle touch of the blunt stylet causes peristalsis, and this motion of the bowel clears the path to the target.

Cutting needles are used to obtain tissue samples for histologic analysis. These needles are further classified as end-cutting or side-cutting, depending on their design. The first-generation end-cutting needles were basically aspiration needles with a sharpened tip for cutting.

Several different needle types were developed with various beveled angles, needle tips, and stylet configurations [28]. The simplest end-cutting needle is a Menghini needle (Dyna Medical Corp., London, Ontario, Canada). It has a sharp, beveled convex tip with a 45° angle (Fig. 1.3). When moved forward into the tumor, it cuts out a cylinder of tissue [31]. The cutting tip of the Franseen needle (Cook) is serrated and has a sawtooth appearance (Fig. 1.4) [32]. With rotation and forward movement, the needle cuts into the tissue, collecting a small core biopsy sample. The Westcott needle (Cardinal Health, Dublin, OH) has a combined side-cutting and end-cutting mechanism. It has a side slot

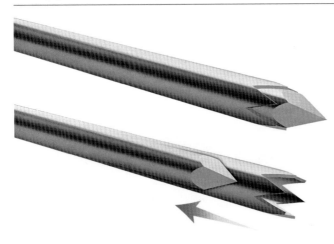

Fig. 1.4 Franseen-type needle has a serrated tip. With rotation and forward movement, the needle cuts into the tissue, collecting a relatively small core biopsy sample

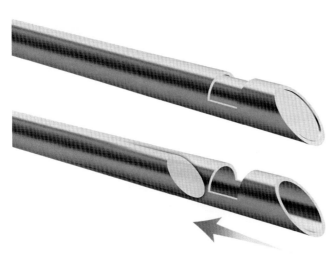

Fig. 1.5 Westcott-type needle has a side slot near the tip of the needle. The dual sampling mechanism consisting of the side slot and the end hole allows for collection of larger amount of tissue compared to other end-cutting core biopsy needles

measuring approximately 2-mm long that is located a few millimeters from the tip of the needle (Fig. 1.5). The combination of the side slot and the cutting tip enables aspiration of a larger amount of tissue when compared to Menghini or Franseen needles [33].

Cope and Abrams biopsy needles are examples of side-cutting needles used in pleural biopsy in patients with pleural effusion [34, 35]. Both of these needles have a notch near the tip. Once the needle assembly is introduced into the pleural cavity, the side-cutting edge of the needle is used to snag the pleura and collect a tissue sample. Multiple passes are often necessary to obtain an adequate sample. Cope and Abrams biopsy needles are often used in "blind" biopsy procedures without the use of imaging guidance. In the United States, blind biopsy procedures have primarily been replaced by image-guided biopsies using semiautomated cutting biopsy needles.

To increase the yield of cutting biopsy needles, a manual side-cutting needle was developed to cut a string of tissue [36]. The initial Tru-Cut needle consisted of an inner stylet fitted with a notch for trapping tissue and an outer beveled cannula for cutting the tissue. To obtain a biopsy sample, one would insert the whole needle into the edge of the targeted tissue, advance the inner stylet into the targeted tissue, and then move the outer cutting cannula manually over the stylet to cut the tissue trapped in the notch of the stylet. This would yield a semicylindrical piece of tissue.

In the more contemporary designs, the function of the Tru-Cut needle is automated in spring-loaded biopsy guns (Fig. 1.6) [37]. The automated devices obtain higher quality and more intact core biopsy samples than obtained with manual needles [37, 38]. Currently, side-cutting biopsy guns are available in a variety of sizes, ranging from 20 gauge (the smallest) to 14 gauge (the largest). The length of the tissue sample is determined by the length of the notch in the stylet, also referred to as the "throw" of the needle. Some automated biopsy devices have a set "throw" (e.g., 1 or 2 cm),

Fig. 1.6 Side-cutting core biopsy gun. QuickCore (Cook, Bloomington, IN) is a semiautomated, side-cutting core biopsy needle system (*arrow*). It may be used with a guide needle (*arrowhead*) during coaxial biopsy procedures (Permission for use granted by Cook Medical Incorporated, Bloomington, Indiana)

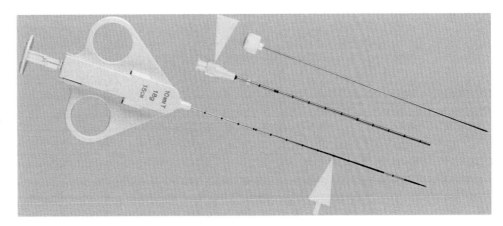

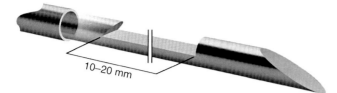

Fig. 1.7 Semiautomated cutting core biopsy needles allow procurement of tissue cores of variable lengths. Some needles have a predetermined throw, whereas others have an adjustable throw

whereas other devices have adjustable "throw" lengths (e.g., 1- and 2-cm options) (Fig. 1.7).

To operate a side-cutting biopsy gun, it has to be loaded prior to inserting it into the targeted tissue. For most devices, this is accomplished by pulling the stylet out until the spring is engaged. For needles with an adjustable throw (e.g., Temno; Cardinal Health, Dublin, OH), the trocar can be pulled until one click is heard for a short tissue sample or until two clicks are heard for a long tissue sample. The needle is then inserted into the edge of the tumor or just short of the targeted area within the organ of interest. In fully automated biopsy guns firing, the biopsy gun thrusts the inner stylet forward, followed almost instantaneously by the outer cannula. The specimen is cut and trapped in the side notch of the trocar. In semiautomated devices (e.g., QuickCore, Cook), the stylet is advanced gently into the tissue. Prior to firing the biopsy gun, additional imaging can be obtained to confirm that the needle is in the appropriate position. While holding the biopsy gun steady, the spring is released and the cutting cannula travels over the stylet, cutting a predetermined length of tissue that is trapped in the side notch of the trocar. The needle is then removed from the tissue. To harvest the specimen, the stylet is pulled back until the spring is engaged. The stylet is advanced gently to expose the sample for retrieval (Fig. 1.8). After retrieving the tissue sample, the needle is ready to be reinserted into the tissue to obtain additional samples.

The automated end-cutting biopsy needle (e.g., BioPince; Angiotech Pharmaceuticals, Vancouver, BC) has two cannulas. The tissue sample is obtained with a strong forward stroke of the cutting cannula. As opposed to the semicylindrical specimen obtained with side-cutting needles, end-cutting needles yield a cylindrical specimen that is slightly larger in diameter and volume for needles of similar gauge. One drawback of the end-cutting needle is a high rate of failure that results in no biopsy sample [39, 40]. This so-called zero biopsy may be more common with devices that have shorter throw lengths. Another disadvantage of automated end-cutting needles is that additional imaging cannot be obtained to confirm that the needle is in the appropriate position just prior to releasing the spring.

Needles larger than 18 gauge have been shown to increase the risk of pneumothorax during intrathoracic biopsy procedures [41]. In this case, a detachable 18-gauge cutting needle allows the largest possible sample to be collected without an

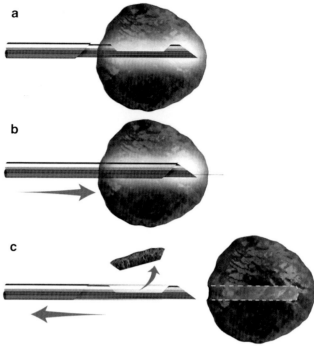

Fig. 1.8 Mechanism of a semiautomated cutting core biopsy needle. The stylet is advanced into the tumor (*top*). The position of the stylet can be confirmed by imaging. Once the biopsy gun is triggered, the cutting cannula travels over the stylet and traps the tissue in the groove of the stylet (*middle*). The biopsy sample is retrieved after removing the needle from the tissue (*bottom*)

increased risk of pneumothorax, potentially increasing the yield [42, 43]. Detachable cutting needles function as both a guide and a cutting needle. The notched stylet containing the specimen can be detached and removed while the cannula remains in place, allowing for multiple passes. However, reattaching the stylet to the cannula has been reported as cumbersome, and therefore these needles have not gained wide acceptance [42].

Transvenous Biopsy Devices

The rationale and technique for transvenous organ biopsy are further discussed in the next section. Briefly, liver biopsies in patients with irreversible coagulopathy or ascites are performed using the transvenous technique to avoid the risk of peritoneal bleeding. Initially, transjugular liver biopsies were performed using reverse-beveled end-cutting needles [44]. Contemporary transvenous biopsy devices use spring-loaded side-cutting needles (Fig. 1.9) [45]. A typical transvenous biopsy set (e.g., Cook) consists of the following essential elements: a multipurpose catheter for selective catheterization of the hepatic vein; a 7-French stiff cannula with an angled tip that can be pointed anterior or posterior; and a 60-cm long, side-cutting semiautomated biopsy needle with a 2-cm throw. Both 18- and 19-gauge needles are available.

Fig. 1.9 Transjugular liver biopsy system. The 7-French stiff cannula is fitted with a hemostatic valve (*white arrowhead*) for introduction of the 18- or 19-gauge side-cutting core biopsy needle (*white arrow*). The distal end of the stiff cannula is gently curved (*black arrowhead*). When the handle is rotated, the tip of the stiff cannula faces the wall of the hepatic vein, which is then pierced by the needle tip (*black arrow*) (Permission for use granted by Cook Medical Incorporated, Bloomington, Indiana)

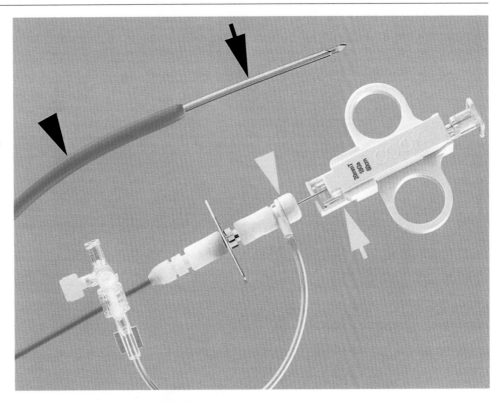

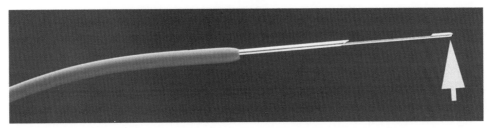

Fig. 1.10 Transjugular renal biopsy system. In comparison to the transjugular liver biopsy set, the core biopsy needle has a blunt tip (*arrow*) to prevent perforation of the renal capsule (Permission for use granted by Cook Medical Incorporated, Bloomington, Indiana)

In addition, a 9-French angled-tip introducer sheath can help stabilize access in the hepatic vein during the procedure. A shorter version of the device is available for use in pediatric patients. A transvenous biopsy set is also available for renal biopsies in patients with irreversible coagulopathy, severe hypertension, or small atrophic kidneys [46]. A transjugular renal biopsy set (Cook) is comparable to the set used in transjugular liver biopsy with some modifications [47]. The stiff cannula is fitted with a decreased curvature to accommodate the renal vein, and the biopsy needle is 70-cm long and has a blunt tip to prevent perforation of the renal capsule (Fig. 1.10).

When access to the hepatic or renal vein is not available using a superior approach, transvenous liver or renal biopsies can be performed from a femoral approach using biopsy forceps (Meditech) [48, 49]. The flexible forceps have oval-shaped, serrated cutting jaws. Biopsy samples are obtained by opening and wedging the jaws of the forceps into the targeted tissue (Fig. 1.11). A bite of tissue is trapped in the forceps when the jaws are closed. To cut the tissue, the catheter is pulled back into the introducer sheath. Once the biopsy forceps are removed from the patient, the jaws are opened to expose the tissue sample for harvesting.

Endoluminal Biopsy Devices

Biopsy of endoluminal lesions or strictures in the bile duct or ureter can be accomplished using biopsy forceps or brush biopsy devices [50, 51]. In the assessment of biliary or ureteral strictures, brush biopsy samples are more cellular than direct bile or urine samples owing to traumatization of the ductal epithelium or urothelium through contact with the abrasive bristles of the brush [52]. The brush biopsy device consists of a blunt-tipped flexible wire with a short, circumferential brush located near the tip of the wire (Fig. 1.12). The brush is contained within a 5-French housing catheter. An introducer sheath is necessary to maintain access in the bile duct or ureter while using the brush biopsy device.

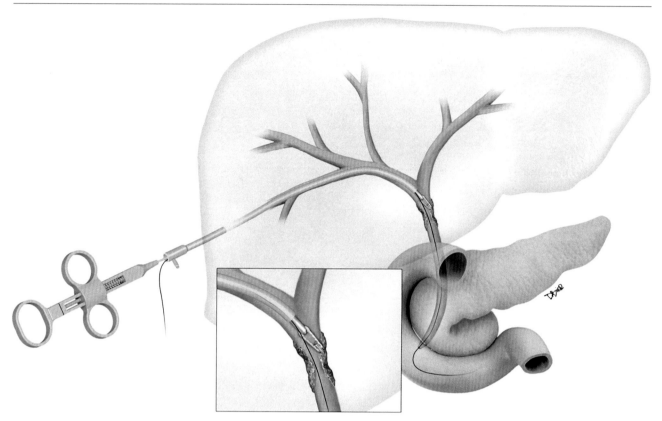

Fig. 1.11 Artist rendition of a forceps biopsy device used for sampling of a bile duct stricture. During the procedure, an introducer sheath is placed over a guidewire. The biopsy device is inserted alongside the guidewire. Once the forceps device is at the intended target, the sheath is withdrawn to expose the forceps. With the wings open, the device is advanced and wedged into the biopsy site. Once the forceps wings are closed, a bite of tissue is trapped. Pulling the device back procures the sample

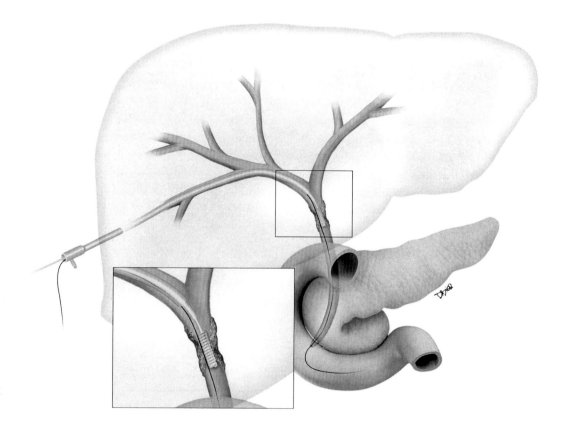

Fig. 1.12 Artist rendition of a brush biopsy device used for sampling of a bile duct stricture

Bone Biopsy Needles and Devices

Osteolytic lesions and tumors that destroy the bone can be biopsied using any of the soft tissue biopsy needles. Both FNA and cutting needles can obtain diagnostic samples. Special bone biopsy needles have been developed for sampling sclerotic bone lesions and for sampling targeted tissue that lies deep to an intact cortical surface. Stronger and possibly larger needles are needed under these circumstances. In general, most of these bone biopsy needles are designed to perform trephine biopsies of bony lesions with sufficient matrix [53]. An inadequate tissue sample volume or excessive fragmentation of the sample may lead to inconclusive pathology results. To sample a sclerotic lesion or to make an opening in the intact cortex of a bone, several needle designs have been evaluated.

The Jamshidi-type needles (Fig. 1.13) have a cannula and a trocar stylet that is fitted with a large sturdy handle to provide the operator with a good grip, allowing for application of pressure or turning of the needle as well as providing a surface where a light hammer can be used. Other bone biopsy needles have a serrated or saw-toothed cutting edge (Fig. 1.14), often used to sample hard sclerotic lesions. These needles are also fitted with a large handle to provide the operator with a good grip. The needle is advanced with the trocar stylet to the surface of the bone. Once the stylet is removed, the needle is turned while applying forward pressure to cut through the cortex or sclerotic bone. One drawback of this system is that to harvest the sample, the needle has to be removed completely from the bone.

The Elson bone biopsy needle (Cook) (Fig. 1.15) is designed for a modified coaxial technique (see below) where a 23-gauge needle with a removable hub is first inserted to the surface of the needle. Subsequently, a combination of a blunt-tipped cannula and a tapered obturator is advanced over the 23-gauge needle. A cutting needle with a serrated tip is advanced in coaxial fashion through the cannula. The cutting needle has a small disc-shaped handle, providing a grip that enables the operator to turn the needle. With this needle, and probably with other trephine biopsy needles, the cortical bone may clog the needle tip [54]. To obtain lesion tissue deep to the cortex, the needle should be unclogged by removing the impacted cortical bone. In this manner, additional biopsies from the lesion deep to the cortex will not lead to an impacted sample.

Other needles have a stylet that is shaped like an eccentric drill (Bonopty; Bone Biopsy System, Apriomed, Londonderry, NH) (Fig. 1.16). The stylet is introduced through the cannula in coaxial fashion and helps cut the cortex; the cannula is then advanced over the stylet to engage the bone (Fig. 1.17). In this fashion, the cannula acts as a guide needle for sampling the deeper tissue.

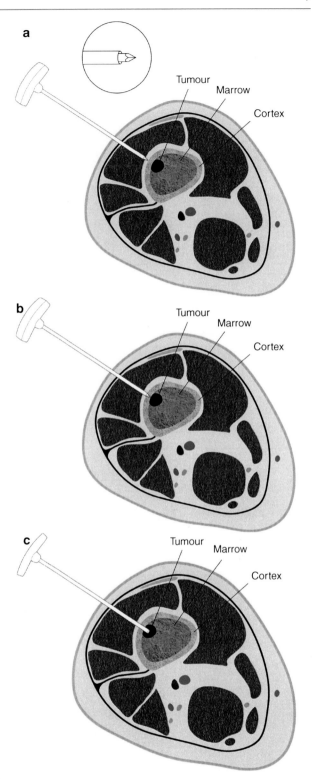

Fig. 1.13 Jamshidi-type needle for bone biopsy. These needles have a trocar stylet and a large sturdy handle (**a**). The needle is driven into the hard bone using a hammer (**b**), necessitating larger and stronger needle shafts. Usually, the smallest of these needles are 13 gauge in size. Once the cannula reaches the lesion deep to the cortex, the stylet is removed providing a conduit for placement of the sampling needle (**c**). If the tumor is lytic and has no bony matrix, any FNA or cutting core biopsy needle can be used for sampling. For sclerotic lesions, a Franseen-type needle with serrated tip can be used to obtain a trephine biopsy sample

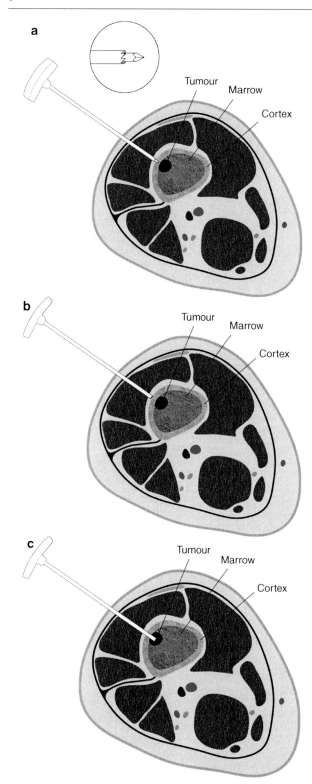

Fig. 1.14 Bone biopsy needle for sclerotic lesions. The cannula in these needles is fitted with a saw-toothed cutting tip. A trocar stylet helps advance the needle through the soft tissues to the surface of the bone (**a**). The stylet is removed, and the needle is advanced by turning it as the serrated tip cuts into the cortex (**b**). As the needle is advanced into the sclerotic bone, the cannula is packed with hard bone (**c**). To harvest the sample, the needle has to be removed from the bone completely

And finally, some needles have a threaded cutting cannula (Ostycut, Bard) (Fig. 1.18). A trocar stylet helps guide the needle to the surface of the bone. Once the stylet is engaged in the sclerotic bone, the cannula is turned to engage the bone. Turning the cannula further advances the needle into the hard bone.

For lesions that lie deep to an intact cortex and for sclerotic bone lesions, a handheld drill may be used to penetrate the bone [55]. Handheld drills are either manual or electrical, usually battery operated. The OnControl Bone Marrow Biopsy System (Vidacare Corporation, Shavano Park, TX) consists of a driver and biopsy needle set (Fig. 1.19) [56]. The battery-powered driver resembles a small handheld drill, weighs 315 g, and fits into a sterile bag fitted with an adaptor. Bone biopsy needles are 11 or 15 gauge and consist of a diamond-tipped stylet and a biopsy cannula with serrated tip. The hub of the needle is designed to fit into the adaptor. The device helps advance the needle with ease into the sclerotic bone.

Treated Needles for Use Under Ultrasound Guidance

Visibility of the needle on ultrasonography may be limited in tissues with increased echogenicity, deeper tissues, or when access is limited by overlying air or bone [57]. A poor angle of sonication (<20°) and a small-gauged needle also contribute to suboptimal visualization of the needle on ultrasonography [57]. Under these circumstances, treated needles facilitate detection and monitoring of the needle tip as it is advanced through the overlying tissues to the targeted tissue. There are several strategies to improve needle visibility under ultrasound visualization. Teflon (Cook) or echogenic polymer coating (Echo-Coat, STS Biopolymers, Inc., Henrietta, NY) on the biopsy needle helps visualize the entire shaft of the needle. One drawback of this technology is that over time the needles lose their coating, presumably owing to resorption of microbubbles by the surrounding fluid during the biopsy. Manufacturers have used dimpled (Fig. 1.20), etched-tipped (Cook), or screw-tipped stylets (Inrad, Grand Rapids, MI) to improve needle visibility ultrasonography. Visibility is usually limited to the last few millimeters of the needle's length. In general, coated needles seem to provide better echogenicity and better visualization than do partially etched or dimpled needles, particularly at small angles of insonication [57]. The diagnostic yield of ultrasound-guided biopsies is similar for treated and untreated needles; but with better visualization of the needle tip, the procedure may take less time and be safer for patients [58].

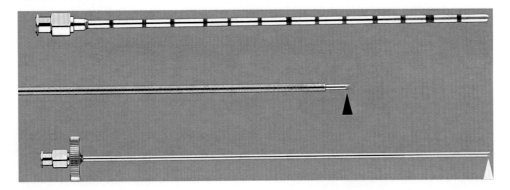

Fig. 1.15 Elson bone biopsy needle (Cook). This needle has three major components. First, a 23-gauge needle (*middle*) fitted with a trocar tip (*black arrowhead*) and a removable hub allows targeting of the tumor. Next, the cannula (*top*) fits over the 23-gauge needle as it is advanced to the edge of the bone. Finally, the biopsy needle (*bottom*) with serrated tip (*white arrowhead*) is advanced through the cannula to obtain a trephine biopsy sample. Multiple samples can be obtained through the cannula (Permission for use granted by Cook Medical Incorporated, Bloomington, Indiana)

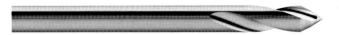

Fig. 1.16 Bonopty-type needles have a stylet that is shaped like an eccentric drill. The needle is driven into the bone by manually rotating it clockwise

MRI-Compatible Needles and Devices

Most biopsy needles are made of stainless steel and are not MRI compatible, as the needles may become projectiles in the presence of a strong magnetic field. Other alloys may be relatively MRI safe but may still create a ferromagnetic susceptibility artifact that is too large and is unacceptable for imaging purposes. As experience with MRI-guided biopsies grows and MRI-guided interventions gain acceptance in the interventional radiology community, more MRI-compatible needles and devices are being introduced on the commercial market. Currently, MRI-compatible needles are usually made of titanium alloys. These needles create minor artifacts, estimated roughly at twice the size of the needle [59]. But the exact thickness of the needle artifact depends on the magnetic field strength and specific imaging parameters [60]. Titanium needles are softer and more pliable, do not track as well as stainless steel needles, and may not be as sharp as their stainless steel counterparts [61]. Both aspiration and semiautomated side-cutting titanium needles are available for MRI-guided biopsies (Invivo, Gainesville, FL). A trephine bone biopsy set is available with a serrated-tipped cannula, allowing biopsy of sclerotic bone lesions (Invivo). An MRI-compatible handheld drill is commercially available to create an opening in the cortical bone and to sample sclerotic bone lesions (Invivo). The drill is operated using a piezoelectric motor and is fully MRI compatible.

Techniques

Various techniques have been described to increase the diagnostic yield and to minimize the complications associated with image-guided biopsies.

Percutaneous Biopsy Techniques

FNA Biopsy

For FNA biopsies, the mechanism of sampling is a rapid to-and-fro movement of the needle within the targeted tissue while maintaining negative pressure using a syringe connected to the hub of the needle. The rapid to-and-fro motion is repeated about 10–15 times or until blood is aspirated in the syringe, at which time the negative pressure is released to prevent further dilution of the sample with blood. In absence of blood filling the syringe, the negative pressure is released prior to removing the needle from the tissue to prevent aspiration of the sample into the syringe.

Several studies have suggested that negative pressure is not required to obtain an adequate specimen when using fine biopsy needles [62, 63]. Alternatively, sampling may rely on the capillary suction within a small needle to obtain a specimen and is referred to by various terms—cytopuncture [64], fine-needle sampling without aspiration [65], nonaspiration fine-needle cytology [66], and fine-needle capillary [67]. The rationale for the capillary technique is that samples may contain less blood or background clot when compared with the conventional suction FNA biopsy samples. Hopper et al. evaluated the effect of needle size and length on cytopathologic specimen quality for capillary and aspiration biopsy techniques [68]. The study demonstrated that the capillary techniques obtained less background blood or clot, although not significantly different from the aspiration technique

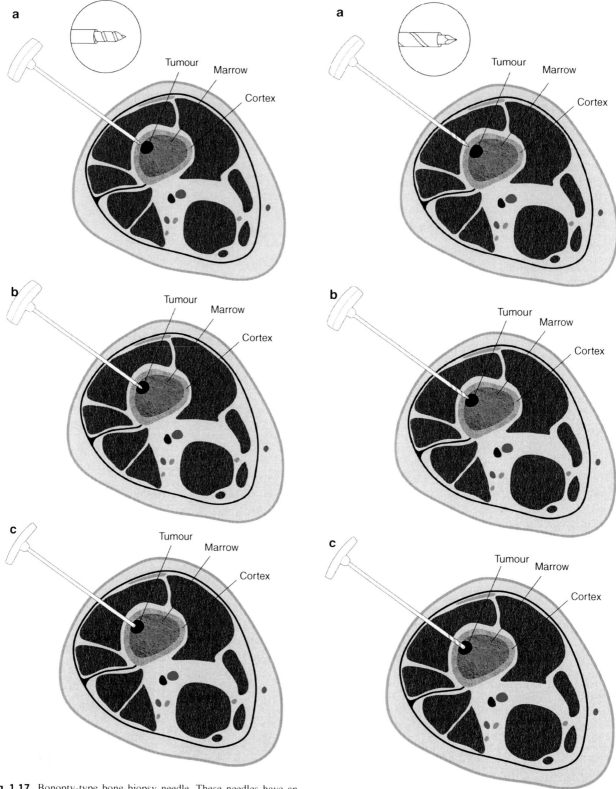

Fig. 1.17 Bonopty-type bone biopsy needle. These needles have an additional trocar stylet (not shown) to help advance the needle through the soft tissues. Once the cannula is positioned against the bone, the trocar is replaced with the drill stylet (**a**). As the whole needle is turned clockwise, the drill bit engages the bone (**b**). The stylet is removed, providing a conduit for coaxial biopsy needles and sampling of the lesion (**c**). The cannula must be removed from the bone carefully to avoid fracturing the tip

Fig. 1.18 Bone biopsy needle with a threaded cannula. These needles have a trocar stylet. The cannula is threaded to engage the cortex (**a**) and to drive the needle into the bone (**b**). Once the tip is deep to the cortex, the stylet is removed (**c**), providing a conduit for biopsy needles

($p = 0.2$). On the other hand, the aspiration technique resulted in significantly more cellular material and significantly better retention of the tissue architecture ($p < 0.01$).

Considering that application of minimal suction may be adequate for FNA biopsy, self-aspirating FNA needles were developed to potentially obviate the need to attach a syringe and apply suction during the biopsy [69]. These needles have an internal sealing diaphragm that creates a negative pressure within the cannula as the stylet is partially withdrawn. The diaphragm helps maintain the vacuum, permitting removal of the specimen without a syringe.

Single-Needle Technique

In the single-needle technique, the biopsy needle is inserted into the tumor to obtain one single biopsy sample (Fig. 1.21). It is unlikely that a single pass will provide adequate tissue for complete characterization of the tumor. Therefore, usually multiple passes are needed. Every needle pass requires image guidance, prolonging the procedure and increasing radiation exposure when CT or fluoroscopy is used. With each pass, the needle traverses the skin and the overlying tissues, resulting in patient discomfort and increased risk of complications such as hemorrhage. At our institution, the single-needle technique is only occasionally used for superficial lesions such as inguinal or cervical lymph nodes targeted under real-time ultrasound guidance.

Tandem-Needle Technique

In the tandem-needle technique, the first needle is inserted into the target under imaging guidance. Additional needles are placed immediately adjacent to and parallel with the initial needle without using image guidance (Fig. 1.22). When compared with the single-needle technique, the tandem-needle technique shortens the duration of the procedure and reduces radiation exposure when ionizing radiation is involved. However, the tandem-needle technique still requires multiple punctures. Moreover, localization of the tip of additional needles is not precisely controlled.

Coaxial-Needle Technique

In the coaxial-needle technique, a thin-walled guide needle is placed under image guidance in or close to the targeted lesion. Biopsy needles—either FNA or cutting needles—can then be advanced in coaxial fashion through the guide needle (Fig. 1.23). The guide needle is slightly larger than the biopsy needle. For example, a 19-gauge guide needle

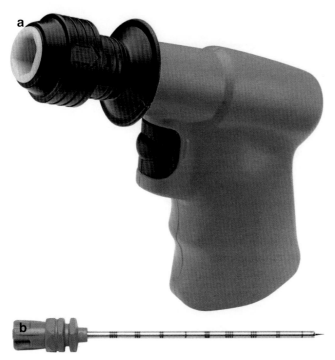

Fig. 1.19 Handheld drill for bone biopsy. The reusable, battery-powered driver of the OnControl Bone Marrow Biopsy System (Vidacare Corporation, Shavano Park, TX) (**a**) is placed in a sterile plastic cover (not shown) for each procedure. The hub of the disposable biopsy needle (**b**) fits into the drill (Published with permission from Vidacare Corporation)

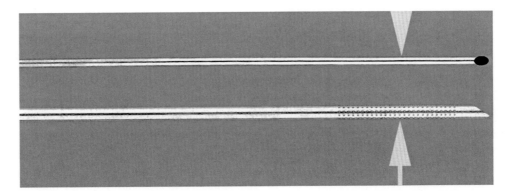

Fig. 1.20 Chiba aspiration biopsy needle with echogenic tip. The distal end of the cannula (*arrow*) is dimpled to improve its visibility under ultrasonography. The Chiba needle has a stylet that matches the 25° angle of the cannula (*arrowhead*) (Permission for use granted by Cook Medical Incorporated, Bloomington, Indiana)

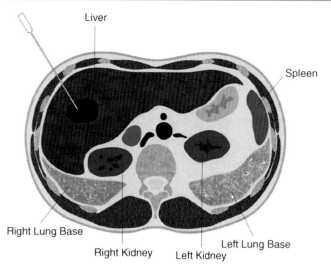

Fig. 1.21 Illustration of the single-needle technique. A biopsy needle is inserted in a liver tumor under image guidance. To procure the sample, the needle must be removed, leaving no access to the tumor. Acquiring more than one sample requires multiple organ punctures

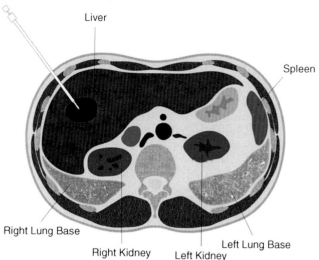

Fig. 1.23 Illustration of coaxial-needle technique. In this technique, a larger thin-walled needle is placed into the target under image guidance. Once the stylet is removed, the cannula provides a conduit for additional FNA or core biopsy needles to obtain multiple samples from the tumor

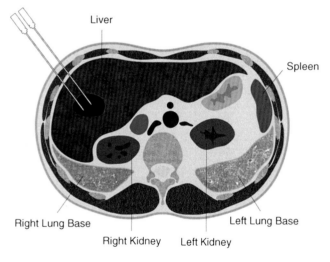

Fig. 1.22 Illustration of tandem-needle technique. The first needle is inserted into a liver tumor under image guidance. The second needle can be inserted immediately adjacent and parallel with the initial needle. Multiple punctures are needed to obtain more than one sample

accommodates 20-gauge and smaller FNA and 20-gauge cutting biopsy needles. The guide needle allows rapid sampling of the tumor using multiple biopsy needles without the need for additional imaging and with no additional discomfort or risk to the patient.

One potential shortcoming of the coaxial-needle technique is that after the first sample is obtained, additional sampling of the same location may yield little additional tumor tissue, and any additional tumor tissue may be diluted with blood. Although in vitro studies have shown that there is no significant drop-off in the quality of cytological specimens among the first, second, and third biop-

sies at a specific site [70], strategies have been developed to allow sampling of different parts of the tumor in coaxial fashion. A side-exiting guide needle may help avoid this potential problem [71]. This special guide needle is fitted with a side hole near the tip, where the 25-gauge FNA needle exits the guide cannula. The guide needle can be rotated incrementally, providing access to different parts of the tumor. A drawback of this system is the small size of the FNA needle (25 gauge), which may decrease the diagnostic yield of the biopsy. Furthermore, core biopsies cannot be obtained through the guide needle.

Alternatively, the beveled tip of FNA needles can be fitted with a gentle curve prior to insertion into the guide needle (Fig. 1.24) [72]. The degree and length of the curvature can be adjusted to match the location and depth of the targeted tissue in relation to the tip of guide needle. The tip of a 22-gauge Chiba needle is curled over a syringe, or it can be gently shaped using a pair of forceps such that the bevel is lined along the convex curvature of the needle. The curved Chiba needle retains its shape when it exits the guide needle and can be directed at different angles. Compared with advancing a straight needle through a guide cannula, the operator feels more resistance when advancing a curved-tip FNA needle in coaxial fashion. As soon as the biopsy needle tip exits the guide needle, the resistance to advancing the needle disappears. Care must be taken while removing the stylet from the curved-tip Chiba needle. There will be some increased resistance, requiring the operator to hold on to the biopsy needle while withdrawing the stylet. Otherwise, the whole needle may be pulled back. Similarly, when removing the curved-tip biopsy needle from the guide nee-

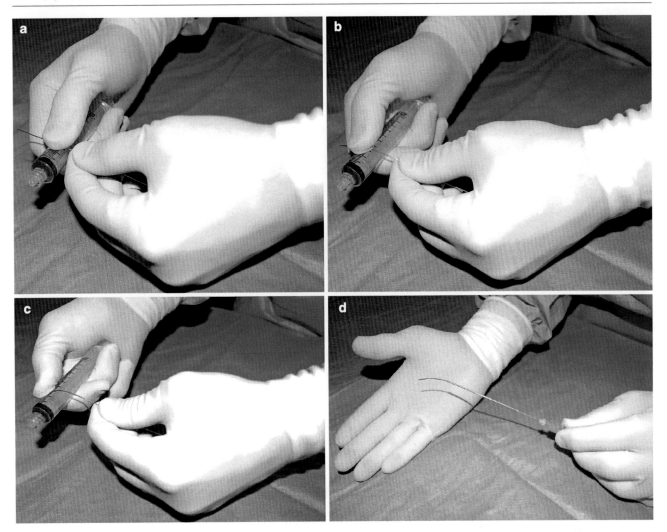

Fig. 1.24 Curved needle technique. A 22-gauge Chiba needle is placed over a syringe with the bevel facing up (**a**). The distal end of the needle is curled over the syringe (**b** and **c**). The bevel is lined along the convex curvature of the needle. The curved biopsy needle is placed through a guide needle (**d**), it retains its shape as it exits the guide needle. The direction of the curved biopsy needle is opposite the notch in the hub of the needles manufactured by Cook Medical and most other manufacturers

dle, the operator should fix the guiding needle in place. Otherwise, the curved-tip biopsy needle may pull the guide needle back as it is withdrawn from the target. Side-cutting automated biopsy needles can be shaped in similar fashion to obtain core biopsies from different parts of the tumor (Fig. 1.25) [73]. An exaggerated curve introduced to the stylet of these needles may lead to lower quality samples (e.g., fragmented) and possibly can lead to bending of the stylet as the cannula travels over the stylet.

If none of these strategies are successful in sampling different areas of the tumor, the guide needle can be repositioned within the tumor to allow redirecting of the biopsy needle. This can be accomplished by pulling the guide needle back, levering the needle, and advancing it to different areas of the tumor. Depending on the depth of the target and the stiffness of the overlying tissues, the guide needle may have to be pulled back a few or several centimeters to allow redirecting into different areas of the tumor. Stiffness of the guide needle is also an important factor. Thinner needles may actually bend as a result of levering rather than redirecting the path of the needle. For example, in a thin individual, an 18-gauge guide needle can be easily redirected in lung tissue by simply torquing the needle, whereas a needle that is inserted into the retroperitoneum through the paraspinal muscles needs to be pulled back nearly to the skin surface before it can be redirected.

A modification of the coaxial-needle technique involves the use of vanSonnenberg needle. Initially, a 23-gauge needle with a detachable hub is placed into the lesion. Once the needle is positioned, the hub is removed, and a 19-gauge needle is inserted over the 23-gauge needle. The small 23-gauge needle is then removed, and the 19-gauge needle

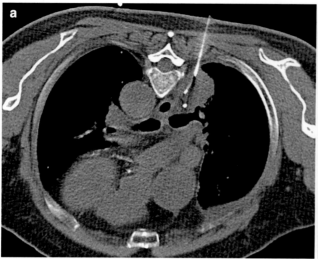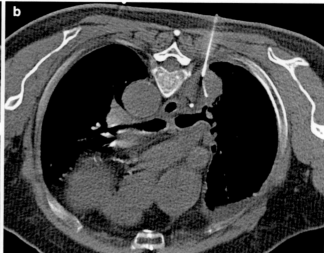

Fig. 1.25 A 68-year-old man with history of non-small cell lung cancer underwent chemoradiation. Follow-up CT demonstrated an enlarging mass in the right lung. During CT-guided biopsy, a 20-gauge core biopsy needle was gently curved and introduced through a 19-gauge guide needle to obtain core biopsy samples from the medial (**a**) and lateral (**b**) aspects of the tumor. Pathology showed squamous cell carcinoma with necrosis

is used as a guide for coaxial placement of FNA or cutting needles [74].

Using a blunt-tipped coaxial introducer needle, access can be established to sample lesions with intervening bowel loops or vascular structures [30]. First, the coaxial introducer is inserted with the sharp stylet into the thoracic or abdominal cavity. Then the blunt-tipped stylet is used to dissect along the tissues without penetrating the intervening organ, bowel, or vessels. Theoretically, the blunt stylet simply bounces off the organs or structures that should not be entered. Alternatively, the needle is used to displace the structure manually by levering the needle.

Transvenous Biopsy Technique

The need for nontarget biopsy of liver parenchyma in high-risk patients including those with irreversible coagulopathy or ascites led to the development of transvenous biopsy techniques [75–78]. To obtain liver samples using a transjugular approach, access is obtained in the right jugular vein. The left jugular vein is also acceptable, but the right is preferred. Using a multipurpose catheter, the right hepatic vein is selected. Use of an angled introducer sheath facilitates the biopsy, helping maintain access into the right hepatic vein. A 7-French stiff cannula with an angled tip is then inserted over the wire. The stiff cannula is turned counterclockwise to point anterior to the right hepatic vein where the liver parenchyma is thickest. A 60-cm side-cutting semi-automated biopsy needle is inserted in coaxial fashion to obtain biopsy samples. The coaxial nature of this procedure allows for collection of multiple samples. The stiff guiding

cannula has a tendency to move with normal respiration. It may disengage from the hepatic vein and retract into the inferior vena cava (IVC). To avoid this, the operator or an assistant should continue to exert gentle forward pressure on the cannula while the other person removes the biopsy needle and collects the specimen.

The right hepatic vein is usually preferred because of its predictable course and location placing abundant liver parenchyma anterior to it for targeting with the counterclockwise turn of the stiff cannula. The middle hepatic and left hepatic veins can also be used for transjugular liver biopsy, but the stiff cannula may have to be turned posteriorly to aim at the thickest portion of the liver.

When hepatic veins can only be accessed from a femoral approach, flexible biopsy forceps are used to obtain biopsy samples [49, 79, 80]. Khosa et al. reported using a long introducer sheath (9 French) that is advanced into the hepatic vein, usually the right hepatic vein [49]. An inferior right hepatic vein or a dorsal sector vein joining the right side of the IVC inferior to the main ostia of the hepatic veins may also be used. This vein provides a less acute angle to the liver and may be more easily accessed. With the tip of the sheath placed in the central liver within the middle third of a main hepatic vein, the biopsy forceps are advanced in coaxial fashion. The jaws are opened and wedged into the hepatic parenchyma. The position of the forceps can be further characterized by oblique or lateral fluoroscopy to avoid liver capsule perforation. Samples are obtained by closing the jaws and pulling the forceps back from the liver. This same technique may also be used to obtain biopsy samples from the kidney and any intravascular tumors [48].

Endoluminal Biopsy Technique

Endoluminal lesions involving the bile ducts or ureters can be biopsied with flexible forceps as described earlier [50]. Alternatively, brush biopsy devices can be used to sample areas of stricture or intraluminal abnormalities [51]. Initially, the stricture is traversed using a guidewire. An introducer sheath is then advanced beyond the stricture. The 5-French catheter containing the biopsy brush is inserted into the sheath and is advanced to the tip; the sheath is then pulled back to uncover the distal end of the housing catheter. Once the position of the biopsy device is optimized within the target area, the housing catheter is pulled back to expose the brush. Repeated to-and-fro movement of the brush within the stricture causes exfoliation of the cells by the abrasive bristles of the brush. The brush is pulled back just inside the 5-French catheter, and the whole assembly is removed from the sheath. The brush is then exposed to prepare touch-prep slides for immediate cytological evaluation. The remainder of the biopsy material can be placed in an appropriate solution, which is then used to prepare cytospin or cell block for further staining and evaluation.

In summary, image-guided biopsy is an essential step in establishing a definitive diagnosis for a variety of different medical conditions. Specific biopsy devices and techniques have been developed to render these procedures safer and more effective than in the past. In planning an image-guided biopsy, the interventional radiologist should carefully select an appropriate device and use the best techniques possible to avoid nondiagnostic biopsies and/or complications.

References

1. Horton KM, Bluemke DA, Hruban RH, Soyer P, Fishman EK. CT and MR imaging of benign hepatic and biliary tumors. Radiographics. 1999;19:431–51.
2. Israel GM, Bosniak MA. An update of the Bosniak renal cyst classification system. Urology. 2005;66:484–8.
3. Bosniak MA, Megibow AJ, Hulnick DH, Horii S, Raghavendra BN. CT diagnosis of renal angiomyolipoma: the importance of detecting small amounts of fat. Am J Roentgenol. 1988;151:497–501.
4. Bosniak MA. Angiomyolipoma (hamartoma) of the kidney: a preoperative diagnosis is possible in virtually every case. Urol Radiol. 1981;3:135–42.
5. Leslie DF, Johnson CD, Johnson CM, Ilstrup DM, Harmsen WS. Distinction between cavernous hemangiomas of the liver and hepatic metastases on CT: value of contrast enhancement patterns. Am J Roentgenol. 1995;164:625–9.
6. Motosugi U, Ichikawa T, Onohara K, Sou H, Sano K, Muhi A, et al. Distinguishing hepatic metastasis from hemangioma using gadoxetic acid-enhanced magnetic resonance imaging. Invest Radiol. 2011;46:359–65.
7. Czernin J, Benz MR, Allen-Auerbach MS. PET/CT imaging: the incremental value of assessing the glucose metabolic phenotype and the structure of cancers in a single examination. Eur J Radiol. 2010;73:470–80.
8. Gemmel F, Rijk PC, Collins JM, Parlevliet T, Stumpe KD, Palestro CJ. Expanding role of 18F-fluoro-D-deoxyglucose PET and PET/CT in spinal infections. Eur Spine J. 2010;19:540–51.
9. Poeppel TD, Krause BJ, Heusner TA, Boy C, Bockisch A, Antoch G. PET/CT for the staging and follow-up of patients with malignancies. Eur J Radiol. 2009;70:382–92.
10. Gupta S. Role of image-guided percutaneous needle biopsy in cancer staging. Semin Roentgenol. 2006;41:78–90.
11. Clark DP. Seize the opportunity: underutilization of fine-needle aspiration biopsy to inform targeted cancer therapy decisions. Cancer. 2009;117:289–97.
12. Mookerjee RP, Lackner C, Stauber R, Stadlbauer V, Deheragoda M, Aigelsreiter A, et al. The role of liver biopsy in the diagnosis and prognosis of patients with acute deterioration of alcoholic cirrhosis. J Hepatol. 2011;55(5):1103–11.
13. Sheth SG, Gordon FD, Chopra S. Nonalcoholic steatohepatitis. Ann Intern Med. 1997;126:137–45.
14. Mahgerefteh SY, Sosna J, Bogot N, Shapira MY, Pappo O, Bloom AI. Radiologic imaging and intervention for gastrointestinal and hepatic complications of hematopoietic stem cell transplantation. Radiology. 2011;258:660–71.
15. Fuiano G, Mazza G, Comi N, Caglioti A, De Nicola L, Iodice C, et al. Current indications for renal biopsy: a questionnaire-based survey. Am J Kidney Dis. 2000;35:448–57.
16. Furness PN, Philpott CM, Chorbadjian MT, Nicholson ML, Bosmans JL, Corthouts BL, et al. Protocol biopsy of the stable renal transplant: a multicenter study of methods and complication rates. Transplantation. 2003;76:969–73.
17. Gazelle GS, Haaga JR. Biopsy needle characteristics. Cardiovasc Intervent Radiol. 1991;14:13–6.
18. Gazelle GS, Haaga JR, Rowland DY. Effect of needle gauge, level of anticoagulation, and target organ on bleeding associated with aspiration biopsy. Work in progress. Radiology. 1992;183:509–13.
19. Okuda K, Tanikawa K, Emura T, Kuratomi S, Jinnouchi S. Nonsurgical, percutaneous transhepatic cholangiography – diagnostic significance in medical problems of the liver. Am J Dig Dis. 1974;19:21–36.
20. Isler RJ, Ferrucci Jr JT, Wittenberg J, Mueller PR, Simeone JF, vanSonnenberg E, et al. Tissue core biopsy of abdominal tumors with a 22 gauge cutting needle. Am J Roentgenol. 1981;136:725–8.
21. Wittenberg J, Mueller PR, Ferrucci Jr JT, Simeone JF, vanSonnenberg E, Neff CC, et al. Percutaneous core biopsy of abdominal tumors using 22 gauge needles: further observations. Am J Roentgenol. 1982;139:75–80.
22. Ferrucci Jr JT, Wittenberg J. CT biopsy of abdominal tumors: aids for lesion localization. Radiology. 1978;129:739–44.
23. Ferrucci Jr JT, Wittenberg J, Mueller PR, Simeone JF, Harbin WP, Kirkpatrick RH, et al. Diagnosis of abdominal malignancy by radiologic fine-needle aspiration biopsy. Am J Roentgenol. 1980;134:323–30.
24. Sundaram M, Wolverson MK, Heiberg E, Pilla T, Vas WG, Shields JB. Utility of CT-guided abdominal aspiration procedures. Am J Roentgenol. 1982;139:1111–15.
25. Yamamoto R, Tatsuta M, Noguchi S, Kasugai H, Okano Y, Okuda S, et al. Histocytologic diagnosis of pancreatic cancer by percutaneous aspiration biopsy under ultrasonic guidance. Am J Clin Pathol. 1985;83:409–14.
26. Hall-Craggs MA, Lees WR. Fine-needle aspiration biopsy: pancreatic and biliary tumors. Am J Roentgenol. 1986;147:399–403.
27. Dickey JE, Haaga JR, Stellato TA, Schultz CL, Hau T. Evaluation of computed tomography guided percutaneous biopsy of the pancreas. Surg Gynecol Obstet. 1986;163:497–503.
28. Andriole JG, Haaga JR, Adams RB, Nunez C. Biopsy needle characteristics assessed in the laboratory. Radiology. 1983;148:659–62.
29. Akins EW, Hawkins Jr IF, Mladinich C, Tupler R, Siragusa RJ, Pry R. The blunt needle: a new percutaneous access device. Am J Roentgenol. 1989;152:181–2.

30. de Bazelaire C, Farges C, Mathieu O, Zagdanski AM, Bourrier P, Frija J, et al. Blunt-tip coaxial introducer: a revisited tool for difficult CT-guided biopsy in the chest and abdomen. Am J Roentgenol. 2009;193:W144–8.

31. Menghini G. One-second needle biopsy of the liver. N Engl J Med. 1970;282:582–5.

32. Franseen CC. Aspiration biopsy, with a description of a new type of needle. N Engl J Med. 1941;224:1054–8.

33. Westcott JL. Direct percutaneous needle aspiration of localized pulmonary lesions: result in 422 patients. Radiology. 1980;137:31–5.

34. Cope C. New pleural biopsy needle; preliminary study. J Am Med Assoc. 1958;167:1107–8.

35. Abrams LD. A pleural-biopsy punch. Lancet. 1958;1:30–1.

36. Littlewood ER, Gilmore IT, Murray-Lyon IM, Stephens KR, Paradinas FJ. Comparison of the Trucut and Surecut liver biopsy needles. J Clin Pathol. 1982;35:761–3.

37. Hopper KD, Abendroth CS, Sturtz KW, Matthews YL, Shirk SJ, Stevens LA. Blinded comparison of biopsy needles and automated devices in vitro: 1. Biopsy of diffuse hepatic disease. Am J Roentgenol. 1993;161:1293–7.

38. Hopper KD, Abendroth CS, Sturtz KW, Matthews YL, Shirk SJ, Stevens LA. Blinded comparison of biopsy needles and automated devices in vitro: 2. Biopsy of medical renal disease. Am J Roentgenol. 1993;161:1299–301.

39. Haggarth L, Ekman P, Egevad L. A new core-biopsy instrument with an end-cut technique provides prostate biopsies with increased tissue yield. BJU Int. 2002;90:51–5.

40. Ozden E, Gogus C, Tulunay O, Baltaci S. The long core needle with an end-cut technique for prostate biopsy: does it really have advantages when compared with standard needles? Eur Urol. 2004;45:287–91.

41. Klein JS, Zarka MA. Transthoracic needle biopsy: an overview. J Thorac Imaging. 1997;12:232–49.

42. Moulton JS, Moore PT. Coaxial percutaneous biopsy technique with automated biopsy devices: value in improving accuracy and negative predictive value. Radiology. 1993;186:515–22.

43. Lucidarme O, Howarth N, Finet JF, Grenier PA. Intrapulmonary lesions: percutaneous automated biopsy with a detachable, 18-gauge, coaxial cutting needle. Radiology. 1998;207:759–65.

44. Colapinto RF, Blendis LM. Liver biopsy through the transjugular approach. Modification of instruments. Radiology. 1983; 148:306.

45. Smith TP, Presson TL, Heneghan MA, Ryan JM. Transjugular biopsy of the liver in pediatric and adult patients using an 18-gauge automated core biopsy needle: a retrospective review of 410 consecutive procedures. Am J Roentgenol. 2003;180: 167–72.

46. Misra S, Gyamlani G, Swaminathan S, Buehrig CK, Bjarnason H, McKusick MA, et al. Safety and diagnostic yield of transjugular renal biopsy. J Vasc Interv Radiol. 2008;19:546–51.

47. Sofocleous CT, Bahramipour P, Mele C, Hinrichs CR, Barone A, Abujudeh H. Transvenous transjugular renal core biopsy with a redesigned biopsy set including a blunt-tipped needle. Cardiovasc Intervent Radiol. 2002;25:155–7.

48. Bilbao JI, Idoate F, Joly MA, Vazquez C, Sangro B, Larrea JA, et al. Renal biopsy with forceps through the femoral vein. J Vasc Interv Radiol. 1995;6:641–5.

49. Khosa F, McNulty JG, Hickey N, O'Brien P, Tobin A, Noonan N, et al. Transvenous liver biopsy via the femoral vein. Clin Radiol. 2003;58:487–91.

50. Jung GS, Huh JD, Lee SU, Han BH, Chang HK, Cho YD. Bile duct: analysis of percutaneous transluminal forceps biopsy in 130 patients suspected of having malignant biliary obstruction. Radiology. 2002;224:725–30.

51. Xing GS, Geng JC, Han XW, Dai JH, Wu CY. Endobiliary brush cytology during percutaneous transhepatic cholangiodrainage in patients with obstructive jaundice. Hepatobiliary Pancreat Dis Int. 2005;4:98–103.

52. Selvaggi SM. Biliary brushing cytology. Cytopathology. 2004;15: 74–9.

53. Kattapuram SV, Rosenthal DI. Percutaneous biopsy of skeletal lesions. Am J Roentgenol. 1991;157:935–42.

54. Roberts CC, Morrison WB, Leslie KO, Carrino JA, Lozevski JL, Liu PT. Assessment of bone biopsy needles for sample size, specimen quality and ease of use. Skeletal Radiol. 2005;34:329–35.

55. Buckley O, Benfayed W, Geoghegan T, Al-Ismail K, Munk PL, Torreggiani WC. CT-guided bone biopsy: initial experience with a commercially available hand held Black and Decker drill. Eur J Radiol. 2007;61:176–80.

56. Cohen SC, Gore JM. Evaluation of a powered intraosseous device for bone marrow sampling. Anticancer Res. 2008;28:3843–6.

57. Culp WC, McCowan TC, Goertzen TC, Habbe TG, Hummel MM, LeVeen RF, et al. Relative ultrasonographic echogenicity of standard, dimpled, and polymeric-coated needles. J Vasc Interv Radiol. 2000;11:351–8.

58. Jandzinski DI, Carson N, Davis D, Rubens DJ, Voci SL, Gottlieb RH. Treated needles: do they facilitate sonographically guided biopsies? J Ultrasound Med. 2003;22:1233–7.

59. Schulz T, Puccini S, Schneider JP, Kahn T. Interventional and intraoperative MR: review and update of techniques and clinical experience. Eur Radiol. 2004;14:2212–27.

60. Weiss CR, Nour SG, Lewin JS. MR-guided biopsy: a review of current techniques and applications. J Magn Reson Imaging. 2008;27:311–25.

61. Adam G, Bucker A, Nolte-Ernsting C, Tacke J, Gunther RW. Interventional MR imaging: percutaneous abdominal and skeletal biopsies and drainages of the abdomen. Eur Radiol. 1999;9: 1471–8.

62. Hueftle MG, Haaga JR. Effect of suction on biopsy sample size. Am J Roentgenol. 1986;147:1014–16.

63. Zajdela A, Zillhardt P, Voillemot N. Cytological diagnosis by fine needle sampling without aspiration. Cancer. 1987;59:1201–5.

64. Santos JE, Leiman G. Nonaspiration fine needle cytology. Application of a new technique to nodular thyroid disease. Acta Cytol. 1988;32:353–6.

65. Zajdela A, de Maublanc MA, Schlienger P, Haye C. Cytologic diagnosis of orbital and periorbital palpable tumors using fine-needle sampling without aspiration. Diagn Cytopathol. 1986;2:17–20.

66. Fagelman D, Chess Q. Nonaspiration fine-needle cytology of the liver: a new technique for obtaining diagnostic samples. Am J Roentgenol. 1990;155:1217–19.

67. Mair S, Dunbar F, Becker PJ, Du Plessis W. Fine needle cytology—is aspiration suction necessary? A study of 100 masses in various sites. Acta Cytol. 1989;33:809–13.

68. Hopper KD, Grenko RT, Fisher AI, TenHave TR. Capillary versus aspiration biopsy: effect of needle size and length on the cytopathological specimen quality. Cardiovasc Intervent Radiol. 1996; 19:341–4.

69. Monsein LH, Kelsey CA, Williams WL, Olson NJ. Fine needle biopsy without syringe aspiration. Cardiovasc Intervent Radiol. 1993;16:11–3.

70. Hopper KD, Abendroth CS, TenHave TR, Hartzel J, Savage CA. Multiple fine-needle biopsies using a coaxial technique: efficacy and a comparison of three methods. Cardiovasc Intervent Radiol. 1995;18:307–11.

71. Kopecky KK, Broderick LS, Davidson DD, Burney BT. Side-exiting coaxial needle for aspiration biopsy. Am J Roentgenol. 1996;167:661–2.

72. Gupta S, Ahrar K, Morello Jr FA, Wallace MJ, Madoff DC, Hicks ME. Using a coaxial technique with a curved inner needle for CT-guided fine-needle aspiration biopsy. Am J Roentgenol. 2002;179:109–12.

73. Singh AK, Leeman J, Shankar S, Ferrucci JT. Core biopsy with curved needle technique. Am J Roentgenol. 2008;191:1745–50.

74. vanSonnenberg E, Lin AS, Casola G, Nakamoto SK, Wing VW, Cubberly DA. Removable hub needle system for coaxial biopsy of small and difficult lesions. Radiology. 1984;152:226.

75. Bull HJ, Gilmore IT, Bradley RD, Marigold JH, Thompson RP. Experience with transjugular liver biopsy. Gut. 1983;24:1057–60.

76. Gamble P, Colapinto RF, Stronell RD, Colman JC, Blendis L. Transjugular liver biopsy: a review of 461 biopsies. Radiology. 1985;157:589–93.

77. Lebrec D, Goldfarb G, Degott C, Rueff B, Benhamou JP. Transvenous liver biopsy: an experience based on 1000 hepatic tissue samplings with this procedure. Gastroenterology. 1982;83:338–40.

78. McAfee JH, Keeffe EB, Lee RG, Rosch J. Transjugular liver biopsy. Hepatology. 1992;15:726–32.

79. Teare JP, Watkinson AF, Erb SR, Mayo JR, Connell DG, Weir IH, et al. Transfemoral liver biopsy by forceps: a review of 104 consecutive procedures. Cardiovasc Intervent Radiol. 1994;17: 252–7.

80. Savader SJ, Prescott CA, Lund GB, Osterman FA. Intraductal biliary biopsy: comparison of three techniques. J Vasc Interv Radiol. 1996;7:743–50.

CT-Guided Biopsy

2

Kamran Ahrar

Early experience with computed tomography (CT)-guided biopsy was based on the use of conventional multisectional CT, consisting of individual scans obtained during separate breath holds. In these early days, respiratory misregistration presented a major obstacle in identifying the biopsy needle tip. Development of spiral CT scanners, which use a continuously rotating detector system and move the patient continuously through the scanner, has helped avoid some of the respiratory misregistration problems by imaging the entire area of interest in a single breath hold [1]. Modern multidetector CT scanners allow for rapid imaging during biopsy procedures during "quiet respiration" (i.e., diaphragmatic respiration). This chapter outlines the equipment, advantages, disadvantages, applications, and techniques used in CT-guided and CT fluoroscopy (CTF)-guided biopsies.

Equipment

CT

CT-guided biopsies can be performed using any diagnostic CT equipment. However, certain features are more desirable for CT-guided interventions. Multidetector CT scanners with wide detector arrays are ideal for imaging large anatomical sections where the intervention is taking place. This imaging of a large anatomical area helps the interventional radiologist recognize needle deviation in cranial and caudal directions

K. Ahrar, MD, FSIR
Department of Interventional Radiology,
Department of Thoracic and Cardiovascular Surgery,
The University of Texas MD Anderson Cancer Center,
1515 Holcombe Boulevard, Unit 1471,
Houston, TX 77030, USA
e-mail: kahrar@mdanderson.org

and adjust the puncture direction if organ shift occurs during the intervention. Also, rapid three-dimensional (3D) reconstruction and viewing of the needle in nonaxial planes are possible with multidetector CT scanners.

The gantry on a typical diagnostic CT scanner is 70 cm in diameter, but CT scanners with large-bore gantries (up to 85 cm) are commercially available and are more suitable for CT-guided interventions. A wider CT gantry allows better access to the patient during needle or device placement and imaging. The procedure room should contain at least one monitor so that the radiologist can review the most recent images while inserting the biopsy needle or device; however, a dual monitor system is ideal because it allows reference or planning images to be projected and maintained on one monitor while the other monitor shows the most recent or real-time CT images.

The CT scanner should have a foot pedal control that allows the radiologist to start and stop sequential scans or CT fluoroscopy from the procedure room. The foot control feature is necessary to perform CT fluoroscopy, but even for sequential imaging during a biopsy, a foot pedal enables the radiologist to be more independent of the technologist in the control room. Similarly, table-side controls for moving the table in and out of the gantry make CT-guided biopsies more efficient by allowing the radiologist to control the table. Most manufacturers offer software packages dedicated to CT-guided biopsies. This software makes it possible for the technologist to quickly set up a small section of anatomy to be imaged during a biopsy procedure.

CT Fluoroscopy

CTF can provide continuous imaging with real-time reconstruction and display of images that allows the radiologist to monitor percutaneous biopsy procedures in near-real-time mode. CTF was initially introduced into clinical practice in 1996 [2]. The first prototype was constructed using a third-generation CT scanner (Xpress/SX; Toshiba, Tokyo, Japan) equipped with a slip ring and an 896-channel solid-state

K. Ahrar, S. Gupta (eds.), *Percutaneous Image-Guided Biopsy*,
DOI 10.1007/978-1-4614-8217-8_2, © Springer Science+Business Media New York 2014

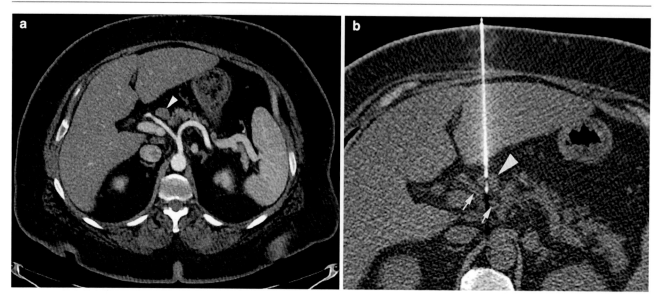

Fig. 2.1 A morbidly obese, 55-year-old woman with endometrial cancer was found to have periportal lymphadenopathy. Diagnostic contrast-enhanced CT image of the abdomen (**a**) shows a 1.5 cm lymph node (*arrowhead*) immediately anterior to the common hepatic artery. Axial CT fluoroscopy image of the abdomen (**b**) shows a transhepatic approach to the lymph node (*arrowhead*). The core biopsy needle is centered within the lesion, anterior to common hepatic artery (*arrows*)

detector array that was modified by adding a high-speed array processor (real-time reconstruction unit) to increase the image reconstruction speed. The CTF prototype unit had a display rate of six images per second with a delay time of 0.17 s [2]. Initially, CTF was performed only in "still mode" without any motion of the patient table or gantry; however, further development of CTF made it possible to perform CTF while sliding the patient table or tilting the gantry.

Currently, all available commercial CTF systems use continuous rotation, fan-beam geometry CT scanners. The high-speed array processor allows image display rates of up to 8 frames per second with an average inter-image spacing of 0.17 s. CTF images are displayed in a "near-real-time" mode on a monitor inside the procedure room to provide immediate feedback to the radiologist.

Demand for CT-guided interventions has increased over the years, and manufacturers have modified CT scanners to include additional hardware and software packages specifically designed to accommodate the needs of interventional radiologists. The wider gantry openings of up to 85 cm provide the radiologist with better patient access during interventional procedures, and ultrafast imaging and near-real-time 3D image reconstruction to help needle path planning and needle artifact prevention have improved the accuracy of interventions. Modern interventional CT units have been designed to obtain optimal imaging while reducing the dose of ionizing radiation to the patient and radiologist. CT scanners with table-side controls have been developed to allow radiologists to control imaging and display during CT-guided interventions.

Advantages

CT provides high-spatial and high-contrast resolution that allows accurate needle-tip localization (Fig. 2.1). CT allows for excellent delineation of intervening vital structures, permitting a safe biopsy path (Fig. 2.2). It also allows for early detection of complications (Fig. 2.3). CT-guided biopsies are associated with a shorter learning curve for the radiologists than are ultrasound-guided biopsies. CT guidance allows the interventional radiologist to target the viable portion of a mass and to avoid areas of necrosis or cystic degeneration [3].

Disadvantages

Density differences between normal tissues and tumors may not be sufficiently large to allow tumor pathology to be distinguished from normal tissue on noncontrast CT images (Fig. 2.4). While contrast-enhanced CT can be performed to help guide the biopsy procedure (Fig. 2.5) [4], contrast enhancement is often transient and may not last for the entire procedure.

Another disadvantage of CT guidance is that CT imaging is limited to an axial plane. As such, the biopsy planning route is often severely restricted. A multidetector CT with automated reconstruction of images in arbitrary planes alleviates some of these limitations (Fig. 2.6).

Another major disadvantage of conventional CT for image-guided biopsies is the lack of real-time imaging.

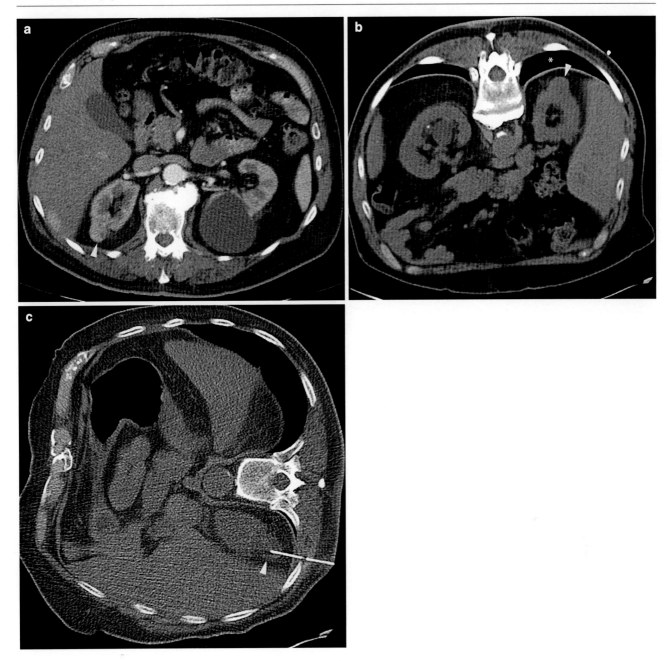

Fig. 2.2 A 78-year-old man was referred for biopsy of a right kidney mass for consideration of percutaneous thermal ablation. Axial CT image of the abdomen (**a**) shows a solid enhancing mass (*arrowhead*) in the upper pole of the right kidney. Axial image of the abdomen in prone position (**b**) shows intervening lung (*asterisk*). When patient was positioned in right lateral decubitus (**c**), the lung volume decreased and a safe window appeared for biopsy of the renal mass (*arrowhead*). A pathologic assessment revealed renal cell carcinoma, clear cell type, nuclear grade 3

Although CTF provides near-real-time imaging, the radiation dose to the patient and operator may prohibit its routine, unrestricted utilization [5–8]. Several studies have documented higher radiation exposure to patients and radiologists from both direct skin exposure and scattered radiation during CTF-guided procedures than during conventional, sequential CT-guided procedures [2, 5–10].

Applications

Although CT can be used to biopsy masses in virtually any part of the body, CT-guided biopsy is most often used for sampling small abdominal (Fig. 2.1), retroperitoneal (Fig. 2.7), thoracic (Fig. 2.8), and musculoskeletal (Fig. 2.9) lesions that are not well visualized on

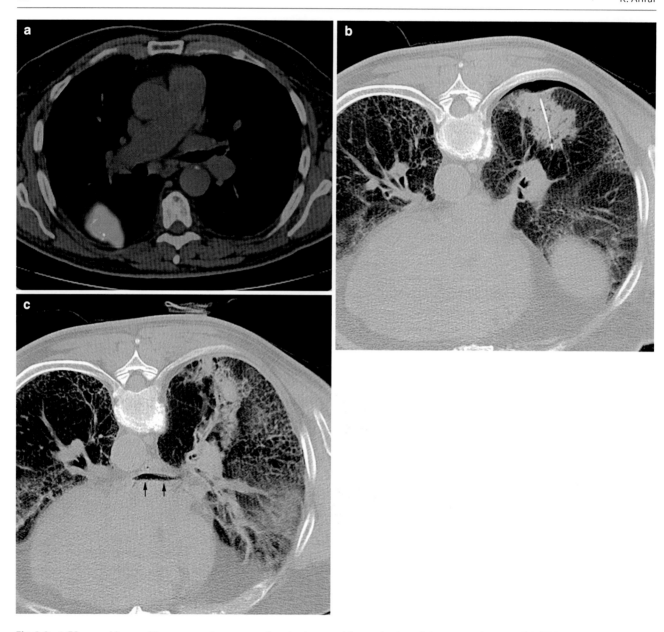

Fig. 2.3 A 75-year-old man with severe emphysema was found to have a mass in the right lower lobe. Axial PET/CT image of the mass (**a**) shows high metabolic activity. CT image of the patient in prone position shows the needle tip within the mass (**b**) and small pneumothorax. After aspiration of the pneumothorax, axial CT image of the chest (**c**) shows air within the left atrium (*arrows*). Systemic air embolism is best treated with hyperbaric oxygen

ultrasonography or fluoroscopy [3]. CTF-guided biopsy has been most commonly used for sampling pulmonary nodules. CTF, with its near-real-time imaging capabilities, allows the interventional radiologist to time the needle puncture with the patient's breathing, which helps in targeting a moving nodule and avoiding ribs during thoracic biopsies. Most studies on the use of CTF-guided biopsy of pulmonary lesions have shown high rates of technical success [11–16]. CTF-guided transthoracic biopsy procedures are associated with shorter procedural times and fewer needle punctures than are conventional CT-guided biopsies [8, 9, 11–17].

In addition, the needle tip and the biopsy target can be visualized during sampling to ensure that the needle tip is indeed within the target. CTF also facilitates placement of the biopsy needle at the edge of a lesion that has a predominantly necrotic center. With CTF, complications are recognized immediately, allowing for rapid institution of appropriate therapy.

Although CTF is not routinely used for abdominal and pelvic biopsies, CTF guidance can be useful in certain circumstances [18, 19]. CTF can be used to guide biopsy of liver lesions that show transient enhancement after intravenous injection of contrast medium, masses with difficult or narrow

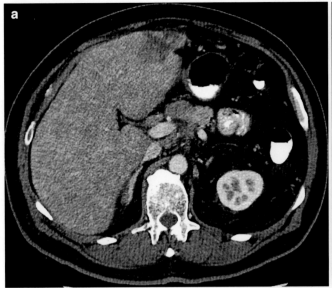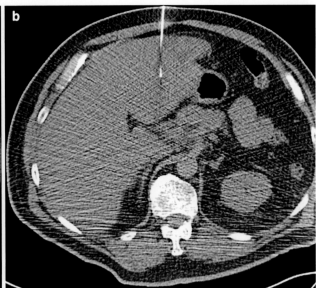

Fig. 2.4 A 65-year-old man with history of Merkel cell carcinoma was referred for liver biopsy. Diagnostic axial CT image of the abdomen after administration of contrast (**a**) shows a lesion in segment II of the liver. A noncontrast axial CT image of the abdomen (**b**) at the time of biopsy did not clearly show the tumor. The lesion was targeted by anatomic landmarks. Immediate assessment of the FNA samples by cytopathologist confirmed metastatic Merkel cell carcinoma. Also note that the diagnostic CT scan (**a**) was performed with the patients arms elevated above his head. Whereas his arms were left on his side during CT-guided biopsy (**b**). The artifact from the arms can hinder visualization of subtle lesions

access routes, and masses close to the diaphragm or critical vascular structures [20, 21]. CTF can assist in needle placement in omental or mesenteric lesions that move with respiration or that may be intermittently surrounded by bowel loops.

Techniques

Setup

For CT-guided biopsies, a sterile field is set up on a movable procedure cart in the CT room. The interventional radiologist reviews existing images, and then the patient is placed in a position that facilitates needle insertion in a safe and efficient manner from the skin surface to the target. Patients can be placed in supine, prone, lateral, or lateral oblique positions as needed, but it is crucial to select a stable and comfortable position for the patient. The patient should remain in the same position after the initial planning images are obtained. Streak artifacts caused by the patient's arms can be reduced by positioning the arms outside the imaging field (Fig. 2.4). Space within the gantry can be maximized by placing the table at the lowest position possible.

A radiopaque marker or grid is placed over the intended area of puncture. Radiopaque grids are commercially available; however, grids can be created on site using various types of catheters that are cut to a length of 10–20 cm, placed parallel at 1- to 2-cm intervals, and taped at the ends.

The simplest radiopaque marker consists of a single piece of angiographic or drainage catheter placed on the patient in longitudinal fashion. Alternatively, one can use the laser lights that are built in the gantry together with the grid which can be displayed on the patient's image to determine the needle puncture site.

For most interventions, a spiral scan of the area of interest is performed, including the marker or grid. In most cases, intravenous administration of contrast medium is unnecessary, but occasionally noncontrast images do not allow differentiation of the target from adjacent vascular structures. Tumors within solid organs may be isodense with their surrounding tissue on noncontrast images, in which case the contrast medium may be given intravenously to delineate the vascular structures or to differentiate the lesion from normal parenchyma (Fig. 2.5) [4].

The interventional radiologist identifies the target and then determines a path for placement of the biopsy needle or device. The needle path depends on the organ of interest and the intervening anatomy. In general, the path should be kept short, but it should also avoid certain anatomic structures such as bone, vessels, bowel, or other organs to render the procedure as safe as possible. Once the needle insertion site is determined, the patient is placed into the gantry. The positioning laser light and the radiopaque marker together provide adequate information to localize the exact site for needle insertion. A small ruler and a skin marker are often necessary to mark the puncture site accurately on the

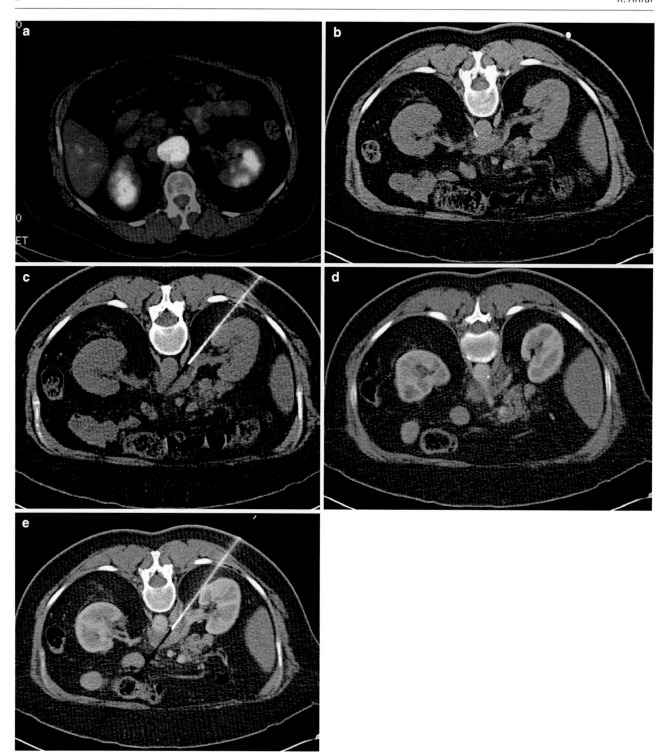

Fig. 2.5 A 62-year-old woman with lymphoma underwent restating PET/CT examination. Axial fused PET/CT image of the abdomen (**a**) shows a metabolically active soft tissue mass encasing the celiac axis. Noncontrast axial CT image of the abdomen in prone position (**b**) shows the soft tissue mass abutting the anterior wall of aorta. A guide needle was advanced to the edge of the lesion (**c**). Immediately before insertion of the core biopsy needle, contrast-enhanced CT images were obtained demonstrating the celiac artery (**d**). The guide needle is identified approximately 10 mm inferior to the celiac artery (**e**). Contrast-enhanced axial CT image of the lesion (**e**) confirms the absence of any major vessels in the path of the needle

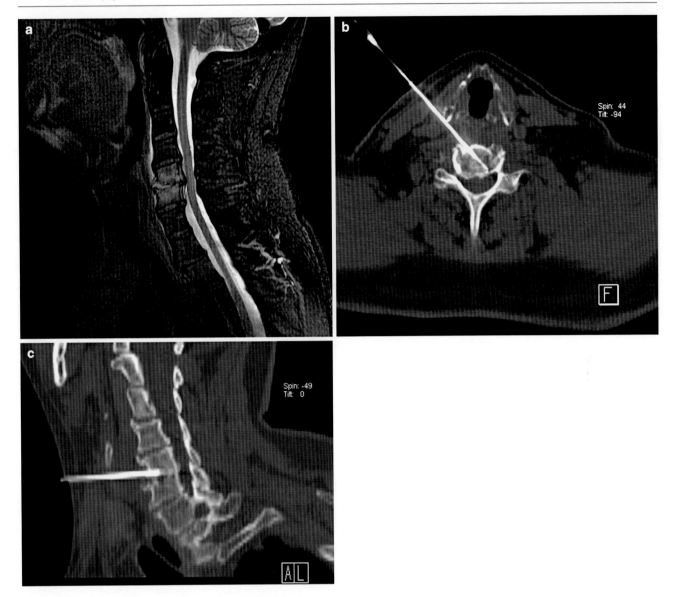

Fig. 2.6 A 53-year-old man with leukemia was referred for biopsy of cervical spine. Sagittal T2 MRI of the cervical spine (**a**) shows high signal intensity in C5 and C6 vertebral bodies with involvement of the disc space. Axial-oblique (**b**) and sagittal-oblique (**c**) multiplanar reformatted images show the position of the needle within the area of interest

skin. The skin is then prepared in a sterile manner, and a keyhole drape is placed over the puncture site. A sterile cover may be applied to the table-side control panel so that the radiologist can operate the CT scanner during the procedure.

Biopsy Technique

Most biopsies are performed under moderate sedation or local anesthesia. The skin entry site is infiltrated with local anesthetic agent (e.g., lidocaine 1 %), and sufficient local anesthetic agent should be injected at the interface of the pleura, peritoneum, or periosteum. A small stab incision is made to help the needle pass through the skin and subcutaneous tissues. CT guidance provides intermittent imaging, and thus the needle is inserted incrementally (1 to a few centimeters at a time) during CT-guided biopsy, and images are obtained after each manipulation to confirm proper advancement of the needle along the desired path.

CTF guidance provides continuous near-real-time imaging that allows monitoring of the needle insertion during CTF-guided biopsy. To avoid excessive radiation to the operator's hand, needle-holding devices may be used [22]. Even with the use of needle-holding devices, radiation exposure to the operator and patient may not warrant real-time continuous-mode CTF. Alternatively, intermittent CTF can be performed after incremental advancement of the needle [23].

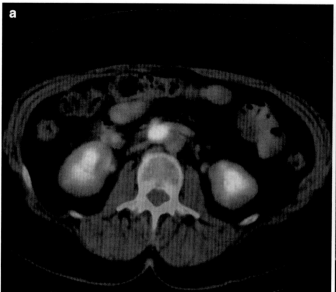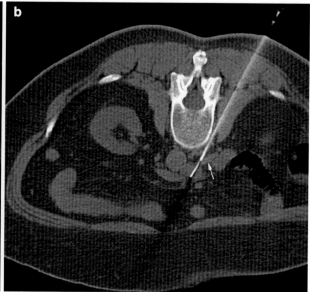

Fig. 2.7 A 56-year-old woman with history of ovarian cancer underwent PET/CT for restaging. Axial PET/CT image of the abdomen (**a**) shows a mass with high metabolic activity in aortocaval space. Axial CT image of the abdomen in prone position (**b**) shows the needle entering the mass from a posterior approach. The *white arrow* shows the inferior vena cava

The operator must be cognizant of two angles when performing CT- or CTF-guided biopsy. Most CT-guided biopsies are performed in a true axial plane. This approach provides the easiest imaging protocol to confirm needle placement. Therefore, the operator has to keep the needle in one axial plane perpendicular to the Z axis. Cranial or caudal angulation of the needle can be detected on sequential CT images, and the path of the needle can be adjusted accordingly. One can take advantage of the laser light of the scanner for alignment of the needle in an axial plane. When the laser light shines on the skin entry site and the hub of the needle, it confirms the positioning of the needle in the imaging plane. The simplest CT-guided biopsy plan is one in which the needle is inserted perpendicular to the skin. However, this approach is not always feasible, depending on the intervening organs or structures that may have to be avoided. Therefore, the second angle that the operator should observe is the steepness of the approach with respect to the skin's surface. Placement of the needle can be guided with the naked eye; however, this is more easily accomplished if the patient is taken out of the gantry and the puncture site is placed directly in front of the operator to avoid issues related to parallax.

Ancillary Techniques

Triangulation Method

The ideal skin entry site may be cranial or caudal to the axial plane containing the target lesion. In these cases, the interventional radiologist can calculate the needle angle using the Pythagorean theorem [24]. This triangulation method is a simple and useful technique that allows the target to be reached without traversing structures directly overlying the target. This technique has been successfully used to reach adrenal lesions without traversing the pleural space. The path of the needle must be followed on sequential axial CT images, and at least one image should be obtained beyond the needle tip to confirm the tip's location (Fig. 2.10).

Angled-Gantry Technique

As discussed above, when the needle path is not in an axial plane, conventional CT images will not show the entire needle in one axial image. Deviation from an axial plane may be necessary to avoid puncturing certain structures, or deviation may develop during the course of biopsy because of patient movement, organ shift, or inaccurate placement of the needle [25, 26]. Sequential axial images have to be reviewed to determine the path of the needle and the location of the needle tip, and localization of the needle tip on sequential axial images requires at least one image to be obtained beyond the needle tip to confirm the tip's position. Alternatively, the interventional radiologist can tilt the gantry cranially or caudally, depending on the angle of the needle path, to view the entire needle in an axial plane (Fig. 2.8). The laser light will shine through the hub of the needle and the skin insertion site when the needle is lined up with the gantry, and the entire needle should be visible in one image. The degree to which the gantry can be tilted depends on two factors: the size of the gantry and the size of the patient. The combination of a large gantry and a small patient allows a greater gantry tilt to

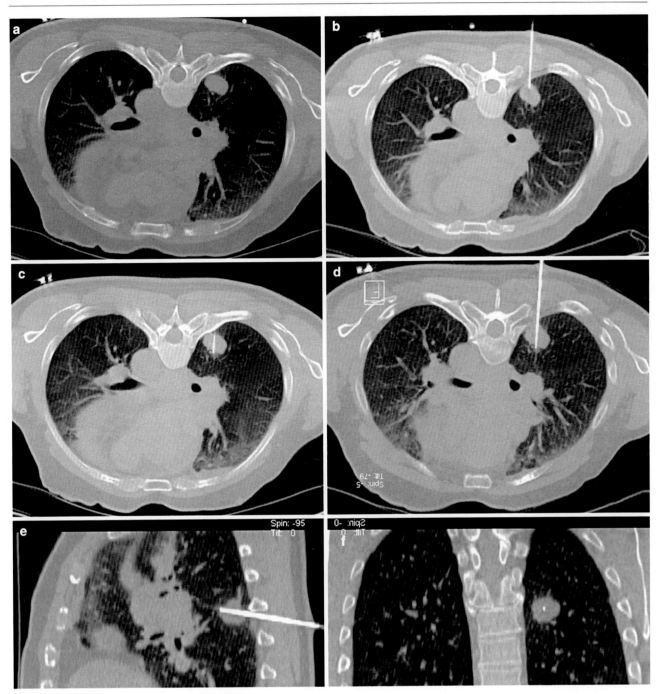

Fig. 2.8 A 57-year-old man with newly diagnosed right lung mass was referred for biopsy. Axial CT image of the chest in prone position (**a**) shows the right lung mass. Overlying rib and costovertebral joint limit access to the lesion in a true axial plane. The gantry was tilted 10° caudo-cranial. Axial-oblique CT fluoroscopy image of the chest (**b**) demonstrates entire length of the needle extending to the posterior border of the tumor. True axial CT image of the chest (**c**) shows only the tip of the needle within the lesion. Multiplanar reformatted images demonstrate entire length of the needle in axial-oblique (**d**) and sagittal-oblique (**e**) planes. A coronal reconstructed image of the patient in prone position (**f**) shows the tip of the needle within the center of the mass

be created. This angled-gantry approach may help overlying ribs to be avoided when performing biopsy of small pleural-based intrathoracic lesions. Another common scenario is avoidance of the lung base while targeting upper pole renal tumors or adrenal tumors [25].

"Salinoma" Creation and Organ Displacement

"Salinoma" refers to an iatrogenic fluid collection that is intentionally created to allow safe passage of a biopsy needle without traversing vital structures (Fig. 2.11). Injection of saline or CO_2 can help displace bowel or bladder to create a

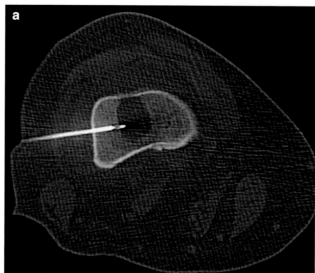

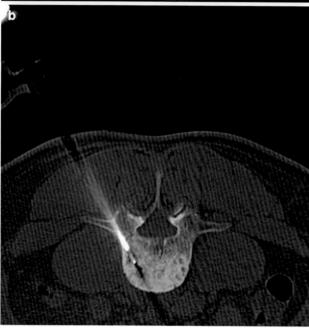

Fig. 2.9 Both lytic (**a**) and sclerotic (**b**) bone lesions can be visualized and targeted for biopsy. Biopsy of the lytic lesion in the distal right femur (**a**) showed metastatic cervical cancer. Biopsy of a sclerotic lumbar vertebral body tumor (**b**) showed metastatic neuroendocrine carcinoma

safe approach to a lesion [27–29], and injection of saline can help widen existing narrow spaces [30, 31]. Paravertebral or paramediastinal spaces can be artificially widened by injection of saline to allow safe placement of a biopsy needle without puncturing the visceral pleura.

Breath-Hold Monitoring and Feedback

Respiratory motion poses a problem in targeting small lesion in the lower thorax and upper abdomen [32]; however, breathing instructions may help avoid this problem in compliant patients [33]. Respiratory gating and breath-hold monitoring and feedback systems have been developed to synchronize intermittent CTF imaging with specific phases of respiration [32, 34, 35]. One such system monitors changes in body-wall girth and provides immediate feedback to patients so that they can adjust their breath-hold levels accordingly [34]. All of these strategies require some degree of patient training and cooperation and are less reliable in sedated patients.

Image Fusion with Positron Emission Tomography (PET)-CT

All cross-sectional modalities, including CT, provide excellent anatomical information about the extent of disease, but they have limited capability in differentiating viable from nonviable tissues. Sampling of nonviable regions within the tumor may lead to false-negative results and delay therapy. Functional imaging with PET using 2-fluoro-2-deoxy-D-glucose (FDG) relies on differences in the metabolic activity of different tissues and allows for more reliable detection of viable tumor tissue [36]. The limited anatomic information provided by PET can be overcome by fusing functional PET data with morphologic CT data; this fusing of PET and CT data is possible with dual modality PET-CT imaging systems [37, 38]. Similarly, PET can be used in patients with multiple lesions to identify the lesions with the highest FDG uptake for sampling. Frequently, a simple review of previously acquired PET-CT images provides sufficient information for CT-guided biopsies based on morphologic findings or anatomic landmarks (Fig. 2.12). In more subtle cases such as smaller targets, previously acquired PET-CT images can be coregistered with intraprocedural CT scans to guide the biopsy [39]. Other investigators have demonstrated the feasibility of PET-CT-guided interventions, taking advantage of PET imaging and CT-guided navigation in the same setting [40]. In very subtle cases, this combination allows for detection of metabolically active lesions and for placement of the needle at the same time.

Methods of Reducing Radiation Exposure from CTF

Several strategies have been developed to make CTF safer by lowering radiation exposure to the operator and patient [5–9, 11]. Dedicated needle holders have been developed to keep the operator's hands away from the primary CT beam [22]. The use of a needle holder is associated with the loss of tactile feedback, resulting in reduced control over the needle, difficulty with needle advancement through resistant tissue planes, artifacts from some metallic needle holders, difficulty in keeping the needle in the scan plane, and a tendency for thin needles to bend during insertion.

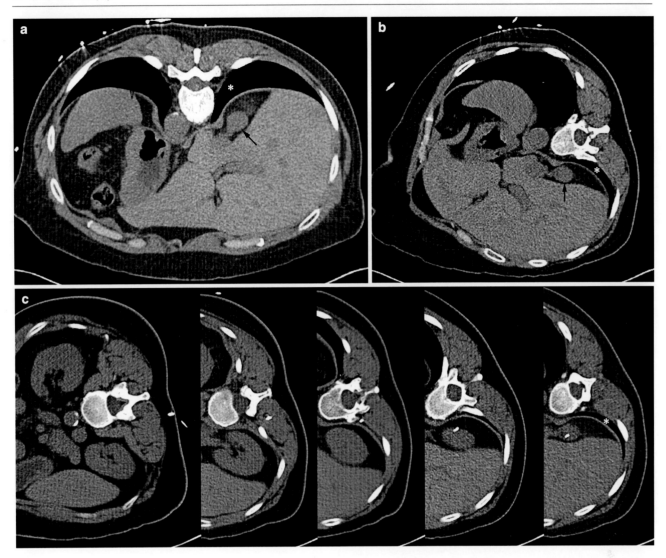

Fig. 2.10 A 56-year-old woman with history of melanoma was referred for a biopsy of right adrenal gland. Axial CT image of the abdomen in prone position (**a**) shows the adrenal mass (*arrow*). Intervening lung parenchyma (*asterisk*) precludes safe needle insertion in this position. Often placing the patient in the ipsilateral decubitus position helps decrease the lung volume and provides a safe path for needle. In this case, axial CT image of the abdomen in right lateral decubitus (**b**) still shows the intervening lung (*asterisk*). A needle insertion site was selected approximately 9 cm inferior to the lesion. Multiple axial images (**c**) show the path of the needle extending cephalad and avoiding the lung base (*asterisk*)

Imaging techniques have been modified using lower tube potential and current and thinner slices. Placement of a lead drape next to the imaging plane helps reduce scatter radiation. Finally, using "quick-check" CTF intermittently between needle advancements instead of continuously during the entire biopsy has been shown to reduce radiation exposure to well within acceptable limits [11, 41].

In summary, CT is well suited to guide percutaneous biopsies. It is widely available, and its high spatial and contrast resolution help detect the targets easily. Although most CT-guided biopsies are performed without the need for administration of intravenous contrast medium, review of a contrast-enhanced diagnostic CT scan is essential for planning a safe and effective biopsy procedure. At times, intravenous contrast medium can be administered immediately prior to the biopsy to help localize the lesion, but the resulting enhancement is often short lived. The learning curve is short, but mastering the art of CT-guided biopsy to target small, mobile, or difficult to reach lesions and to obtain viable and adequate samples requires attention to details, use of various ancillary techniques, and practice.

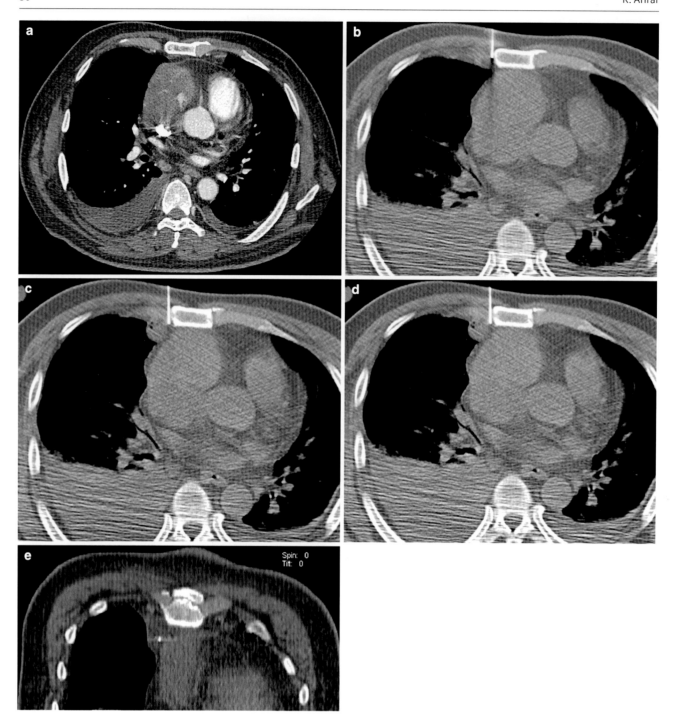

Fig. 2.11 A 53-year-old man was referred for biopsy of a mediastinal mass (**a**). Axial CT image of the chest shows the path of the biopsy needle traversing the pleura (**b**). After injection of 10 mL of saline (**c**), the mediastinal window was widened to advance the needle without traversing the pleura (**d**). A coronal reformatted image shows the lung displaced laterally and the needle traversing the "salinoma" (**e**)

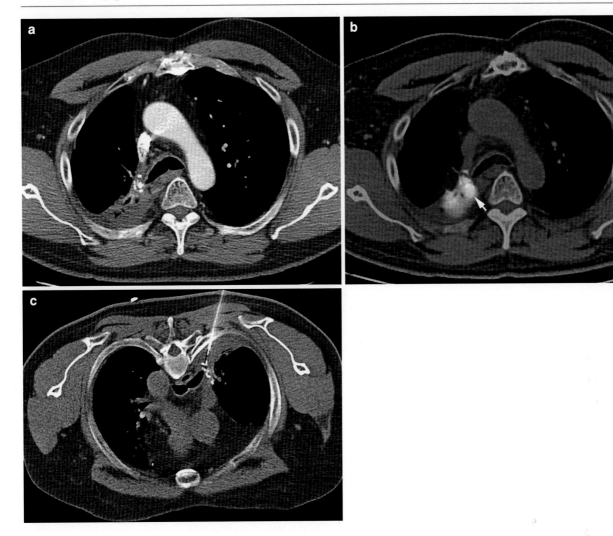

Fig. 2.12 A 72-year-old man with history of non-small cell lung cancer and right upper lobectomy underwent surveillance CT imaging. Axial CT image of the chest (**a**) shows a new soft tissue mass in the posterior aspect of the right chest. PET/CT image of the same area (**b**) shows a focal area of high metabolic activity (*arrow*). This particular spot was targeted for CT-guided biopsy based on anatomical and surgical landmarks (**c**). Pathology showed recurrent adenocarcinoma

References

1. Silverman SG, Bloom DA, Seltzer SE, Tempany CM, Adams DF. Needle-tip localization during CT-guided abdominal biopsy: comparison of conventional and spiral CT. Am J Roentgenol. 1992; 159:1095–7.
2. Katada K, Kato R, Anno H, Ogura Y, Koga S, Ida Y, et al. Guidance with real-time CT fluoroscopy: early clinical experience. Radiology. 1996;200:851–6.
3. Gupta S. Role of image-guided percutaneous needle biopsy in cancer staging. Semin Roentgenol. 2006;41:78–90.
4. Collins JM, Kriegshauser JS, Leslie KO. CT-guided biopsy of perivascular tumor encasement using simultaneous IV contrast enhancement. Am J Roentgenol. 2009;193:W283–7.
5. Kato R, Katada K, Anno H, Suzuki S, Ida Y, Koga S. Radiation dosimetry at CT fluoroscopy: physician's hand dose and development of needle holders. Radiology. 1996;201:576–8.
6. Paulson EK, Sheafor DH, Enterline DS, McAdams HP, Yoshizumi TT. CT fluoroscopy–guided interventional procedures: techniques and radiation dose to radiologists. Radiology. 2001;220:161–7.
7. Nawfel RD, Judy PF, Silverman SG, Hooton S, Tuncali K, Adams DF. Patient and personnel exposure during CT fluoroscopy-guided interventional procedures. Radiology. 2000;216:180–4.
8. Daly B, Templeton PA. Real-time CT fluoroscopy: evolution of an interventional tool. Radiology. 1999;211:309–15.
9. Froelich JJ, Wagner HJ. CT-fluoroscopy: tool or gimmick? Cardiovasc Intervent Radiol. 2001;24:297–305.
10. Nishizawa K, Uruma T, Takiguchi Y, Kuriyama T, Yanagawa N, Matsumoto M, et al. Dose evaluation and effective dose estimation from CT fluoroscopy-guided lung biopsy. Igaku Butsuri. 2001; 21:233–44.
11. Irie T, Kajitani M, Yoshioka H, Matsueda K, Inaba Y, Arai Y, et al. CT fluoroscopy for lung nodule biopsy: a new device for needle placement and a phantom study. J Vasc Interv Radiol. 2000; 11:359–64.
12. de Mey J, Op de Beeck B, Meysman M, Noppen M, De Maeseneer M, Vanhoey M, et al. Real time CT-fluoroscopy: diagnostic and therapeutic applications. Eur J Radiol. 2000;34:32–40.
13. Froelich JJ, Ishaque N, Regn J, Saar B, Walthers EM, Klose KJ. Guidance of percutaneous pulmonary biopsies with real-time CT fluoroscopy. Eur J Radiol. 2002;42:74–9.

14. Kirchner J, Kickuth R, Laufer U, Schilling EM, Adams S, Liermann D. CT fluoroscopy-assisted puncture of thoracic and abdominal masses: a randomized trial. Clin Radiol. 2002;57:188–92.

15. Muehlstaedt M, Bruening R, Diebold J, Mueller A, Helmberger T, Reiser M. CT/fluoroscopy-guided transthoracic needle biopsy: sensitivity and complication rate in 98 procedures. J Comput Assist Tomogr. 2002;26:191–6.

16. White CS, Meyer CA, Templeton PA. CT fluoroscopy for thoracic interventional procedures. Radiol Clin North Am. 2000;38: 303–22, viii.

17. Gianfelice D, Lepanto L, Perreault P, Chartrand-Lefebvre C, Milette PC. Value of CT fluoroscopy for percutaneous biopsy procedures. J Vasc Interv Radiol. 2000;11:879–84.

18. Silverman SG, Tuncali K, Adams DF, Nawfel RD, Zou KH, Judy PF. CT fluoroscopy-guided abdominal interventions: techniques, results, and radiation exposure. Radiology. 1999;212:673–81.

19. Liermann D, Kickuth R. CT fluoroscopy-guided abdominal interventions. Abdom Imaging. 2003;28:129–34.

20. Schweiger GD, Brown BP, Pelsang RE, Dhadha RS, Barloon TJ, Wang G. CT fluoroscopy: technique and utility in guiding biopsies of transiently enhancing hepatic masses. Abdom Imaging. 2000;25:81–5.

21. Schweiger GD, Yip VY, Brown BP. CT fluoroscopic guidance for percutaneous needle placement into abdominopelvic lesions with difficult access routes. Abdom Imaging. 2000;25:633–7.

22. Daly B, Templeton PA, Krebs TL, Carroll K, Wong-You-Cheong JJ. Evaluation of biopsy needles and prototypic needle guide devices for percutaneous biopsy with CT fluoroscopic guidance in simulated organ tissue. Radiology. 1998;209:850–5.

23. Kim GR, Hur J, Lee SM, Lee HJ, Hong YJ, Nam JE, et al. CT fluoroscopy-guided lung biopsy versus conventional CT-guided lung biopsy: a prospective controlled study to assess radiation doses and diagnostic performance. Eur Radiol. 2011;21:232–9.

24. vanSonnenberg E, Lin AS, Casola G, Nakamoto SK, Wing VW, Cubberly DA. Removable hub needle system for coaxial biopsy of small and difficult lesions. Radiology. 1984;152:226.

25. Hussain S. Gantry angulation in CT-guided percutaneous adrenal biopsy. Am J Roentgenol. 1996;166:537–9.

26. Yueh N, Halvorsen Jr RA, Letourneau JG, Crass JR. Gantry tilt technique for CT-guided biopsy and drainage. J Comput Assist Tomogr. 1989;13:182–4.

27. Haaga JR, Beale SM. Use of CO_2 to move structures as an aid to percutaneous procedures. Radiology. 1986;161:829–30.

28. Langen HJ, Jochims M, Gunther RW. Artificial displacement of kidneys, spleen, and colon by injection of physiologic saline and CO_2 as an aid to percutaneous procedures: experimental results. J Vasc Interv Radiol. 1995;6:411–16.

29. Langen HJ, Klose KC, Keulers P, Adam G, Jochims M, Gunther RW. Artificial widening of the mediastinum to gain access for extrapleural biopsy: clinical results. Radiology. 1995;196:703–6.

30. Carlson P, Crummy AB, Wojtowycz M, McDermott JC. A safe route for deep pelvic biopsy with distention of the iliacus muscle. J Vasc Interv Radiol. 1991;2:277–8.

31. Karampekios S, Hatjidakis AA, Drositis J, Gourtsoyiannis N. Artificial paravertebral widening for percutaneous CT-guided adrenal biopsy. J Comput Assist Tomogr. 1998;22:308–10.

32. Carlson SK, Felmlee JP, Bender CE, Ehman RL, Classic KL, Hoskin TL, et al. CT fluoroscopy-guided biopsy of the lung or upper abdomen with a breath-hold monitoring and feedback system: a prospective randomized controlled clinical trial. Radiology. 2005;237:701–8.

33. Schaefer PJ, Schaefer FK, Heller M, Jahnke T. CT fluoroscopy guided biopsy of small pulmonary and upper abdominal lesions: efficacy with a modified breathing technique. J Vasc Interv Radiol. 2007;18:1241–8.

34. Carlson SK, Felmlee JP, Bender CE, Ehman RL, Classic KL, Hu HH, et al. Intermittent-mode CT fluoroscopy-guided biopsy of the lung or upper abdomen with breath-hold monitoring and feedback: system development and feasibility. Radiology. 2003;229:906–12.

35. Tomiyama N, Mihara N, Maeda M, Johkoh T, Kozuka T, Honda O, et al. CT-guided needle biopsy of small pulmonary nodules: value of respiratory gating. Radiology. 2000;217:907–10.

36. Reading CC, Charboneau JW, James EM, Hurt MR. Sonographically guided percutaneous biopsy of small (3 cm or less) masses. Am J Roentgenol. 1988;151:189–92.

37. Aquino SL, Asmuth JC, Alpert NM, Halpern EF, Fischman AJ. Improved radiologic staging of lung cancer with 2-[18 F]-fluoro-2-deoxy-D-glucose-positron emission tomography and computed tomography registration. J Comput Assist Tomogr. 2003;27:479–84.

38. Schwartz DL, Ford E, Rajendran J, Yueh B, Coltrera MD, Virgin J, et al. FDG-PET/CT imaging for preradiotherapy staging of head-and-neck squamous cell carcinoma. Int J Radiat Oncol Biol Phys. 2005;61:129–36.

39. Tatli S, Gerbaudo VH, Mamede M, Tuncali K, Shyn PB, Silverman SG. Abdominal masses sampled at PET/CT-guided percutaneous biopsy: initial experience with registration of prior PET/CT images. Radiology. 2010;256:305–11.

40. Klaeser B, Mueller MD, Schmid RA, Guevara C, Krause T, Wiskirchen J. PET-CT-guided interventions in the management of FDG-positive lesions in patients suffering from solid malignancies: initial experiences. Eur Radiol. 2009;19:1780–5.

41. Carlson SK, Bender CE, Classic KL, Zink FE, Quam JP, Ward EM, et al. Benefits and safety of CT fluoroscopy in interventional radiologic procedures. Radiology. 2001;219:515–20.

Radiation Protection During CT-Guided Interventions

3

A. Kyle Jones

Patient Dose in CT-Guided Interventions

During a CT procedure, dose is deposited within a patient in a fundamentally different manner than during an angiography procedure. In angiography, the x-ray field is large and irradiates a patient from a single projection, resulting in an entrance dose that is much higher than the exit dose (Fig. 3.1). A large volume of the patient is exposed to the primary x-ray beam. In CT, the x-ray source rotates around the patient, resulting in a relatively uniform distribution of dose on the surface of the patient. A very small volume of the patient is exposed to the primary x-ray beam during each rotation, but a large volume of the patient is exposed to scattered radiation. This difference is exaggerated during CT-guided interventions, as the table remains stationary and the same volume of the patient is continuously irradiated. The dose distribution within a patient depends on the patient size. Small patients experience a dose that is relatively uniform throughout the volume irradiated by the primary beam, while large patients experience doses that are much higher near the surface of the patient compared to within the patient (Fig. 3.2).

During CT-guided interventions, the entrance air kerma rate (EAKR) is approximately equal to the $CTDI_{100}$[1] rate for a typical patient [1]. However, manufacturers typically display the $CTDI_{vol}$ rate or accumulated $CTDI_{vol}$, not $CTDI_{100}$, on the scanner. Based on the relationship between $CTDI_{100}$

and $CTDI_{vol}$, the EAKR for a typical patient is equal to approximately $0.6 \times CTDI_{vol}$ [2]. Typical entrance air kerma rates during CT-guided interventions range from 1.5 to 8 mGy/s, depending on the operating mode and scanner hardware. If we consider an EAKR of 5 mGy/s, 400 s of imaging would be required to reach an ESAK of 2,000 mGy (2 Gy). While the ESAK is not equal to the actual skin dose, it is a reasonable quantity to use for monitoring the progress of a procedure. Also, the ratio of the EAKR to the CTDI rate will vary with patient size and beam width [1]. Tables 3.1 and 3.2 provide some helpful information regarding radiation dose to the patient during CT-guided interventions.

Operator Dose in CT-Guided Interventions

Operators face unique radiation protection challenges when working with CT. In angiography, exposure to intense backscattered radiation can be avoided by maintaining the x-ray tube beneath the patient table or by standing by the image receptor end of the C-arm when using oblique or lateral projections. In CT, some exposure to backscattered radiation is unavoidable, as the x-ray tube is not stationary but instead rotates around the patient. In addition, the intensity of stray radiation in CT is higher by approximately a factor of 10 compared to the angiography lab.

Protection of the Patient

Interventional CT procedures utilize a different workflow from diagnostic CT procedures. A typical procedure involves the acquisition of high-quality planning data, followed by the biopsy procedure and its associated scans, and often ends with the acquisition of another set of high-quality post-procedure data. The technical factors used during the different phases of the procedure should be tailored to the goals of each individual phase. In particular, the biopsy portion of the procedure should use lower techniques than the

[1] The computed tomography dose index (CTDI) can be measured in several ways. $CTDI_{100}$ refers to the dose measured in an acrylic phantom using a 100 mm ionization chamber during a single axial scan. $CTDI_{vol}$ is a calculated quantity equal to $1/3 \times CTDI_{100}$ measured along the central axis of the phantom plus $2/3 \times CTDI_{100}$ measured along the peripheral axis of the phantom, 1 cm below the surface. Modern CT scanners display the $CTDI_{vol}$ on the scan console.

A.K. Jones, PhD
Department of Imaging Physics,
The University of Texas MD Anderson Cancer Center,
1400 Pressler, Unit 1472, Houston, TX 77030, USA
e-mail: kyle.jones@mdanderson.org

K. Ahrar, S. Gupta (eds.), *Percutaneous Image-Guided Biopsy*,
DOI 10.1007/978-1-4614-8217-8_3, © Springer Science+Business Media New York 2014

Fig. 3.1 Distribution of dose within a patient undergoing an angiographic procedure using a PA projection

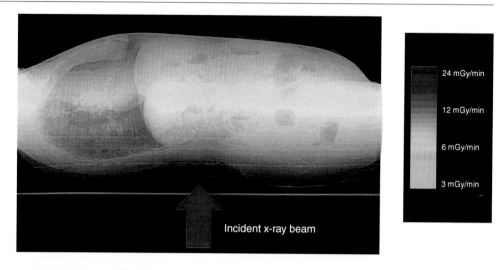

Fig. 3.2 Distribution of dose within a patient undergoing a CT procedure. (**a**) Small patient, (**b**) large patient

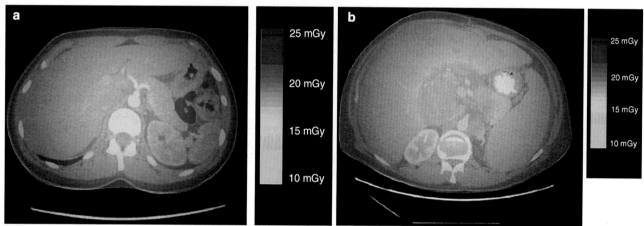

Table 3.1 Variations in ESAK rate in CT with changes in kVp and mA

kVp	Adjustment factor	
80	0.4	ESAK changes linearly with mA. Doubling the mA doubles ESAK, halving the mA halves the ESAK for the same time
100	0.7	
120	1.0	
140	1.4	

For example, if changing from 120 kVp, 50 mA to 80 kVp, 90 mA the dose would change from the typical rate (5 mGy/s) to 5 mGy/s × 0.4 × 90/50 = 3.6 mGy/s

Table 3.2 CT fluoroscopy time required to reach specific skin dose levels

kVp	mA	Time to reach threshold (s)	
		1,000 mGy	2,000 mGy
80	75	435	869
80	100	328	656
80	150	195	392
120	50	184	357
120	100	86	173

Data adapted from Nawfel et al. [3]. A 20 cm PMMA phantom was used in this study

pre- and post-procedure scans. This is especially important considering the fact that the patient is likely to be scanned multiple times at the same location. The use of excessive technical factors for the biopsy phase may put the patient at risk for deterministic radiation injuries such as erythema or epilation [4]. High-contrast anatomical landmarks can be used to navigate on the biopsy scans, or an external electromagnetic guidance system can be used in conjunction with the planning data to guide the intervention.

Appropriate Technical Factors for CT-Guided Interventions

The key to maintaining appropriate patient doses during CT-guided interventions is the selection of appropriate technical factors. A CT-guided intervention is not a diagnostic imaging procedure. While high-quality pre-procedure planning data and post-procedure assessment data may be needed, the CT guidance for the actual procedure can in most cases be performed with greatly reduced technical factors

Table 3.3 Typical technical factors for CT examinations

Procedure	kVp	mAs	CTDI$_{vol}$[a](mGy)	Scan length (cm)	Number of scans in same location	Effective dose (mSv)
Diagnostic abdomen CT	120	200	15	40	One	9
Biopsy planning CT	120	150	11	10	One	2
Biopsy CT guidance	120	50	4	2	Multiple	1–10

[a]Volume computed tomography dose index (CTDI$_{vol}$) is a CT-specific dosimetric quantity. See footnote on page 33

Fig. 3.3 Illustration of the function of HandCARE™

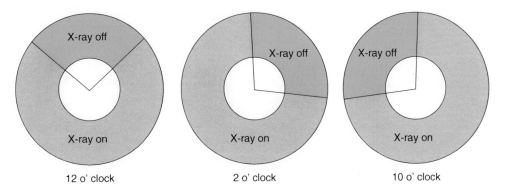

(Table 3.3) [5]. Externally placed markers and internal landmarks can be used for navigation. In addition, some modern ultrasound systems offer navigation options that fuse the ultrasound images with prior CT images, and several companies manufacture guidance systems that use prior CT images for navigation.

Special Patient Concerns

Certain types of patients present unique concerns for radiation protection. CT-guided interventions performed on pediatric patients should use child-sized techniques. The Image Gently campaign is an excellent resource for information on pediatric CT [6]. The glandular breast tissue of female patients is especially radiosensitive. Avoiding direct frontal irradiation of the breast tissue greatly reduces the effective dose to female patients resulting from CT-guided interventions in the lung. This can be accomplished in two ways. First, disposable, sterile lead-free drapes can be used. These shields protect the breast tissue from direct AP irradiation, and the breast tissue is exposed only to radiation that has already passed through the body. However, these shields may interfere with the biopsy itself and cause artifacts in CT images and, depending on how the scanner is used, may in some cases result in little to no dose reduction. Siemens offers a radiation protection feature, designed for the operator, that removes power from the x-ray tube during a certain angular range. The original purpose of this option (HandCARE™) was to reduce dose to the hands of the operator, but it is also useful for reducing dose to female breast tissue. This feature de-energizes the x-ray tube through a 100° range centered at 10 o'clock, 12 o'clock (AP), or 2 o'clock (Fig. 3.3). While a 100° range does

not completely avoid direct irradiation of the breast tissue, it does provide a substantial reduction. Reductions in breast dose of up to 47 % have been reported using this technique [7]. Siemens has recently adapted this technique to diagnostic CT examinations across a wider angular range. Philips' implementation of CT fluoroscopy energizes the x-ray tube only during the 240° of rotation during which the x-ray tube is located under the patient table. One important note is that mA is increased at the angles for which the x-ray tube is energized when angular beam modulation techniques.

Concerns also vary based on the body habitus of the patient. The skin of large patients is closer to the x-ray source than the skin of small patients, which means that large patients are at greater risk for tissue effects. However, small patients have less tissue shielding their internal organs than a large patient, so organ doses, and therefore the effective dose, will be higher for small patients compared to large patients. The CT system will not, however, increase technical factors during CT fluoroscopy in response to changing body habitus, which is in contrast to how angiography equipment operates.

Other Tools for Ensuring Patient Safety

Manufacturers who offer CT fluoroscopy often include constraints on the total number of scans or the cumulative scan time that can be utilized during a single patient study. In addition, some manufacturers include a "dose progress bar" that displays the accumulated CTDI resulting from CT fluoroscopy procedures (Fig. 3.4). This value is not measured, but is instead calculated based on the technical factors used. Recently, the National Electrical Manufacturer's Association (NEMA) has developed safeguards that will notify the

Fig. 3.4 Dose progress bar displays remaining scan time and accumulated CTDI$_{vol}$

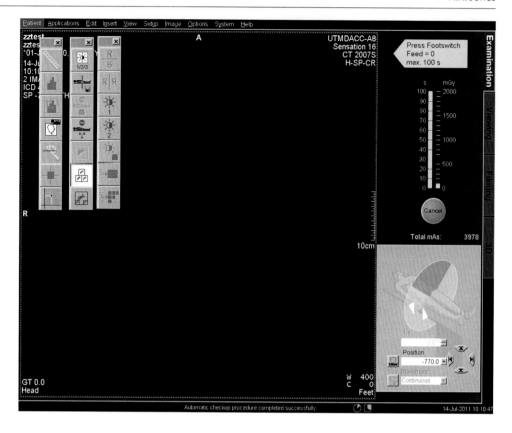

operator, and optionally require a password-protected override, when the total volume CTDI (CTDI$_{vol}$) accumulated at the same z-axis (table) location exceeds a certain value that is preprogrammed by the user [8]. While this was originally intended as a response to overdoses resulting from CT perfusion studies, it may also be useful for CT fluoroscopy and CT-guided biopsy procedures, which employ an irradiation pattern that is very similar to CT perfusion.

Protection of the Operator

The operator enjoys maximum radiation protection when he stands outside the CT lab at the control console. Structural shielding is used in the walls of labs containing radiation-producing equipment, and this shielding, combined with a long distance from the patient, reduces stray radiation exposure to minimal levels. Standing in the open doorway of the CT lab, however, provides only the protection offered by distance from the patient. Stray radiation levels in CT are highest along the patient table (Fig. 3.5), and the operator can be exposed to significant amounts of radiation when standing in the open doorway. Standing in the shadow of the CT gantry offers excellent protection, as the detectors, associated hardware, and the gantry itself attenuate much of the primary and

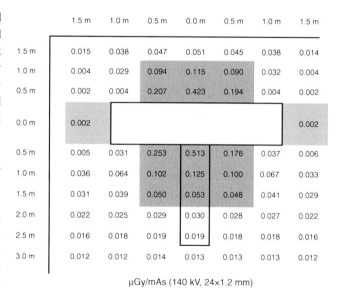

	1.5 m	1.0 m	0.5 m	0.0 m	0.5 m	1.0 m	1.5 m
1.5 m	0.015	0.038	0.047	0.051	0.045	0.038	0.014
1.0 m	0.004	0.029	0.094	0.115	0.090	0.032	0.004
0.5 m	0.002	0.004	0.207	0.423	0.194	0.004	0.002
0.0 m	0.002						0.002
0.5 m	0.005	0.031	0.253	0.513	0.176	0.037	0.006
1.0 m	0.036	0.064	0.102	0.125	0.100	0.067	0.033
1.5 m	0.031	0.039	0.050	0.053	0.048	0.041	0.029
2.0 m	0.022	0.025	0.029	0.030	0.028	0.027	0.022
2.5 m	0.016	0.018	0.019	0.019	0.018	0.018	0.016
3.0 m	0.012	0.012	0.014	0.013	0.013	0.013	0.012

μGy/mAs (140 kV, 24×1.2 mm)

Fig. 3.5 Stray radiation isodose plot for a typical CT scanner. Note highest stray radiation intensity along table and lowest intensity in shadow of gantry

scattered radiation in this direction [9]. This is also more convenient, reducing the total time required to complete a CT-guided intervention.

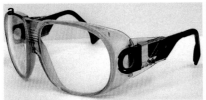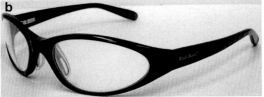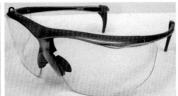

Fig. 3.6 Styles of lead eyewear. (**a**) Traditional, (**b**) sport wrap, (**c**) panoramic (Photos courtesy of Beth Schueler, Ph.D.)

Should an intervention require that continuous CT fluoroscopy be used while a needle or probe is advanced, special precautions should be taken to reduce the dose to the operator. In all cases, the operator and any other personnel remaining in the room should wear lead or lead-equivalent protective garments with a minimum lead equivalence of 0.35 mm [10]. Protection should be provided throughout the entire garment, not just where double layers are created by overlap. Options for additional protection include suspended "face" shields and lead-free sterile drapes that can be placed on the patient to attenuate much of the scattered radiation that is directed at the operator. Mobile lead barriers are a good alternative for protection for persons who are stationary during the procedure, for example, anesthesia support personnel who remain in the room or are positioned in the open doorway of the room.

Hand Protection

Needle holders or forceps offer additional protection to the hands of the operator by increasing the distance between the primary beam and the operator's hands, at the cost of reduced sensitivity and tactile feedback. Hand dose reductions of up to 98 % have been reported when needle holders are used [11]. Sterile lead-free gloves offer some protection at CT energies but at a substantial cost per use. Those opting for sterile lead-free gloves should be cautious about protection specifications, as in general CT x-ray beams are of higher energy and are more penetrating than fluoroscopic x-rays beams. A better alternative, at least initially, is for physicians who are concerned about hand dose to request a ring badge from their radiation safety office. The feedback from the ring badge may alleviate concerns and if not can be used to initiate practice changes or justify the cost of additional protection for the hands. Siemens' CT fluoroscopy package includes a feature (HandCARE™) where the x-ray tube can be shut off across certain angular ranges within the gantry (Fig. 3.3). Reductions in hand dose ranging from 27 to 72 % have been reported when this technology is used, the magnitude of the reduction depending on the location of the

operator's hands along the z-axis of the scanner [7]. Implementations of CT fluoroscopy where the x-ray tube is energized only during the 240° of rotation under the patient, such as that from Philips, will also result in lower doses to the hands of the operator.

Eye Protection

Lead eyewear affords excellent protection to the wearer, but the amount of protection provided depends on both the lead content of the lenses as well as the design of the eyewear. It is usually the case that the lightest eyewear affords the least protection, and the heaviest eyewear affords the most protection. The use of traditional goggle-type eyewear (Fig. 3.6a) reduces lens dose by approximately 80 %, while the use of sport-wrap type eyewear (Fig. 3.6b) results in a reduction of approximately 50 %. This is similar to the reduction experienced when using panoramic-type eyewear (Fig. 3.6c) [12]. While panoramic eyewear wraps far around the side of the face, the lead content of the lenses is typically much lower than sport-wrap or traditional eyewear. A final consideration is the use of prescription lead eyewear. Prescription eyewear is more comfortable than an overshield, but sport-wrap style eyewear with highly curved lenses may not accept prescription lenses.

The operator should always wear lead eyewear when using continuous CT fluoroscopy. The operator should also wear lead eyewear when using biopsy mode while not using additional protection, such as standing in the gantry shadow, behind a mobile lead barrier, or using a suspended shield. Lens doses to ancillary personnel who are positioned behind barriers or outside the lab are generally low enough such that the use of lead eyewear is not required, even if occasional excursions are made outside the protected zone.

Use of the hand dose reduction technology discussed previously will result in a further reduction of the dose to the eyes and face of the operator. For example, an operator standing on the left side of a supine patient could select an option that removes power from the x-ray tube over a 100° range centered at the 2 o'clock position in the gantry, reducing his exposure to intense backscattered radiation. Implementations of CT fluoroscopy where the x-ray tube is energized only during the 240° of rotation under the patient also reduce doses to the lenses of the eye.

References

1. Lucas PA, Dance DR, Castellano IA, Vano E. Estimation of the peak entrance surface air kerma for patients undergoing computed tomography-guided procedures. Radiat Prot Dosimetry. 2005;114:317–20.

2. Leng S, Christner JA, Carlson SK, Jacobsen M, Vrieze TJ, Atwell TD, McCollough CH. Radiation dose levels for interventional CT procedures. Am J Roentgenol. 2011;197:W97–103.

3. Nawfel RD, Judy PF, Silverman SG, Hooton S, Tuncali K, Adams DF. Patient and personnel exposure during CT fluoroscopy-guided interventional procedures. Radiology. 2000;216: 180–4.

4. Balter S, Hopewell JW, Miller DL, Wagner LK, Zelefsky MJ. Fluoroscopically guided interventional procedures: a review of radiation effects on patients' skin and hair. Radiology. 2010;254: 326–41.

5. Lucey BC, Varghese JC, Hochberg A, Blake MA, Soto JA. CT-guided intervention with low radiation dose: feasibility and experience. Am J Roentgenol. 2007;188:1187–94.

6. The Alliance for Radiation Safety in Pediatric Imaging. The image gently and step lightly campaigns. http://www.pedrad.org/associations/5364/ig/. Accessed Jan 2013.

7. Hohl C, Suess C, Wildberger JE, Honnef D, Das M, Muhlenbruch G, Scahller A, Gunther RW, Mahnken AH. Dose reduction during CT fluoroscopy: phantom study of angular beam modulation. Radiology. 2008;246:519–25.

8. National Electrical Manufacturers Association (NEMA). XR 25-2010, computed tomography dose check. http://www.nema.org/stds/xr25.cfm. Accessed Jan 2013.

9. Jones AK. Is it safe? A look at exposures in the shadow of MDCT scanner gantries. Med Phys. 2008;35:2656.

10. National Council on Radiation Protection and Measurements (NCRP). NCRP Report 168. Radiation dose management for fluoroscopically-guided interventional medical procedures. NCRP, Bethesda, MD, 2011.

11. Kato R, Katada K, Anno H, Suzuki S, Ida Y, Koga S. Radiation dosimetry at CT fluoroscopy: physician's hand dose and development of needle holders. Radiology. 1996;201:576–8.

12. Schueler B, Sturchio G, Landsworth R, Magnuson D. Does new lightweight leaded eyewear provide adequate radiation protection for fluoroscopists? Med Phys. 2009;36:2747–8.

Ultrasound-Guided Biopsy

Judy U. Ahrar and Kamran Ahrar

Introduction

Ultrasound-guided biopsy has become an essential diagnostic technique in radiology [1]. It is safe and accurate and is often used for confirmation of suspected malignancy and characterization of other lesions throughout the body. Initially, ultrasound-guided biopsies were restricted to large, superficial cystic lesions. Improvements in imaging technology and biopsy techniques now allow even small masses located deep within the body to be imaged and targeted for sampling under ultrasound guidance. This chapter outlines the equipment, advantages, disadvantages, applications, and techniques used in ultrasound-guided biopsies.

Equipment

Any ultrasonography unit that can image and localize a lesion within the body can also be used to guide a biopsy of that lesion. In general, the transducer that is most suitable for imaging of the organ of interest is also used to guide the biopsy. High-frequency linear transducers are appropriate for targeting more superficial lesions (Fig. 4.1), whereas low-frequency curved array transducers are more appropriate for targeting lesions that are located deep within the body (Fig. 4.2) (e.g., liver tumors). Needle-guidance systems are available for use with various ultrasonography units and transducers. The guidance system consists of an adaptor that attaches directly to the transducer (Fig. 4.3). Once attached to the transducer, the predicted needle path is displayed on the screen. The depth and angle of needle insertion can be adjusted by choosing from the available predetermined choices. The adaptor has a groove or slot to allow passage of the biopsy needle. The needle should be held firmly in place to avoid deviation from the predetermined path. Therefore, different sizes of needle guides are available to be inserted into the groove or slot of the adaptor. The guidance system helps maintain the needle path in the plane of the ultrasound beam, simplifying ultrasound-guided biopsies. On the other hand, the inability to operate the transducer and the needle separately from one another takes away some of the flexibility of the freehand needle-insertion technique (Fig. 4.4).

Advantages

Ultrasonography is appealing as an image-guidance modality for several reasons. Ultrasonography is readily available, relatively inexpensive, and portable. It allows multiplanar imaging in any conventional or arbitrary plane. Unlike computed tomography (CT), ultrasonography does not use ionizing radiation. Most importantly, ultrasound guidance provides real-time visualization and monitoring of the needle tip as it is advanced into the skin, through the overlying soft tissues, and into the biopsy target. This visualization of the needle tip allows precise needle placement while avoiding damage to the nearby structures. Color flow Doppler imaging can help identify the vascular nature of the mass and the adjacent vascular structures (Fig. 4.1) [2, 3]. The imaging plane can be adjusted to exclude vessels from the path of the needle. Watching the needle tip during the sampling process in real time helps ensure that the needle tip does not extend outside the mass and that the biopsy is obtained from the lesion of interest (Fig. 4.5).

J.U. Ahrar, MD
Department of Interventional Radiology,
The University of Texas MD Anderson Cancer Center,
1515 Holcombe Boulevard, Unit 1471, Houston, TX 77030, USA
e-mail: judy.ahrar@mdanderson.org

K. Ahrar, MD, FSIR (✉)
Department of Interventional Radiology,
Department of Thoracic and Cardiovascular Surgery,
The University of Texas MD Anderson Cancer Center,
1515 Holcombe Boulevard, Unit 1471,
Houston, TX 77030, USA
e-mail: kahrar@mdanderson.org

K. Ahrar, S. Gupta (eds.), *Percutaneous Image-Guided Biopsy*,
DOI 10.1007/978-1-4614-8217-8_4, © Springer Science+Business Media New York 2014

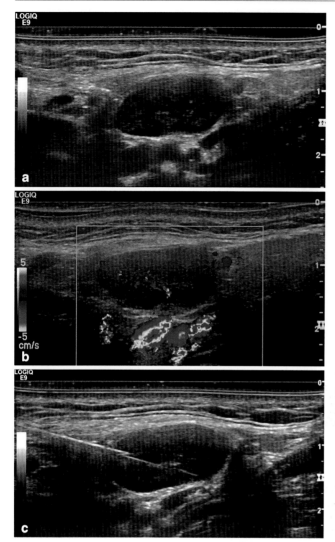

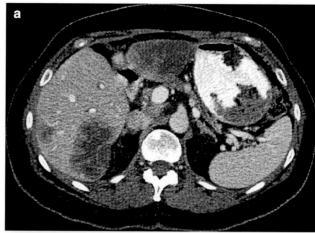

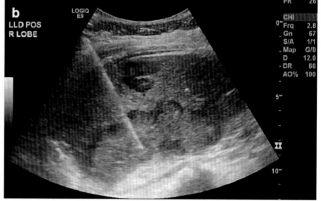

Fig. 4.2 A 68-year-old woman with a history of metastatic breast cancer was referred for a biopsy prior to enrollment in a clinical trial. An axial CT image of the liver (**a**) revealed a 6-cm mass in the medial aspect of segment VI. A smaller (2 cm) mass is seen more superficially closer to the liver capsule. With the patient in the left lateral decubitus position, real-time ultrasound guidance was used to target the medial lesion for sampling (**b**). When possible, the target liver lesion and biopsy path should be selected such that the needle traverses a segment of normal liver before entering the tumor. This may reduce the risk of bleeding and tumor seeding after the biopsy

Fig. 4.1 A 51-year-old man with a history of lymphoma was referred for biopsy of an enlarged right cervical lymph node. A high-frequency (6–15 MHz) linear transducer was used to image this superficial lesion (**a**). Duplex Doppler sonography revealed some vascularity in the lesion and larger vascular structures deeper to the lesion (**b**). An 18-gauge core biopsy needle was used to obtain several core biopsy samples (**c**). A trajectory was chosen to obtain the longest possible core biopsy sample. Pathologic evaluation revealed mantle cell lymphoma, diffuse pattern

Another major advantage of ultrasound guidance is that the patient can be placed in various positions and that steep out-of-axial-plane angles can be used for needle guidance. Flexibility in the positioning of the patient also adds to the patient's comfort during the biopsy. For example, the head of the bed may be elevated or the patient may be allowed to move slightly during the biopsy to get into a more comfortable position to relieve back or joint pain.

Compared to CT-guided biopsies, ultrasound-guided biopsies require less time to perform and can be more cost effective [4–6]. Some studies have suggested that ultrasound-guided biopsies are more accurate and have lower false-negative rates than CT-guided biopsies [6, 7].

Disadvantages

Not all lesions can be well visualized on ultrasonography. Ultrasound guidance is optimal for targeting lesions that are located superficially or at a moderate depth in a thin- to moderate-sized patient. Ultrasound guidance is of limited use in identifying and targeting lesions in obese patients or lesions located deep within the body. Similarly, ultrasound-guided biopsy may not be possible when lesions are located

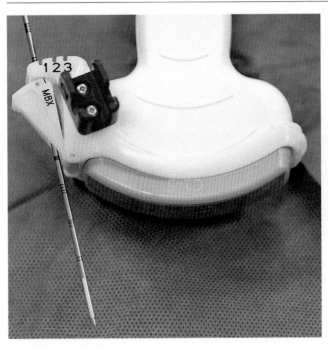

Fig. 4.3 In this photograph, the curved transducer is fitted with an adaptor with several predetermined angle settings. With this technique, the needle and the transducer work as a unit. The adaptor fits the needle and guides it to the target while preventing deviation of the needle from the set course

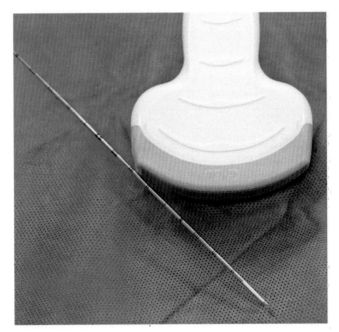

Fig. 4.4 In the "freehand technique," the needle and the transducer are operated separately from one another. The needle can be inserted at any angle. One can also choose an insertion site that is not directly in the imaging plane, but maintaining the needle tip in the imaging plane of the transducer is more challenging and requires experience

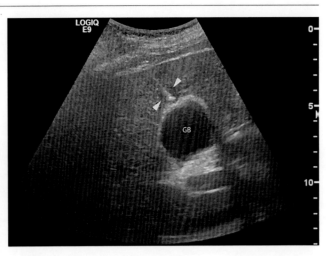

Fig. 4.5 A 54-year-old man with history of prostate cancer was referred for biopsy of a small liver lesion. Gray-scale sonographic image of the liver during the biopsy revealed a 1-cm hypoechoic tumor (*arrowheads*) adjacent to the gallbladder (*GB*). The echogenic needle is seen in the tumor. Real-time monitoring of the needle tip during fine-needle aspiration biopsy ensured safe, selective sampling of the small lesion without inadvertent puncture of the gallbladder

behind a reflective surface such as bone or gas-filled bowel and when the transducer cannot be positioned to look from a different angle.

Applications

Any mass that is well visualized on ultrasonography can be targeted for biopsy. This includes any superficial soft tissue mass, head and neck lesion, breast tumor, or solid or cystic mass in the liver, kidney, or spleen [8–14]. Ultrasound guidance is commonly used to perform liver biopsies. This may include biopsy of specific lesions within the liver or biopsy of liver parenchyma to investigate the cause and severity of liver failure. The left lobe of the liver can often be reached from an anterior subcostal approach. The sagittal imaging plane can be helpful for lesions closer to the dome of the liver, although a steep-angle approach may be necessary. Lesions in the inferior aspect of the right lobe of the liver may be approached by a lateral subcostal route. Frequently, lesions in the right lobe of the liver are approached through an intercostal route with the patient placed in left lateral decubitus or supine position. Ultrasound-guided biopsy of a renal mass can be performed if the patient is not morbidly obese and the kidney can be adequately imaged on ultrasonography (Fig. 4.6). Ultrasonography can also be used to guide core biopsies of native and transplanted renal parenchyma to determine the etiology of parenchymal disease. Other abdominal and retroperitoneal organs such as the pancreas and adrenal gland may

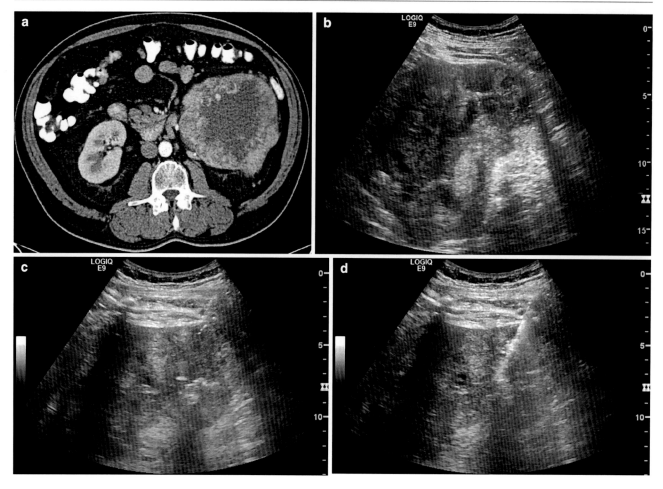

Fig. 4.6 An axial CT image of the abdomen (**a**) in a 53-year-old man revealed a large left renal mass with central necrosis. A gray-scale sonographic image (**b**) revealed a large mass with heterogeneous echogenicity. During ultrasound-guided biopsy (**c**), a 16-gauge guide needle is visualized with difficulty. When the stylet is replaced by the core biopsy needle, microbubbles introduced into the guide needle greatly enhance the echogenicity of the guide needle (**d**) and allow better visualization of the needle in the target

be targeted with ultrasound for biopsy [15, 16]. Ultrasound guidance can be used to biopsy lung, mediastinal, and pleural masses that abut the chest wall [17]. Some musculoskeletal lesions can be targeted using ultrasound guidance (Fig. 4.7) [18–20]. For retroperitoneal lesions, an anterior approach is preferred. Using specialized transducers, pelvic organs can be reached by transvaginal or transrectal approaches [21–23].

Techniques

Prior to ultrasound-guided biopsy, a limited ultrasound is performed to localize the lesion, select a suitable transducer, and plan the needle's path. The distance between the puncture site and the target is measured to help select an appropriate biopsy needle. In some practices, a sonographer is responsible for imaging the patient during the biopsy, while the physician advances the needle to the target. Experienced interventional radiologists do not require a sonographer's assistance, as the interventional radiologist will hold the transducer in one hand and the biopsy needle in the other hand. In this manner, hand-eye coordination is optimized.

Biopsy procedures are performed under sterile conditions. The transducer is covered with a sterile plastic cover. To prevent image degradation, ultrasound gel is placed inside the sterile cover to provide acoustic coupling. In addition, sterile gel is placed on the skin's surface. Others prefer to clean the transducer with alcohol and place it directly on the skin [24], and no increase in post-biopsy infection rates has been reported [25].

Ultrasound-guided biopsies are performed under continuous real-time visualization of the biopsy needle as it is advanced to the target. If a needle-guidance system is used,

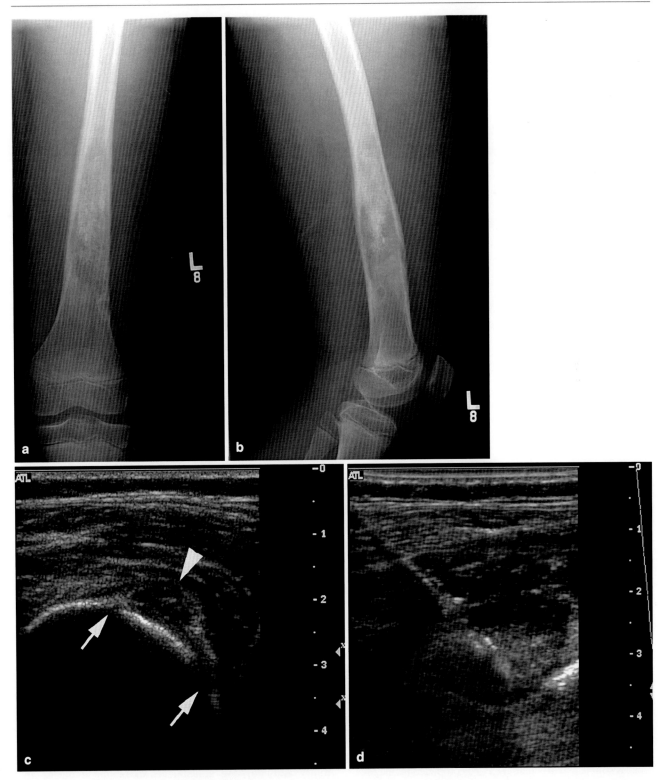

Fig. 4.7 An 11-year-old boy presented with pain and discomfort in the left thigh. Anteroposterior (**a**) and lateral (**b**) radiographs of the left femur revealed an expansile lesion of the distal femoral diaphysis, with osteoid matrix, suspicious for osteosarcoma. The radiographs do not reveal a significant soft tissue component. He was referred for image-guided biopsy. Transverse gray-scale ultrasound of the left femur (**c**) revealed a rind of soft tissue thickening, with a nodular component (*arrowhead*) with underlying cortical breakdown (*arrows*). The soft tissue component of the tumor was targeted for biopsy (**d**) using a 14-gauge semiautomatic core biopsy needle. Four samples were obtained. A pathologic review revealed high-grade osteoblastic osteosarcoma

Fig. 4.8 Illustration of the freehand technique. (**a**) In this frontal view of the transducer, the target lesion and needle are in the imaging plane. The insertion angle is adjusted so that the needle penetrates the lesion. In the lateral (**b**) and superior (**c**) views, the artist demonstrates how the needle can deviate (*arrow*) from the imaging plane and potentially miss the target

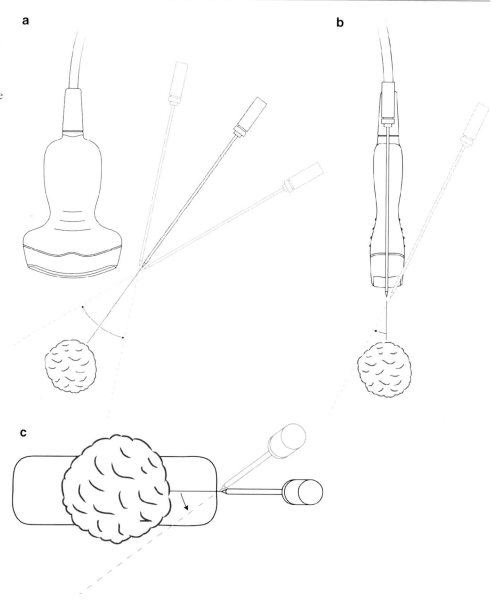

a scanning plane is chosen so that the target lesion is lined up with the needle path. The depth of the needle insertion can be adjusted by choosing from the available predetermined angle choices. A needle guide of the correct size is attached or inserted into the transducer guide prior to insertion of the needle. The entire shaft of the needle can be constantly visualized when using a guidance system, making the needle-insertion process simple and efficient. It can be completed in one breath hold if needed. On the other hand, there is limited flexibility with the plane of imaging when using a rigid guidance system. Also, the needle must be placed close to the transducer and cannot be inserted at a more remote puncture site.

Experienced radiologists prefer to use a freehand technique without a needle guide [24, 26]. The operator holds the transducer in one hand and the needle in the other. With experience, one can use either hand as the needle or operating hand and avoid crossing hands, which may lead to difficulties in orientation. In this technique, the needle is freely inserted into the view of the transducer, providing great flexibility and allowing adjustments to be made during the biopsy. On the other hand, improper alignment of the needle tip and the plane of imaging (transducer) may lead to suboptimal visualization or nonvisualization of the needle tip (Fig. 4.8).

Needle visualization may be enhanced by increasing the reflective or scattering properties of the biopsy needle [27–29]. This can be accomplished by dimpling or etching of the needle tip, using a screw-tip needle or coating the needle with Teflon or other reflective substances [30]. Jiggling the needle as it is advanced in the tissue, jiggling the stylet in and out of the needle, and keeping the bevel of the needle up may improve visualization of the needle [31]. Large-gauge needles cause brighter reflections and are more easily visualized than are small-gauge needles. Using the highest frequency possible improves visualization of the needle. Color flow Doppler imaging may also help visualize the needle tip [32, 33]. Needles are more difficult to visualize at shallow insertion angles [34]. When the needle is inserted nearly parallel to the ultrasound beam, the major portion of the ultrasound beam is reflected away from the transducer face, making it more difficult to visualize the needle. If the needle is inserted nearly perpendicular to the ultrasound beam, more of the beam is reflected back to the transducer face, allowing excellent needle visualization. Needles are more easily detected in fluid and tissues with low echogenicity than in highly echogenic tissues. Treated needles are most helpful in echogenic tissues.

A linear high-frequency transducer is optimal for targeting superficial lesions such as structures in the head and neck or superficial lymph nodes throughout the body (Fig. 4.1). A curved array transducer is often used to target lesions that are located at a moderate depth from the skin surface (Fig. 4.2). For example, lesions in the liver or kidney are often targeted using a curved array transducer (1- to 5-MHz). The ultrasound parameters should be optimized for visualization of the target lesion. The depth of the imaging is set to the depth of the lesion, and the focal zone is placed in the near field or just at the level of the lesion for better needle visualization. A single focal zone is preferred because multiple focal zones may decrease the frame rate.

Ideally, the interventional radiologist can visualize the needle and the target on the same image on the screen and can watch the needle as it is advanced toward the target. If the needle and the lesion are both visible on one image, but the angle of the needle is such that it would miss the target, the angle needs to be corrected (Fig. 4.8a). If the needle is already beyond the subcutaneous tissues, levering of the needle may not lead to the desired change in the angle of the trajectory. Oftentimes, the needle has to be withdrawn to just below the skin and reinserted at the desirable angle. When the needle deviates from the imaging plane, the tip will not be seen as it is advanced into the body (Fig. 4.8b, c). If not recognized, this may lead to injury of adjacent structures. First, the operator should visually inspect the relationship of the transducer and the needle on the patient. The transducer might have slipped on the skin and turned away from the puncture site. This can be easily corrected by realigning the transducer along the needle path. On the other hand, if the needle has deviated from the desirable imaging plane and is off target, the operator needs first to locate the needle tip by angling the transducer from side to side. Once the position of the needle tip relative to the target is determined (e.g., medial or cephalad), the needle is withdrawn and reinserted after slight correction toward the target (e.g., lateral or caudad). Occasionally, a firm mass located superficially in the subcutaneous tissues may be pushed out of the way by the needle tip. To secure the target, the operator can apply firm pressure, fixing the lesion in place while puncturing it with the biopsy needle. Also during biopsy of abdominal lesions, the operator may press the transducer firmly toward the lesion to reduce the skin-to-lesion distance and to displace any overlying loops of bowel [35]. Care must be taken to make sure the bowel loop is actually displaced out of the needle path and is not compressed between the transducer and the target.

In recent years, more sophisticated ultrasound units are fitted with software packages that allow fusion of previously obtained cross-sectional images with the real-time ultrasound examination (Fig. 4.9). This feature allows more confident sampling of the lesion and targeting of lesions that may be hard to visualize with ultrasound alone.

In summary, ultrasound guidance is an effective and efficient technique to target lesions or organs during biopsy procedures. Use of needle-guidance systems facilitates the procedure, but mastering the freehand technique allows the maximum flexibility during ultrasound-guided biopsies.

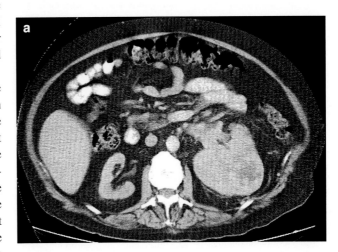

Fig. 4.9 An axial CT image of the abdomen (**a**) revealed a large ill-defined, infiltrative mass involving the lower pole of the left kidney. Ultrasound-guided biopsy was performed in the prone position (**b**) after fusion of the previously acquired CT images (*right*) with the real-time ultrasound image (*left*). The software allows real-time reconstruction of previously acquired CT images in any arbitrary plane, corresponding to that of the ultrasound transducer

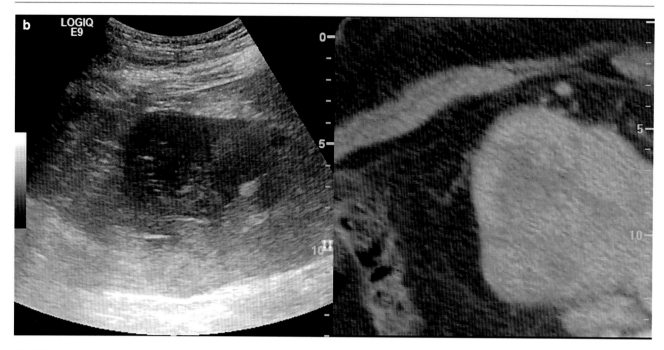

Fig. 4.9 (continued)

References

1. Charboneau JW, Reading CC, Welch TJ. CT and sonographically guided needle biopsy: current techniques and new innovations. Am J Roentgenol. 1990;154:1–10.
2. Longo JM, Bilbao JI, Barettino MD, Larrea JA, Pueyo J, Idoate F, et al. Percutaneous vascular and nonvascular puncture under US guidance: role of color Doppler imaging. Radiographics. 1994; 14:959–72.
3. McGahan JP, Anderson MW. Pulsed Doppler sonography as an aid in ultrasound-guided aspiration biopsy. Gastrointest Radiol. 1987;12:279–84.
4. Kliewer MA, Sheafor DH, Paulson EK, Helsper RS, Hertzberg BS, Nelson RC. Percutaneous liver biopsy: a cost-benefit analysis comparing sonographic and CT guidance. Am J Roentgenol. 1999;173:1199–202.
5. Sheafor DH, Paulson EK, Kliewer MA, DeLong DM, Nelson RC. Comparison of sonographic and CT guidance techniques: does CT fluoroscopy decrease procedure time? Am J Roentgenol. 2000;174:939–42.
6. Sheafor DH, Paulson EK, Simmons CM, DeLong DM, Nelson RC. Abdominal percutaneous interventional procedures: comparison of CT and US guidance. Radiology. 1998;207:705–10.
7. Dameron RD, deLong DM, Fisher AJ, Dodd LG, Nelson RC. Indeterminate findings on imaging-guided biopsy: should additional intervention be pursued? Am J Roentgenol. 1999;173: 461–4.
8. Cho HW, Kim J, Choi J, Choi HS, Kim ES, Kim SH, et al. Sonographically guided fine-needle aspiration biopsy of major salivary gland masses: a review of 245 cases. Am J Roentgenol. 2011;196:1160–3.
9. Copel L, Sosna J, Kruskal JB, Kane RA. Ultrasound-guided percutaneous liver biopsy: indications, risks, and technique. Surg Technol Int. 2003;11:154–60.
10. Handa U, Tiwari A, Singhal N, Mohan H, Kaur R. Utility of ultrasound-guided fine-needle aspiration in splenic lesions. Diagn Cytopathol. 2011 [Epub ahead of print].
11. Johnson PT, Nazarian LN, Feld RI, Needleman L, Lev-Toaff AS, Segal SR, et al. Sonographically guided renal mass biopsy: indications and efficacy. J Ultrasound Med. 2001;20:749–53; quiz 55.
12. Jung AS, Sharma G, Maceri D, Rice D, Martin SE, Korostoff AB, et al. Ultrasound-guided fine needle aspiration of major salivary gland masses and adjacent lymph nodes. Ultrasound Q. 2011;27: 105–13.
13. Povoski SP, Jimenez RE, Wang WP. Ultrasound-guided diagnostic breast biopsy methodology: retrospective comparison of the 8-gauge vacuum-assisted biopsy approach versus the spring-loaded 14-gauge core biopsy approach. World J Surg Oncol. 2011;9:87.
14. Tang S, Li JH, Lui SL, Chan TM, Cheng IK, Lai KN. Free-hand, ultrasound-guided percutaneous renal biopsy: experience from a single operator. Eur J Radiol. 2002;41:65–9.
15. Brandt KR, Charboneau JW, Stephens DH, Welch TJ, Goellner JR. CT- and US-guided biopsy of the pancreas. Radiology. 1993;187:99–104.
16. Tikkakoski T, Taavitsainen M, Paivansalo M, Lahde S, Apaja-Sarkkinen M. Accuracy of adrenal biopsy guided by ultrasound and CT. Acta Radiol. 1991;32:371–4.
17. Sheth S, Hamper UM, Stanley DB, Wheeler JH, Smith PA. US guidance for thoracic biopsy: a valuable alternative to CT. Radiology. 1999;210:721–6.
18. Ahrar K, Himmerich JU, Herzog CE, Raymond AK, Wallace MJ, Gupta S, et al. Percutaneous ultrasound-guided biopsy in the definitive diagnosis of osteosarcoma. J Vasc Interv Radiol. 2004;15:1329–33.
19. Saifuddin A, Mitchell R, Burnett SJ, Sandison A, Pringle JA. Ultrasound-guided needle biopsy of primary bone tumours. J Bone Joint Surg Br. 2000;82:50–4.
20. Yeow KM, Tan CF, Chen JS, Hsueh C. Diagnostic sensitivity of ultrasound-guided needle biopsy in soft tissue masses about superficial bone lesions. J Ultrasound Med. 2000;19:849–55.

21. O'Neill MJ, Rafferty EA, Lee SI, Arellano RS, Gervais DA, Hahn PF, et al. Transvaginal interventional procedures: aspiration, biopsy, and catheter drainage. Radiographics. 2001;21:657–72.

22. Pinto PA, Chung PH, Rastinehad AR, Baccala Jr AA, Kruecker J, Benjamin CJ, et al. Magnetic resonance imaging/ultrasound fusion guided prostate biopsy improves cancer detection following transrectal ultrasound biopsy and correlates with multiparametric magnetic resonance imaging. J Urol. 2011;186:1281–5.

23. Roy D, Kulkarni A, Kulkarni S, Thakur MH, Maheshwari A, Tongaonkar HB. Transrectal ultrasound-guided biopsy of recurrent cervical carcinoma. Br J Radiol. 2008;81:902–6.

24. Reading CC, Charboneau JW, James EM, Hurt MR. Sonographically guided percutaneous biopsy of small (3 cm or less) masses. Am J Roentgenol. 1988;151:189–92.

25. Caturelli E, Giacobbe A, Facciorusso D, Villani MR, Squillante MM, Siena DA, et al. Free-hand technique with ordinary antisepsis in abdominal US-guided fine-needle punctures: three-year experience. Radiology. 1996;199:721–3.

26. Matalon TA, Silver B. US guidance of interventional procedures. Radiology. 1990;174:43–7.

27. Heckemann R, Seidel KJ. The sonographic appearance and contrast enhancement of puncture needles. J Clin Ultrasound. 1983;11:265–8.

28. McGahan JP. Laboratory assessment of ultrasonic needle and catheter visualization. J Ultrasound Med. 1986;5:373–7.

29. Reading CC, Charboneau JW, Felmlee JP, James EM. US-guided percutaneous biopsy: use of a screw biopsy stylet to aid needle detection. Radiology. 1987;163:280–1.

30. Culp WC, McCowan TC, Goertzen TC, Habbe TG, Hummel MM, LeVeen RF, et al. Relative ultrasonographic echogenicity of standard, dimpled, and polymeric-coated needles. J Vasc Interv Radiol. 2000;11:351–8.

31. Bisceglia M, Matalon TA, Silver B. The pump maneuver: an atraumatic adjunct to enhance US needle tip localization. Radiology. 1990;176:867–8.

32. Cockburn JF, Cosgrove DO. Device to enhance visibility of needle or catheter tip at color Doppler US. Radiology. 1995;195:570–2.

33. Hamper UM, Savader BL, Sheth S. Improved needle-tip visualization by color Doppler sonography. Am J Roentgenol. 1991;156:401–2.

34. Nichols K, Wright LB, Spencer T, Culp WC. Changes in ultrasonographic echogenicity and visibility of needles with changes in angles of insonation. J Vasc Interv Radiol. 2003;14:1553–7.

35. Fisher AJ, Paulson EK, Sheafor DH, Simmons CM, Nelson RC. Small lymph nodes of the abdomen, pelvis, and retroperitoneum: usefulness of sonographically guided biopsy. Radiology. 1997;205:185–90.

MRI-Guided Biopsy

5

Kamran Ahrar and R. Jason Stafford

Radiology departments are equipped with fluoroscopy, computed tomography (CT), and ultrasound units, which are used for both diagnostic and interventional purposes. Depending on the location, size, and imaging characteristics of a mass, any one or more of these imaging modalities may be used to guide the biopsy procedure. More recently, owing to its unique soft-tissue contrast capability, the use of magnetic resonance imaging (MRI) guidance for percutaneous biopsy has gained popularity [1]. For instance, MRI has been increasingly incorporated into the assessment of breast disease. The need to biopsy MRI findings that could not be visualized on ultrasound resulted in the development of biopsy techniques, hardware, and software that has made MRI-guided breast biopsies a ubiquitous procedure in standard 1.5 T cylindrical bore scanners [2, 3].

However, owing to the superficial placement of the breast and ability to stabilize the gland, the breast is a unique case where access for biopsy is fairly easy in the MRI environment. Other areas of the body are much more challenging in conventional, cylindrical bore scanners. Although biopsies can be performed in conventional diagnostic MRI units, direct access to the patient during image acquisition is limited by the length of the bore (generally >150 cm), and small bore apertures place challenging limits on the tradeoffs between patient size and the placement of needles and devices in the bore of the magnet [4]. Because of these limitations, the primary clinical development of MRI-guided biopsies in the body has been in MRI units with an open design and a low magnetic field gradient (<1.0 T) [5, 6].

The availability of MRI units with high magnetic field ($\geq$1.0 T), and a more open design that is more accommodating to the needs of the interventional radiologist without sacrificing signal-to-noise ratio or speed, and the increasing availability of MRI-compatible equipment for interventions are spurring the creation of dedicated interventional MRI (iMRI) suites at various medical centers throughout the United States. The wider availability of MRI systems for guidance in the interventional environment allows the interventional radiologist to employ the benefits of this non-ionizing, real-time modality, such as superior soft-tissue contrast and tumor conspicuity and multislice imaging in arbitrarily oriented planes, in the interventional patient population.

Equipment

Through proper equipment selection and careful patient selection, MRI-guided biopsies of many anatomical sites can be performed in practically any conventional MRI cylindrical system. Admittedly, these diagnostic magnets often have a small diameter bore ($\leq$60 cm) and are quite long (>150 cm). Under such circumstances, image guidance is restricted to intermittent imaging updates in which the patient is moved out of the unit for needle manipulation and back into the unit for imaging [7]. The introduction of compact-length large-bore magnets facilitates better access to the patient and better placement of the needles and devices using either an intermittent imaging technique or real-time MRI fluoroscopy (Fig. 5.1) [8]. The signal requirements of high-resolution MRI requires placement of radiofrequency coils over the desired body segment for reception. Current surface coil designs provide suboptimal access to the patient; surface coils that are specifically designed and

K. Ahrar, MD, FSIR (✉)
Department of Interventional Radiology,
Department of Thoracic and Cardiovascular Surgery,
The University of Texas MD Anderson Cancer Center,
1515 Holcombe Boulevard, Unit 1471,
Houston, TX 77030, USA
e-mail: kahrar@mdanderson.org,

R.J. Stafford, PhD
Department of Imaging Physics,
The University of Texas MD Anderson Cancer Center,
1400 Pressler Street, Unit 1472,
Houston, TX 77064, USA
e-mail: jstafford@mdanderson.org

K. Ahrar, S. Gupta (eds.), *Percutaneous Image-Guided Biopsy*,
DOI 10.1007/978-1-4614-8217-8_5, © Springer Science+Business Media New York 2014

Fig. 5.1 The interventional MRI unit at The University of Texas MD Anderson Cancer Center is equipped with a short (125 cm) expanded diameter (70 cm) bore in a 1.5-T MRI scanner (Magnetom Espree, Siemens Medical Solutions, Erlangen, Germany). In-room monitors are available for the radiologist to use while performing an intervention

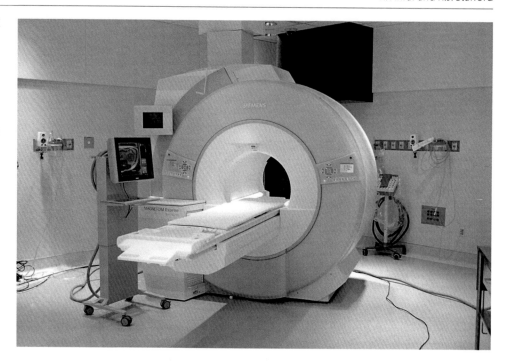

Fig. 5.2 A standard Siemens large-loop coil has a diameter of 17 cm. This coil provides good image quality for superficial lesions

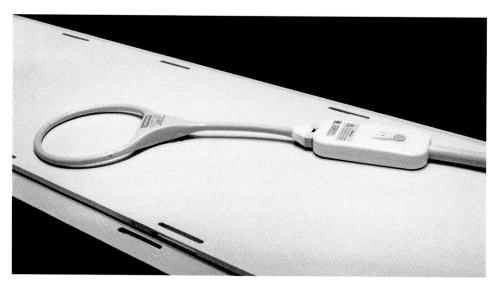

manufactured for interventional procedures, similar to those designed specifically for breast imaging and intervention, are needed to overcome the logistical hurdles of this technological limitation. Most standard diagnostic surface coils have one or more openings that can be placed over the area of interest, providing adequate, albeit small, access to the biopsy site. Single-loop coils provide the largest aperture for patient access, but these coils suffer from decreased signal-to-noise ratio at depth (Fig. 5.2). Array coils have superior image quality but limited aperture size based on the number of coil elements (Fig. 5.3). Often, as MRI systems increase in the number of independent channels, the aperture of the standard multi-element array coils decreases in size as more elements are added for image quality. An important consideration when investigating an MRI system for use in interventions is the availability of array coils that

facilitate reasonable access to the patient as well as reasonable image quality.

Positioning of the coils, equipment, and patient within the bore must be performed by experienced MRI personnel so as to minimize risk of excessive heating from the radiofrequency excitation pulses used during imaging. Additionally, because of the radiofrequency pulses and high magnetic field in the room, safety regulations require screening of patients and staff. During real-time imaging, the rapidly switched gradients result in high noise levels in the room so that hearing protection must be worn by patient and staff alike. Dedicated MRI-compatible communication systems are very useful for communicating with staff during real-time imaging (Fig. 5.4). Additionally, all ancillary equipment that will be used on the patient in the suite needs to be safe for the MRI environment. MRI-compatible

Fig. 5.3 A standard Siemens body array coil has six elements and provides better image quality for deeper targets than does the large-loop coil. On the other hand, the body coil has small openings (10 cm) that limit access to the patient and the biopsy site

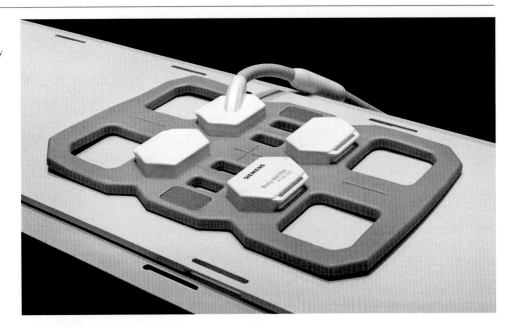

Fig. 5.4 During a typical MRI-guided intervention, the radiologist stays in the MRI suite during imaging. Ear protection and communication is accomplished using an MRI-compatible fiber-optic communication system (IMROC, OptoAcoustics Ltd., Or-Yehuda, Israel). An in-room monitor provides updated images in real time for the radiologist to view

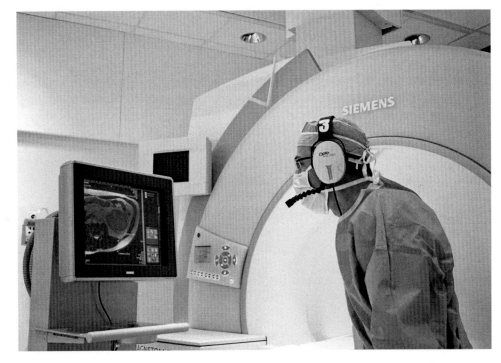

patient-monitoring devices are required to perform interventional procedures in the MRI suite. Fortunately, these devices are widely available in most MRI suites as some patients may require sedation during imaging and therefore require hemodynamic monitoring [9]. Similarly, MRI-compatible anesthesia equipment is commercially available.

Finally, several ancillary devices can be extremely helpful in facilitating MRI-guided interventions. First, a tableside monitor located in the MRI suite may be used by the operator to review images immediately prior to or subsequent to any needle manipulation (Figs. 5.1 and 5.4). Such equipment has become an

option with most major MRI manufacturers and is an essential component for executing real-time MRI-guided biopsies. Additionally, tableside control buttons to perform simple tasks, such as starting and stopping a prescribed imaging sequence or quickly moving the patient in and out of the bore of the magnet during intermittent imaging, can markedly improve the workflow for the interventional radiologist (Fig. 5.5).

At the University of Texas MD Anderson Cancer Center, our initial experience with MRI-guided biopsies began with the use of a 1.5 T conventional cylindrical MRI unit (Signa Excite, GE Healthcare, Waukesha, WI). This system is an older magnet

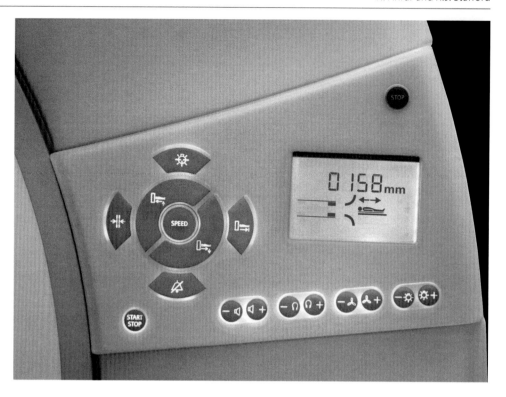

Fig. 5.5 Tableside controls allow the radiologist to perform simple tasks without the assistance of the technologist. Two of the most important functions are moving the patient in and out of the unit and starting and stopping an imaging sequence

design with a bore length of 175 cm and a high-performance gradient package (Cardiac Resonance Module: maximum amplitude of 40 mT/m and slew rate of 150 T/m/s) resulting in a smaller than average bore diameter of 55 cm. These dimensions precluded any real-time access to the patient within the bore of the magnet. Imaging was performed with the patient at the isocenter of the magnet, and needle manipulation was performed with the patient moved back to landmark outside the bore of the magnet after reviewing the acquired images.

Conventional receive-only radiofrequency coils (13-cm diameter surface coil or 4-channel torso array) were used for biopsy. The 4-channel torso array coil had a reasonably large (17.0×10.5 cm) aperture for adequate patient access and good signal-to-noise ratio at depth compared with the surface coil. The torso array consisted of anterior and posterior components that worked together to provide good signal-to-noise ratio across the target region. To mark the needle insertion site on the patient, we used the existing patient localizer light in front of the magnet. Patients were first positioned in a manner most conducive to performing the intervention based on prior imaging studies, then the region of interest was imaged using a fast, balanced steady-state free-precession sequence for T2-like contrast. Planning was usually performed using the axial plane. Once the most appropriate plane of approach was identified, the patient couch was brought out of the scanner and that plane brought to the landmark location illuminated by the light. Fiducials placed on the patient were used to localize the entry point in the lateral direction. Planning from a sagittal plane was similar but required using the lateral localizer light as a point of

reference. Because of the dependence on the localizer lights, the accuracy of these lights was incorporated into the scanners daily quality assurance routine.

Patients were monitored using standard hemodynamic monitoring equipment (Magnitude 3150 MRI, Invivo Corporation, Orlando, FL). One major drawback of working on this particular MRI system was the lack of a tableside monitor for the operator to review the most recent images prior to manipulation of the needle. Another limitation was the lack of a communication system between the operator in the MRI suite and the personnel in the control room. These limitations, in concert with limited access to the patient, severely limited procedural workflow, the types of procedures that could be performed, and patient selection. This made it difficult and time consuming for the interventional radiologist to effectively triage patients for procedures in this room.

Experience using an existing 1.5 T clinical MRI for interventional procedures guided our prospective specification of a new system that was to be dedicated for interventions. Our current iMRI suite is equipped with a short (125 cm), expanded diameter (70 cm) bore in a 1.5 T MRI scanner (Magnetom Espree, Siemens Medical Solutions, Erlangen, Germany). This system features gradients with maximum amplitude of 33 mT/m and slew rates of 170 T/m/s and the Siemens 18-channel total imaging matrix technology running the B17 software platform (Fig. 5.1). Two in-room MRI consoles facilitate in-room visualization and access to MRI controls during procedures (Fig. 5.4). Additional control buttons are located at three locations around the magnet, allowing the operator to start and stop imaging or to move the patient in and out of the magnet as needed (Fig. 5.5). The MRI suite also features an integrated, floor-mounted fluoroscopy unit (Axiom Artis, Siemens Medical Solutions) located outside the 5-gauss line and a specially designed patient transfer table that moves the patient smoothly between MRI and angiography (MR-Miyabi, Siemens).

At our center, standard Siemens radiofrequency coils are used during biopsy procedures. For most procedures, the patient is placed atop the spine coil, the signal of which is combined with the surface coil placed on the opposite side of the patient. The primary coils used on the surface of the patient where needle entry is planned include a six-element phased-array body coil and a large-loop surface coil (Figs. 5.2 and 5.3). The body coil has four small openings that can be positioned immediately over the biopsy site. The openings of the body coil are small (10×10 cm), which somewhat impedes access to the biopsy site. The access granted by the large-loop coil (17-cm diameter) is more amenable to biopsy procedures; however, image quality at depth is inferior compared with the body array coil. These coils are not sterilized for each procedure; instead, they are placed between two sterile "keyhole" drapes.

Real-time image-guided interventions require the operator to remain in the iMRI suite. Ear protection and communication is accomplished using an MRI-compatible fiber-optic communication system (IMROC, OptoAcoustics LTD, Or Yehuda, Israel) (Fig. 5.4). The system has six channels—one channel for the patient and five channels for the staff in the iMRI suite. The microphones have noise cancellation capabilities to minimize the noise from the scanner and to accentuate voices. The headphones provide 30-dB passive noise reduction. The lines of communication can be controlled between the operators, the patient, and the control room using a mixing box that is positioned in the MRI control room. From the control room, the MRI operator can listen or speak to anyone on the system. One limitation of the system is the fiber-optic cables that tether each individual to the system and complicate movement around the suite; however, a wireless system has become available recently.

Needles are visualized on MRI because of their magnetic susceptibility artifact, which depends on the raw material of which the needle is made, the size and shape of the needle, and the field strength of the magnet (Fig. 5.6) [7, 10–12].

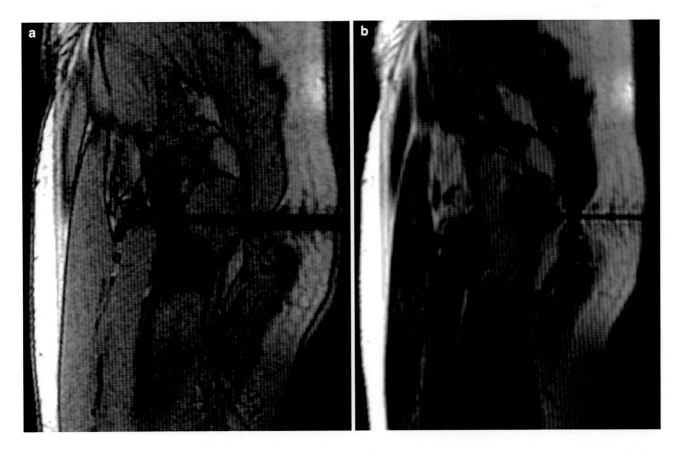

Fig. 5.6 A 61-year-old man with a history of unclassified sarcoma presented with a lytic lesion involving the proximal left femur. A biopsy was performed under MRI guidance, using a 12-gauge guide needle so that 14-gauge core biopsy samples could be obtained. An out-of-phase, T1-weighted GRE image (**a**) in the sagittal plane reveals a larger needle artifact and a lower signal-to-noise ratio than do the T1-weighted TSE (**b**) and bSSFP (**c**) images. In this case, the T2-weighted contrast of bSSFP provided better contrast and a higher signal-to-noise ratio than did the T2-weighted HASTE image (**d**). On the other hand, the tip of the biopsy needle is more sharply identified on the HASTE image (**d**). Suppression of the bright fat signal in the bSSFP (**e**) and HASTE (**f**) images further increases the conspicuity of the needle and the lesion against the background

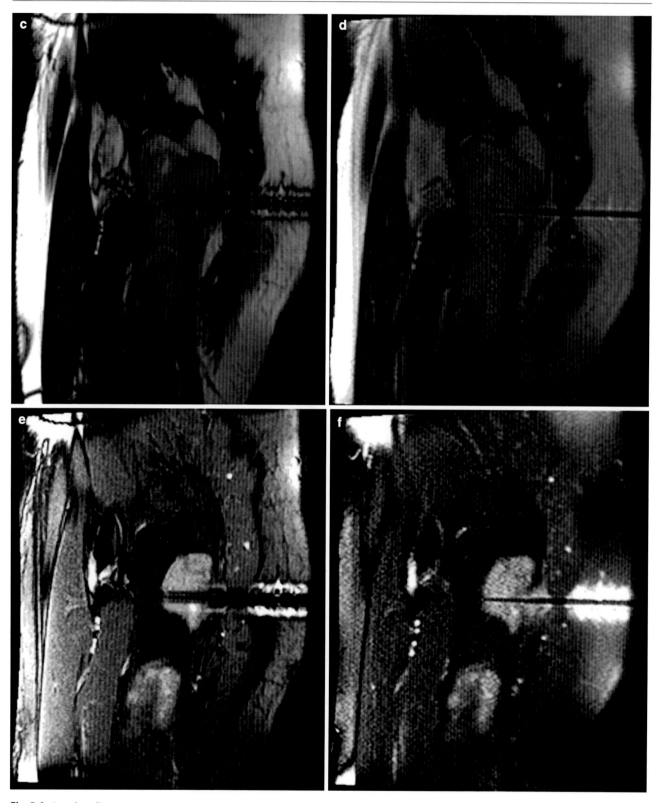

Fig. 5.6 (continued)

Relatively inexpensive alloys such as high-nickel, high-chromium, and stainless steel may create an acceptable susceptibility artifact for a 0.2 T magnet, but the artifact may be quite large for 1.5 T magnets. With the current trend toward higher magnetic fields, most MRI-compatible needles are made of titanium or nitinol. In the United States, there are only a few companies that market MRI-compatible needles, and most MRI-compatible needles are geared toward breast biopsy procedures, limiting their length and caliber. The Invivo Corporation provides the largest selection of needles for aspiration and core tissue biopsies. Some bone biopsy needles are also available through the Invivo Corporation. MRI-compatible fine-needle aspiration biopsy needles are also available through Cook Medical (Bloomington, IN).

Advantages

There are several advantages in using MRI to guide percutaneous biopsies. First, MRI provides excellent soft-tissue contrast and exquisite anatomic detail. MRI helps localize tumors that may not be easily detected with CT or ultrasound, and MRI visualizes the anatomy surrounding the biopsy target

(Figs. 5.7, 5.8, and 5.9) [6, 13, 14]. This is particularly important in detecting and targeting bone and soft-tissue tumors for which CT and ultrasound may be inadequate [15]. The use of different pulse sequences during MRI-guided interventions allows the operator to elicit different tissue characteristics within the biopsy target and the surrounding structures (Figs. 5.7 and 5.9). The use of T1- and T2-weighted pulse sequences and the application of fat suppression-, perfusion-, and diffusion-weighted images can help direct the intervention to the most relevant location within the tumor (Fig. 5.10). Easy detection and continuous visualization of vascular structures during the procedure without the need for intravenous contrast medium helps reduce the risk of hemorrhagic complications. The multiplanar imaging capability of MRI is highly desirable to guide biopsies of tumors that are in difficult locations (Figs. 5.11 and 5.12). For example, tumors in the dome of the liver can be targeted using any of the sagittal, coronal, or double-oblique imaging planes. Imaging in any conceivable plane allows on-the-fly adjustments such that the entire biopsy needle and the target tissue are simultaneously visualized on one image. When compared to CT, MRI has no ionizing radiation, which is particularly important in pediatric patients, in women of childbearing age, and to

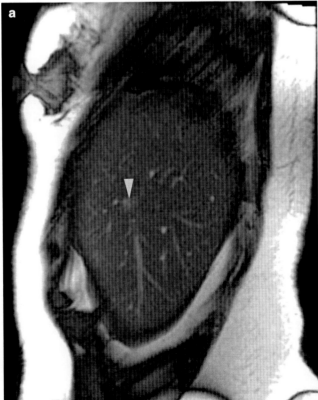
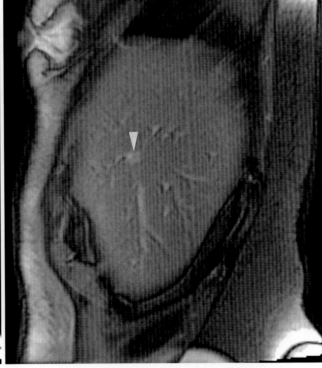

Fig. 5.7 A 60-year-old woman with a history of breast cancer and pancreatic neuroendocrine tumor was found to have a sub-centimeter liver lesion. A sagittal trueFISP image (**a**) of the liver reveals a small ill-defined lesion (*arrowhead*). After suppression of the fat signal (**b**), the tumor is better visualized (*arrowhead*). Real-time MRI guidance was used in the sagittal plane, with no breath-hold instructions. A montage of three sequential sagittal images (**c**) reveals the tip of the guide needle at the edge of the tumor in the *center image*. A pathologic evaluation revealed a metastatic neuroendocrine tumor

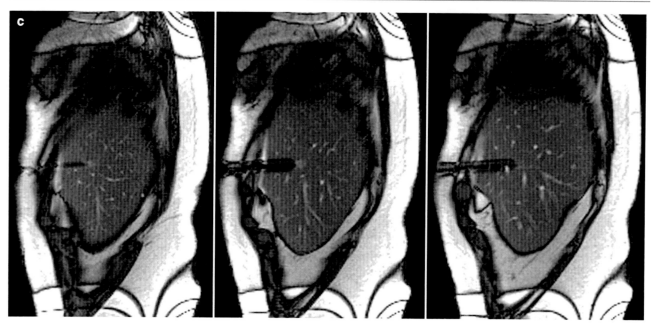

Fig. 5.7 (continued)

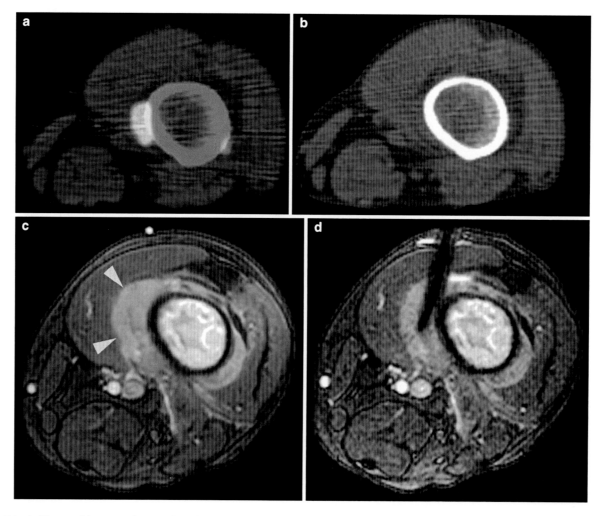

Fig. 5.8 A 70-year-old man underwent PET-CT imaging. A fused PET-CT image (**a**) reveals two focal areas of increased FDG uptake in the soft tissues surrounding the distal left femur but no abnormal uptake in the bone. A CT image of the femur from the same study (**b**) reveals no morphologic abnormality that could be targeted for biopsy. An axial bSSFP image (**c**) of the distal left femur reveals a soft-tissue mass (*arrowheads*) surrounding the distal femur. An MRI-guided biopsy (**d**) revealed high-grade B-cell lymphoma

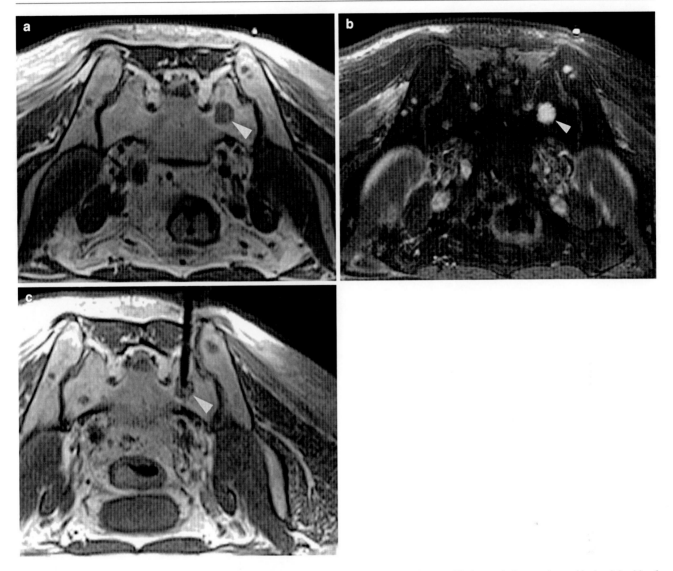

Fig. 5.9 A 61-year-old man with a history of rectal cancer was referred for biopsy of small bone lesions in the pelvis. Axial (**a**) T1- and (**b**) T2-weighted images of the pelvis in the prone position reveal multiple small bone lesions. These nodules had a low signal on T1- and high signal on T2-weighted images. The largest lesion was located in the right side of the sacrum (*arrowheads*) and measured 1.5 cm in diameter. To reduce ferromagnetic susceptibility artifacts from the 3-mm bone biopsy needle, a fast T1-weighted sequence was used during MRI-guided biopsy (**c**)

physicians and their staff who may be exposed to radiation during CT or fluoroscopic procedures. Long imaging acquisition times were once a major limitation of MRI-guided interventions such as biopsies. Ultrafast imaging sequences with high signal-to-noise ratio and soft-tissue contrast are now available, allowing fast imaging of the biopsy needle position after each manipulation.

Disadvantages

Until recently, appropriately equipped and designed MRI units were not widely available to interventional radiologists. MRI is more costly than other imaging modalities and requires more rigid quality assurance, maintenance, and safety monitoring. As such, MRI use has traditionally been limited to diagnostic studies. MRI-compatible equipment and devices such as in-room monitors and communication systems have recently become available and are still quite expensive. MRI-compatible needles are often made of titanium to allow their use inside the magnetic field with little ferromagnetic artifact; however, the quality of titanium needles is perceived to be lower than the quality of their stainless steel counterparts [4, 16, 17]. The selection of MRI-compatible needles is more limited compared with those made of stainless steel. MRI provides many opportunities to optimize images for better detection and targeting of lesions, but patient setup and imaging protocol setup and execution

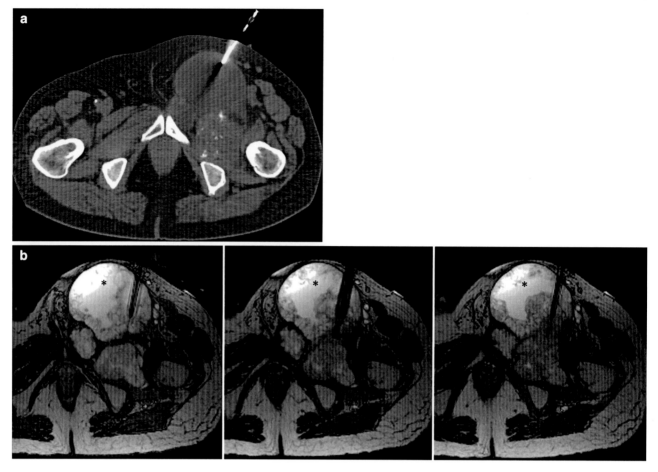

Fig. 5.10 A 76-year-old man underwent a CT-guided biopsy (**a**) at another institution. The pathologic results were inconclusive. A sequential axial bSSFP MRI (**b**) during biopsy reveals high signal intensity in the cystic or degenerated part of the tumor (*). The solid, viable component of the tumor was targeted under real-time MRI guidance. A pathologic evaluation revealed chondrosarcoma

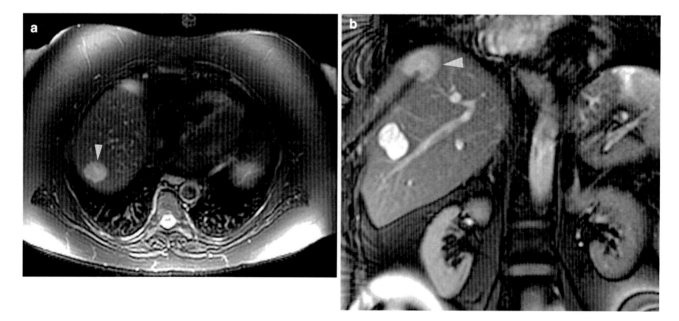

Fig. 5.11 A 57-year-old woman with a history of adrenal cortical carcinoma was found to have a liver lesion. An axial diagnostic T2-weighted image (**a**) of the liver reveals a lesion in the dome of the liver (*arrowhead*). A biopsy was performed under MRI guidance using the coronal imaging plane (**b**) to allow steep angulation of the biopsy needle

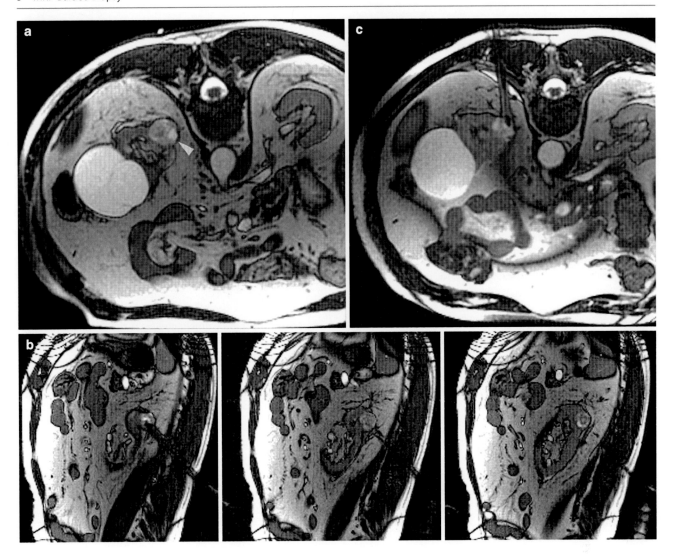

Fig. 5.12 A 67-year-old man with a history of prostate cancer and lymphoma was found to have a new solid enhancing mass in the upper pole of the left kidney. Because of his comorbidities, he was referred for percutaneous ablation. Prior to MRI-guided cryoablation, a biopsy was obtained. An axial bSSFP image (**a**) of the left kidney with the patient in the prone position reveals a 2.2-cm mass (*arrowhead*) in the medial upper pole of the left kidney. A biopsy was performed in the sagittal plane under real-time MRI guidance using the BEAT IRTTT sequence. During the real-time intervention, (**b**) three sequential images were repeatedly updated (medial to lateral) to show the needle as it was advanced toward the target. An oblique axial bSSFP image (**c**) of the left kidney was obtained along the path of the needle (47° cranial) to confirm accurate placement of the needle in the target. A biopsy revealed renal cell carcinoma, clear cell type, nuclear grade 2

for most procedures tend to require more time than those performed under CT or ultrasound guidance.

Applications

At our institution, once a request for biopsy is received, it is reviewed by an interventional radiologist for appropriateness and is scheduled for image-guided biopsy using one of the imaging modalities that may be suitable, including CT, ultrasound, fluoroscopy, or MRI. MRI guidance has been used to biopsy osseous lesions that cannot be visualized by other imaging modalities. Similarly, most soft-tissue tumors in the musculoskeletal system are more easily detected and better characterized by MRI than by other imaging modalities. At our center, the majority of musculoskeletal and soft-tissue biopsies are preferably assigned to iMRI. Liver lesions that are poorly visualized by ultrasound or CT can be targeted with MRI [18, 19]. MRI, with its sagittal and coronal imaging capabilities, facilitates biopsy of hepatic dome lesions that would require an angled or double-oblique approach with CT guidance [14, 20]. Intraparenchymal renal tumors and other renal tumors with large areas of necrosis appear to be another good application for MRI-guided biopsy using sagittal or multiple orthogonal views. When ultrasound cannot visualize deep lesions in the head and neck regions and

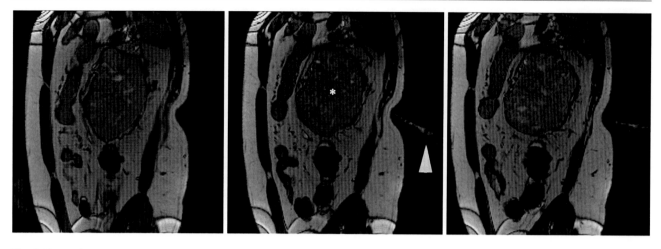

Fig. 5.13 A 58-year-old man with a retroperitoneal mass (*) was referred for biopsy. Real-time imaging with a trueFISP sequence provided a montage of three sequential sagittal images. The operator's finger (*arrowhead*) marks the needle insertion site in the *center image*

CT would require intravenous contrast administration and a double-oblique approach, MRI can help guide these challenging biopsies [21, 22]. The elimination of beam hardening artifacts inherent in CT also supports the use of MRI for guidance of skull base and high cervical spine procedures [23, 24]. MRI-guided breast biopsies have made a significant impact in the management of patients with suspicious breast lesions visible on MRI [2, 3]. MRI-guided prostate biopsy has been demonstrated as helpful in patients with focal prostate lesions but negative transrectal ultrasound biopsies [25]. Additionally, because of the lack of ionizing radiation, MRI-guided biopsies are preferred for pediatric patients and potentially for obstetric applications.

Technique

At our center, nearly all MRI-guided biopsies are performed under moderate sedation and occasionally under general anesthesia. The expanded diameter of the Espree magnet (Siemens Medical Solutions) facilitates the positioning of patients in a number of positions including supine, prone, oblique, or lateral decubitus [8]. During the procedures, patients are monitored using MRI-compatible, wireless monitoring devices (Precess, InVivo Corporation). An MRI-compatible ventilator is available in the iMRI suite at all times.

Initial imaging of the biopsy site includes a three-plane localizer usually followed by T2-weighted fast imaging with steady-state precession (trueFISP) images of the region of interest in any one of the conventional planes (axial, sagittal, or coronal). The T2-like contrast of this balanced steady-state free-precession sequence is usually sufficient for identifying the lesion of interest. The biopsy site can be marked in similar fashion to CT-guided biopsies. The visualization

software for the Espree unit can identify the exact coordinates of a desired skin entry site relative to the existing laser lights, which are checked for accuracy daily. When using sagittal images for guidance, one may use the existing laser lights to measure the coordinates of a desired skin entry site. Alternatively, a combination of the laser light and an external skin marker may be used to mark the skin entry site if axial imaging is used for planning the biopsy. When using coronal plane images for guiding needle placement, a combination of coordinates, external markers, and existing laser lights are used to mark the desired skin entry site. Alternatively, the skin entry point may be located using a fingertip or a syringe filled with water for T2-weighted image guidance (Figs. 5.13 and 5.14) [26]. This can be performed when real-time imaging and tableside monitors are available. With the patient placed at the isocenter of the magnet, initial imaging is performed to localize the most appropriate plane and slice of imaging for needle insertion. With repetitive imaging of the desired plane, the operator moves an object (a finger or a syringe) on the patient skin surface until the object comes into the field of view. The skin entry site can be adjusted in the plane of imaging to avoid overlying and intervening structures such as ribs.

The biopsy site is prepared in sterile fashion and a key-hole drape is placed over the puncture site. The surface coil is then placed over the sterile drape with the opening of the coil positioned directly over the skin insertion site. A second keyhole drape is then placed over the coil to sandwich the non-sterile coil between the two sterile key-hole drapes. The sterility of the field is maintained in this fashion.

Advancing the biopsy needle to the target lesion can be accomplished in one of the two ways: using intermittent imaging or using real-time imaging. With the patient outside the bore of the magnet, the operator can engage the needle in the subcutaneous soft tissues at an appropriate angle and

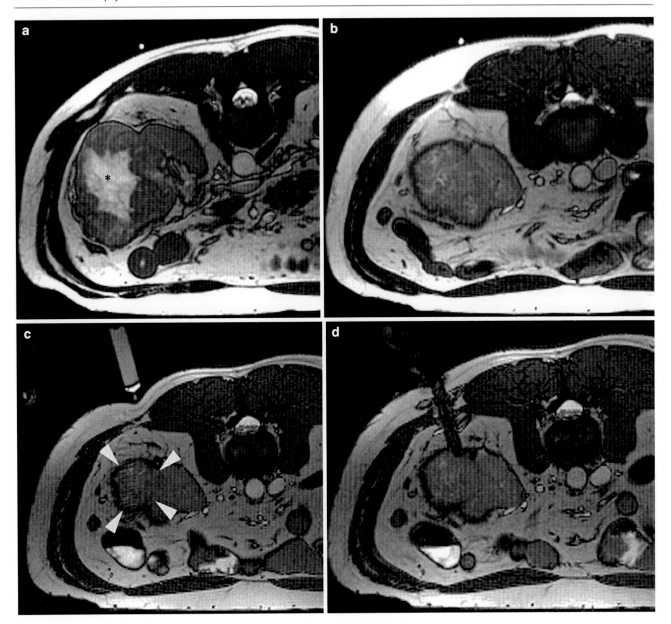

Fig. 5.14 A 58-year-old man was found to have a large left renal mass. An axial bSSFP image of the left kidney (**a**) in the prone position revealed a large exophytic mass with central necrosis (*). A solid, non-necrotic portion of the mass along the lower pole of the kidney (**b**) was chosen for biopsy. The puncture site and angle of needle insertion were selected under real-time imaging with a bSSFP sequence. The operator held a syringe filled with saline, (**c**) marked the insertion site, and selected an angle that allowed targeting of the periphery of the mass (*arrowheads*). The biopsy needle was inserted under real-time imaging (**d**) at the selected insertion site and angle

advance the needle incrementally with intermittent imaging of the needle, making appropriate adjustments in the trajectory of the needle after each set of images is obtained. Alternatively, the operator can reach into the bore of the magnet and advance the needle under real-time MRI guidance. When feasible and appropriate, this is an elegant and efficient method for performing MRI-guided biopsies.

Other than needle composition, several factors may impact the visualization of biopsy needles during MRI-guided procedures. These include the needle caliber, strength of the magnetic field, orientation of the needle relative to the main magnetic field (B0), pulse sequences used, pulse sequence sampling bandwidth, and frequency encoding direction [1]. In general, the apparent width of the needle on MRI is larger for large caliber needles, with higher magnetic field strength, and when the needle is placed perpendicular to the orientation of the main magnetic field (B0); under these circumstances, the susceptibility artifact is enhanced [11]. Rapid gradient-recalled echo sequences such as FISP, trueFISP, and PSIF are often used for MRI-guided interventions because they provide near real-time imaging with high signal-to-noise ratio [1]. However, these sequences create a larger susceptibility artifact from needles when compared with the often slower spin-echo-based pulse sequences such as turbo-spin echo or single-shot fast spin-echo techniques like half-Fourier acquisition single-shot turbo-spin echo (HASTE). When using a large caliber needle in a sensitive area adjacent to neurovascular structures, minimizing the susceptibility artifact is desirable to avoid inadvertent damage to critical neighboring structures. Under these circumstances, rapid gradient-recalled echo sequences can be used for initial navigation followed by turbo-spin-echo pulse sequences to confirm the needle-tip position. Additional adjustments of some imaging parameters can be made to decrease the needle susceptibility artifact. For example, increasing the sampling bandwidth and setting the frequency encoding direction parallel to the needle can help reduce the needle artifact.

For intermittent imaging, we often utilize trueFISP imaging. A series of 3–5 images can be obtained in less than 5 s. A quick review of these images on the in-room tableside monitor provides sufficient information about the trajectory of the needle and appropriate adjustments can be immediately implemented. For liver lesions, the stronger T2-weighting of HASTE images has often been useful for providing optimal tumor conspicuity.

For real-time imaging, we routinely utilize trueFISP images. A single repetitive image or, more often, a series of three sequential parallel images in rapid succession may be used for this purpose. We have also had success using a prototype balanced steady-state free-precession sequence from Siemens optimized for interventional use (BEAT IRTTT), which provides rapid, real-time imaging with high resolution and good soft-tissue differentiation as well as a mechanism to display a montage of the three slices on the monitor in near real time (Figs. 5.7, 5.12, and 5.13). The sequence allows interactive real-time manipulation of the scan planes, which when used in conjunction with existing static orthogonal slices on the scanner, can be used to adjust slice group orientation and position by the technologist to better track the needle and observe surrounding anatomy. The BEAT IRTTT images can also be automatically sent to an external workstation where prototype real-time software from Siemens (Interactive Front End) can visualize up to six multiple orthogonal planes as well as interact with the sequence to facilitate real-time prescription of scan location and orientation based on the dynamically acquired images.

In summary, there are several advantages to using iMRI to guide biopsies. Subtle tumors are more easily identified and distinguished from adjacent structures, lesions can be approached in nearly any conceivable imaging plane, and real-time imaging without ionizing radiation is possible. On the other hand, iMRI suites and MRI-compatible devices are not readily available and are often more expensive than for other imaging modalities. With advances in technology and the increasing availability of short, wide-bore, high-field magnets and MRI-compatible needles and devices, MRI-guided biopsies will become more widely accepted in the future.

References

1. Weiss CR, Nour SG, Lewin JS. MR-guided biopsy: a review of current techniques and applications. J Magn Reson Imaging. 2008; 27:311–25.
2. Kuhl CK, Morakkabati N, Leutner CC, Schmiedel A, Wardelmann E, Schild HH. MR imaging–guided large-core (14-gauge) needle biopsy of small lesions visible at breast MR imaging alone. Radiology. 2001;220:31–9.
3. Perlet C, Heywang-Kobrunner SH, Heinig A, Sittek H, Casselman J, Anderson I, et al. Magnetic resonance-guided, vacuum-assisted breast biopsy: results from a European multicenter study of 538 lesions. Cancer. 2006;106:982–90.
4. Langen HJ, Kugel H, Landwehr P. MR-guided core biopsies using a closed 1.0 T imager. First clinical results. Eur J Radiol. 2002;41: 19–25.
5. Lewin JS, Petersilge CA, Hatem SF, Duerk JL, Lenz G, Clampitt ME, et al. Interactive MR imaging-guided biopsy and aspiration with a modified clinical C-arm system. Am J Roentgenol. 1998;170: 1593–601.
6. Silverman SG, Collick BD, Figueira MR, Khorasani R, Adams DF, Newman RW, et al. Interactive MR-guided biopsy in an open-configuration MR imaging system. Radiology. 1995;197: 175–81.
7. Mueller PR, Stark DD, Simeone JF, Saini S, Butch RJ, Edelman RR, et al. MR-guided aspiration biopsy: needle design and clinical trials. Radiology. 1986;161:605–9.
8. Stattaus J, Maderwald S, Baba HA, Gerken G, Barkhausen J, Forsting M, et al. MR-guided liver biopsy within a short, wide-bore 1.5 Tesla MR system. Eur Radiol. 2008;18:2865–73.
9. Keeler EK, Casey FX, Engels H, Lauder E, Pirto CA, Reisker T, et al. Accessory equipment considerations with respect to MRI compatibility. J Magn Reson Imaging. 1998;8: 12–8.
10. Frahm C, Gehl HB, Melchert UH, Weiss HD. Visualization of magnetic resonance-compatible needles at 1.5 and 0.2 Tesla. Cardiovasc Intervent Radiol. 1996;19:335–40.
11. Lewin JS, Duerk JL, Jain VR, Petersilge CA, Chao CP, Haaga JR. Needle localization in MR-guided biopsy and aspiration: effects of field strength, sequence design, and magnetic field orientation. Am J Roentgenol. 1996;166:1337–45.
12. Lufkin R, Teresi L, Hanafee W. New needle for MR-guided aspiration cytology of the head and neck. Am J Roentgenol. 1987;149: 380–2.
13. Rofsky NM, Yang BM, Schlossberg P, Goldenberg A, Teperman LW, Weinreb JC. MR-guided needle aspiration biopsies of hepatic masses using a closed bore magnet. J Comput Assist Tomogr. 1998; 22:633–7.
14. Schmidt AJ, Kee ST, Sze DY, Daniel BL, Razavi MK, Semba CP, et al. Diagnostic yield of MR-guided liver biopsies compared with CT- and US-guided liver biopsies. J Vasc Interv Radiol. 1999;10: 1323–9.
15. Smith KA, Carrino J. MRI-guided interventions of the musculoskeletal system. J Magn Reson Imaging. 2008;27:339–46.
16. Adam G, Bucker A, Nolte-Ernsting C, Tacke J, Gunther RW. Interventional MR imaging: percutaneous abdominal and skeletal biopsies and drainages of the abdomen. Eur Radiol. 1999;9: 1471–8.
17. Zangos S, Eichler K, Wetter A, Lehnert T, Hammerstingl R, Diebold T, et al. MR-guided biopsies of lesions in the retroperitoneal space: technique and results. Eur Radiol. 2006;16: 307–12.
18. Genant JW, Vandevenne JE, Bergman AG, Beaulieu CF, Kee ST, Norbash AM, et al. Interventional musculoskeletal procedures performed by using MR imaging guidance with a vertically open MR unit: assessment of techniques and applicability. Radiology. 2002; 223:127–36.

19. Ueno S, Yokoyama S, Hirakawa H, Yabe H, Suzuki Y, Atsumi H, et al. Use of real-time magnetic resonance guidance to assist bone biopsy in pediatric malignancy. Pediatrics. 2002;109:E18.

20. Lu DS, Lee H, Farahani K, Sinha S, Lufkin R. Biopsy of hepatic dome lesions: semi-real-time coronal MR guidance technique. Am J Roentgenol. 1997;168:737–9.

21. Hathout G, Lufkin RB, Jabour B, Andrews J, Castro D. MR-guided aspiration cytology in the head and neck at high field strength. J Magn Reson Imaging. 1992;2:93–4.

22. He Y, Zhang Z, Tian Z, Zhang C, Zhu H. The application of magnetic resonance imaging-guided fine-needle aspiration cytology in the diagnosis of deep lesions in the head and neck. J Oral Maxillofac Surg. 2004;62:953–8.

23. Lewin JS. Interventional MR, imaging: concepts, systems, and applications in neuroradiology. AJNR Am J Neuroradiol. 1999;20: 735–48.

24. Lewin JS, Nour SG, Duerk JL. Magnetic resonance image-guided biopsy and aspiration. Top Magn Reson Imaging. 2000;11:173–83.

25. Lawrentschuk N, Fleshner N. The role of magnetic resonance imaging in targeting prostate cancer in patients with previous negative biopsies and elevated prostate-specific antigen levels. BJU Int. 2009;103:730–3.

26. Stattaus J, Maderwald S, Forsting M, Barkhausen J, Ladd ME. MR-guided core biopsy with MR fluoroscopy using a short, wide-bore 1.5-Tesla scanner: feasibility and initial results. J Magn Reson Imaging. 2008;27:1181–7.

Fluoroscopy-Guided Biopsy

6

Kamran Ahrar

Prior to the development and acceptance of using computed tomography (CT) and ultrasonography to guide percutaneous biopsies of abdominal and retroperitoneal lesions, fluoroscopy was the main imaging modality used to guide these procedures. Tumors were marked by contrast-enhanced examination of the affected or nearby organs [1]. For example, renal, suprarenal, and other retroperitoneal masses affecting the urinary system were marked by intravenous urography. Pancreatic masses were biopsied during arteriography, and lymph nodes were marked by lymphography. Biopsies were performed under frontal plane fluoroscopic guidance, while horizontal beam radiography in the lateral projection was used to verify the depth of the needle. Although today all these biopsies are performed under cross-sectional imaging guidance using ultrasonography, CT, or magnetic resonance imaging (MRI), fluoroscopy remains a viable imaging modality to guide biopsies of certain lesions involving the lung or bone [2–4]. Fluoroscopy is also the preferred imaging modality for guiding endoluminal biopsies of bile ducts and ureters [5, 6] and is the modality of choice for guiding transjugular liver and renal biopsies [7, 8]. This chapter outlines the current equipment, advantages, disadvantages, applications, and techniques used in fluoroscopy-guided biopsies.

Equipment

The minimum requirement for fluoroscopy-guided biopsy is a C-arm unit that allows frontal, oblique, and lateral imaging of the target lesion (Fig. 6.1) [9]. Additional desirable options include flexible collimation, image magnification, and the ability to angle the C-arm in cranial and caudal directions. At many institutions, the angiography equipment is also used to perform nonvascular interventions such as biopsies. As such, C-arm cone-beam CT (CBCT) may be available to enhance image guidance during interventions [10]. CBCT is an advanced three-dimensional (3D) imaging technology that allows the acquisition of multiple 2D fluoroscopic projection images in a circular trajectory that covers approximately 200° around the patient to create a 3D volumetric imaging dataset. After processing the dataset, images can be reconstructed and displayed in any desirable plane (Fig. 6.1). CBCT images resemble those acquired by spiral CT scans, but axial CBCT images have lower spatial and contrast resolution.

Unlike fluoroscopy, which provides real-time guidance, CBCT images require up to 8 s for acquisition and up to 1 min for reconstruction and thus, CBCT alone cannot be used for real-time needle guidance. Dedicated needle path-planning software has been developed to complement CBCT for needle guidance. The needle trajectory is planned in the 3D dataset, which is then coregistered with real-time fluoroscopy. The desired needle insertion site and the calculated trajectory are displayed over real-time fluoroscopic images, guiding accurate needle placement [11, 12].

Advantages

The main advantage of fluoroscopy over other imaging modalities for guiding percutaneous biopsies is the real-time nature of the technology. In addition, fluoroscopy is readily available, is relatively inexpensive compared with CT and MRI, and provides easy access to the patient during the procedure. If available, CBCT can be used to confirm the exact position of the biopsy needle that is inserted under real-time fluoroscopic guidance. When used with image-overlay software, CBCT allows accurate localization and targeting of certain structures and lesions.

K. Ahrar, MD, FSIR
Department of Interventional Radiology,
Department of Thoracic and Cardiovascular Surgery,
The University of Texas MD Anderson Cancer Center,
1515 Holcombe Boulevard, Unit 1471,
Houston, TX 77030, USA
e-mail: kahrar@mdanderson.org

K. Ahrar, S. Gupta (eds.), *Percutaneous Image-Guided Biopsy*,
DOI 10.1007/978-1-4614-8217-8_6, © Springer Science+Business Media New York 2014

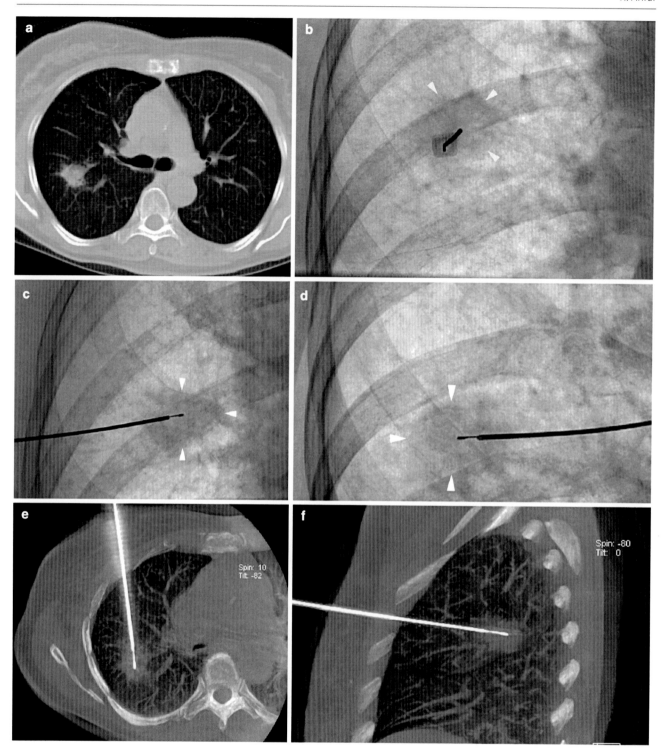

Fig. 6.1 Fluoroscopic-guided lung biopsy. A 63-year-old woman with newly diagnosed right upper lobe lung lesion was referred for biopsy. Axial CT image of the chest (**a**) shows a 2.3 cm mass in the right upper lobe. Biopsy was performed under real-time fluoroscopic guidance (**b**). The C-arm was angled caudal approximately 10° to place the lesion (*arrowheads* in **b**) in between the anterior ribs. The needle was then advanced parallel to the x-ray beam into the lesion under real-time fluoroscopy. Two orthogonal images (right anterior oblique [**c**] and left anterior oblique [**d**]) were acquired to confirm the depth of the biopsy needle and appropriate position of the biopsy needle within the mass (*arrowheads*). C-arm cone-beam CT images were acquired and reconstructed in axial (**e**), sagittal (**f**), and coronal (**g**) planes to confirm the position of the biopsy needle within the tumor. Pathology showed non-small cell lung cancer

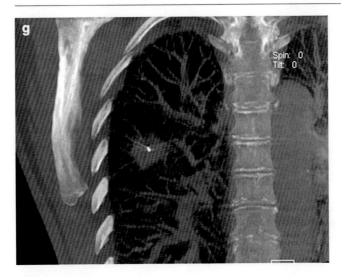

Fig. 6.1 (continued)

Disadvantages

Fluoroscopy is limited to imaging in a single plane. Fluoroscopy flattens a volume of tissue to a single two-dimensional image and is not capable of characterizing tissue traversed by the needle as it travels to the target. Fluoroscopy also has limited soft-tissue contrast resolution. Therefore, only tumors or structures that have density that is markedly different from that of their surroundings can be targeted for biopsy under real-time fluoroscopy. For example, a relatively small (about 2 cm) solid tumor within an aerated lung has a density that is adequately different from its surrounding tissue to be visualized under fluoroscopy, whereas a large soft-tissue mass in the retroperitoneum may not be adequately detected or targeted with fluoroscopy.

CBCT and image overlay may help alleviate some of fluoroscopy's shortcomings in certain cases; however, at the time of this writing, the resolution of CBCT images was suboptimal compared with other cross-sectional imaging modalities used to guide complex biopsies of deep-seated structures within the abdomen or retroperitoneum [13].

Applications

Fluoroscopy is a viable imaging modality for guiding biopsies of certain lesions of the lung or bone. Fluoroscopy is also the preferred imaging modality for guiding endoluminal biopsies of bile ducts and ureters and for guiding transjugular liver and renal biopsies.

Although CT is the modality of choice for guiding percutaneous lung biopsies [14], lesions in the lower lobes are affected by respiratory motion and can be difficult to target with CT. CT fluoroscopy, with or without respiratory control, can help target some of these lesions [15, 16]. However, some radiologists prefer fluoroscopy-guided lung biopsies for lesions that can be easily identified on chest radiography [4]. A review of diagnostic CT images can help select patients appropriately and can help determine the optimal patient position and biopsy approach [17].

Sclerotic (Fig. 6.2) and lytic (Fig. 6.3) bone tumors often create adequate changes in density under fluoroscopy to allow visualization and targeting for biopsy [3, 18]. Transpedicular vertebral body biopsy is a simple and effective sampling technique when the vertebra is diffusely involved by a pathological process [2, 19]. Biopsy of lesions in the small bones of a hand or foot may be more easily accomplished under real-time fluoroscopic guidance, which allows more flexibility for positioning the affected area.

Endoluminal brush or forceps biopsy of strictures within the bile ducts or ureters (Fig. 6.4) requires fluoroscopic examination of the biliary or urinary tract [5, 6]. Finally, transjugular liver or kidney biopsy requires fluoroscopy to identify and select the appropriate veins (Fig. 6.5) [7, 8]. Endoluminal or transvenous biopsy devices are manipulated under real-time fluoroscopy and positioned appropriately to optimize the biopsy yield.

Technique

Fluoroscopy-guided biopsy of lung tumors is best planned after a review of the diagnostic CT scan [17]. The location of the tumor, fissures, and vascular structures help determine the best way to position the patient and the most suitable approach for needle insertion. The length of the needle insertion is measured on CT images. Under real-time fluoroscopic guidance, a pair of forceps is used to mark the skin site for needle insertion. A small stab incision is made, and the needle is inserted just below the skin using a pair of forceps. The needle is then aligned parallel to the direction of the x-ray beam (Fig. 6.1b). At this time, the image of the needle should appear as a small radiopaque point projected over the tumor. When properly aligned, this image should resemble a "bull's eye" or target sign. Keeping the image of the needle to a barely perceptible length (nearly a point), the needle is advanced toward the tumor. Once the needle is inserted to the predetermined length, putting the needle close to or within the lesion, the C-arm is rotated 30–90° in one and then the other lateral oblique projection (Fig. 6.1c, d). Orthogonal images will depict the depth and position of the needle tip with respect to the tumor.

The needle can be advanced or pulled back to place the needle tip within the desired location for sampling. This may be the center of the tumor or the anterior or posterior margin.

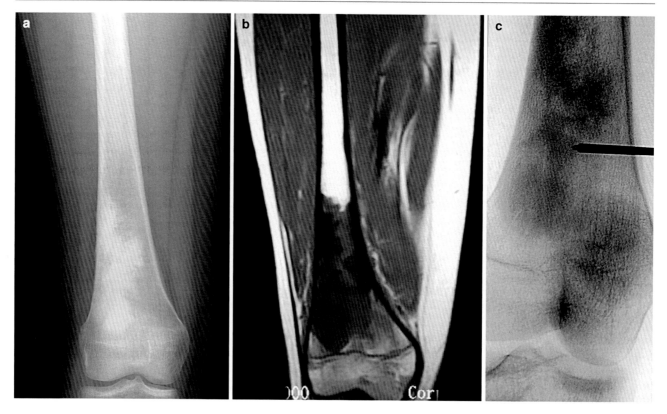

Fig. 6.2 Fluoroscopic-guided biopsy of sclerotic bone lesion. A 16-year-old girl complained of pain in the right distal thigh. AP radiograph of the right femur (**a**) showed a dense sclerotic lesion. Coronal T1-weighted image of the femur (**b**) showed abnormal signal in the distal femur with no associated soft-tissue mass. Biopsy of the distal femur was performed under fluoroscopic guidance (**c**). Pathology showed osteosarcoma

While performing a fine-needle aspiration biopsy, the to-and-fro motion of the needle can be visualized in real time, and the depth of the insertion can be kept to a limit such that the needle tip remains within the tumor during the sampling process. The same technique is applied for fluoroscopy- guided bone and transpedicular vertebral biopsies.

For endoluminal biopsies, the conduit (e.g., bile duct, ureter, or hepatic vein) is opacified with contrast material (Figs. 6.4c and 6.5a). Once the desired position for sampling is identified, devices such as biopsy brush, forceps, or needles are placed through introducer sheaths or catheters and manipulated to gather the appropriate biopsy samples. Real-time fluoroscopy allows safe and precise positioning of the devices.

Although cross-sectional imaging has replaced fluoroscopic guidance for many biopsy procedures, there remain several applications for real-time fluoroscopic guidance. Further developments in CBCT technology may help revive the role of fluoroscopy in guiding nonvascular interventions, including biopsy procedures, in the future.

Fig. 6.3 Fluoroscopic-guided biopsy of lytic bone lesion. A-19-year-old man presented with pain involving the left hip. AP radiograph of the left femur (**a**) shows a lytic lesion involving the greater trochanter of the left femur with sclerotic border extending medially. Axial T1-weighted image of the pelvis (**b**) confirms mixed lytic-sclerotic bone lesion involving the proximal left femur (*). The lytic lesion in the greater trochanter was sampled under fluoroscopic guidance (**c**). Pathology showed osteosarcoma

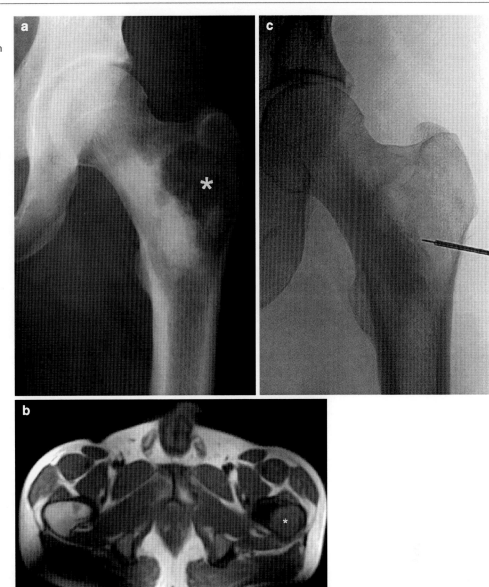

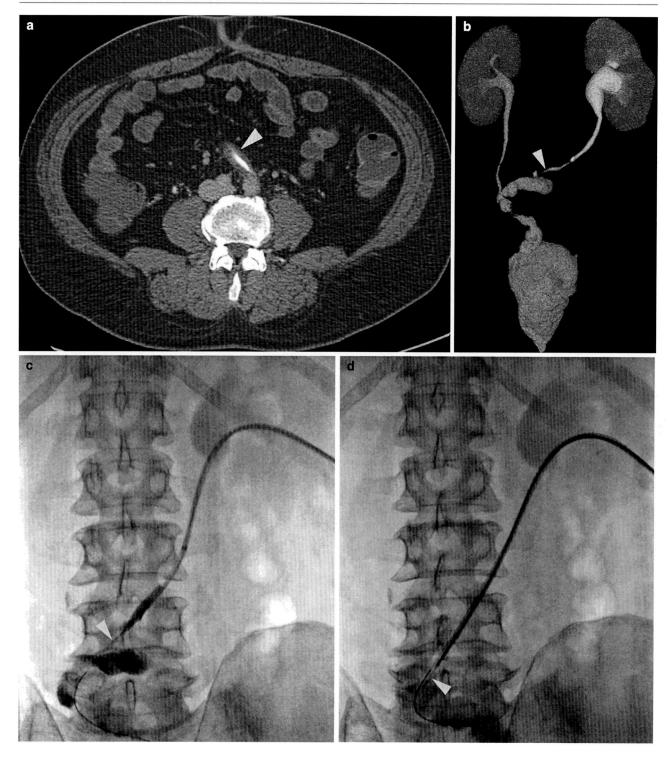

Fig. 6.4 Ureteral brush biopsy. A 57-year-old man underwent radical cystoprostatectomy for transitional cell carcinoma of the bladder. Four years later, axial CT image of the abdomen (**a**) shows soft-tissue thickening involving the distal left ureter (*arrowhead*). CT urography (**b**) confirms a stricture of the distal left ureter (*arrowhead*) and left hydronephrosis. Patient was referred for endoluminal brush biopsy. Fluoroscopic image of the left ureter (**c**) at the time of biopsy shows the area of stricture (*arrowhead*). (**d**) A brush biopsy device was placed in the stricture to obtain samples of the urothelial lining. Cytology showed high grade urothelial carcinoma

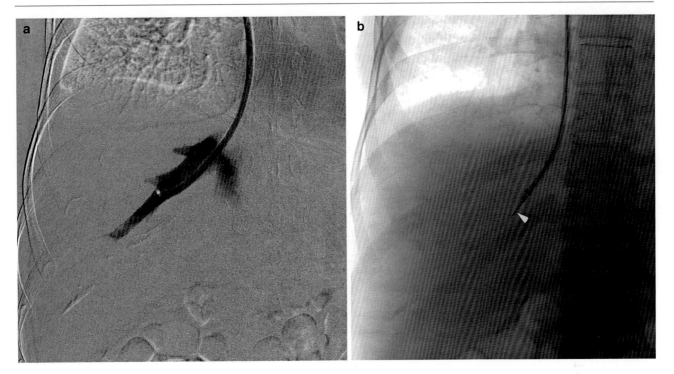

Fig. 6.5 Transjugular liver biopsy. A 41-year-old woman with acute lymphocytic leukemia was referred for biopsy to determine the etiology of her liver insufficiency. She had thrombocytopenia, and a transjugular liver biopsy rather than a percutaneous biopsy was recommended. After selective catheterization of the right hepatic vein under real-time fluoroscopy, venogram (**a**) confirms placement of the introducer sheath in the right hepatic vein. The curved stiff cannula from the biopsy set is turned anterior within the right hepatic vein (**b**), a core biopsy needle (*arrowhead*) is advanced under fluoroscopy into the liver parenchyma to obtain a biopsy sample

References

1. Pereiras RV, Meiers W, Kunhardt B, Troner M, Hutson D, Barkin JS, et al. Fluoroscopically guided thin needle aspiration biopsy of the abdomen and retroperitoneum. AJR Am J Roentgenol. 1978;131:197–202.
2. Jelinek JS, Kransdorf MJ, Gray R, Aboulafia AJ, Malawer MM. Percutaneous transpedicular biopsy of vertebral body lesions. Spine (Phila Pa 1976). 1996;21:2035–40.
3. Jelinek JS, Murphey MD, Welker JA, Henshaw RM, Kransdorf MJ, Shmookler BM, et al. Diagnosis of primary bone tumors with image-guided percutaneous biopsy: experience with 110 tumors. Radiology. 2002;223:731–7.
4. Kurban LA, Gomersall L, Weir J, Wade P. Fluoroscopy-guided percutaneous lung biopsy: a valuable alternative to computed tomography. Acta Radiol. 2008;49:876–82.
5. Jung GS, Huh JD, Lee SU, Han BH, Chang HK, Cho YD. Bile duct: analysis of percutaneous transluminal forceps biopsy in 130 patients suspected of having malignant biliary obstruction. Radiology. 2002;224:725–30.
6. Xing GS, Geng JC, Han XW, Dai JH, Wu CY. Endobiliary brush cytology during percutaneous transhepatic cholangiodrainage in patients with obstructive jaundice. Hepatobiliary Pancreat Dis Int. 2005;4:98–103.
7. McAfee JH, Keeffe EB, Lee RG, Rosch J. Transjugular liver biopsy. Hepatology. 1992;15:726–32.
8. Misra S, Gyamlani G, Swaminathan S, Buehrig CK, Bjarnason H, McKusick MA, et al. Safety and diagnostic yield of transjugular renal biopsy. J Vasc Interv Radiol. 2008;19:546–51.
9. Smith DF, Doust BD. Angulated fluoroscopy for needle biopsy localization. AJR Am J Roentgenol. 1982;138:765–7.
10. Wallace MJ, Kuo MD, Glaiberman C, Binkert CA, Orth RC, Soulez G. Three-dimensional C-arm cone-beam CT: applications in the interventional suite. J Vasc Interv Radiol. 2009;20:S523–37.
11. Braak SJ, van Strijen MJ, van Leersum M, van Es HW, van Heesewijk JP. Real-time 3D fluoroscopy guidance during needle interventions: technique, accuracy, and feasibility. AJR Am J Roentgenol. 2010;194:W445–51.
12. Tam AL, Mohamed A, Pfister M, Chinndurai P, Rohm E, Hall AF, et al. C-arm cone beam computed tomography needle path overlay for fluoroscopic guided vertebroplasty. Spine (Phila Pa 1976). 2010;35:1095–9.
13. Kroeze SG, Huisman M, Verkooijen HM, van Diest PJ, Ruud Bosch JL, van den Bosch MA. Real-time 3D fluoroscopy-guided large core needle biopsy of renal masses: a critical early evaluation according to the IDEAL recommendations. Cardiovasc Intervent Radiol. 2012;35:680–5.
14. Wu CC, Maher MM, Shepard JA. CT-guided percutaneous needle biopsy of the chest: preprocedural evaluation and technique. AJR Am J Roentgenol. 2011;196:W511–14.
15. Carlson SK, Felmlee JP, Bender CE, Ehman RL, Classic KL, Hoskin TL, et al. CT fluoroscopy-guided biopsy of the lung or upper abdomen with a breath-hold monitoring and feedback system: a prospective randomized controlled clinical trial. Radiology. 2005;237:701–8.
16. Hiraki T, Mimura H, Gobara H, Iguchi T, Fujiwara H, Sakurai J, et al. CT fluoroscopy-guided biopsy of 1,000 pulmonary lesions

performed with 20-gauge coaxial cutting needles: diagnostic yield and risk factors for diagnostic failure. Chest. 2009;136: 1612–17.

17. Cohan RH, Newman GE, Braun SD, Dunnick NR. CT assistance for fluoroscopically guided transthoracic needle aspiration biopsy. J Comput Assist Tomogr. 1984;8:1093–8.

18. Datir A, Pechon P, Saifuddin A. Imaging-guided percutaneous biopsy of pathologic fractures: a retrospective analysis of 129 cases. AJR Am J Roentgenol. 2009;193:504–8.

19. Moller S, Kothe R, Wiesner L, Werner M, Ruther W, Delling G. Fluoroscopy-guided transpedicular trocar biopsy of the spine–results, review, and technical notes. Acta Orthop Belg. 2001;67:488–99.

Advanced Tools and Devices: Navigation Technologies, Automation, and Robotics in Percutaneous Interventions

Aradhana M. Venkatesan and Bradford J. Wood

Introduction

The development and maturation of percutaneous image-guided biopsy techniques over the past three decades has enabled these procedures to supplant open surgical biopsy for a variety of anatomic sites. However, at present conventional techniques have limitations in the amount of pre-biopsy imaging data that may be taken into the interventional suite for real-time guidance [1]. Typically, the optimal use of three-dimensional imaging information is limited by the operator's own mental approximations of needle and target location derived from two-dimensional imaging data [1]. Currently, many minimally invasive biopsies are performed in the CT suite [1]. However, these procedures often require significant CT scanner time (and measurable radiation), are limited to only axial images, and do not directly link images to the needle to enable real-time guidance during insertion and repositioning [1].

Novel tools and devices, including navigation platforms, advanced image-processing software, and robotic needle guidance, have the potential to enable or further enhance the accuracy of percutaneous image-guided biopsy. In certain cases such as PET-guided biopsy, procedures may not have been able to be performed at all without these novel technologies. Navigation and guidance systems have been deployed clinically but primarily in the setting of radiation therapy, brachytherapy, and open surgery such as neurosurgery,

orthopedics, or otolaryngology [2]. Minimally invasive image-guided biopsy and tumor ablation procedures have become integral interventions, particularly in the care of the oncology patient. Thus, there is an ongoing need for ever more sophisticated methods of successful targeting of technically challenging or otherwise subtle lesions [3]. Novel navigation platforms facilitating these image-guided interventions offer several advantages. Navigation platforms enable real-time referencing of tracked devices throughout an intervention, as opposed to only intermittent displays of needle angle and position during conventional CT-guided biopsy. Novel image-processing algorithms enable displays of multiplanar, multimodality co-registered imaging data that can offer the interventional radiologist real-time imaging data about multiple modalities (e.g., ultrasound, CT, MRI, PET) simultaneously during a biopsy. Robotic needle guidance may potentially reduce inter-operator variability and procedure time. Use of these technologies has the potential to not only simplify complex spatial relationships for the interventional radiologist but potentially improve lesion targeting and patient care. Tissue characterization via advanced biopsy techniques has the potential to facilitate drug discovery, by enabling assessment of up- or downregulation of biomarker targets, susceptibility to specific pharmacologic regimens, and risk of toxicities based upon genetic variation in drug metabolism. Biopsy guided by metabolic and functional imaging could transform the minimally invasive characterization of human disease, which is of increasing importance as the "personalization" of medical care permeates oncology. Biopsy navigation is anticipated to play an increasingly important role in the evolution of cancer therapies in the future.

A.M. Venkatesan, MD (✉)
Department of Radiology and Imaging Sciences
and Center for Interventional Oncology,
NIH Clinical Center, 10 Center Dr., Bldg. 10,
Rm. 1C369, MSC 1182, Bethesda, MD 20892, USA
e-mail: venkatesana@cc.nih.gov

B.J. Wood, MD
Department of Radiology and Imaging Sciences,
Center for Interventional Oncology, Interventional Radiology,
NIH Clinical Center, 10 Center Dr., Bldg. 10,
Rm. 1C369, MSC 1182, Bethesda, MD 20892, USA
e-mail: bwood@cc.nih.gov

Technical Considerations

The use of novel navigation platforms, image-processing algorithms, and medical robots necessitates knowledge of a basic lexicon of key terms, when using these advanced tools

K. Ahrar, S. Gupta (eds.), *Percutaneous Image-Guided Biopsy*,
DOI 10.1007/978-1-4614-8217-8_7, © Springer Science+Business Media New York 2014

Table 7.1 Glossary of key terms relevant to device tracking, image fusion, and robotics [4–8]

Term	Definition
Medical global positioning system (GPS)	Localization of a device or image in relation to prior pre-procedural imaging. The electromagnetic field generator is the "satellite" and the needle tip is the "car"
Multimodality or image fusion	Overlapping visual display of multiple imaging modalities during a percutaneous biopsy
Electromagnetic tracking	Mechanism to locate a needle (or ultrasound plane) within a 3D volume of imaging data (like CT, MR, or PET) or to locate a 2D ultrasound plane within a 3D volume
Tracking error/target to registration Error (TRE)	Difference between the real and virtual needle positions. How accurate is the location of the "virtual needle" as displayed on the images?
Registration error (root mean square/RMS)	How well two sets of imaging data or selected anatomic points on each of two imaging modalities match up (ideally <2 mm)
Placement error	How close the needle is placed to the target point
Dynamic reference	Patch or sensor placed on patient that corrects for patient or generator motion. Without this, patient must remain in exact position throughout body intervention
Registration	Matches two (or more) sets of imaging data, or matches image space to "magnetic space"
Rigid registration	Matches two (or more) sets of imaging data based upon fixed anatomic landmarks; it does not, on its own, account for organ shift or tissue deformation between image sets or during the procedure
Deformable/elastic registration	Matches two (or more) sets of imaging data based upon common anatomic landmarks but can deform/warp image sets to account for organ shift or deformation between different images or due to imaging at different times
Medical robot	Mechanical manipulator connected by joints that allow relative motion from one link to another
Robotic arm	Part of the robot that orients the end effectors and/or sensors
End effector	Any attachment on the end of a robot that interacts with the environment, such as a device to lift and position a needle; the robotic "hand" at the end of the robot arm
Degrees of freedom	Axes of movement; reflect the flexibility of an instrument (robot) to achieve positions and orientations. Six degrees of freedom are required for a robotic device to reach, position, and orient an instrument at any point in space. The seventh degree of freedom is inherent to the procedure itself (e.g., cutting, grasping)

and devices. Table 7.1 summarizes some definitions relevant to body interventions employing device tracking, image fusion, and robotic assistance.

Device Tracking

The primary methods for real-time device tracking include electromagnetic tracking and optical tracking. Electromagnetic (EM) and optical tracking are standard techniques used to register devices to preoperative images during neurosurgery and orthopedic surgery, but these technologies have not been widely applied in interventional radiology [3]. Medical devices like needles, catheters, and guidewires may be tracked via placement of minute electromagnetic sensor coils within their tips (PercuNav Image Fusion and Instrument Navigation, Philips Healthcare, Cleveland, Ohio). Tracking of these sensor coils provides spatial information on internal device location in real time during a biopsy, relative to preoperative imaging anatomy (CT, MR, PET). This tracking is analogous to a miniaturized global positioning system (GPS) [3, 9]. The minute size of EM sensor coils allows localization and tracking of internalized medical devices; at present, these can be fitted within coaxial biopsy introducers, stylets, and hollow cannulas as small in diameter as 22 gauge [3]. Optical and infrared tracking of devices requires either optical or infrared cameras, which require direct line of sight

that is less practical in the setting of image-guided biopsy [9]. Electromagnetic tracking requires a small EM field generator and software to detect and display the tracked devices (Fig. 7.1). Registration between tracking space and image space may be performed by using reference markers attached to the skin near the planned needle entry point ("fiducials"). These may be either passive fiducial markers or actively tracked fiducials (or patches) with sensors integrated directly inside the fiducial. After identifying the fiducials on intraprocedural CT, the corresponding tracking coordinates may be obtained automatically (or alternatively by pointing the tracked needle to each of the fiducials during the breath hold and averaging the tracking signal for several seconds until a stable reading is obtained). A rigid registration transformation between tracking coordinates and CT image coordinates is computed, and the root-mean-square distance (fiducial registration error) between the CT image coordinates of the fiducials and the transformed tracking coordinates of the fiducials is displayed. The registration with the lowest fiducial registration error is used, typically with a fiducial registration error (FRE) smaller than 2 mm. Sensor coil placement upon an ultrasound probe can also enable tracking of the US transducer. Correction for the moving liver may be attempted with tracking of the hepatic biopsy needle itself or other gating methods. The interventional radiologist is essentially provided with a road map to facilitate needle placement and repositioning, by having information about biopsy needle

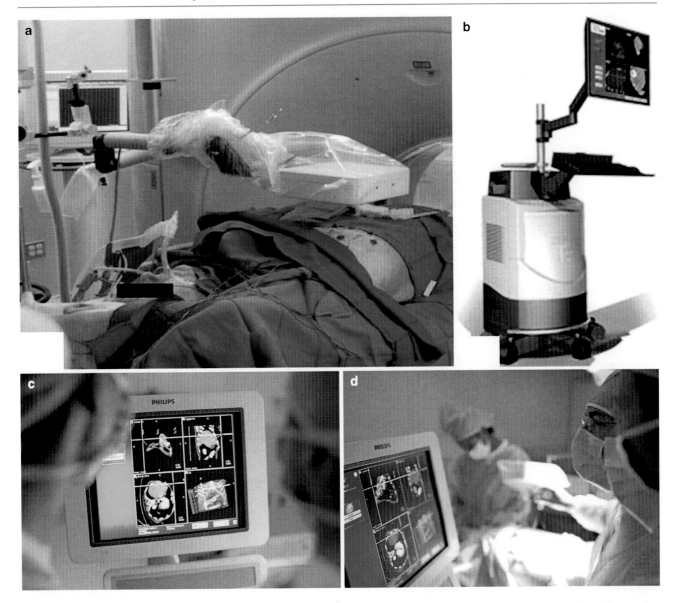

Fig. 7.1 Components for electromagnetic needle tracking during percutaneous biopsy. (**a**) An electromagnetic field generator, sterilely draped, is placed near the working space, directed toward the target and path of needle entry to facilitate image co-registration and device tracking. (**b**) Navigation workstation that enables display of co-registered images and tracked needle during biopsy (PercuNav Image Fusion and Instrument Navigation, Philips Healthcare, Cleveland, Ohio). (**c**) Custom software with display of tracked needle superimposed on multiplanar CT images co-registered to real-time ultrasound. (**d**) Use of needle tracking and multimodality image display facilitates percutaneous biopsy (Image **a** reprinted with permission from Venkatesan et al. [10], Radiological Society of North America (RSNA). Images **b**–**d** reprinted with permission from Philips Healthcare, Cleveland, Ohio)

location, referenced within pre-procedural imaging. Use of this technology has the potential to be superior to the use of conventional biopsy technique, particularly for lesions whose intra-procedural visualization is suboptimal relative to pre-acquired images, e.g., tumors that are only briefly seen during arterial-phase CT (Fig. 7.2).

Early clinical trials suggest good spatial accuracy and feasibility of electromagnetic needle tracking. Kruecker et al. evaluated the spatial accuracy of electromagnetic needle tracking and demonstrated the feasibility of US to CT fusion during CT- and US-guided biopsy and radiofrequency ablation (RFA) procedures, performing a 20-patient clinical trial to investigate electromagnetic needle tracking during interventional procedures [11]. Eight patients underwent RFA; the remainder underwent needle biopsy of sites in the liver, kidney, lung, chest wall, and retroperitoneum [11]. Needles were positioned by using CT and US guidance, and an electromagnetic tracking system was used consisting of internally tracked needles and software to record needle positions relative to previously obtained CT scans (Philips Healthcare,

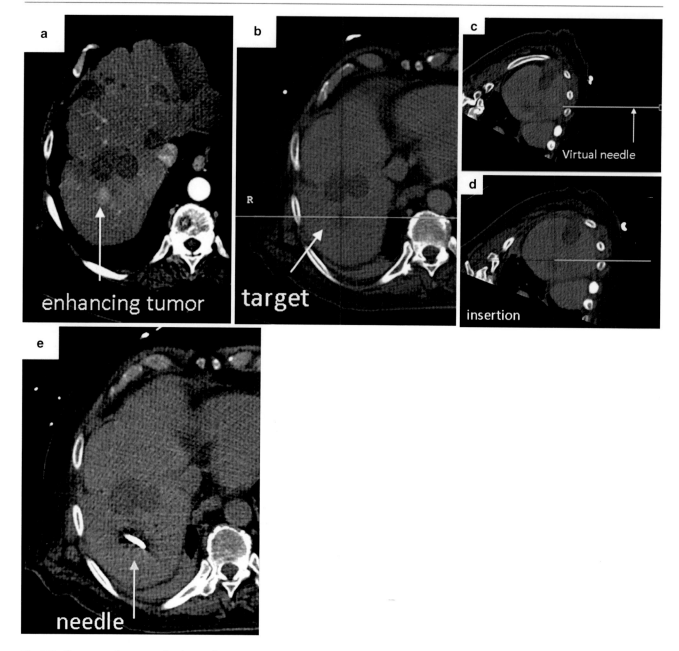

Fig. 7.2 Representative case using image fusion and needle tracking to facilitate percutaneous biopsy. (**a**) Pre-procedural imaging demonstrates the target, a briefly apparent 1 cm arterially enhancing lesion that was not well seen on non-contrast CT, venous phase CT or ultrasound. (**b**) Intra-procedural CT with selected location of target highlighted as a *red dot* on the navigation workstation. The location and orientation of the tracked needle is displayed as a *blue* "virtual needle." (**c** and **d**) Serial images demonstrate location and position of tracked needle relative to target during needle insertion. (**e**) Intra-procedural CT confirms needle tip within location of target. Percutaneous biopsy of this small (1 cm) nodule yielded a diagnosis of hepatocellular carcinoma (Reprinted with permission from Wood et al. [8])

Cleveland, Ohio, formerly Traxtal, Inc., Toronto, CA and Philips Research, Briarcliff, NY) [11]. The electromagnetic field generator was mounted on an articulated mechanical arm, which was attached to a stereotactic frame connected to the CT gantry or simply mounted on a nearby structure such as the ultrasound itself or table [11]. Position tracking data were acquired to evaluate the tracking error [11]. Registration between tracking space and image space was obtained by using reference fiducial markers (or patches) attached to the skin [11]. The US transducer was tracked to demonstrate real-time US-CT fusion for imaging guidance, where the needle is displayed on the ultrasound as well as the pre-procedural CT image [11]. The basic tracking error was 3.5 mm ± 1.9 with use of nonrigid registrations that used previous internal needle positions as additional fiducials reference markers and more recently was found to be 2.7 ± 1.6 mm in a more recent

35-patient study [11, 12]. Fusion of tracked US with CT was successful; patient motion and distortion of the tracking system by the CT table and gantry were identified as sources of error [11]. The spatial tracking accuracy of this system was sufficient to display clinically relevant pre-procedural imaging information during needle-based procedures. Particular benefit was noted for virtual needles displayed within pre-procedural images of transiently apparent targets, such as arterial-phase enhancing liver lesions, or during thermal ablations when obscuring gas is released [11].

Santos et al. evaluated an electromagnetic (EM) navigation system (Veran Medical Technologies Inc, St. Louis, MO) to assess its potential to reduce the number of skin punctures and instrument adjustments during CT-guided percutaneous ablation and biopsy of small (<2 cm) lung nodules [12]. Nineteen EM interventions were performed, including 6 biopsies, 9 radiofrequency ablations (RFAs), 1 combined biopsy with an RFA, and 3 microwave ablations [12]. Median nodule diameter was 1.95 cm (range, 1.2–2.4 cm), and median distance from the skin to lesion was 7.6 cm (2–18 cm) [12]. When an EM-guided biopsy was performed, the intervention was done immediately prior to ablation. For all 19 EM interventions, only one skin puncture was required. The mean number of instrument adjustments required was 1.2 (range, 0–2) [12]. The mean time for each EM intervention was 5.2 min (range, 1–20 min) [12]. Pneumothorax occurred in five patients (50 %), with only the number of instrument adjustments being significantly related to the pneumothorax rate ($p \leq 0.005$) [12]. The authors concluded that the EM navigation is feasible and a useful aid for image-guided biopsy and ablation of small pulmonary tumors [12]. Their experience suggests the EM navigation system might require fewer skin punctures and instrument adjustments for lung biopsies than using CT fluoroscopy guidance alone [12].

The use of fusion-guided biopsy and ablation has demonstrated improvement over conventional CT and US guidance in terms of improved angle selection compared to conventional technique. Kruecker et al. reported that the addition of needle and ultrasound tracking improved needle path "off-target error" from 17.8 ± 17.1 mm to 3.3 ± 3.1 mm and changed insertion angle by $13.3° \pm 6.5°$. This added accuracy has the potential to translate into improved outcomes, particularly for biopsy or ablation of occult targets, where targeting accuracy is crucial [13].

A recent clinical study has evaluated this potential, by assessing the feasibility of combined electromagnetic device tracking and computed tomography (CT)/ultrasonography (US)/fluorine-18 fluorodeoxyglucose (FDG) positron-emission tomography (PET) fusion for real-time feedback during percutaneous and intraoperative biopsies and hepatic radiofrequency ablation [10]. Targets demonstrated heterogeneous FDG uptake or were not well seen or were totally inapparent at conventional imaging and were thus considered technically challenging or impossible to target using conventional imaging guidance [10]. In this study, pre-procedural FDG-PET scans were rigidly registered using a semiautomatic method to intra-procedural CT. Real-time US scans were registered through a fiducial-based method, allowing US scans to be fused with intra-procedural CT and pre-acquired FDG-PET scans. A visual display of US-CT image fusion with overlaid co-registered FDG-PET targets was used for guidance [10]. Navigation software enabled real-time biopsy needle and needle electrode navigation and feedback, employing coaxial biopsy needle introducer tips and RF ablation electrode guider needle tips containing electromagnetic sensor coils spatially tracked through an electromagnetic field generator [10]. Successful fusion of real-time US to co-registered CT and FDG-PET scans was achieved in all patients, with 31 of 36 biopsies being diagnostic and one case of RF ablation resulting in resolution of targeted FDG avidity, with no local treatment failure over a short follow-up period [10].

Additional Navigation Tools for Device Tracking

Additional tools facilitating needle tracking for percutaneous biopsy include mechanical devices, optical devices, and rotational CT-based tools. Mechanical devices include commercial needle stabilizers, which may be fixed to a patient's skin via adhesive and which contain a central needle guide, into which a biopsy needle may be inserted, with the initial biopsy needle angle selected by the operator being able to be "locked" into position within the stabilizer, enabling maintenance of the same needle angle throughout the process of needle insertion to the desired target. Commercial devices facilitating needle angle precision include the SeeStar (St. Jude Medical, formerly Radi Medical Systems, St. Paul, MI) and the Simplify (NeoRad, Oslo, Norway) (Fig. 7.3).

Optical tracking devices for percutaneous biopsy involve optical sensors which may be mounted on needles or probes that may be paired with custom software enabling multiplanar display of patient anatomy, including the location of the desired target in relation to the needle during needle insertion, thereby potentially minimizing the number of serial CT scans required to perform a biopsy, reducing procedure time and radiation dose. The CT-Guide® optical guidance system (approved for marketing in USA, China, Europe, Canada, and Israel) is one example of an optical guidance system for use in CT-guided needle procedures (ActiViews Ltd., Haifa, Israel). Components of this system include a disposable, miniature video camera that may be mounted on any commercial needle or probe, fiducial markers printed on a flexible adhesive pad, and a custom computer graphical user interface. The pre-procedural CT images with overlying

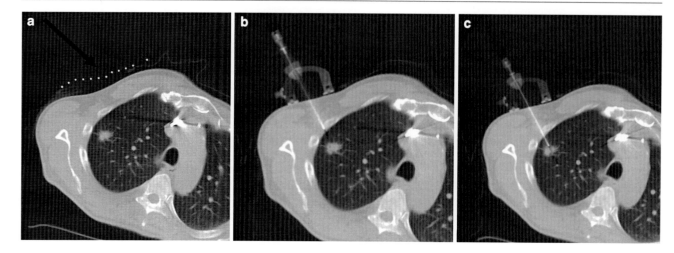

Fig. 7.3 Representative images during percutaneous lung biopsy using the Simplify (NeoRad, Oslo, Norway). (**a**) Grid placement and initial CT scan confirms right upper lobe lung nodule for biopsy. A grid is placed on the overlying skin to mark the target at the level of the skin

(*black arrow*). (**b**) Simplify placed on the skin enables maintenance of initial needle angle throughout needle insertion. (**c**) Successful percutaneous needle biopsy of the targeted lesion

fiducial markers are imported into the custom planning software and used for target and angle selection and real-time guidance (see Fig. 7.4).

Rotational CT for navigation may be referred to by many terms, including cone-beam CT (CBCT), C-arm CT, cone-beam volume CT, angiographic CT, flat-panel CT, rotational angiography CT, rotational fluoro CT, and C-arm CBCT. These systems can function in at least two modes: conventional CT intermittent guidance and a fluoroscopy overlay tool that overlays the intended pathway over a live fluoroscopy image. In one iteration, a live triplanar needle guidance image tool creates overlays of live fluoroscopy with triplanar CT displays which provide information on planned needle path and target not available with the use of fluoroscopic guidance alone. Real-time advancement of needle may be performed based on a planned needle trajectory, with live feedback provided by intra-procedural rotational CT images. Advantages of rotational CT compared to multi-detector CT include the lack of requirement for a CT gantry and no need to transfer patients between CT and a fluoroscopy table, as well as lower radiation dose [14, 15]. Drawbacks include much smaller field of view, less control over parameters like mAs and kVp, higher scatter radiation, lower spatial and contrast resolution, and longer acquisition time [14]. Commercial examples of rotational CT navigation platforms include Xper Guide (Philips Healthcare, Best, Netherlands), the iGuide system (Siemens, Erlangen, Germany), and the InnovaCT (GE Healthcare, Waukesha, WI).

Early studies have described the feasibility of using CBCT for common interventions. Hirota et al. have reported the feasibility of employing CBCT angiography during abdominal interventions, including trans-arterial chemoembolization (TACE), splenic embolization, and implantation of intra-arterial port systems [15]. More recent investigations describe the potential for CBCT to facilitate technically challenging interventions, including successful biopsy of technically challenging FDG-PET avid targets [16]. The ability of CBCT to enable real-time, intra-procedural assessment of the effectiveness of TACE has also been described [17]. A recent study described the integration of CBCT with PET/CT for biopsy and ablation in seven patients, who underwent a total of two ablations and six biopsies without the need for additional specialized hardware [16]. Loffroy et al. describe the ability of intra-procedural dual-phase CBCT to predict tumor response at 1-month follow-up in 29 patients with 50 targeted hepatocellular carcinoma lesions undergoing TACE with doxorubicin-eluting beads, when compared against 1-month posttreatment MRI [17]. The decrease in tumor enhancement observed with dual-phase cone-beam CT after TACE showed a linear correlation with MR findings, assessed according to European Association for the Study of the Liver (EASL) guidelines. A significant relationship between tumor enhancement at cone-beam CT after TACE and complete and/or partial tumor response at MR imaging was found for both arterial (odds ratio, 0.95; 95 % confidence interval [CI], 0.91, 0.99; $p = .023$) and venous (odds ratio, 0.96; 95 % CI, 0.93, 0.99; $p = .035$) phases using a multivariate logistic regression model [16]. As the authors note, the ability of intra-procedural C-arm dual-phase CBCT to predict future tumor response may be especially beneficial, given that treatment response has been identified as an independent predictor of survival [17, 18].

Image Fusion/Co-registration Methods

Multimodality image fusion, including US, CT, MRI, and FDG-PET, has the potential to enhance the utility and indications for biopsy and may be superior to conventional imaging guidance in specific settings. Co-registration between patient anatomy and pre- and intra-procedural data enables simultaneous display of multiplanar anatomic details from CT and MRI and the functional imaging of FDG-PET

while providing real-time anatomic data obtained from US [3]. The operator has the useful imaging information available from each modality when he or she needs it most.

Use of a single imaging modality for guidance may not be ideal during image-guided biopsy. This can be especially true for targets seen only fleetingly during contrast-enhanced CT and/or targets that are in proximity to large blood vessels, where real-time sonographic information about vulnerable anatomy is useful [3]. Registration and fusion of real-time US

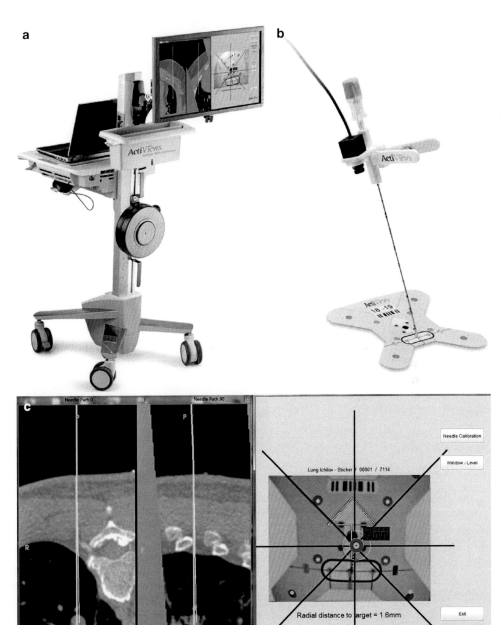

Fig. 7.4 Representative images of the CT-Guide® (ActiViews Ltd, Haifa, Israel) optical guidance system. (**a**) Custom computer with graphical user interface enables target and angle selection and real-time guidance. (**b**) Biopsy needle with miniature video camera (*black square*) clipped to needle hub. (**c**) Close-up of custom graphical user interface with display of tracked needle superimposed on multiplanar CT images, providing the operator with real-time feedback based upon selection of initial skin entry site and target location. (**d**) Use of optical needle tracking and image display facilitates during percutaneous biopsy (Images reprinted with permission from Activiews Ltd., Haifa, Israel)

Fig. 7.4 (continued)

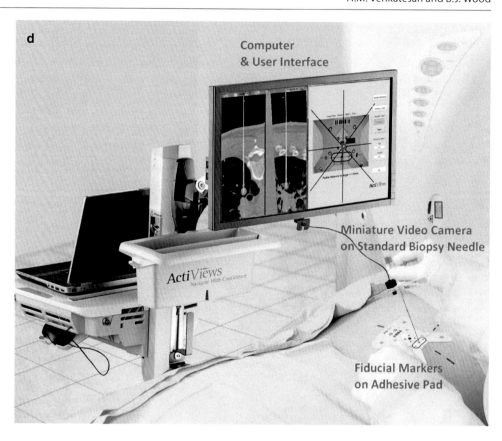

imaging with a pre-acquired 3D image such as CT address these technical challenges [3]. Combining these two modalities also increases the likelihood of target lesion visualization, as the contribution of several modalities can be adjusted and blended to maximize lesion contrast [3]. Superimposing a display of the real-time image of the needle within the larger, higher-resolution CT image may also assist in using other internal anatomic landmarks for navigation even if the target lesion cannot be visualized well with either modality during biopsy [3]. Real-time US and CT image fusion is enabled by electromagnetic tracking of the US probe. The two-dimensional (2D) US image is superimposed with variable opacity and windowing with blending onto the corresponding slice in the CT volume. Alignment of the two image data sets is maintained as the US transducer is moved with real-time updating of fused US and CT images to visualize lesions in both modalities. In this fashion, the ultrasound transducer becomes a "multiplanar reconstruction (MPR) 2D plane selector," and the MPRs are updated in real time with the needle location displayed on all images. Sonography systems for which a pre-acquired CT or MRI may be displayed and co-registered with ultrasound are commercially available from an increasing number of vendors (Hitachi Real-time Virtual Sonography (HI-RVS), Hitachi Medical Systems, Tokyo, Japan; PercuNav Image Fusion and Instrument Navigation, Philips Medical Systems, Cleveland, Ohio; Virtual Navigator, Esaote, Genoa, Italy; Veran ig4

Navigation System, Veran Medical Technologies, St. Louis, Missouri; SonixGPS, Medical Corporation; Logiq E9 Ultrasound System, General Electric Healthcare, Little Chalfont, Buckinghamshire, UK, Milwaukee, WI).

Indications and Patient Selection

Multimodality image fusion and needle tracking are particularly useful to facilitate percutaneous biopsy of lesions that are not consistently seen across imaging modalities. Examples of targets that are very difficult to target with conventional technique include lesions apparent only on a single (e.g., T2-weighted) MR pulse sequence and lesions seen only as a focus of FDG abnormality on FDG-PET scan or only momentarily seen during an arterial-phase CT and occult on ultrasound. Successful biopsy is sometimes enabled by co-registering the images that demonstrate the target lesion in relation to the patient's intra-procedural imaging and anatomy [13]. Lesions that are heterogeneous in their imaging appearance can also be difficult to successfully target with conventional technique, such as tumors with heterogeneous FDG uptake where biopsy of the highest PET activity should relate to validity and integrity of the tissue sample (or biomarker), including diagnostic material-yielding genomic and proteomic data, which is key information in today's era of personalized targeted therapies. These abnormalities can be successfully biopsied with tracking and image fusion; the image fusion technology can display the location of focal areas of FDG avidity, and real-time device tracking can display needle position in relation to the desired target. Tracking and image fusion are also useful when CT, MR, or FDG-PET imaging is not available in the procedure room for real-time intra-procedural guidance. It can also be used to facilitate training or potentially even compensate for lack of experience, normalizing the operator for variabilities in experience or broadening the capabilities of the less experienced operator.

Robotics

In contrast to the aforementioned device tracking and multi-modality image fusion techniques, the use of medical robots to facilitate IR procedures is, at present, far more experimental, albeit promising. Medical robots are typically mechanical device manipulators connected by joints that allow active or passive motion from one link to another [4, 5]. The use of medical robots to assist or to perform intraoperative procedures has been motivated by goals of patient safety, enhanced precision and accuracy, and reduced inter-operator variability and procedure time. It is important to point out that typical "medical procedural robots" are often thought of in the surgical tele-robotics setting, where the surgeon sits at a nearby console and performs the surgery through laparoscopic manipulators and end effectors (arms and hands), such as with the *da Vinci* Surgical System (Intuitive Surgical Inc., Sunnyvale, CA). Robots have been used in neurosurgery, orthopedics, and urology; however, their use is still not considered as a standard of care practice [5], although urological applications for prostatectomy and certain cardiac procedures have seen broadened use of the *da vinci* Surgical System in particular (Intuitive Surgical Inc., Sunnyvale, CA). It is important to note that these surgical robots are quite different and significantly more expensive from any robot that might be used in CT or MRI *da vinci* Surgical System. IR robots that may become standard for CT-guided procedures someday are distinct entities, potentially very inexpensive and directly integrated to the CT software and CT imaging data. The potential for medical robots to facilitate percutaneous interventions remains an area of ongoing research, with relatively little clinical experience to date. As noted by Cleary et al, there remain ongoing challenges to implement a robot in the clinical setting, with medical robots needing to adhere to strict safety and application requirements [5, 19].

There is promising preclinical research demonstrating the ability of medical robots to facilitate percutaneous biopsy. Kettenbach et al. developed a robotic system for ultrasound (US)-guided biopsy and validated its feasibility, accuracy, and efficacy using phantoms [20]. The authors conclude that robotic-assisted biopsies in vitro using US guidance are feasible with high accuracy [20].

Sun et al. have also described in vitro use of a robotic end effector for driving needles during simulated image-guided liver biopsy [21]. This design involves a single articulating arm mounted on a stereotactic frame with a needle gripper on its distal tip that tenses and relaxes based on electronic signals conveyed to it via operator instructions. Operators are able to control not only needle angle and insertion but also two activation states, rigid mode and relaxed mode, to be used throughout the duration of the procedure [21]. Actual needle driving and gripping utilizes the rigid activation state, during which the articulating arm of the end effector is locked to inhibit non-controlled movement [21]. In the relaxed mode, the articulations along the length of the end effector facilitate concurrent movements of the engaged needle with the liver along the craniocaudal axis and potentially any other axes that the liver may travel during respiration [21]. Any shear injury to the liver and adjacent soft tissues would be eliminated as the end effector adjusts its position in accordance with respiration-induced liver motion [21]. A simulation study was performed to define these processes using tissue phantoms with mechanical properties in the range of hepatic tissue and the overlying abdominal wall. A series of tests using a moving bovine liver sample compared performances during the flaccid and rigid modes, demonstrating the design's ability to accommodate soft tissue and organ motion in a single direction [21]. The flexibility offered by the flaccid state of the end effector was found to effectively eliminate the tearing that could occur if a rigid needle-driving end effector was used alone [21]. As the authors conclude, such a switchable and flexible mode for a robotic arm could overcome existing limitations of automated needle placement within a mobile target, minimizing sheer stress upon organ capsules and thereby enhancing patient safety [21].

Several CT- and MRI-compatible robots are being developed for percutaneous image-guided interventions within the existing environments of the CT gantry and closed-bore magnet. Melzer et al. describe development of a CT- and MRI-compatible robotic system, termed "INNOMOTION" (Synthes Inc., formerly Innomedic, Oberdorf, Switzerland) [22]. This pneumatic robotic system consists of a robot arm which can be manipulated in six degrees of freedom, with the device has carefully optimized for use in closed-bore MRI scanners and the CT gantry [5, 22]. The robot arm is attached to a 260° arch that is mounted to the patient table of the scanner and can be passively repositioned on either side of the arch at 0°, 30°, and 60° to the vertical according to the region of interest (e.g., spine, liver, kidney, breast) [5]. Active positioning measurements are achieved via fiber optic coupled switches, along with rotational and linear incremental sensors [5]. The mobile arch can be fixed to the patient table of the MR system [5]. A module for application of coaxial probes (e.g., cannulas for biopsies) provides two degrees of freedom in X and Z axes and is attached to a robotic arm with five degrees of freedom [5]. This design assures stable positioning of the instrument. A pneumatic drive enables controlled insertion of the cannula in incremental steps of 1–20 mm [5]. A graphical user interface provides trajectory planning directly on the MRI images [5].

Chellaturai et al. describe the clinical use of an automated guiding apparatus for CT-guided interventions, which calculates coordinates on DICOM images from a CT scanner and guides physician needle placement [23]. The system includes an electromechanical robotic guide arm that provides five degrees of freedom, a computer console for receiving CT images and calculating coordination, and an interface for data communication between the guide arm and computer console (PIGA-CT, Perfint Healthcare Pvt. Ltd, Chennai, India) [23]. After the physician operator selects skin entry and target points, the apparatus positions itself over the patient and aligns its needle guide accordingly. The needle is subsequently inserted via the guide by the operator [23].

Stoianovici et al. describe the development of a fully automated MRI-compatible robot, termed the "MrBot." This robot has been optimized specifically for transperineal access during MRI-guided prostate biopsy and is fully MRI compatible, with components that are nonmagnetic and dielectric [24]. As the homogeneity of the magnetic field is not affected by the presence of MrBot in the scanner's bore, spectral data from tissues can also be acquired and incorporated into precise targeting of focal metabolic abnormalities [24]. Fitted with optical sensors, the robot operates independently of an electrical source [24]. Its robotic needle possesses six degrees of freedom—five for positioning and orienting and one degree of freedom for setting the depth of needle insertion [24]. In addition, the needle driver presents several additional degrees of freedom for operating the needle, stylet, and loading the markers and can automatically place brachytherapy seeds [24]. The robot is constructed in the form of a platform supported by articulated linear actuators in a five-degree-of-freedom parallel link structure, with significant rigidity inherent within this structure facilitating targeting precision [24]. Although the MrBot is invisible in MRI, a high-contrast marker is built in the robot to enable registration. The accuracy of registration demonstrates targeting errors due to registration to be as low as 0.3 mm [24]. This robot has been tested on a canine model with images acquired for registration, organ visualization, and target specification [24]. Needle targeting error using this experimental model was less than 1 mm [24]. Robotic targeting tests are currently underway using this device to target simulated cancer lesions and to pursue a pilot clinical feasibility study for MRI-guided biopsy [24].

Early clinical experience using robots for percutaneous interventions has been promising. Su et al. evaluated the efficiency, accuracy, and safety of robotic percutaneous access to the kidney (PAKY) for percutaneous nephrolithotomy compared to conventional manual technique [25]. Intraoperative access variables including the number of access attempts, time to successful access, estimated blood loss and complications of 23 patients who underwent robotic PAKY with a remote center of motion device (PAKY-RCM) were compared with the same data from a series of 23 patients who underwent conventional manual percutaneous access to the kidney [25]. The PAKY-RCM incorporates a robotic arm with an axial loading system to accurately position and insert a standard 18-gauge needle percutaneously into the kidney [25]. When comparing PAKY-RCM with standard techniques, no significant difference was noted in the mean number of attempts to biopsy nor in the estimated blood loss score; the difference in the time to access the target approached statistical significance, being lower with use of the robotic system (10.4 ± 6.5 min vs. 15.1 ± 8.8 min ($p = 0.06$) [19]. The PAKY-RCM was successful in obtaining access in 87 % (20 of 23) of cases. The other three patients (13 %) required conversion to manual technique [25]. No major intraoperative complications were observed in either group, suggesting that this robotic system is a feasible, safe, and efficacious method of obtaining renal access for nephrolithotomy, demonstrating a number of attempts and time to access that was comparable to those of standard manual percutaneous access techniques [24]. As noted by Su et al, these data support the prospect of a completely automated robot-assisted percutaneous renal access device [25].

Chokkappan et al. describe the feasibility and preliminary efficacy of the PIGA-CT automated guiding apparatus in the performance of CT-guided lung biopsy as compared with conventional technique in a cohort of 72 consecutive CT-guided biopsies, 36 each performed with manual planning vs. the automated biopsy system [26]. Fewer mean needle repositionings were observed with the assistance platform (1.3) compared to conventional technique (2.9) ($p < 0.001$). Twenty-five biopsies yielded sufficient tissue for pathologic evaluation using the assistance platform vs. 23 using conventional technique ($p = 1.00$). Average number of verification scans was significantly lower with the use of the assistance platform (1.3) compared to conventional technique (3.6) ($p < 0.001$). Procedure time was also notably reduced with the assisted approach (30.8 min) compared to conventional technique (58.7 min) ($p < 0.001$). Complication rates were not statistically significant ($p = 0.15$) [26]. The authors conclude that both manual and automated planning offer comparable diagnostic yield and incidence of complications, with the assisted approach facilitating fewer needle passes, reduced procedure time, number of check scans, and hence the patient's radiation dosage [26]. Promising preliminary results such as these, employing robotic assistance platforms, remain of ongoing interest for future clinical investigation. Additional prospective randomized clinical studies in the future are anticipated to further define the specific benefits of these technologies.

Summary

Many novel tools and devices are available or being investigated to facilitate percutaneous image-guided interventions. These include software for image registration and fusion, electromagnetic tracking, mechanical, optical, and rotational CT-based methods of device tracking, multimodality imaging, and semiautomated robotic needle guidance integrated to the CT. The use of these innovative device tracking techniques and CT robot systems has the potential to improve patient safety and procedural efficiency while potentially reducing procedure time, radiation dose, and inter-operator variability. Many of these novel tools are available to the interventional radiologist, and prospective clinical studies should soon further define the specific clinical benefits of these technologies.

Acknowledgments This work was supported by the NIH Intramural Research Program and the NIH Center for Interventional Oncology. NIH may have intellectual property in the area. The NIH and Philips Healthcare (Best, Netherlands) have a Cooperative Research and Development Agreement (CRADA). The written opinions are those of the authors alone and do not necessarily reflect official positions of the NIH or the US government. The content of this publication does not necessarily reflect the views or policies of the Department of Health and Human Services, nor does mention of trade names, commercial products, or organizations imply endorsement by the U.S. Government.

References

1. Solomon S, Magee C, Acker D, Venbrux A. Experimental nonfluoroscopic placement of inferior vena cava filters: use of an electromagnetic navigation system with previous CT data. J Vasc Interv Radiol. 1999;10:92–5.
2. Varro Z, Locklin J, Wood B. Laser navigation for radiofrequency ablation. Cardiovasc Intervent Radiol. 2004;27:512–17.
3. Wood B, Locklin J, Viswanathan A, et al. Technologies for guidance of radiofrequency ablation in the multimodality interventional suite of the future. J Vasc Interv Radiol. 2007;18:9–24.
4. Craig J. Introduction to robotics. 2nd ed. Reading: Addison-Wesley; 1985.
5. Cleary K, Melzer A, Watson V, Kronreif G, Stoianovici D. Interventional robotic systems: applications and technology state-of-the-art. Minim Invasive Ther Allied Technol. 2006;15(2):101–13.
6. Wood B, Venkatesan A, Abi-Jaoudeh N. Navigation tools and video games in IR and interventional oncology. Society for Interventional Radiology, 2010, Tampa, Florida; 2010.
7. National Aeronautics and Space Administration. Education brief: humans and robots. EB-2001-04-004-JSC. REI Systems Inc.; 2004. p. 1–4.
8. Wood BJ, Kruecker J, Abi-Jaoudeh N, Locklin JK, Levy E, Xu S, Solbiati L, Kapoor A, Amalou H, Venkatesan AM. Navigation systems for ablation. J Vasc Interv Radiol. 2010;21(8 Suppl):S25–63.
9. Wood B, Zhang H, Durrani A, et al. Navigation with electromagnetic tracking for interventional radiology procedures: a feasibility study. J Vasc Interv Radiol. 2005;16(4):493–505.
10. Venkatesan AM, Kadoury S, Abi-Jaoudeh N, et al. Real-time FDG PET guidance during biopsies and radiofrequency ablation using multimodality fusion with electromagnetic navigation. Radiology. 2011;260(3):848–56.
11. Kruecker J, Xu S, Glossop N, et al. Electromagnetic tracking for thermal ablation and biopsy guidance: clinical evaluation of spatial accuracy. J Vasc Interv Radiol. 2007;18(9):1141–50.
12. Santos R, Gupta A, Ebright M, et al. Electromagnetic navigation to aid radiofrequency ablation and biopsy of lung tumors. Ann Thorac Surg. 2010;89:265–8.
13. Kruecker J, Venkatesan A, Xu S, et al. Clinical utility of real-time fusion guidance for biopsy and ablation. J Vasc Interv Radiol. 2011;22(4):515–24.
14. Orth R, Wallace M, Kuo MD. C-arm cone-beam CT: general principles and technical considerations for use in interventional radiology. J Vasc Interv Radiol. 2008;19(6):814–20.
15. Hirota S, Nakao N, Yamamoto S, et al. Cone-beam CT with flat-panel detector digital angiography system: early experience in abdominal interventional procedures. Cardiovascl Intervent Radiol. 2006;29:1034–8.
16. Abi-Jaoudeh N, Mielekamp P, Noordhoek N, et al. Cone-beam computed tomography fusion and navigation for real-time positron emission tomography-guided biopsies and ablations: a feasibility study. J Vasc Interv Radiol. 2012;23:737–43.
17. Loffroy R, Lin M, Yenokyan G, et al. Intraprocedural C-arm dual-phase cone beam CT: can it be used to predict short-term response to TACE with drug-eluting beads in patients with hepatocellular carcinoma? Radiology. 2013;266(2):636–48.
18. Llovet JM, Real MI, Montana X, et al. Arterial embolisation or chemoembolisation versus symptomatic treatment in patients with unresectable hepatocellular carcinoma: a randomised controlled trial. Lancet. 2002;359(9319):1734–9.
19. Cleary K, Davies B, Fichtinger G, Troccaz J, Lueth T, Watson V. Medical robotics workshop-MRWS. Comput Aided Surg. 2004;9(4):167–70.
20. Kettenbach J, Kronreif G, Figl M, Furst M, Birkfellner W, Hanel R, et al. Robot-assisted biopsy using ultrasound guidance: initial results from in vitro tests. Eur Radiol. 2004;15:765–71.
21. Sun D, Willingham C, Durrani A, King P, Cleary K, Wood B. A novel end-effector design for robotics in image guided needle procedures. Int J Med Robot Comput Assist Surg. 2006;2(1):91–7.
22. Melzer A, Schurr M, Kunert W, Buess G, et al. Intelligent surgical instrument system ISIS. Concept and preliminary experimental application of components and prototypes. Endosc Surg Allied Technol. 1993;1:165–70.
23. Chellaturai A, Kanhirat S, Chokkappan K, et al. Technical note: CT-guided biopsy of lung masses using an automated guiding apparatus. Indian J Radiol Imaging. 2009;19(3):206–7.
24. Stoianovici D, Song D, Petrisor D, et al. "MRI stealth" robot for prostate interventions. Minim Invasive Ther Allied Technol. 2007;16:241–8.
25. Su L, Stoianovici D, Jarrett T, et al. Robotic percutaneous access to the kidney: comparison with standard manual access. J Endourol. 2002;16(7):471–7.
26. Chokkappan K, Swaminathan TS, Kulasekaran N, et al. Scrutinizing the efficacy of automated method over manual methods in CT guided biopsies. Electronic poster presentation, European Society of Radiology March 6–9, 2009, Vienna, Austria.

Pathologic Evaluation of Tissues Obtained by Interventional Radiology Techniques

Savitri Krishnamurthy

Fine Needle Aspiration Biopsy (FNAB)

FNAB is a minimally invasive procedure that is performed using a 21-, 23-, or 25-gauge needle attached to a 10 cm³ syringe. The needle is introduced into the lesion and moved several times, dislodging cells, which are aspirated and deposited onto glass slides. Direct smears are made manually and fixed in alcohol for staining using the Papanicolaou or hematoxylin and eosin (H&E) method and then air-dried for staining using the Diff-Quik method for conventional cytological examination [1]. By changing the direction of the needle during aspiration, different sites in the target area can be evaluated.

Direct smears stained using the Papanicolaou method are valuable for studying the details of the nucleus; the nuclear chromatin, in particular, is useful for cytologically categorizing lesions. Air-dried smears stained using the Diff-Quik method are helpful for studying cytoplasmic characteristics, including intracellular and extracellular secretory material. Interpreting FNAB findings requires expertise and training in cytopathology and is based on evaluating cytomorphological characteristics of the cells. The entire staining process can be completed in approximately 10 min, after which the aspirate is available for immediate interpretation. Immediate assessment is valuable for helping the interventional radiologist determine the adequacy of the specimen for optimal interpretation and the accuracy of lesion localization.

The success of FNAB depends on the operator's skill, the nature of the lesion, and good communication between the interventional radiologist and pathologist. Many lesions can be diagnosed using the cytomorphological features of the constituent cells on direct smears, with no knowledge of the tissue architecture or results of ancillary studies. Figure 8.1

shows a Papanicolaou-stained direct smear of a lung mass with tumor cells that exhibit melanin pigment, indicating metastatic melanoma; in this case, diagnosis is based on the cytomorphological features of the tumor cells alone. Lesions that do not yield diagnostic material on repeated FNAB must be investigated by core needle biopsy (CNB).

The needle used for aspiration can be rinsed in solutions such as RPMI medium 1640 (Gibco, Invitrogen) or CytoLyt solution (Hologic Corp.) immediately after the aspirate has been added to glass slides; this approach is useful for preparing tissue blocks, also referred to as cell blocks. Cell blocks are useful for collecting any remaining cells and tissue fragments in the needle and syringe that can be used for additional cytopathologic evaluation. The RPMI or CytoLyt solution is then centrifuged to obtain a sediment containing the cellular material. A small amount of sediment is used to prepare one or two cytospin smears, which can be stained similarly to a direct smear. Cell blocks can be prepared if

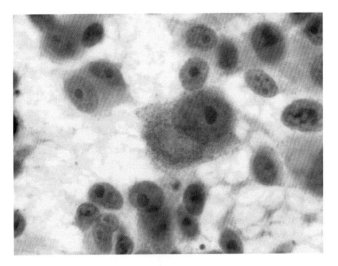

Fig. 8.1 Direct smear prepared from FNAB sample of a lung mass and stained using the Papanicolaou method. Note the presence of many tumor cells with prominent nucleoli. The presence of melanin pigment in one tumor cell confirms the diagnosis of metastatic melanoma

S. Krishnamurthy, MD
Department of Pathology,
The University of Texas MD Anderson Cancer Center,
Houston, TX, USA
e-mail: skrishna@mdanderson.org

K. Ahrar, S. Gupta (eds.), *Percutaneous Image-Guided Biopsy*,
DOI 10.1007/978-1-4614-8217-8_8, © Springer Science+Business Media New York 2014

sufficient sediment is available. Different methods are used to prepare cell blocks [2–5]. One of the most common methods includes wrapping the sediment in Shark Skin Filter Paper (Whatman); this is then placed in a plastic cassette, fixed in formalin, and subjected to routine processing. After processing, the cell blocks are embedded in paraffin wax to create tissue blocks, which are cut at 5-μm intervals and stained using the H&E method for pathologic interpretation. These cell blocks are a valuable resource for generating additional unstained sections for ancillary studies using methods such as immunocytochemical analysis, in situ hybridization, or polymerase chain reaction (PCR) or next generation sequencing.

Core Needle Biopsy (CNB)

CNB is performed using a 14–21-gauge, coaxial, automated cutting needle biopsy system (Cook). Usually, 2–4 cores of tissue are obtained from the lesion. For conventional pathological examination, the samples are fixed in formalin, routinely processed, and embedded in paraffin. The paraffin blocks are then cut at 5 μm and stained with H&E for final histopathological interpretation. The advantage of CNBs over FNAB is the availability of tissue architecture; this facilitates the rendering of a specific diagnosis on the basis of histopathologic examination, alone or in conjunction with ancillary testing. The entire process, from fixing the sample in formalin to the availability of tissue sections for pathologic interpretation, can take a mean of 6–24 h. Therefore, CNBs are not available for immediate assessment, unlike FNAB, in which direct smears are available within a few minutes of the procedure to determine specimen adequacy, localization accuracy, and a preliminary diagnosis. However, in centers in which immediate evaluation by cytopathologists or cytotechnologists is available, touch imprints of CNBs can be prepared by gently touching the cores on glass slides. These touch imprints can be fixed in alcohol for Papanicolaou or H&E staining and air-dried for Diff-Quik staining, similarly to direct FNAB smears, for immediate assessment of specimen adequacy and to determine whether the CNB represents the target lesion [6, 7].

FNAB and CNB are complimentary techniques for evaluating the lesion of interest; both have distinct advantages and limitations. In centers in which immediate assessment of the specimen is possible, direct FNAB smears or touch imprints can contribute to the overall success of obtaining diagnostic material from the target lesion. Direct smears may be more useful than touch imprints for rendering a preliminary diagnosis within a few minutes of the biopsy. FNAB is the preferred method in technically challenging sites such as those close to major blood vessels or neurovascular bundles. In addition, FNAB is the preferred method for obtaining material for microbiologic culture studies from lesions that are thought to be infectious on the basis of clinical history, radiologic images, the results of direct FNAB smears, or CNB touch imprints. In cases of suspected hematopoietic neoplasms, FNAB is better than CNB for obtaining material for immunophenotyping by flow cytometry for establishing the clonality of the lymphoid cells [8]. The cytomorphological features alone are sufficient to render a specific diagnosis in many cases. The availability of tissue architecture in FNAB cell blocks aids in generating a specific diagnosis. However, tissue architecture in larger CNB fragments eases interpretation and the rendering of a definite and specific diagnosis. CNB samples invariably contain more tissue than do FNAB samples, making ancillary studies possible. In selected cases, either technique alone can be used, but both are preferable because both have distinct diagnostic advantages. Figure 8.2 shows a case of CT-guided biopsy of a 2.5 cm lung mass; diagnostic material was found on an FNAB direct smear and cell block and on CNB. Figure 8.3 illustrates a case of sonography-guided FNAB and CNB of an enlarged neck lymph node for which CNB, but not FNAB, provided diagnostic material.

Several investigators have compared the performance of FNAB and concurrent CNB for evaluating target lesions in selected organs [9–18]. Most of these studies concluded that both these techniques are generally complementary. The diagnostic yield may be similar for both techniques, but in a small number of patients, diagnostic material can only be obtained using one or the other method. Therefore, overall diagnostic accuracy can be increased using both techniques, if possible, in any given patient. In most cases, the combination of FNAB and CNB can obviate the need for incisional biopsy or other invasive procedures, such as mediastinoscopy, thoracoscopy, or laparoscopy; all of these procedures are performed under general anesthesia and are generally associated with higher morbidity and cost than are preoperative biopsies performed in radiology or pathology suites.

Ancillary Testing

Ancillary tests, when used in conjunction with conventional cytopathological or histopathological examination, increase the specificity of the pathologic diagnosis. The different ancillary tests that can be used in anatomic pathology are described in the sections below.

Immunohistochemical Analysis

Immunohistochemical analysis is the most commonly used ancillary test in the work-up of specimens; it plays a valuable role in rendering a specific pathologic diagnosis. The technique

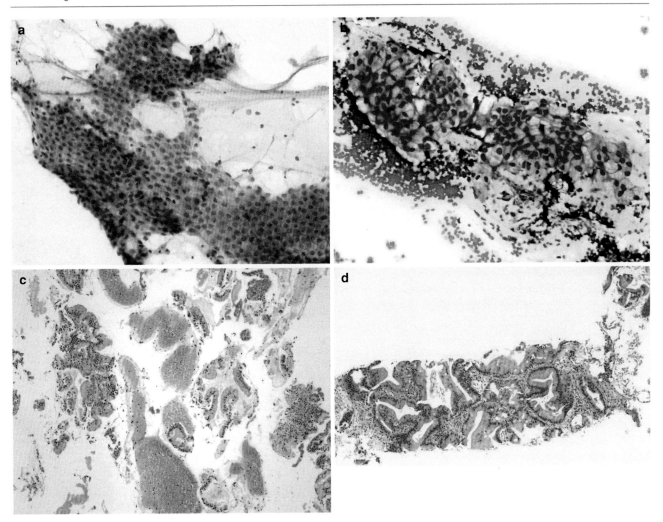

Fig. 8.2 Direct smears prepared from FNAB of a lung mass, stained using the Papanicolaou (**a**) and Diff-Quik (**b**) methods, reveal mucin-containing tumor cell fragments in the cytoplasm. The corresponding cell block section (**c**) reveals several fragments of tumor cells that are consistent with mucinous bronchioloalveolar carcinoma. The core needle biopsy of the lung mass is shown in (**d**). Note that the concurrently obtained CNB sample demonstrates the same tumor in a larger continuous tissue fragment

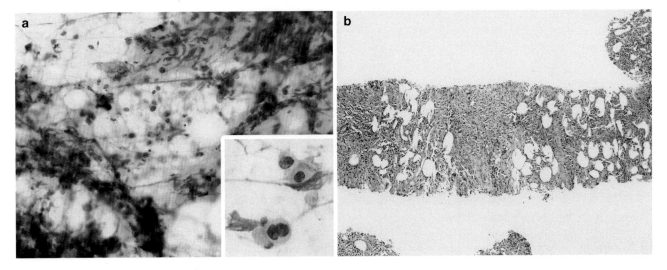

Fig. 8.3 Direct smears prepared from FNAB of an enlarged neck lymph node stained using the Papanicolaou method (**a**) reveal a prominent crush artifact, with only a few scattered atypical cells. The corresponding CNB sample (**b**) reveals adequate diagnostic material that permits accurate pathologic evaluation of the tissue

entails the use of antibodies specific to pertinent epitopes in cells. The antibody binds to the epitope, which, if present in the tissue, can be visualized using different types of chromogens [9]. Immunostaining can be performed using tissue obtained by CNB or FNAB, provided the tissue contains adequate material. Because more representative tissue is available on CNB than on FNAB, CNB is preferred for immunostaining. However, with good-quality cell blocks that contain adequate representative tissue, the results of immunostaining with FNAB cell block sections can be equivalent to those of CNB sections. Cell blocks are the optimal FNAB preparation for immunostaining, but alcohol-fixed or air-dried smears and formalin-fixed direct smears can be used when cell blocks, or CNB samples are not available. Because the positive control used for immunostaining of smears is usually formalin-fixed tissue and not a similarly prepared direct smear, careful interpretation of the results is generally recommended. Similarly fixed direct smears should be used as positive controls to validate antibodies' performance in direct smears compared with formalin-fixed, paraffin-embedded tissue; this should be established before the direct smears are used for immunostaining.

Common applications of immunohistochemical analysis include detecting infectious agents; categorizing and typing tumors; determining the site of origin of metastatic tumors, including those with multiple or unknown primaries; and evaluating prognostic and predictive tumor markers for targeted therapy. Antibodies against the intermediate filaments of cells, namely, cytokeratins in epithelial cells and vimentin in mesenchymal cells, facilitate the categorization of poorly differentiated tumors, as carcinoma when positive for the former marker and as sarcoma when positive for the latter. The expression patterns of different types of low- and high-molecular weight cytokeratins are specific and consistent with respect to organs. Primary antibodies developed against specific cytokeratins are valuable for phenotyping benign and malignant tissues to determine the organ of origin. The use of a panel of two cytokeratins, CK7 and CK20, can help in determining the site of origin of many epithelial tumors [19]. The organs and their corresponding tumors that are positive for CK7 but negative for CK20 include the lungs, breasts, and ovaries; those that are positive for CK20 but negative for CK7 include the colorectum and urinary bladder; those positive for both markers include selected instances of tissues from the stomach and pancreaticobiliary tract; and those negative for both include the kidneys, adrenal gland, and liver. In addition, several specific antibodies are available to help further characterize tumors.

Tissue specific markers include thyroid transcription factor 1, surfactant apoprotein A, and Napsin A for lung adenocarcinoma; mammaglobin, gross cystic disease fluid protein 15 (GCDFP15), and estrogen and progesterone receptor expression for mammary tumors; HePar1 and glypican 3 for hepatocellular carcinoma; prostate-specific antigen, prostate-specific acid phosphatase, and prostein for prostate disease; parathyroid hormone for the parathyroid gland; thyroglobulin and thyroid transcription factor 1 for the thyroid gland; renal cell carcinoma marker and CD10 for renal cell carcinoma; and calretinin, D2-40, and mesothelin for mesothelial cells [20–22]. Markers for confirming neuroendocrine differentiation include chromogranins, synaptophysin, and CD56 [23]. Markers for diagnosing melanoma include S-100 protein, MART1, Melan A, HMB45, and tyrosinase [24]. Prognostic and predictive markers that can be evaluated by immunohistochemical analysis include estrogen and progesterone receptors and human epidermal receptor 2 (HER2)/neu in breast carcinomas and c-kit in gastrointestinal stromal tumors [25–27]. Figure 8.4 shows a poorly differentiated carcinoma on a sonography-guided CNB of a 2.5-cm mass in the liver that is positive for estrogen receptor and demonstrates HER2/neu protein overexpression on immunohistochemical analysis.

Leukocyte common antigen is an immunomarker for hematopoietic cells [28, 29]. CNB is optimal for immunostaining in hematopoietic lesions; however, selected immunostains can be performed on cytospin FNAB smears to characterize lymphoid cells. The most common B cell markers are CD19, CD20, CD79, PAX5, and kappa and lambda light chains; T-cell markers include CD2, CD3, CD5, CD7, CD4, and CD8. For typing lymphomas, useful markers are bcl2 for follicular lymphoma, cyclin D1 for mantle cell lymphoma, ALK1 for anaplastic lymphoma, and CD138 for plasma cell tumors [28, 29]. CNB is preferred for diagnosing non-Hodgkin's lymphoma; FNAB can be equivalent using a multiparametric approach, including cytomorphological evaluation and ancillary immunophenotyping by flow cytometry [30]. Figure 8.5 shows the results of ancillary immunostains performed on unstained CNB sections of the case in Fig. 8.3. The tumor cells are positive for leukocyte common antigen, CD20, and lambda light chain. The overall cytomorphological features, in conjunction with ancillary immunostains, are consistent with high-grade malignant B cell lymphoma. It is to be noted that in patients with Hodgkin disease, CNB is optimal because fibrosis makes it difficult to obtain cells and because a panel of immunostains is needed to establish the diagnosis.

Flow Cytometry Analysis

Immunophenotyping by flow cytometry analysis is routinely performed on all suspected hematopoietic lesions to characterize the cells comprising the lesion and to establish clonality. While both CNB and FNAB samples can be used, but the latter is preferred because the cells are already in suspension [8]. However, with FNAB, it is important to ensure that the aspirate contains an adequate number of cells. Immediate

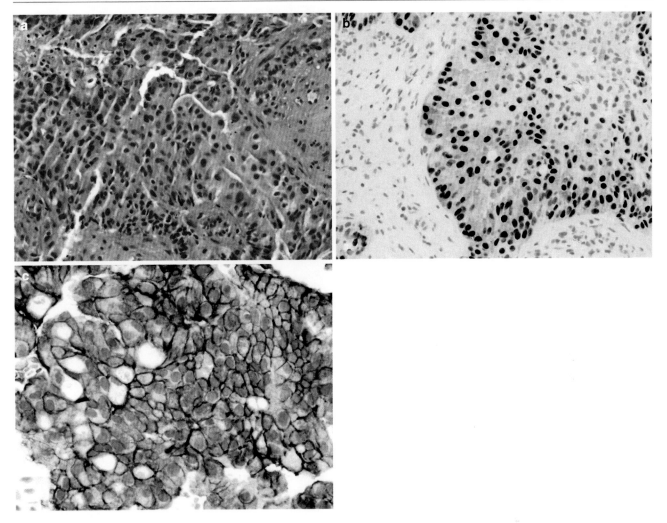

Fig. 8.4 Tissue section prepared from CNB of a liver mass stained using the H&E method (**a**) demonstrate features of a poorly differentiated adenocarcinoma. The tumor cells are positive for estrogen receptor (**b**) and HER2/neu on immunohistochemical staining (**c**). The overall findings support the diagnosis of metastatic breast carcinoma

assessment of direct smears for the presence of the cells of interest and the extent of blood contamination can be useful for determining the quality of the aspirate for successful immunophenotyping. However, counting the lymphoid cells in an RPMI suspension using a cell counter can provide more definite proof. Approximately 5–10 million cells are generally adequate for flow cytometry analysis of a variety of T and B lymphocytic or myeloid cell panels that can be tested on the basis of the preliminary diagnosis of direct smears or CNB touch preparations.

are preferred for molecular tests such as in situ hybridization, PCR, sequencing, and transcriptional profiling on preoperative tissue obtained under imaging guidance. However, FNAB samples, including alcohol-fixed, air-dried direct smears; aspirate in any transport media; and unstained sections of formalin- or alcohol-fixed, paraffin-embedded cell blocks can also be used provided they demonstrate adequate cellularity. The details of the molecular tests and the optimal specimen needed for each test are summarized in the sections below.

Molecular Testing

Several molecular tests are performed as the standard of care to arrive at a definite diagnosis or to select patients for or predict response to targeted therapy. The list of molecular markers that can be tested is rapidly evolving. CNB specimens

Diagnosis of Soft Tissue Tumors

Molecular testing is often performed on soft tissue tumors for a definite preoperative diagnosis. Translocations that lead to recombination of coding sequences of different genes and expression of pathologic gene fusion products are common

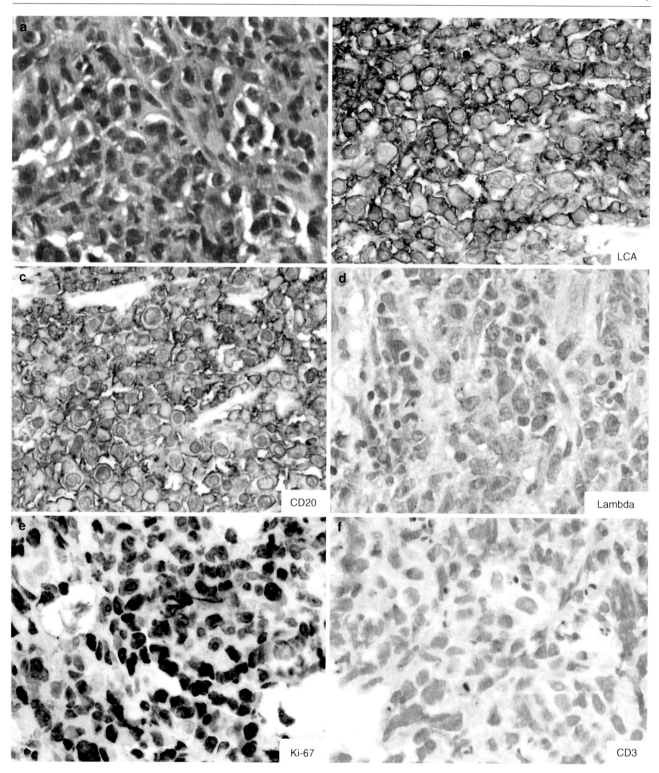

Fig. 8.5 Ancillary immunostains performed on the CNB of the case in Fig. 8.3. H&E stain shows large cell lymphoma involving the lymph node (**a**). The tumor cells are positive for leukocyte common antigen (**b**), CD20 (**c**), and lambda light chain (**d**) and negative for CD3 (**f**). Note the high proliferative index, as demonstrated by Ki67 labeling, in almost all tumor cells (**e**). The overall findings are consistent with high-grade malignant B cell lymphoma

and specific in soft tissue sarcomas. Recognition of these specific cytogenetic alterations can be achieved on molecular analysis and is valuable for making an accurate diagnosis. Specific cytogenetic alterations in soft tissue tumors can be detected using karyotypic analysis, PCR, or fluorescence in situ hybridization (FISH) [31]. FISH is the most commonly used technique for this purpose; the preferred specimens for this test are formalin-fixed, paraffin-embedded CNB sections. When CNB samples are not available, cell block sections and direct FNAB smears can be used [32]. When

Fig. 8.6 Illustration of a case of synovial sarcoma reveals spindle cell proliferation on an H&E-stained CNB tissue section (**a**) and on a Papanicolaou-stained direct FNAB smear (**b**). FISH using dual-color break-apart in an SYT 18 q11.2 probe reveals *yellow fusion signals*, indicating t(x;18) (p11;q11) chromosomal translocation (**c**)

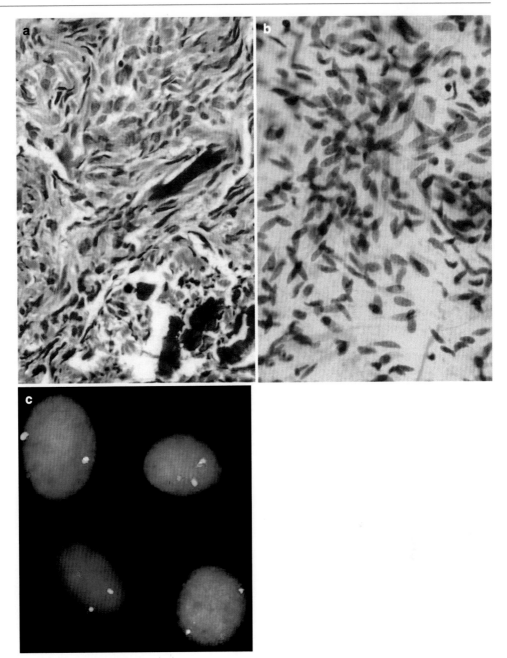

karyotypic analysis or PCR is required, dedicated FNAB or CNB passes can be used for both techniques; unstained tissue sections of formalin-fixed, paraffin-embedded CNB or FNAB cell blocks can be used for latter technique.

The chromosomal translocation t(11;22)(q24;q12) is specific for Ewing sarcoma, peripheral neuroepithelioma, and Askin tumor. This cytogenetic alteration rearranges and fuses the EWS gene on chromosome 11 and the FLI1 genes of the ETS transcription family on chromosome 22; it is a sensitive and specific molecular test for diagnosing these tumors [31]. The EWS gene, fused with genes belonging to other members of the ETS transcription family, is specific for other soft tissue tumors. When fused with the ATF-1 gene, resulting in t(12;22)(q13;q12), it is specific for clear cell sarcoma; when fused with the WT1 gene in t(11;22)(p13;q12), it is specific

for desmoplastic small round cell tumor; when fused with the CHN gene in t(9;22)(q22;q12), it is specific for myxoid chondrosarcoma. Alveolar rhabdomyosarcoma is characterized by two tumor-specific translocations, t(2;13)(q35;q14) and t(1;13) (p36;q14), resulting in fusions of the PAX3 and PAX7 genes, which are members of the PAX transcription family. Synovial sarcoma is characterized by a specific t(X;18)(p11;q11) translocation involving the SYT gene on chromosome 18 and one of the SSX genes on chromosome X, leading to functional fusion (SYT-SSX). Figure 8.6 shows a spindle cell tumor on a H&E-stained CNB tissue section (a) and a Papanicolaou-stained FNAB direct smear (b). The presence of yellow fusion signals by FISH using the dual-color break-apart SYT 18 q11.2 probe indicates chromosomal translocation t(x;18)(p11;q11) in tumor cells, which confirms the diagnosis of synovial sarcoma.

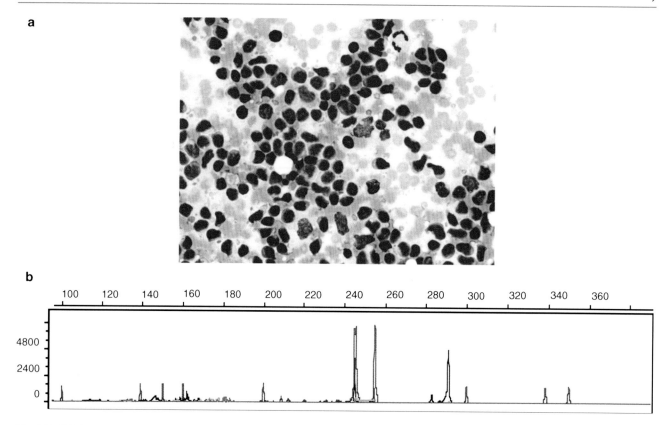

Fig. 8.7 FNAB sample of T-cell malignant lymphoma reveals small lymphoid cells in a Diff-Quik-stained direct smear (**a**) and the results of a T-cell receptor gamma chain PCR analysis, detected by capillary electrophoresis in (**b**). The large red peaks represent biallelic clonal T-cell receptor gamma rearrangement

Diagnosing Hematopoietic Tumors

Molecular tests are used in selected cases of hematopoietic lesions when cytomorphological evaluation, histopathological examination, and ancillary immunophenotyping by flow cytometry and immunohistochemistry are unable to generate a definite diagnosis. In such cases, molecular tests, such as FISH and PCR, can be used to determine the clonality of suspected hematopoietic lesions. PCR is the most widely used method to detect immunoglobulin heavy chain gene rearrangement for tumors arising from B lymphoid cells and T-cell receptor gene rearrangements for those derived from T lymphoid cells [28, 29].

These tests can be performed using FNAB or CNB. In FNAB, the aspirated material is collected in RPMI under sterile conditions. The lymphoid cells present in the RPMI solution are counted using a cell counter. Counts of at least one million cells in 1 ml are optimal for a successful molecular analysis using at least 10 ml of the RPMI solution, with the lymphoid cells in suspension. Figure 8.7 shows an FNAB sample from a lymph node with small lymphoid cells in a Diff-Quik-stained (a) direct smear; also shown are the results of a T-cell receptor gamma chain PCR analysis detected by capillary electrophoresis. The large red peaks represent biallelic clonal T-cell receptor gamma rearrangement, which confirms the diagnosis of malignant T-cell lymphoma. Fresh CNB cores fixed directly in RNAlater solution or tissue sections of formalin-fixed, paraffin-embedded CNB sections can also be used for testing.

Molecular tests such as FISH and PCR can be used to demonstrate relatively specific chromosomal abnormalities that are useful for diagnosis when flow cytometry and immunostaining produce equivocal results or when insufficient material is available for these tests. The FISH assay is useful for demonstrating the t(14;18)(q32;q21) translocation for diagnosing follicular lymphoma; the t(11;14)(q13;q32) translocation for mantle cell lymphoma, with the probes at 14q32 and 11q13 (cyclin D1) loci; and the ALK1 breakpoints to demonstrate t(2;5)(p23;q35) for diagnosing T-null anaplastic lymphoma patients with a favorable prognosis [28].

Carcinoma of Unknown Primary

Carcinomas of unknown primary (CUP) comprise approximately 2–5 % of all cancer diagnoses. The organ of origin cannot be determined in most of these tumors using immunohistochemical phenotyping with the currently available antibodies. Improved diagnostic methods that help us identify

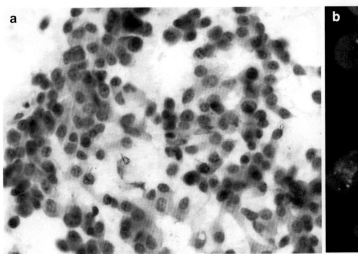

Fig. 8.8 Sonography-guided FNAB sample of an enlarged axillary lymph node reveals features of a poorly differentiated carcinoma in a Papanicolaou-stained direct smear (**a**). FISH using the PathVysion HER2/neu probe (**b**) reveals marked HER2/neu gene amplification, with many *orange signals* (HER2/neu) and 2–4 *green signals* (CEP17) in the nuclei of tumor cells, indicating HER2/neu gene amplification

the tissue of origin of these tumors would facilitate the selection of specific therapy. Recent advances in gene expression profiling using reverse transcription PCR or oligonucleotide microarray have enabled researchers to develop expression profiles unique to a wide variety of well-characterized primary cancers and compare these unique signatures with those of unknown primary tumors. As the gene expression profile is frequently conserved when the tumor metastasizes, it is possible to determine the organ of origin of the metastatic tumor. Various commercially available tests are available to determine the organ of origin of CUP; these tests can be performed using formalin-fixed, paraffin-embedded, or fresh-frozen tissue and have an accuracy of 76–89 % [33]. Prospective clinical trials are ongoing to determine whether therapies based on the results of gene expression profiling to determine the organ of origin of CUP improve patient prognosis. CNB specimens are optimal for these tests because sufficient tissue is available for multiple molecular tests.

Detecting Targets for Targeted Therapy

Determining HER2 gene amplification in breast tumors is routinely performed using fluorescence or chromogenic in situ hybridization (FISH, CISH) [34, 35]. HER2/neu is a proto-oncogene located on the long arm of chromosome 17 and is an important prognostic and predictive factor in patients with invasive breast cancer. Its overexpression is closely related to gene amplification and is seen in 25–30 % of patients with invasive breast cancer [36]. HER2/neu status is valuable for selecting patients for treatment with adjuvant or neoadjuvant trastuzumab, a humanized monoclonal antibody that targets the HER2/neu receptor [37]. HER2/neu is

evaluated in all newly diagnosed patients and in most of those with distant metastasis or recurrence. The FISH/CISH assay for HER2/neu in a primary tumor is usually performed on tissue sections obtained from formalin-fixed, paraffin-embedded CNB of the primary tumor and not on FNAB samples because of the inability to distinguish in situ from invasive breast carcinoma on FNAB. However, in metastatic tumors, both CNB and FNAB specimens can be used for HER2/neu testing. When using FNAB specimens for HER2/neu testing of metastatic tumors, cell block tissue sections or air-dried direct smears, unstained or stained with Diff-Quik, can be used for FISH testing. Figure 8.8 illustrates a case of metastatic breast carcinoma in an axillary lymph node that has features of a poorly differentiated carcinoma on Papanicolaou-stained direct smear and marked HER2/neu gene amplification on FISH. The results of HER2/neu using direct smears have been reported to be similar to those of tissue sections. HER2/neu status is occasionally determined in other carcinomas, such as those in the pancreas, esophagus, lungs, stomach, and ovaries, to determine eligibility for trastuzumab therapy.

Epidermal growth factor receptor (EGFR) has emerged as a leading target for the treatment of colorectal carcinoma and non-small cell lung carcinoma with EGFR inhibitors. Detecting EGFR mutations allows us to select patients with lung adenocarcinoma for EGFR tyrosine kinase inhibitor therapy [38–40]. The EGFR mutations include in-frame deletion in exon 19 or point mutations in exon 21 that occur in approximately 10 % of non-small cell lung carcinomas. These mutations are commonly observed in lung adenocarcinomas in women of Asian ethnicity with no smoking history. The effectiveness of EGFR inhibitors can be determined by detecting KRAS mutations [41]. The KRAS gene is the human homolog of the Kirsten rat sarcoma 2 virus oncogene that encodes a small GTP binding protein that acts as a signal transducer in response to EGFR ligand binding. Activating mutations in codons 12 and 13 of exon 2 are predictive of failure to respond to anti-EGFR therapy in lung and colon cancers. Patients with mutated KRAS do not experience a response to anti-EGFR therapy or bevacizumab (anti-vascular endothelial growth factor).

BRAF mutations occur in a small percentage of patients with melanoma and other solid tumors and are predictive of response to BRAF inhibitors [42]. KRAS/BRAF mutations are predictive of sensitivity to mitogen-activated protein kinase inhibitor therapy [43]. cKIT belongs to the receptor tyrosine kinase family and is important in the development and progression of gastrointestinal stromal tumors, some melanomas, and some small cell lung carcinomas [44]. A mutational analysis of cKIT by sequencing or PCR can be used to predict the response of these tumors to tyrosine kinase inhibitor therapy

Because of the amount of tissue obtained, CNB specimens are optimal for mutational analyses of targets, such as via PCR and sequencing, to select patients for targeted therapy. Dedicated cores introduced into RNAlater or formalin-fixed, paraffin-embedded CNB sections are generally used for molecular testing. However, dedicated FNAB passes directly introduced into RNAlater solution, unstained tissue cell block sections, or cells scraped from alcohol-fixed direct smears can also be used, provided the cellularity is sufficient. The suitability of FNAB specimens is determined on a case-by-case basis after thorough evaluation of the aspirated material for overall cellularity.

References

1. Frable WF. Fine needle aspiration biopsy techniques. In: Bibbo M, Wilbur D, editors. Comprehensive cytopathology. 3rd ed. Philadelphia: Saunders, Elsevier; 2008. p. 579–98.
2. Birge RF, McMullen T, Davis SK. A rapid method for paraffin section study of exfoliated neoplastic cells in body fluids. Am J Clin Pathol. 1948;18:754.
3. Carson CP, Valdes DA. Coagulated plasma as an embedding medium in the cytologic study of body fluids. Am J Clin Pathol. 1951;21:96–8.
4. Fahey C, Bedrosian UK. Collodion bag: a cell block technique for enhanced cell collection. Lab Med. 1993;74:94–6.
5. Akalin A, Lu D, Woda B, et al. Rapid cell blocks improve accuracy of breast FNAs beyond that provided by conventional cell blocks regardless of immediate adequacy evaluation. Diagn Cytopathol. 2008;36:523–9.
6. Hahn PF, Eisenberg PJ, Pitman MB, et al. Cytopathologic touch preparations (imprints) from core needle biopsies: accuracy compared with that of fine-needle aspirates. Am J Roentgenol. 1995;165:1277–9.
7. Chandan VS, Zimmerman K, Baker P, et al. Usefulness of core roll preparations in immediate assessment of neoplastic lung lesions. Chest. 2004;126:739–43.
8. Jorgensen JL. State of the art symposium: flow cytometry in the diagnosis of lymphoproliferative disorders by fine needle aspiration. Cancer. 2005;105:443–51.
9. Bennert KW, Abdul-Karim FW. Fine needle aspiration cytology vs needle core biopsy of soft tissues tumors. A comparison. Acta Cytol. 1994;38:381–4.
10. Ayala AG, ROJ Y, Fanning CV, et al. Core needle biopsy and fine-needle aspiration in the diagnosis of bone and soft tissue lesions. Hematol Oncol Clin North Am. 1995;9:633–51.
11. Koscick RL, Petersilge CA, Makley JT, et al. CT-guided fine needle aspiration and needle core biopsy of skeletal lesions. Complementary diagnostic techniques. Acta Cytol. 1998;42:697–702.
12. Cochand-Priollet B, Chagnon S, Ferrand J, et al. Comparison of cytologic examination of smears and histologic examination of tissues cores obtained by fine needle aspiration biopsy of the liver. Acta Cytol. 1987;31:476–80.
13. Stewart CJ, Coldewey J, Stewart IS. Comparison of fine needle aspiration cytology and needle core biopsy in the diagnosis of radiologically detected abdominal lesions. J Clin Pathol. 2002;55(2):93–7.
14. Gong Y, Sneige N, Guo M, et al. Transthoracic fine-needle aspiration vs concurrent core needle biopsy in diagnosis of intrathoracic lesions: a retrospective comparison of diagnostic accuracy. Am J Clin Pathol. 2006;125:438–44.
15. Aviram G, Greif J, Man A, et al. Diagnosis of intrathoracic lesions: are sequential fine- needle aspiration (FNA) and core needle biopsy (CNB) combined better than either investigation alone? Clin Radiol. 2007;62:221–6.
16. Kraft M, Laeng H, Schmuziger N, et al. Comparison of ultrasound-guided core-needle biopsy and fine-needle aspiration in the assessment of head and neck lesions. Head Neck. 2008;30:1457–63.
17. Kupnick D, Sztajer S, Kordek R, et al. Comparison of core and fine needle aspiration biopsies for diagnosis of liver masses. Hepatogastroenterology. 2008;55:1710–15.
18. Taylor CR, Shi SR, Barr NJ. Techniques of immunohistochemistry: principles, pitfalls, and standardization. In: Dabbs DJ, editor. Diagnostic immunohistochemistry. 3rd ed. Philadelphia: Saunders, Elsevier; 2009. p. 1–41.
19. Chu P, Wu E, Weiss LM. Cytokeratin 7 and cytokeratin 20 expression in epithelial neoplasms: a survey of 435 cases. Mod Pathol. 2000;13(9):962–72.
20. Bhargava R, Dabbs DJ. Immunohistology of metastatic carcinomas of unknown primary. In: Dabbs DJ, editor. Diagnostic immunohistochemistry. 3rd ed. Philadelphia: Saunders, Elsevier; 2009. p. 206–55.
21. Jagirdar J. Application of immunohistochemistry to the diagnosis of primary and metastatic carcinoma to the lung. Arch Pathol Lab Med. 2008;132(3):384–96.
22. Krishna M. Diagnosis of metastatic neoplasms: an immunohistochemical approach. Arch Pathol Lab Med. 2010;134:207–15.
23. Delellis RA, Shin SJ, Treaba DO. Immunohistology of endocrine tumors. In: Dabbs DJ, editor. Diagnostic immunohistochemistry. 3rd ed. Philadelphia: Saunders, Elsevier; 2009. p. 291–339.
24. Wick MR. Immunohistology of melanocytic neoplasms. In: Dabbs DJ, editor. Diagnostic immunohistochemistry. 3rd ed. Philadelphia: Saunders, Elsevier; 2009. p. 189–205.
25. Allred DC, Harvey JM, Berardo M, Clark GM. Prognostic and predictive factors in breast cancer by immunohistochemical analysis. Mod Pathol. 1998;II:155–68.
26. Gown AM. Current issues in ER and HER2 testing by IHC in breast cancer. Mod Pathol. 2008;21 Suppl 2:S8–15.
27. Letcher CD, Bermar JJ, Corless C, et al. Diagnosis of gastrointestinal stromal tumors: a consensus approach. Hum Pathol. 2002;33:459–65.

28. Martin AW. Immunohistology of non-Hodgkin lymphoma. In: Dabbs DJ, editor. Diagnostic immunohistochemistry. 3rd ed. Philadelphia: Saunders, Elsevier; 2009. p. 156–88.

29. Swerdlow SH, Campo E, Harris NL, et al., editors. Mature B-cell neoplasms. WHO classification of tumors of haematopoietic and lymphoid tissues. 4th ed. Lyon: IARC Press; 2008. p. 180–266.

30. Meda BA, Buss DH, Woodruff RD, et al. Diagnosis and subclassification of primary and recurrent lymphoma: the usefulness and limitations of combined fine needle aspiration cytomorphology and flow cytometry. Am J Clin Pathol. 2008;113:688–99.

31. Ladanyi M, Antonescu CR, Dal Cin P. Cytogenetic and molecular genetic pathology of soft tissue tumors. In: Weiss SW, Goldblum JR, editors. Enzinger and Weiss's soft tissue tumors. 5th ed. Philadelphia: Mosby, Elsevier; 2008.

32. Krishnamurthy S. Application of molecular techniques to fine-needle aspiration biopsy. Cancer. 2007;111(2):106–22.

33. Bender RA, Erlander MG. Molecular classification of unknown primary cancer. Semin Oncol. 2009;36:38–43.

34. Wolff AC, Hammond MEH, Schwartz JN, et al. American Society of Clinical Oncology/College of American Pathologists guideline recommendations for human epidermal growth factor receptor 2 testing in breast cancer. J Clin Oncol. 2007;25:118–45.

35. Penault-Llorca F, Bilous M, Dowsett M, et al. Emerging technologies for assessing HER2 amplification. Am J Clin Pathol. 2009;132:539–48.

36. Slamon DJ, Clark GM, Wong SG, et al. Human breast cancer: correlation of relapse and survival with amplification of the HER2/neu oncogene. Science. 1987;235:177–82.

37. Paik S, Bryant J, Park C, et al. erbB2 and response to doxorubicin in patients with axillary lymph node-positive hormone receptor-negative breast cancer. J Natl Cancer Inst. 1998;90:1361–70.

38. Sequist LV, Joshi VA, Janne PA, et al. Epidermal growth factor receptor mutation testing in the care of lung cancer patients. Clin Cancer Res. 2006;12:44035–85.

39. Mitsudoni T, Yatabe Y. Mutations of the epidermal growth factor receptor gene and related genes as determinants of epidermal growth factor receptor tyrosine kinase inhibitor sensitivity in lung cancer. Cancer Sci. 2007;98:1817–24.

40. Girard N, Deshpande C, Azzoli CG, et al. Use of EGFR/KRAS mutation testing to define clonal relationships among multiple lung adenocarcinomas: comparison with clinical guidelines. Chest. 2010;137:46–52.

41. Raponi M, Winkler H, Dracopoli CN. KRAS mutations predict response to EGFR inhibitors. Curr Opin Pharmacol. 2008;8:413–18.

42. Smalley KS, Nathanson KL, Flaherty KT. Genetic subgrouping of melanoma reveals new opportunities for targeted therapy. Cancer Res. 2009;69:3241–4.

43. Wee S, Jagani Z, Xiang KX, et al. PI3K pathology activation mediates resistance to MEK inhibitors in KRAS mutant cancer. Cancer Res. 2009;69:4286–93.

44. Demetri GD, von Mehron M, Blarke CD, et al. Efficacy and safety of imatinib mesylate in advanced gastrointestinal stromal tumors. N Engl J Med. 2002;347:472–80.

Biopsy of Head and Neck Lesions

Sanjay Gupta

Background

Percutaneous needle biopsy with imaging guidance is a well-established technique for the diagnosis of head and neck lesions [1–8]. Percutaneous needle biopsies of deep-seated head and neck lesions are challenging because major vessels, nerves, osseous structures, or the airway often block the projected needle path. Therefore, a thorough knowledge of the complex cross-sectional anatomy of this region is essential in planning a safe access route for a needle biopsy. In this article, we will review the various approaches used for computed tomography (CT)-guided percutaneous needle biopsies of head and neck lesions, focusing on the relevant anatomy, technical aspects, advantages, and limitations of each approach.

Technique

Image Guidance

Sonographic guidance is routinely used for biopsies of thyroid lesions, parotid gland lesions, and superficial cervical lymph nodes [9–11]. However, the lack of an adequate acoustic window because of overlying bony structures (such as the maxilla, mandible, mastoid, and the styloid process) and the presence of air-containing spaces preclude the use of sonographic guidance for many deep-seated head and neck lesions. Although fluoroscopically guided needle placement can be used for biopsy of cervical spine and skull base lesions, the inability to visualize the intervening structures increases the risk of complications. With its high-spatial and high-contrast resolution, CT is the imaging modality of choice for biopsies of deep-seated head and neck lesions [1, 3, 5, 8, 12–14]. CT allows for excellent delineation of intervening vital structures, permitting safe planning of the biopsy path. Magnetic resonance imaging (MRI) guidance also has been used for biopsies of head and neck lesions [4, 6, 15]. The potential advantages of MRI as a guidance modality include its high-contrast resolution, its multiplanar imaging capacity (allowing the use of double oblique approaches), and its ability to visualize vessels without a contrast agent. However, the limited availability of the open-configuration MRI systems as well as MRI's high cost, longer acquisition times, and need for MRI-compatible needles has prevented more widespread use of MRI guidance for head and neck biopsies.

Needle Selection

Percutaneous biopsies of head and neck lesions are usually performed with the coaxial needle technique, which involves the initial placement of an 18- or 19-gauge thin-wall guide needle close to the target lesion; the biopsy needle is then advanced through this guide needle to obtain tissue samples. We use a 20- to 22-gauge needle to obtain aspirates for cytology and, if necessary, 20-gauge cutting needles to obtain tissue cores for histologic evaluation. The small-caliber cutting needles now available consistently provide high-quality specimens that are in most cases adequate to enable a histologic diagnosis without increasing the complication rate. The coaxial technique has the advantage of allowing multiple samples of tissue to be obtained without the need for additional passes through overlying tissues, thus decreasing the procedure time, number of images required, risk of complications, and patient discomfort. Additionally, the use of a Hawkins-Akins (Meditech, Westwood, MS) needle with a blunt trocar may reduce the risk of injury to major vessels and nerves in the needle path [16, 17].

S. Gupta, MD, DNB
Department of Interventional Radiology,
Department of Diagnostic Radiology,
The University of Texas MD Anderson Cancer Center,
1515 Holcombe Blvd., Unit 1471, Houston, TX 77030, USA
e-mail: sgupta@mdanderson.org

K. Ahrar, S. Gupta (eds.), *Percutaneous Image-Guided Biopsy*,
DOI 10.1007/978-1-4614-8217-8_9, © Springer Science+Business Media New York 2014

Relevant Anatomic Considerations

The head and neck area can be divided into suprahyoid and infrahyoid regions [18, 19]. The axial cross-sectional anatomy extending from the skull base to the cervicothoracic junction is shown in our schematic illustrations (Fig. 9.1a–h). The important fascial spaces in the suprahyoid region include the parapharyngeal, masticator, parotid, carotid, pharyngeal mucosal, retropharyngeal, and perivertebral spaces. In the infrahyoid neck, apart from the inferior extensions of the carotid, retropharyngeal, and perivertebral spaces, three other spaces (namely, the visceral, posterior, and anterior cervical spaces) can be identified.

The parapharyngeal space (Fig. 9.1a–e) extends from the hyoid bone inferiorly to the skull base superiorly. The parapharyngeal space is bounded anteriorly by the masticator space, laterally by the deep parotid space, medially by the pharyngeal mucosal space, posteriorly by the carotid space, and posteromedially by the lateral extension of the retropharyngeal space. The major structures that are located in the parapharyngeal space include the internal maxillary, middle meningeal, and ascending pharyngeal arteries; the pterygoid venous plexus; and branches of the mandibular nerve. The pharyngeal mucosal space (Fig. 9.1a–e) is located on the airway side of the buccopharyngeal fascia in the nasopharynx and oropharynx and contains mucosa, lymphoid tissue, minor salivary glands, and pharyngeal constrictor muscles.

The masticator space (Fig. 9.1a–e) can be divided into two components: the infratemporal fossa below the zygomatic arch and the temporal fossa above the arch. The masticator space is bordered by the buccal space anteriorly, the parotid space posteriorly, and the parapharyngeal space posteromedially. Apart from the musculoskeletal structures (the medial and lateral pterygoid, masseter, temporalis muscles, and mandible), the inferior alveolar branch of the mandibular nerve and the inferior alveolar vessels traverse the masticator space.

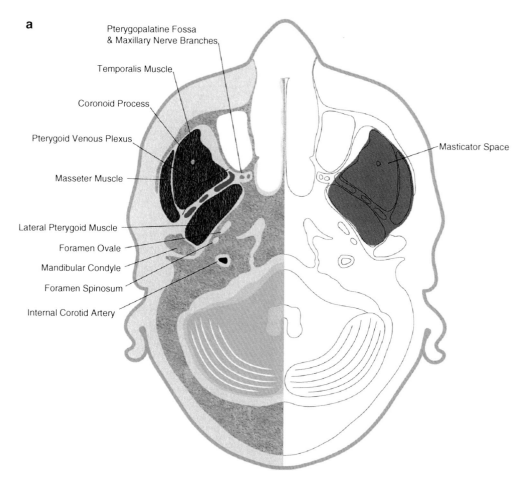

Fig. 9.1 (**a–h**). Schematic drawings showing axial cross-sectional anatomy at various levels in the head and neck region. In each figure, the anatomic structures are shown on the *left* and the spaces on the *right*. (**a**) Skull base level. (**b**) Upper maxillary antrum level. (**c**) Lower maxillary antrum level. (**d**) Alveolar ridge level. (**e**) Mandibular level. (**f**) C4 vertebral level. (**g**) C6 vertebral level. (**h**) C7 vertebral level

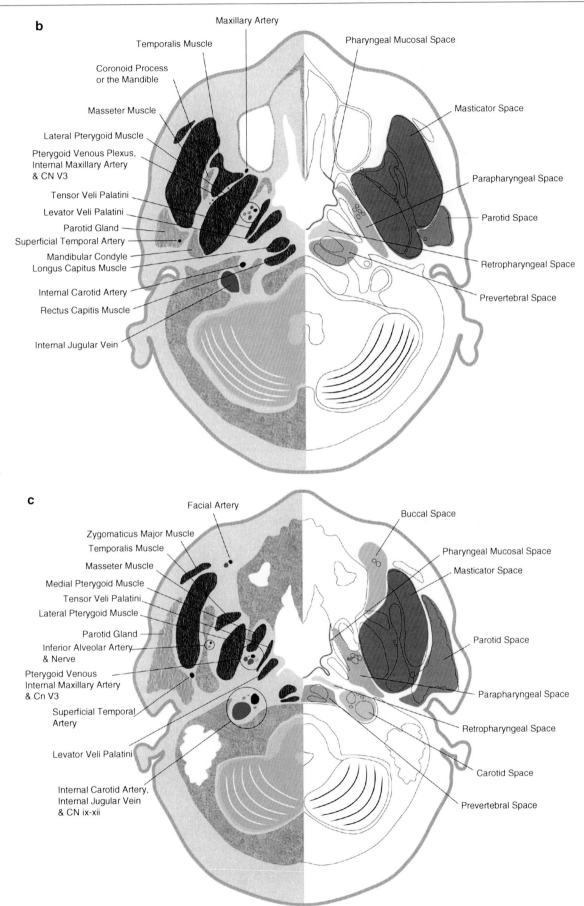

Fig. 9.1 (continued)

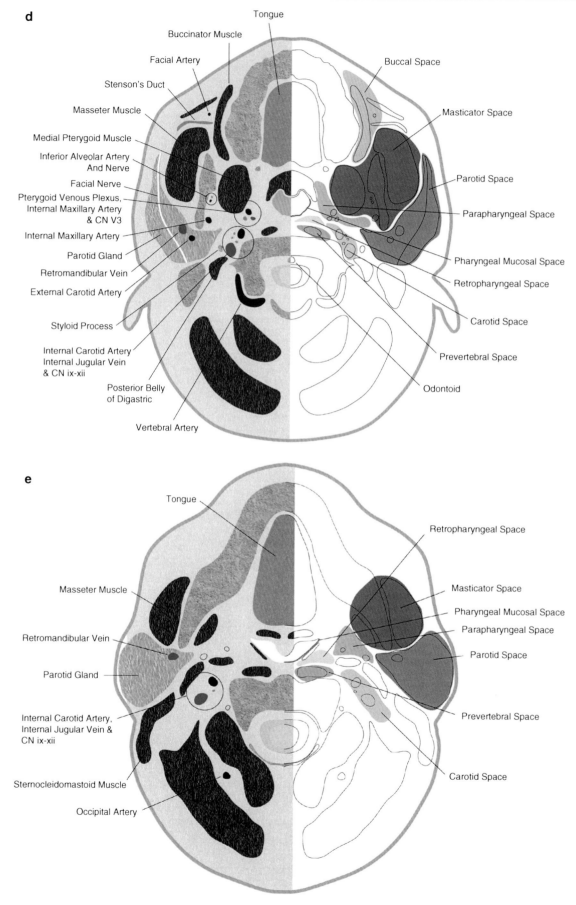

Fig. 9.1 (continued)

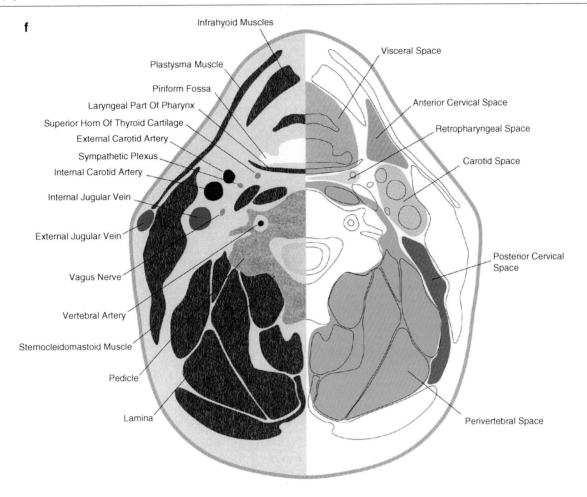

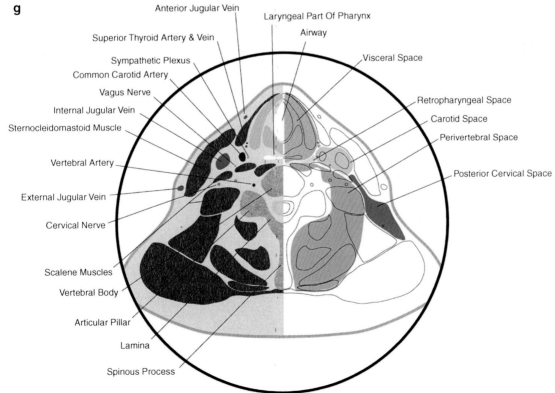

Fig. 9.1 (continued)

Fig. 9.1 (continued)

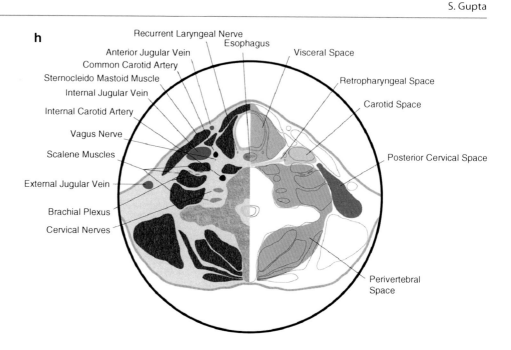

The contents of the carotid space (Fig. 9.1a–h) include the common or the internal carotid artery (depending on the level); the internal jugular vein; sympathetic plexus; cranial nerves IX, X, XI, and XII in the nasopharyngeal portion; cranial nerve X in the oropharyngeal and infrahyoid neck; and lymph nodes.

The parotid space (Fig. 9.1b–e) is located directly lateral to the parapharyngeal space and posterolateral to the masticator space, extending from the level of the external auditory canal down to the angle of the mandible. The posterior belly of the digastric muscle separates the medial portion of the parotid space from the anterolateral aspect of the carotid space. The parotid space contains the parotid gland, facial nerve, external carotid artery, retromandibular vein, and lymph nodes.

The retropharyngeal space (Fig. 9.1a–h) is a midline space that contains fat and lymph nodes only. This space is bordered by the pharyngeal mucosal space anteriorly, the carotid space laterally, and the prevertebral portion of the perivertebral space posteriorly. The perivertebral space (Fig. 9.1a–h) lies beneath the deep layer of deep cervical fascia and can be divided into the prevertebral and paravertebral portions. The prevertebral portion contains the prevertebral muscles, the vertebral artery and vein, the scalene muscles, the brachial plexus, the phrenic nerve, and the vertebral body, transverse process, and pedicle. The paravertebral portion of this space contains the paravertebral muscles and posterior elements of the cervical vertebrae.

In the infrahyoid neck (Fig. 9.1f–h), the visceral space is bounded by the middle layer of the deep cervical fascia and contains the thyroid and parathyroid glands, larynx,

hypopharynx, esophagus, trachea, recurrent laryngeal nerve, and lymph nodes. The posterior cervical space is located posterior to the carotid space and lateral to the perivertebral space and contains the spinal accessory nerve and the preaxillary portion of the brachial plexus. No important structure is present in the anterior cervical space, which is located lateral to the visceral space and anterior to the carotid space.

Approaches for Skull Base, Head, and Suprahyoid Neck Lesions

Subzygomatic (Infratemporal, Transcondylar, Sigmoid Notch) Approach

The subzygomatic approach is ideally suited for the biopsy of lesions in different parts of the masticator space. This approach can also be used for sampling lesions in the parapharyngeal, pharyngeal mucosal, and retropharyngeal spaces and for the prevertebral portion of the perivertebral space. Lesions in the suprazygomatic portion (temporal fossa) of the masticator space and skull base, including the pterygopalatine fossa region, can also be accessed using this approach.

In the subzygomatic approach, the needle is inserted below the zygomatic arch and advanced through the intercondylar (mandibular) notch between the coronoid process anteriorly, the mandibular condyle posteriorly, and the superior border of the mandibular ramus inferiorly (Fig. 9.2). The needle can be angulated in various (anterior, posterior, cranial, or caudal) directions, allowing access to multiple target sites (Figs. 9.3 and 9.4). The needle traverses the masticator

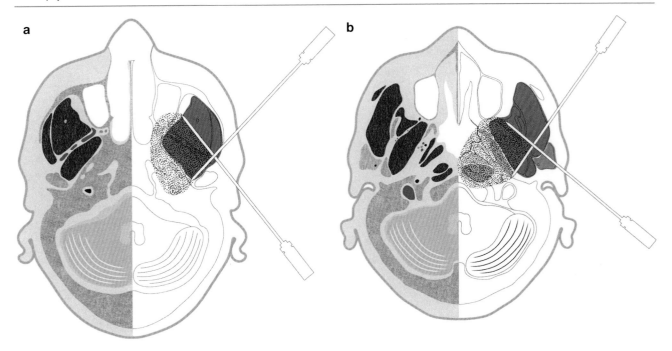

Fig. 9.2 Schematic drawing showing possible needle trajectories for subzygomatic approach at the (**a**) skull base level and (**b**) upper nasopharyngeal level

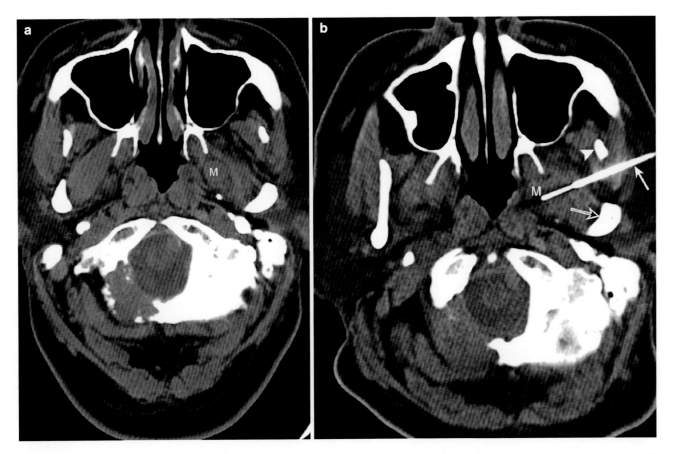

Fig. 9.3 Subzygomatic approach. (**a**) Computed tomography (*CT*) scan shows a soft-tissue mass (*M*) in the parapharyngeal space. (**b**) CT scan shows the biopsy needle (*arrow*) that was advanced between the coronoid process (*arrowhead*) and mandibular condyle (*open arrow*) into the parapharyngeal mass (*M*)

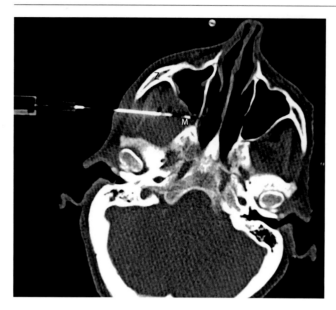

Fig. 9.4 Subzygomatic approach. CT scan shows the biopsy needle advanced under the zygoma (Z) for biopsy of a soft-tissue mass in the pterygomaxillary space (M)

and the parapharyngeal spaces during biopsies of lesions located in the pharyngeal mucosal, retropharyngeal, and pre-vertebral spaces and skull base.

Cranial needle angulation allows the subzygomatic approach to be used for accessing lesions in the skull base and the suprazygomatic portion of the masticator space. Using a triangulation method, the physician estimates the needle angle from contiguous axial CT scans obtained from the level of the planned skin entry site to the level of the target lesion. The needle is inserted below the level of the zygomatic arch and advanced cranially and medially in small increments; axial CT scans are obtained to check the needle tip position and angulation (Fig. 9.5). Alternatively, a change in the degree of neck flexion can bring the target lesion and the skin entry site into the same axial plane, allowing visualization of the entire needle length in a single axial CT image.

It has been suggested that having the patient keep his or her mouth open, preferably with a bite block, can help open up the space between the mandible and the zygomatic arch, thus facilitating needle insertion; however, in our experience, as in that of others [2], this is rarely necessary.

With the sybzygomatic approach, there is a theoretical risk of injury to the mandibular branch of the trigeminal nerve, the internal maxillary artery and its branches (including the middle meningeal artery), and the pterygoid venous plexus. The maxillary artery arises posterior to the neck of the mandible and is embedded in the parotid gland. The mandibular part runs horizontally forward along the medial surface of the ramus and passes between the neck of the mandible and the sphenomandibular ligament. The pterygoid part ascends obliquely forward and medially, either

superficially or deep to the lateral pterygoid muscle, to enter the pterygopalatine fossa through the pterygomaxillary fissure. The middle meningeal artery arises from the mandibular part of the internal maxillary artery and ascends in the posterior part of the sigmoid notch deep to the lateral pterygoid muscle to enter the foramen spinosum. The mandibular nerve exits the cranial cavity through the foramen ovale and descends in the posterior part of the intercondylar notch; the mandibular nerve runs downward medially to the lateral pterygoid muscle and a little anteriorly to the neck of the mandible to enter the inner surface of the mandibular ramus. The pterygoid venous plexus of veins is located partly between the temporalis and lateral pterygoid and partly between the two pterygoid muscles. However, as mentioned earlier, the risk of major injury to the vessels or the nerves is extremely low. A needle inserted posteriorly close to the mandibular condyle and directed anteriorly may occasionally pass through a small anterior portion of the parotid gland, but this usually does not cause problems (Fig. 9.2b).

Retromandibular (Transparotid) Approach

Lesions in the deep parotid space, parapharyngeal space, pharyngeal mucosal space, and lower part of the retropharyngeal space are amenable to biopsy with a retromandibular approach. This approach can also be used for sampling lesions in the carotid sheath if the vessels are displaced medially by the mass.

With the patient in the supine position and his or her head turned to the contralateral side, the needle is inserted posterior to the mandible and anterior to the mastoid process and advanced through the parotid gland (which is located behind the mandible, extending from the external auditory canal to the level of the mandibular angle) toward the target lesion (Fig. 9.6). Care should be taken to identify and avoid the external carotid artery and the retromandibular vein, which are both located within the parotid gland immediately posterior to the mandibular ramus (Fig. 9.6). The external carotid artery is medial of the two vessels. Approximately midway between the tip of the mastoid process and the angle of the mandible, the external carotid artery turns laterally from the carotid sheath and passes anterior to the posterior belly of the digastric muscle to reach the posteromedial surface of the parotid gland. Within the substance of the parotid gland, the external carotid artery ascends behind the condyle and divides into its terminal branches, the superficial temporal and maxillary arteries. The seventh cranial nerve passes just lateral to the retromandibular vein (Fig. 9.1d). The styloid process serves as a useful bony landmark; keeping the needle anterior to the styloid process avoids injury to the internal carotid artery, which is located in a plane posterior to the styloid process (Fig. 9.7). Occasionally, however, medial displacement of the carotid vessels by mass lesions may allow the needle to be advanced posterior to the styloid process.

The presence of surrounding structures, such as the styloid process, internal carotid artery, mastoid process, and mandible,

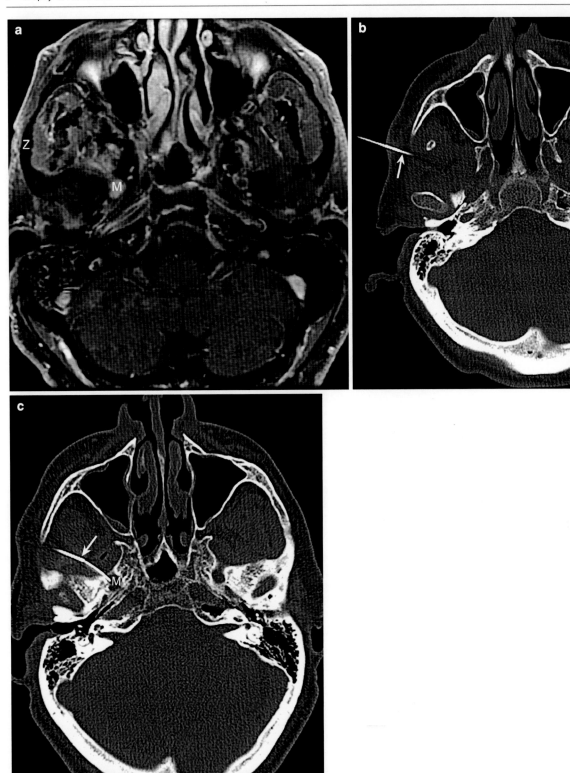

Fig. 9.5 Subzygomatic approach. (**a**) Magnetic resonance image shows a soft-tissue mass (*m*) in the right foramen ovale. A direct lateral approach is precluded by the zygomatic arch (*Z*). (**b**) Computed tomography (*CT*) scan shows the biopsy needle (*arrow*) inserted at a level caudal to the zygomatic arch. The needle was advanced in a cranial direction using the triangulation method. (**c**) CT scan at a more cranial level shows a curved 22-gauge needle (*arrow*) advanced through the guide needle and into the mass (*M*)

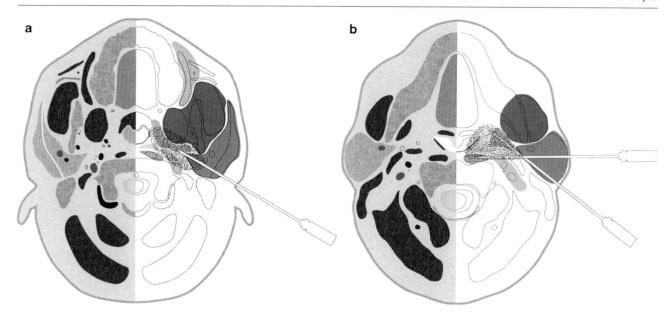

Fig. 9.6 Schematic drawing showing possible needle trajectories for the retromandibular approach at (**a**) alveolar ridge level and (**b**) mandibular level

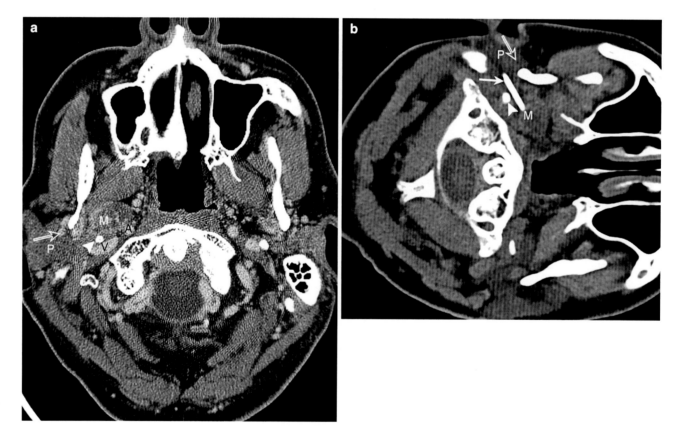

Fig. 9.7 Retromandibular approach. (**a**) Computed tomography (*CT*) scan shows a right parapharyngeal mass (*M*). Note the presence of the external carotid artery and retromandibular vein (*open arrow*) in the anterior portion of the parotid gland (*P*). The carotid artery (*A*) and jugular vein (*V*) are located posterior to the styloid process (*arrowhead*). (**b**) CT scan shows the biopsy needle (*arrow*) inserted through the parotid gland (*P*) posterior to the vessels (*open arrow*). The needle passes anterior to the styloid process (*arrowhead*) into the mass (*M*)

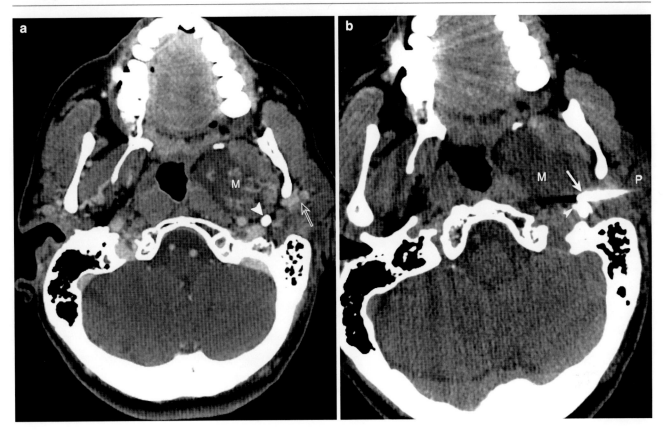

Fig. 9.8 Retromandibular approach. (**a**) Computed tomography (*CT*) scan shows parapharyngeal mass (*M*) located anterior to the styloid process (*arrowhead*). Note the presence of the external carotid artery and retromandibular vein (*open arrow*) in the anterior portion of the parotid gland. (**b**) Presence of vessels in the parotid gland (*P*) and the styloid process (*arrowhead*) limits the needle (*arrow*) angulation, restricting access to the mass (*M*)

does not allow much room for needle angulation. Thus, it is difficult to access the skull base, the prevertebral space, the cervical spine, and portions of the retropharyngeal space with this approach (Fig. 9.8). The potential risk of injury to the facial nerve, which courses through the parotid gland, limits the size of the biopsy needle that can be used with this approach. The use of thin needles precludes the option of obtaining a core specimen. For a biopsy of deeper lesions, the needle passes through the parapharyngeal space, and there is a potential risk of injury to the mandibular nerve branches and branches of the internal maxillary artery, such as the middle meningeal and ascending pharyngeal arteries. Yousem et al. [20] pointed out that a transparotid biopsy may occasionally yield salivary gland tissue, which may be confused with a salivary gland neoplasm of the parapharyngeal space. However, we have not encountered this problem in any of our patients.

Paramaxillary (Retromaxillary, Buccal Space) Approach

The paramaxillary approach offers safe access to lesions in the infrazygomatic portion of the masticator space, the posterior portions of the parapharyngeal and pharyngeal mucosal spaces, the carotid sheath space, and the deep portion of the parotid space [21, 22]. This approach is particularly useful for

lesions in the lateral part of the retropharyngeal (e.g., lateral retropharyngeal node of Rouviere) space and prevertebral portion of the perivertebral space because these lesions are difficult to access by other approaches. The paramaxillary approach can also be used for sampling lesions involving the anterior arch of the first cervical vertebra (C1) and the odontoid and body of the second (C2). In addition, this approach can be used to access the foramen ovale and other skull base lesions by using a cranial needle angulation [23].

For the transfacial paramaxillary approach, the patient is placed in the supine position with his or her head turned to the contralateral side, and the needle is inserted through the buccal space inferior to the zygomatic process of the maxilla and advanced posteriorly between the maxilla (alveolar ridge or sinus) and mandible (Fig. 9.9). It is important to avoid the facial artery, which is easy to identify as it courses in the buccal space (Fig. 9.9). For biopsy of lesions in the masticator and parapharyngeal spaces, the needle passes through the buccinator muscle or anterior portion of the masseter muscle or between them (Fig. 9.10). The needle is advanced through the lateral and medial pterygoid muscles and the parapharyngeal space to biopsy lesions in the retropharyngeal (Fig. 9.11) and carotid space (Fig. 9.12) and C1 and C2 lesions (Fig. 9.13). This approach can also be used to access foramen ovale and

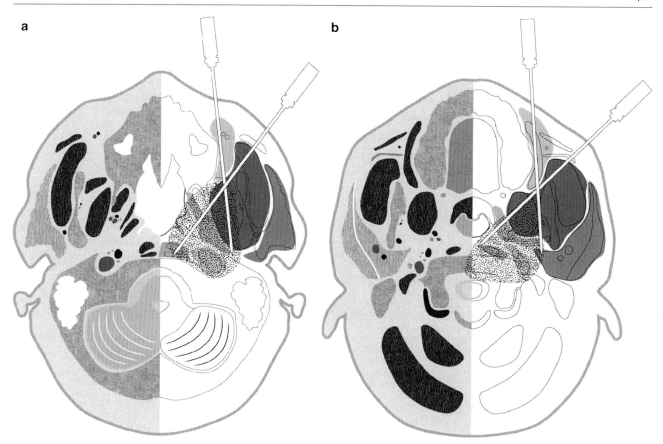

Fig. 9.9 Schematic drawing showing possible needle trajectories for the paramaxillary approach at (**a**) maxillary antrum level and (**b**) alveolar ridge level

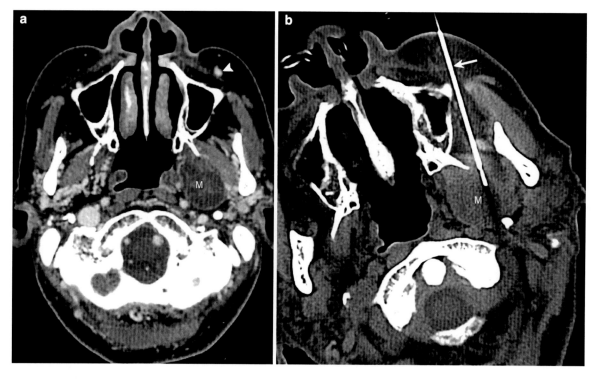

Fig. 9.10 Paramaxillary approach. (**a**) Computed tomography (*CT*) scan shows parapharyngeal mass (*M*). Note the facial artery (*arrowhead*) in the buccal space. (**b**) CT scan shows the biopsy needle (*arrow*) passing through the buccal space into the mass (*M*)

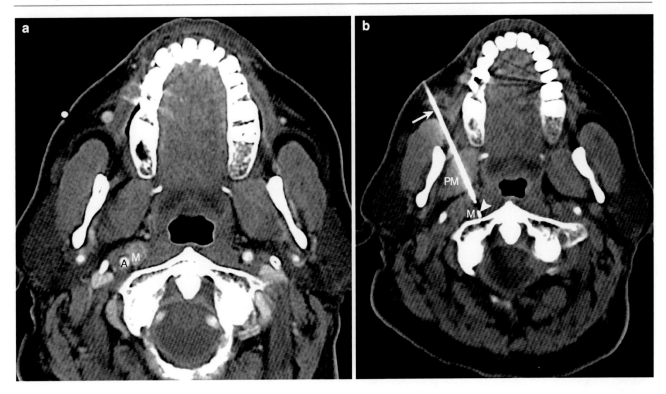

Fig. 9.11 Paramaxillary approach. (**a**) Computed tomography (*CT*) scan shows lateral retropharyngeal node (*M*) immediately medial to carotid artery (*A*). (**b**) CT scan shows an 18-gauge Hawkins needle (*arrow*) passing through the pterygoid muscle (*PM*) and a 20-gauge core biopsy needle (*arrowhead*) advanced coaxially through the guide needle into the mass (*M*)

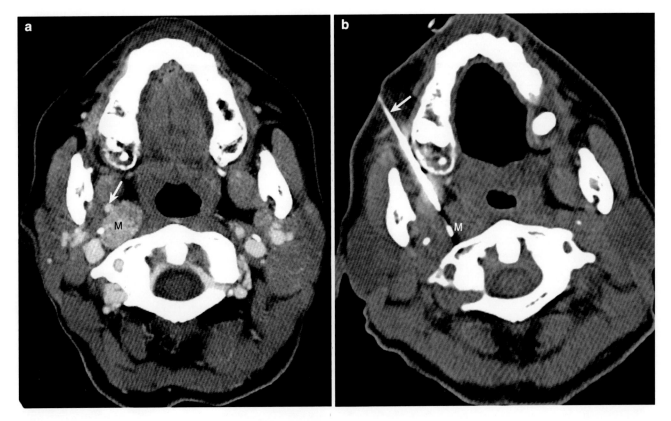

Fig. 9.12 Paramaxillary approach. (**a**) Computed tomography (*CT*) scan shows an enhancing mass (*M*) in the left carotid space displacing the carotid artery (*arrow*) anteriorly. (**b**) CT scan shows the needle (*arrow*) passing through the masticator and parapharyngeal spaces into the mass (*M*)

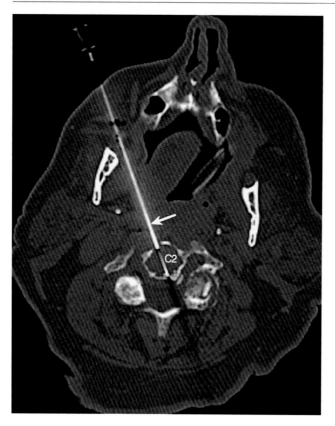

Fig. 9.13 Paramaxillary approach. Computed tomography scan shows the biopsy needle (*arrow*) advanced through the masticator and parapharyngeal spaces and through the prevertebral muscles into a lytic lesion involving C2 vertebral body

other skull base lesions by using cranial needle angulation (Fig. 9.14). Effecting mild hyperextension of the neck by placing padding under the patient's shoulders brings the skull base lesions and the skin entry site into the same axial plane and makes needle placement and visualization simple.

The needle trajectory and angulation with the paramaxillary approach is limited by the shape and size of the adjacent bones (such as the posterolateral wall of the maxillary antrum, the alveolar ridge, the lateral pterygoid plate, and the anterior margin of the mandibular ramus), which all limit access to the anterior and medial portions of the parapharyngeal and pharyngeal mucosal spaces and the medial portions of the retropharyngeal and prevertebral space lesions. In patients with a large maxillary antrum, the space between the maxilla and the mandible may be very narrow, limiting needle placement.

The pterygoid plates prevent inadvertent injury to the maxillary nerve and its main branches, which descend into the pterygopalatine fossa after exiting the foramen rotundum. Care should be taken to identify and avoid the carotid artery, especially during biopsy of lesions in the carotid sheath space, the retropharyngeal and prevertebral spaces, and C1 and C2. Other structures that could be injured with this approach include the branches of the mandibular and maxillary nerves in the masticator space, the pterygoid venus plexus, the internal maxillary artery and its branches in the masticator and parapharyngeal spaces, and the external carotid artery, which courses laterally deep to the lateral pterygoid muscle on its way to the

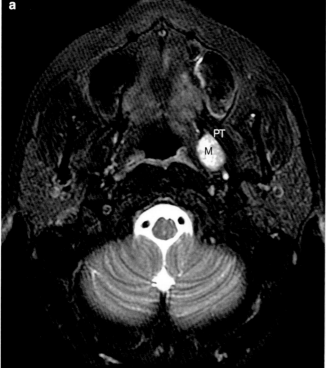

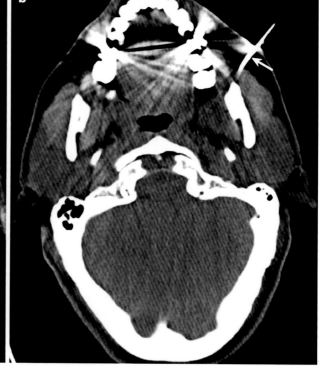

Fig. 9.14 Paramaxillary approach. (**a**) Magnetic resonance image shows a soft-tissue mass (*M*) in the left parapharyngeal space. A direct approach is precluded by the pterygoid plate (*PT*). (**b**) Computed tomography (*CT*) scan shows the biopsy needle (*arrow*) inserted at a level caudal to the pterygoid plate and the mass. The needle was advanced in a cranial direction using the triangulation method. (**c**) CT scan at a more cranial level shows the needle tip (*arrow*) within the mass (*M*)

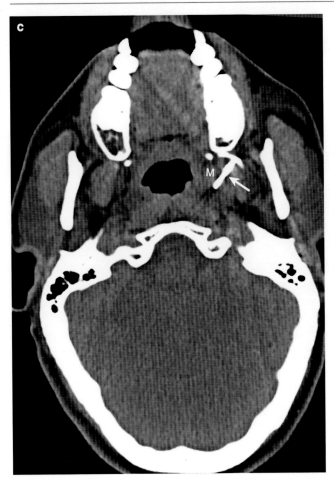

Fig. 9.14 (continued)

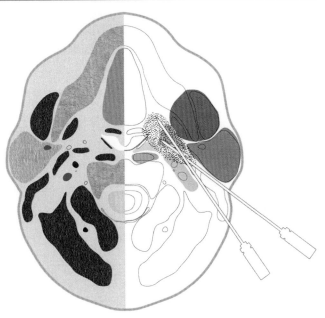

Fig. 9.15 Schematic drawing showing needle trajectory for the submastoid approach

C2 before it enters the C1 foramen. The artery then exits the C1 foramen and turns posteriorly to course along the upper surface of the C1 lamina. The use of contrast medium can improve visualization of the vertebral artery and can thus be a useful adjunct for needle path planning. Because the carotid and vertebral arteries are in the needle path, using the submastoid approach for a biopsy of deeper lesions located in the pharyngeal mucosal, parapharyngeal, or retropharyngeal spaces is not possible unless those vessels are displaced by the lesion.

Transoral Approach

The transoral approach is a well-established open surgical procedure for accessing the atlantoaxial region [24]. This approach can also be used for percutaneous biopsy of lesions in the posterior pharyngeal mucosal space, the retropharyngeal space, and the prevertebral part of the perivertebral space and also for biopsy of lesions involving the anterior portions of the C1 and C2 vertebrae, including the odontoid [25]. A posterior or lateral approach to this region is associated with risk of injury to the vertebral artery.

The use of the transoral approach requires general anesthesia. With the patient in the supine position, a mouth opener is applied after the patient is anesthetized. A trajectory between the tongue and uvula is chosen, and the uvula is pushed away with a retractor or a nasal tube. The intended site of needle puncture in the posterior pharyngeal wall is sprayed and infiltrated with local anesthetic. The needle is then advanced through the patient's open mouth, inserted through the posterior pharyngeal mucosa, and advanced posteriorly through the retropharyngeal space and prevertebral muscles toward the target lesion (Fig. 9.17). This is a relatively safe approach because no important structure lies between the posterior pharyngeal

parotid gland. Using a Hawkins-Akins needle (Meditech) with a blunt tip stylet as the outer guiding needle decreases the risk of injury to the vessels and nerves in these spaces.

Submastoid (Retroparotid) Approach

The submastoid approach is suitable for biopsy of carotid sheath lesions that displace the carotid vessels medially, lesions in the anterolateral portion of the perivertebral space that displace the carotid sheath anteriorly, and occasionally lesions in the parapharyngeal space.

The patient is placed in a prone position or in a supine position with his or her head turned to the contralateral side. The needle is inserted at a variable distance inferior to the mastoid tip and advanced through the sternocleidomastoid muscle (Fig. 9.15). Because the needle is then passed posterior to the parotid gland, there is no risk of damage to that gland, intraparotid vessels, or the facial nerve with this approach. The needle is advanced anteriorly and medially and occasionally cranially toward the lesion (Fig. 9.16).

One must carefully avoid the vertebral artery, especially during biopsy of anterior or lateral perivertebral lesions at the C1–C2 level (Fig. 9.1d, e). After emerging from the C2 foramen, the vertebral artery turns outward to reach the lateral aspect of the lateral mass of C2 and runs cranially along the lateral mass of

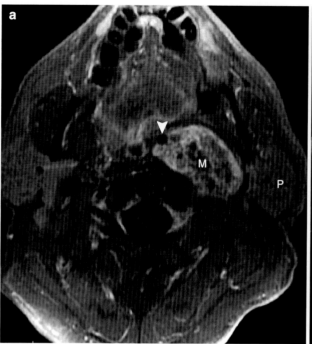

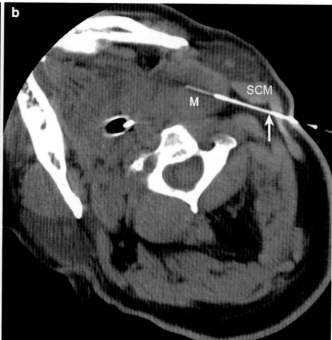

Fig. 9.16 Submastoid approach. (**a**) Magnetic resonance image shows large mass (*M*) in the left carotid space with medial displacement of the carotid artery (*arrowhead*). The parotid gland (*P*) is immediately lateral to the mass. (**b**) Computed tomography scan with the patient's head turned to the contralateral side shows the biopsy needle (*arrow*) passing through the sternocleidomastoid muscle (*SCM*) into the mass (*M*). The needle was inserted at a level 1 cm below the tip of the mastoid process (not seen in the image)

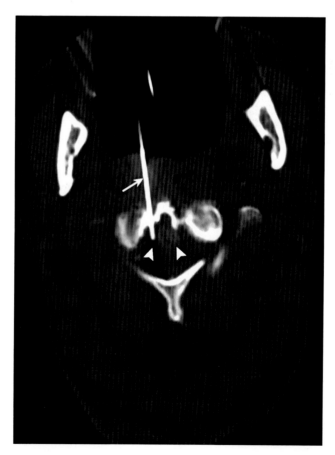

Fig. 9.17 Transoral approach. Computed tomography scan shows the needle (*arrow*) inserted through an open mouth and advanced through the retropharyngeal and prevertebral tissues into a soft-tissue mass (*arrowheads*) involving the tip of the odontoid and the anterior arch of atlas

wall and the bone. Because maintaining a sterile field is often a problem with the transoral approach and because of the inherently contaminated nature of these biopsies, use of antibiotics is recommended. During biopsy of lesions in the anterior arch of the atlas or the odontoid process, care should be taken to avoid any slip because of the proximity to the spinal cord.

Retromastoid Approach

The retromastoid approach can also be used occasionally for biopsy of carotid sheath lesions. With the patient in a prone position or in a supine position and the head turned to the contralateral side, the needle is inserted posterior to the mastoid and advanced in an anterior and medial direction (Fig. 9.18). Care should be taken to avoid injury to the vertebral and carotid arteries.

Posterior Approach

The posterior approach is used for percutaneous biopsies of lesions involving the spinous process, lamina, and articular pillar of the upper cervical vertebrae (Fig. 9.19). This approach is also used for biopsy of occipital condylar lesions and masses located in the posterior and lateral portions of the perivertebral space. Occasionally, this approach can also be used for sampling lateral masses involving C1 and C2, provided care is taken to identify and avoid the vertebral artery (Fig. 9.20).

A posterior-approach needle biopsy is performed with the patient in a prone or decubitus position. The needle is advanced through the posterior neck muscles in an anterior

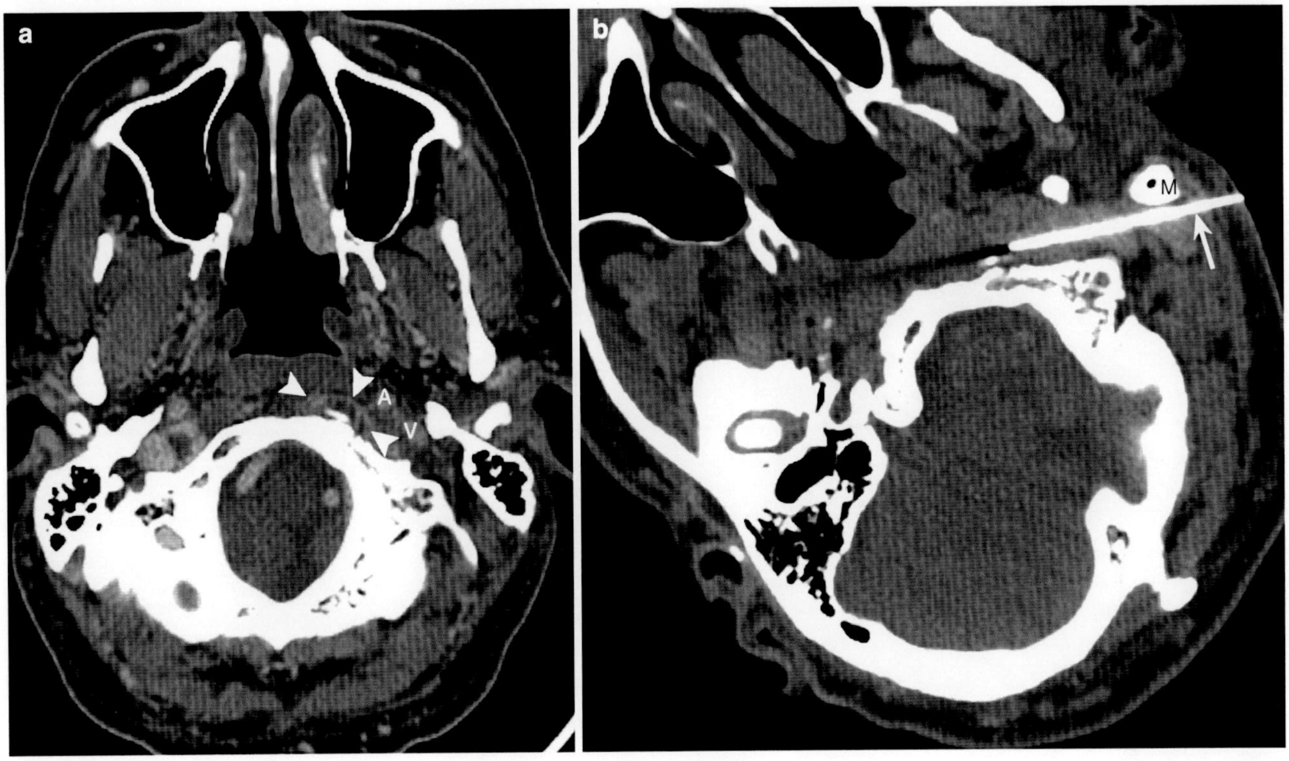

Fig. 9.18 Retromastoid approach. (**a**) Contrast-enhanced computed tomography (*CT*) scan shows mass (*arrowheads*) in the prevertebral space. Note location of the carotid artery (*A*) and jugular vein (*V*). (**b**)

CT scan shows needle (*arrow*) inserted posterior to the mastoid (*M*) to sample the mass

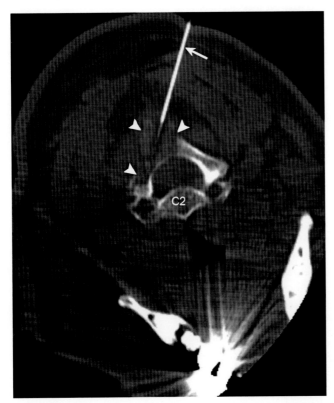

Fig. 9.19 Posterior approach. Computed tomography scan with the patient in the prone position shows the needle (*arrow*) passing through the posterior paravertebral into a lytic process (*arrowheads*) involving the lamina, articular pillar, and pedicle of the C3 vertebra

direction toward the target lesion. For sampling lesions that involve a lateral mass of C1 using a posterior approach, the needle should be advanced under the lamina, not above it. The vertebral artery, after exiting the C1 foramen, courses posteriorly along the upper surface of the C1 lamina. If necessary, intravenous administration of contrast medium can be used to help identify and avoid the vertebral artery (Fig. 9.20).

Approaches for Infrahyoid Neck Lesions

The approaches for biopsy of lesions in the infrahyoid neck and lower cervical vertebrae [14, 26–28] include the anterolateral approach (the needle advanced between the carotid sheath and airway), the posterolateral approach (the needle advanced posterior to the carotid sheath), and the posterior approach (Fig. 9.21).

Anterolateral Approach (Between the Carotid Sheath and Airway)

The anterolateral approach allows access to lesions in the retrotracheal, paraesophageal, and anterior perivertebral spaces (Fig. 9.22). The needle is inserted anterior to the sternocleidomastoid muscle and advanced posteromedially between the visceral space and the carotid space (Figs. 9.21 and 9.22). Care should be taken to avoid the hypopharynx

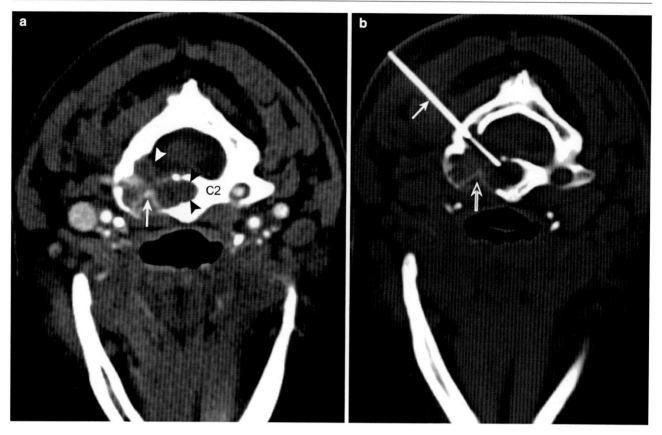

Fig. 9.20 Posterior approach. (**a**) Contrast-enhanced computed tomography (*CT*) scan with the patient in a prone position shows a lytic lesion (*arrowheads*) involving the body and lateral mass of C2 vertebra. Note the vertebral artery (*arrow*) encased and narrowed by the lesion. (**b**) CT scan shows the biopsy needle (*arrow*) passing through the anterior portion of the lamina into the lesion, posterior to the expected location of the vertebral artery (*open arrow*)

and especially the pyriform fossa and the esophagus. For biopsy of lesions in the lower neck, the needle may have to be advanced through the thyroid gland, but transgression of thyroid tissue with a small-caliber needle is generally considered safe [29].

As the needle is pushed posteriorly toward the vertebral body, the vertebral artery may be damaged. From the subclavian artery, the vessel goes upward toward the foramen in the base of the transverse process of the sixth cervical vertebra and then passes upward through the canal in the transverse processes. Between the foramina, the vertebral artery is located lateral to the mid or posterior part of the vertebral body or disc (Fig. 9.1g); care should be taken to avoid the lateral aspect of the vertebral body. Because the needle is directed posteriorly and medially in this approach, the spinal canal theoretically could be penetrated through the neural foramina, which are directed anterolaterally (Fig. 9.1g). However, the use of intermittent CT scans to check the position and trajectory of the needle tip can protect against this problem and prevent possible damage to vascular and neural structures. Furthermore, the presence of the carotid sheath tends to keep the needle pointed medi-

ally and away from the neural foramen and the vertebral artery (Fig. 9.21).

Other important structures could be in the needle path when the anterolateral approach is used: the superior and middle thyroid vessels, the superior and inferior laryngeal nerves, the loop of the hypoglossal nerve, and the cervical ganglia of the sympathetic nervous system (Fig. 9.1f–h). However, the small-caliber needles used for the biopsy are unlikely to cause serious damage to the blood vessels or nerves.

Posterolateral Approach (Posterior to the Carotid Sheath)

The posterolateral approach is used for sampling lesions in the prevertebral and lateral paraspinal portions of the perivertebral space, retropharyngeal space, and posterior cervical space (Fig. 9.23).

With the patient in the supine, prone, or lateral decubitus position, the needle is inserted through the sternocleidomastoid muscle and the posterior cervical space and then advanced posterior to the carotid sheath (Fig. 9.21). Depending on the axial level in the neck (upper vs. lower infrahyoid), the patient's position, and the size and location

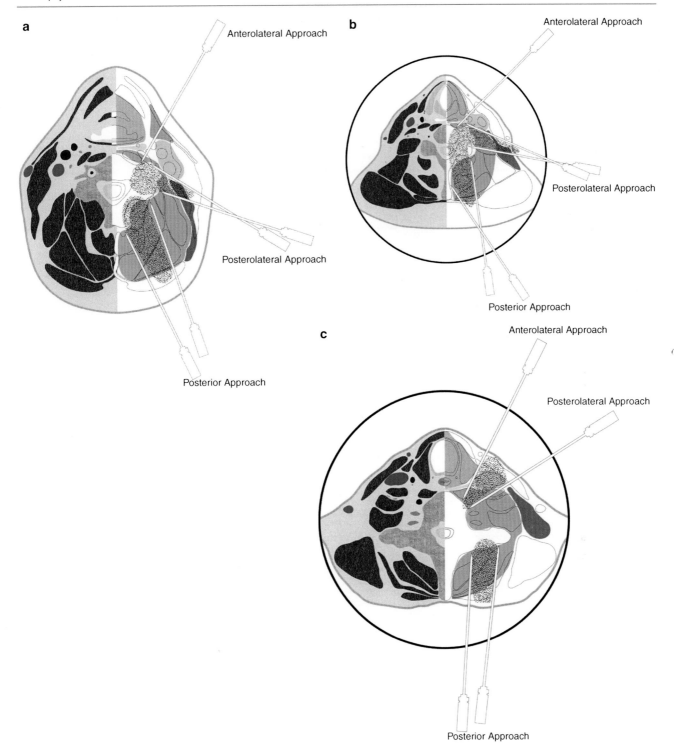

Fig. 9.21 Schematic drawings showing the needle trajectories for the anterolateral, posterolateral, and posterior approaches in the infrahyoid neck region at the (**a**) C4, (**b**) C6, and (**c**) C7 vertebral levels

of the carotid sheath, the needle may be advanced anteromedially or posteromedially. The soft tissues overlying the clavicles and shoulder may interfere with needle placement in the lower neck, particularly in patients with prominent clavicles and short necks. An out-of-plane angled approach with

a caudal needle angulation can be used in this situation; the needle is inserted in a plane cranial to the level of the target lesion and advanced caudally and medially (Fig. 9.23).

The vertebral artery is the structure most vulnerable to injury during biopsy using the posterolateral approach,

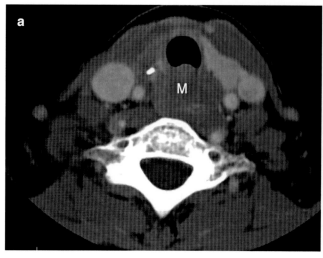

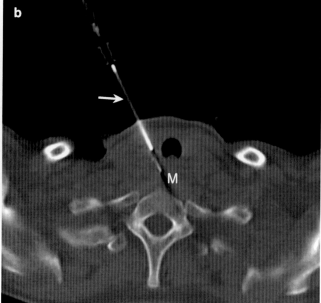

Fig. 9.22 Anterolateral approach. (**a**) Computed tomography (*CT*) scan shows a retrotracheal mass (*M*). Note absence of right lobe of thyroid gland related to previous surgery. (**b**) CT scan shows needle (*arrow*) advanced between the trachea and carotid vessels and through the surgical bed into the mass (*M*)

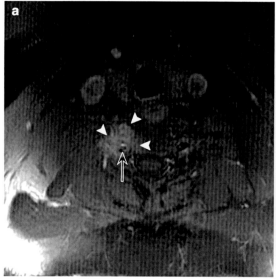

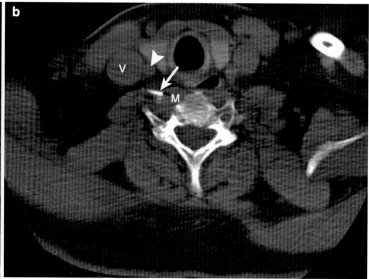

Fig. 9.23 Posterolateral approach. (**a**) Magnetic resonance image shows a hyperintense lesion (*arrowheads*) involving the right transverse process of the C6 vertebra extending into the prevertebral space. The vertebral artery (*arrow*) is immediately posterior to the mass. (**b**) Computed tomography scan shows the needle tip (*arrow*) in the prevertebral portion of the mass. The needle was inserted at a more cranial level, directed caudally, and advanced posterior to the internal jugular vein (*v*) and the common carotid artery (*arrowhead*)

especially at levels between the transverse foramina, where the vessel is located lateral to the vertebral body and disc (Fig. 9.1g). Also, a needle inserted behind the carotid sheath and advanced posteromedially toward a lesion involving the seventh cervical vertebra can poten-tially injure the vertebral artery. Using contrast medium to identify the vertebral artery can reduce the risk of injury. Because the intervertebral foramina run from the spinal canal in an oblique medial-to-lateral and posterior-to-anterior direction, needle penetration of the spinal

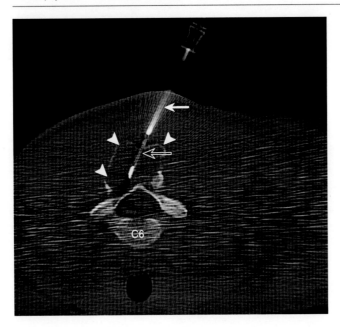

Fig. 9.24 Posterior approach. Computed tomography scan with the patient in the prone position shows the guide needle (*arrow*) that was placed in the posterior soft tissues. A core biopsy needle (*open arrow*) was advanced coaxially through the guide needle for biopsy of an expansile lytic lesion (*arrowheads*) involving the spinous process of the C6 vertebra

canal with this approach is not possible [28]. Furthermore, a small-caliber needle puncture of the brachial or cervical plexus is not dangerous, although it may cause transient pain [28].

Posterior Approach

The posterior approach is used for biopsy of lesions involving the spinous process, lamina, and articular pillars and processes of the lower cervical vertebrae as well as for biopsy of lesions in the posterior and lateral paraspinal portions of the perivertebral space (Fig. 9.24).

With the patient in the prone or lateral decubitus position, the needle is advanced through the posterior paraspinal muscles toward the target lesion. The risk of injury to major vessels or nerves with this approach is extremely low. During biopsy of lesions involving the laminae, care should be taken to ensure that the needle does not penetrate the spinal canal.

Complications

Major complications with CT-guided biopsy procedures of the head and neck are extremely rare [1–8]. Minor complications include pain, vasovagal reaction, minor infection, and minor bleeding. Familiarity with the cross-sectional anatomy of the head and neck region and with the location of major

vessels therein and careful planning of the needle pathway minimize the chances of a clinically significant hemorrhage. Walker et al. [30] reported the case of a patient with an internal maxillary artery pseudoaneurysm formation who developed an oral hemorrhage 3 months after a CT-guided biopsy of the masticator space. According to that study's authors, prior radical neck surgery and radiation therapy increase the risk for vascular complications. Injury to cranial nerves and branches in the head and neck region with subsequent sensory and/or motor loss remains a theoretical concern; however, many large studies have failed to demonstrate any such risk [1–8].

Summary

Depending on location, deep head and neck lesions may be accessed via a variety of percutaneous approaches, each with its own set of advantages and limitations. The location and extent of the lesions and their relationship to adjacent structures influence the choice of the needle trajectory. Familiarity with head and neck anatomy and careful planning of the procedure are necessary to ensure a biopsy that is both precise and safe.

References

1. Abemayor E, Ljung BM, Ward PH, Larsson S, Hanafee W. CT-directed fine needle aspiration biopsies of masses in the head and neck. Laryngoscope. 1985;95:1382–6.
2. Abrahams JJ. Mandibular sigmoid notch: a window for CT-guided biopsies of lesions in the peripharyngeal and skull base regions. Radiology. 1998;208:695–9.
3. DelGaudio JM, Dillard DG, Albritton FD, Hudgins P, Wallace VC, Lewis MM. Computed tomography–guided needle biopsy of head and neck lesions. Arch Otolaryngol Head Neck Surg. 2000;126:366–70.
4. Fried MP, Hsu L, Jolesz FA. Interactive magnetic resonance imaging-guided biopsy in the head and neck: initial patient experience. Laryngoscope. 1998;108:488–93.
5. Gatenby RA, Mulhern Jr CB, Strawitz J. CT-guided percutaneous biopsies of head and neck masses. Radiology. 1983;146:717–19.
6. Merkle EM, Lewin JS, Aschoff AJ, et al. Percutaneous magnetic resonance image-guided biopsy and aspiration in the head and neck. Laryngoscope. 2000;110:382–5.
7. Sack MJ, Weber RS, Weinstein GS, Chalian AA, Nisenbaum HL, Yousem DM. Image-guided fine-needle aspiration of the head and neck: five years' experience. Arch Otolaryngol Head Neck Surg. 1998;124:1155–61.
8. Sherman PM, Yousem DM, Loevner LA. CT-guided aspirations in the head and neck: assessment of the first 216 cases. AJNR Am J Neuroradiol. 2004;25:1603–7.
9. Screaton NJ, Berman LH, Grant JW. US-guided core-needle biopsy of the thyroid gland. Radiology. 2003;226:827–32.
10. Screaton NJ, Berman LH, Grant JW. Head and neck lymphadenopathy: evaluation with US-guided cutting-needle biopsy. Radiology. 2002;224:75–81.
11. Ridder GJ, Technau-Ihling K, Boedeker CC. Ultrasound-guided cutting needle biopsy in the diagnosis of head and neck masses. Laryngoscope. 2005;115:376–7.

12. Kornblum MB, Wesolowski DP, Fischgrund JS, Herkowitz HN. Computed tomography-guided biopsy of the spine. A review of 103 patients. Spine. 1998;23:81–5.

13. Ljung BM, Larsson SG, Hanafee W. Computed tomography-guided aspiration cytologic examination in head and neck lesions. Arch Otolaryngol. 1984;110:604–7.

14. Tampieri D, Weill A, Melanson D, Ethier R. Percutaneous aspiration biopsy in cervical spine lytic lesions. Indications and technique. Neuroradiology. 1991;33:43–7.

15. Lewin JS, Nour SG, Duerk JL. Magnetic resonance image-guided biopsy and aspiration. Top Magn Reson Imaging. 2000;11:173 83.

16. Akins EW, Hawkins Jr IF, Mladinich C, Tupler R, Siragusa RJ, Pry R. The blunt needle: a new percutaneous access device. AJR Am J Roentgenol. 1989;152:181–2.

17. Mukherji SK, Turetsky D, Tart RP, Mancuso AA. A technique for core biopsies of head and neck masses. AJNR Am J Neuroradiol. 1994;15:518–20.

18. Harnsberger HR, Osborn AG. Differential diagnosis of head and neck lesions based on their space of origin. 1. The suprahyoid part of the neck. AJR Am J Roentgenol. 1991;157:147–54.

19. Smoker WR, Harnsberger HR. Differential diagnosis of head and neck lesions based on their space of origin. 2. The infrahyoid portion of the neck. AJR Am J Roentgenol. 1991;157:155–9.

20. Yousem DM, Sack MJ, Scanlan KA. Biopsy of parapharyngeal space lesions. Radiology. 1994;193:619–22.

21. Esposito MB, Arrington JA, Murtagh FR, Ridley MB, Endicott JN, Silbiger ML. Anterior approach for CT-guided biopsy of skull base and parapharyngeal space lesions. J Comput Assist Tomogr. 1996;20:739–41.

22. Tu AS, Geyer CA, Mancall AC, Baker RA. The buccal space: a doorway for percutaneous CT-guided biopsy of the parapharyngeal region. AJNR Am J Neuroradiol. 1998;19:728–31.

23. Dresel SH, Mackey JK, Lufkin RB, et al. Meckel cave lesions: percutaneous fine-needle-aspiration biopsy cytology. Radiology. 1991;179:579–82.

24. Menezes AH, VanGilder JC. Transoral-transpharyngeal approach to the anterior craniocervical junction. Ten-year experience with 72 patients. J Neurosurg. 1988;69:895–903.

25. Patil AA. Transoral stereotactic biopsy of the second cervical vertebral body: case report with technical note. Neurosurgery. 1989;25:999–1001; discussion 1001–1002.

26. Kang M, Gupta S, Khandelwal N, Shankar S, Gulati M, Suri S. CT-guided fine-needle aspiration biopsy of spinal lesions. Acta Radiol. 1999;40:474–8.

27. Kattapuram SV, Rosenthal DI. Percutaneous biopsy of the cervical spine using CT guidance. AJR Am J Roentgenol. 1987;149:539–41.

28. Ottolenghi CE, Schajowicz F, Deschant FA. Aspiration biopsy of the cervical spine. Technique and results in thirty-four cases. J Bone Joint Surg Am. 1964;46:715–33.

29. Gupta S, Henningsen JA, Wallace MJ, et al. Percutaneous biopsy of head and neck lesions with CT guidance: various approaches and relevant anatomic and technical considerations. Radiographics. 2007;27:371–90.

30. Walker AT, Chaloupka JC, Putman CM, Abrahams JJ, Ross DA. Sentinel transoral hemorrhage from a pseudoaneurysm of the internal maxillary artery: a complication of CT-guided biopsy of the masticator space. AJNR Am J Neuroradiol. 1996;17:377–81.

Sanjay Gupta

Introduction

Image-guided percutaneous needle biopsy of mediastinal masses is a safe and effective technique for obtaining tissues for pathologic evaluation [1–3]. Percutaneous mediastinal biopsies are usually performed with computed tomography (CT) and/or ultrasound (US) guidance [4–13]. However, the presence of the major vessels, the bones, the lung, and the trachea often precludes a direct approach to mediastinal lesions. This article reviews the various approaches used for image-guided percutaneous mediastinal needle biopsy and discusses the anatomic and technical aspects, advantages, limitations, and potential complications of each technique as well as briefly describing several alternative methods for accessing mediastinal lesions.

Technique

Patient Preparation and Lesion Localization

Image-guided percutaneous mediastinal needle biopsies are usually performed on an outpatient basis and rarely require general anesthesia. Before the biopsy, prothrombin time, partial thromboplastin time, and platelet counts should be obtained to exclude the possibility of a bleeding disorder. Although some biopsies can be performed without intravenous sedation, we perform all mediastinal biopsies after induction of conscious sedation using midazolam and fentanyl citrate and also administer local anesthesia with continuous pulse oximetry and noninvasive blood pressure monitoring.

Patients are positioned in the supine, prone, or lateral decubitus position depending on the lesion location and the biopsy approach planned. For CT-guided procedures, preliminary 3- or 5-mm-thick contiguous axial slices are obtained to confirm the location of the target lesion and to determine the optimal entry site for the needle. Non-contrast-enhanced CT alone is sufficient for safe biopsy planning in most patients who have had previous contrast-enhanced CT or magnetic resonance imaging (MRI) for diagnostic purposes. Occasionally, intravenous administration of a contrast medium may be required during the procedure to help delineate the mediastinal blood vessels in the projected needle path and differentiate blood vessels from lymph nodes. For US-guided procedures, a preliminary diagnostic US study is performed to localize the lesion and to identify a safe path for the needle. Depending on the thickness of soft tissues and the depth of the target lesion under the skin, a 3.5- to 7.5-MHz convex-array or sector transducer can be used. Color Doppler imaging may be required to identify and avoid major blood vessels.

Patients should be observed for 1–3 h after biopsy to ensure their hemodynamic stability and monitor their respiratory status. Expiratory chest radiographs are obtained both immediately and 3 h after biopsy in patients in whom the needle traverses a pleural surface.

Biopsy Needle Selection

A variety of biopsy needles differing in caliber and mechanism of sample acquisition are available. Biopsy needles can be classified as small-caliber (20- to 25-gauge) or large-caliber (14- to 19-gauge) needles and as aspiration or cutting needles. Aspiration needles are 20- to 23-gauge needles that provide specimens suitable for cytologic evaluation. Cutting needles provide core specimens for histologic evaluation and are available in various calibers ranging from 14 to 20 gauge.

Both FNAB and core biopsy are accepted techniques for obtaining tissues for pathologic evaluation from mediastinal

S. Gupta, MD, DNB
Department of Interventional Radiology,
Department of Diagnostic Radiology,
The University of Texas MD Anderson Cancer Center,
1515 Holcombe Blvd., Unit 1471, Houston, TX 77030, USA
e-mail: sgupta@mdanderson.org

K. Ahrar, S. Gupta (eds.), *Percutaneous Image-Guided Biopsy*,
DOI 10.1007/978-1-4614-8217-8_10, © Springer Science+Business Media New York 2014

lesions. Needle selection depends on a number of factors, including the size and location of the target lesion, all intervening structures in the planned needle path, the experience and preferences of the interventional radiologist, the availability of on-site cytopathologists for immediate assessment, the suspected diagnosis, and the estimated amount of tissue needed.

FNAB of the mediastinum using 20- or 22-gauge needles has a high diagnostic accuracy for epithelial metastatic cancer, with a reported sensitivity ranging from 84 to 100 % [2, 14]. FNAB is also useful for aspiration of fluid from cystic lesions. The role of FNAB in the diagnosis and staging of lymphoma remains controversial, despite recent advances in cytopathologic techniques, such as cytospin preparations, flow cytometry, immunohistochemical phenotyping, and gene rearrangement studies. In general, although FNAB is considered adequate for staging and detecting recurrent or residual disease following treatment, core biopsy remains the preferred choice for initial diagnosis and typing of lymphoma [2, 15]. While the reported sensitivity of FNAB for lymphoma ranges from 42 to 82 %, a core biopsy can correctly diagnose mediastinal lymphoma in up to 91 % of cases [2, 15]. Core biopsies are also preferred for some other histologic types of disease, such as thymomas and germ cell, neurogenic, and benign tumors.

The small-caliber (18- to 20-gauge) automated cutting needles now available consistently provide high-quality histopathologic specimens adequate for histologic diagnosis in most cases, without increasing the complication rate. Several investigators have safely used larger (14- to 16-gauge) cutting needles for mediastinal biopsies in selected patients [16]. However, large-caliber needles should not be used if the projected needle path involves traversal of lung tissue, when the lesions are located adjacent to great blood vessels, or when highly vascular lesions are suspected.

Percutaneous mediastinal needle biopsies can be performed with either single-needle or coaxial techniques. The single-needle technique involves making multiple passes and using a new needle for each pass. The disadvantages of this technique include the need for image guidance for needle localization with each pass, resulting in longer procedure durations, and the need to traverse intervening structures again with each pass, increasing the risk of complications. Thus, the preferred technique for mediastinal biopsies is the coaxial technique, which involves the initial placement of a guide needle close to the target lesion followed by advancing the biopsy needle through the guide needle to obtain tissue samples. In our practice, we use an 18- or 19-gauge thin-wall needle as the guide needle, through which we advance a 20- to 22-gauge needle for obtaining FNABs for cytologic and microbiologic analysis. If indicated, 20-gauge core biopsies for histologic evaluations can also be performed through the same guide needle.

Image Guidance

Percutaneous mediastinal needle biopsies, which were initially performed under fluoroscopic guidance, are now performed primarily under CT guidance, as it allows precise localization of the biopsy needle and target lesion and documentation of the site sampled. CT guidance allows for excellent delineation of intervening vital structures and thus allows accurate planning of a safe needle path.

US guidance can be used for biopsy of large mediastinal masses in contact with the chest wall. The advantages of US guidance include real-time continuous monitoring of the needle during advancement and biopsy, the availability of oblique needle paths, and the ability to perform the biopsy at the bedside of critically ill patients. Additionally, patients with dyspnea who cannot tolerate a supine position can be placed in semi-sitting positions during the biopsy.

Anterior mediastinal lesions that extend to the anterior parasternal chest wall can be accessed by a parasternal approach using US guidance. US guidance can also be used for biopsy of superior mediastinal lesions performed through the suprasternal approach. Ultrasonography performed with the transducer placed in the subxiphoid region and angled cranially allows visualization of and access to posterior mediastinal lesions via a transhepatic approach. Occasionally, US guidance also can be used for accessing mediastinal lesions through large pleural effusions.

Anatomic and Technical Considerations

Extrapleural or Direct Mediastinal Approaches

A direct mediastinal approach involves placement of the biopsy needle through an extrapleural space medial to the lung to avoid traversal of the lung and the pleura. The needle can be advanced through or lateral to the sternum, through the posterior paravertebral space, through the suprasternal notch, or through the subxiphoid space.

Parasternal Approach

In the parasternal approach (Fig. 10.1), the needle is inserted lateral to the sternum and advanced through the parasternal muscles and mediastinal fat into the target lesion. The internal mammary blood vessels are located on either side of the sternum; the artery is usually situated lateral to the vein. The distances from the edge of the sternum range from 0.42 to 1.66 cm for the medial blood vessels and from 0.98 to 2.42 cm for the lateral blood vessels [17]. Three internal mammary vessels (two veins and one artery)

Fig. 10.1 Schematic of a parasternal approach to a mediastinal biopsy on a transverse CT section through the thorax at the level of the aortic arch. The needles are inserted lateral to the sternum and advanced into the mediastinal masses (*M*)

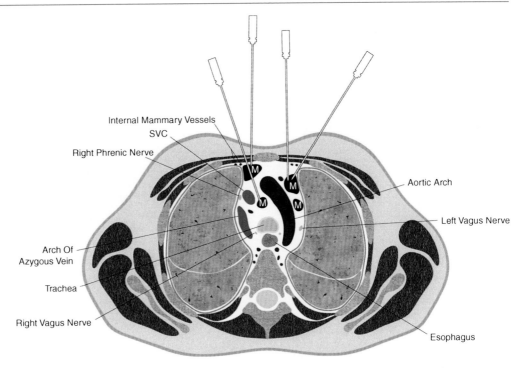

Internal Mammary Vessels
SVC
Right Phrenic Nerve
Aortic Arch
Left Vagus Nerve
Arch Of Azygous Vein
Trachea
Right Vagus Nerve
Esophagus

are present in approximately 20 % of patients. These internal mammary vessels can be easily identified on CT scans, even without intravenous administration of a contrast medium, and should be identified and avoided when planning the needle's path. The biopsy needle can be advanced either medial or lateral to the internal mammary vessels (Fig. 10.1).

Occasionally, the space between the lateral edge of the sternum and the internal mammary vessels may be too small to allow safe parasternal needle placement. Placing the patient in a lateral decubitus position may cause the mediastinum to shift laterally toward the dependent side, bringing the lesion or the mediastinal fat into direct contact with the parasternal chest wall and allowing the needle access to the lesion (Fig. 10.2) [2, 5]. Alternatively, saline solution or dilute contrast medium can be injected to create an artificial extrapleural path for needle placement (Fig. 10.3) [9]. Under CT guidance, a 22-gauge needle is advanced into the extrapleural space to inject the saline solution and create a "salinoma" window. After creation of this safe extrapleural window, the 22-gauge needle is removed and a large-bore (18-gauge or larger) guide needle is advanced through the salinoma to the lesion. Subsequently, using a coaxial technique, FNAB and core biopsies can be obtained through the guide needle. Alternatively, a 22-gauge needle with a removable hub can be used for initial localization, allowing advancement of the guide needle over the 22-gauge needle. It is important to remember that the degree of contact between the mediastinum and the parasternal chest wall may alter with the patient's breathing during the biopsy procedure,

precluding the use of the parasternal approach or resulting in inadvertent traversal of the lung or pleural space (Fig. 10.4). Breathing can also cause a small mediastinal lesion to move out of the biopsy plane.

For a US-guided parasternal biopsy (Fig. 10.5), the parasternal access window should be large enough to allow space for the transducer face and for simultaneous needle placement; hence, the use of US guidance is generally limited to biopsies of large anterior mediastinal lesions. Because of the small size of the access window, a small-footprint transducer is used, and a freehand technique is preferred over needle-attachment guides. It is essential to identify and avoid the major mediastinal blood vessels, including the internal mammary vessels; if needed, color Doppler imaging can be used for this purpose [11]. In some patients, curvature of the anterior ribs or costal cartilage may not allow enough space for the US transducer and the biopsy needle.

The parasternal approach also is appropriate for biopsies of anterior or middle mediastinal lesions. Although the parasternal approach is used mostly for needle biopsy of prevascular lesions or masses in the aortopulmonary window (Fig. 10.6), pretracheal or paratracheal lesions can also be accessed with this approach by advancing the needle between the major vessels (Fig. 10.7). Traversal of the brachiocephalic veins or superior vena cava with thin (e.g., 22-gauge) needles for biopsy of middle mediastinal lesions has been safely performed without complications [3, 7, 12]. Occasionally, a left parasternal approach may be used to access a lesion in the right mediastinum (Fig. 10.8).

Fig. 10.2 Schematic showing the use of decubitus positioning for a parasternal approach. (**a**) In the supine position, aerated lung is interposed between the mass (*M*) and the chest wall. (**b**) In the left lateral decubitus position, the mediastinum shifts to the left, creating a mediastinal window for needle placement

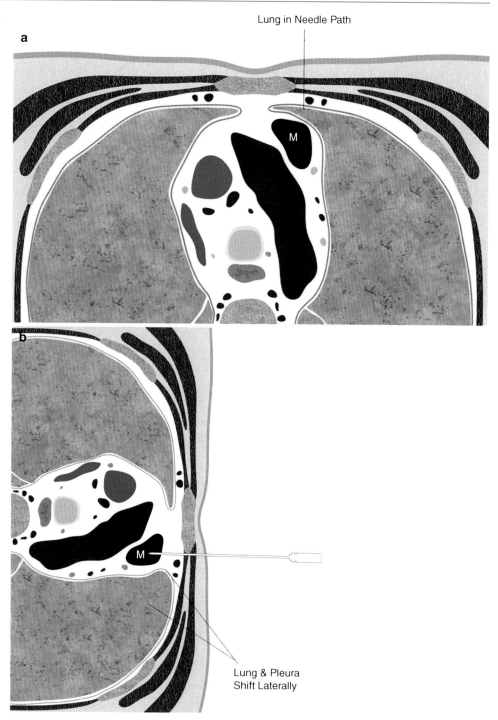

Paravertebral Approach

For the paravertebral approach, the patient is generally placed in the prone position; patients who are unable to lie prone may be placed in a prone oblique or lateral decubitus position. The needle is advanced immediately lateral to the vertebral body between the endothoracic fascia and the parietal pleura. The endothoracic fascia, located outside the parietal pleura, lines the walls of the thorax and merges with the prevertebral fascia posteromedially. In some patients, the paravertebral extrapleural space may be wide enough to allow needle biopsy without traversing the pleura. However, in most patients, an injection of saline solution or a dilute iodinated contrast medium is required to displace the mediastinal parietal pleura and gain extrapleural access (Fig. 10.9) [5, 9].

An 18-gauge blunt-tip needle or cannula is used for creation of the extrapleural window; the same needle can be

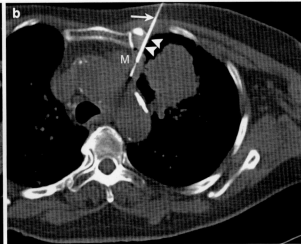

Fig. 10.3 Artificial widening of mediastinum for parasternal approach. (**a**) A CT scan shows an anterior mediastinal mass (*M*) and a narrow parasternal mediastinal window (*arrowheads*). (**b**) A CT scan shows the mediastinum widened by the injection of saline solution (*arrowheads*), allowing for extrapleural placement of the biopsy needle (*arrow*)

used as the guide needle for performing the biopsy with a coaxial technique (Fig. 10.10). Alternatively, a 22-gauge needle may be introduced initially to inject fluid and subsequently be exchanged for an 18-gauge needle to perform the biopsy [9]. In most patients, injection of 10–20 mL of saline solution is sufficient to achieve adequate mediastinal widening; however, larger volumes may be required [18]. Insufficient widening can occur when the needle tip lies outside the endothoracic fascia, in a blood vessel, or in the pleural space. The injection of saline solution also displaces mediastinal structures, such as the azygos vein, esophagus, nerves, and vertebral blood vessels, from the needle's path, thereby reducing the risk of inadvertent injury to these structures. Needle advancement and biopsy must be performed expeditiously because the mediastinal widening regresses along with the redistribution of fluid. The needle should be inserted medial to the pleural surface at the head of the ribs. Administration of saline through a needle placed lateral to the transverse process may not achieve mediastinal widening because of the fixation of the endothoracic fascia and parietal pleura at this location [5, 9]. The biopsy needle should be placed along the superior edge of the rib and above the transverse process to avoid injury to the intercostal nerve and artery. Some investigators recommend oral administration of a contrast medium if the esophagus is not identified on non-contrast-enhanced CT scans [5, 9]. In some patients, the presence of large osteophytes or the orientation of the transverse process may preclude paravertebral extrapleural access [19].

The paravertebral approach allows access to posterior mediastinal lesions and is used mostly for biopsy of subcarinal lesions from the right side (Fig. 10.10). Occasionally, a saline injection may cause sufficient displacement of the descending aorta to allow retroaortic access from the left side (Fig. 10.11) for biopsy of subcarinal, periesophageal, or left paratracheal masses. To avoid inadvertent injury to the aorta, only a blunt-tip guide needle should be used with this approach. The right paravertebral approach can also sometimes be used for accessing middle mediastinal lesions located in the pre- or paratracheal spaces, especially cranial to the level of the arch of the azygos vein [19].

Transsternal Approach

The transsternal approach involves needle placement through the sternum (Fig. 10.12). Any of the commonly available 18-gauge guide needles (Chiba [Cook Inc., Bloomington, IN] or Hawkins-Akins [Meditech, Westwood, MS]) are adequate to penetrate the sternum. Although an 18-gauge hypodermic needle can also be used to penetrate the sternum, it precludes the insertion of a coaxial 20-gauge core-biopsy needle to obtain larger specimens when needed [8]. If necessary, larger-caliber bone biopsy systems and drill bits can be used to gain transsternal access.

Transsternal needle insertion performed with local anesthesia and intravenous sedation is well tolerated by most patients. Injection of a local anesthetic into the periosteum of the anterior and posterior sternal cortices minimizes the discomfort associated with the procedure. A non-contrast-enhanced CT study obtained immediately before the procedure should be sufficient for safe biopsy planning in most patients who have had previous diagnostic contrast-enhanced CT scans; rarely, intravenous administration of a contrast agent may be needed during the procedure to help differentiate among mediastinal structures.

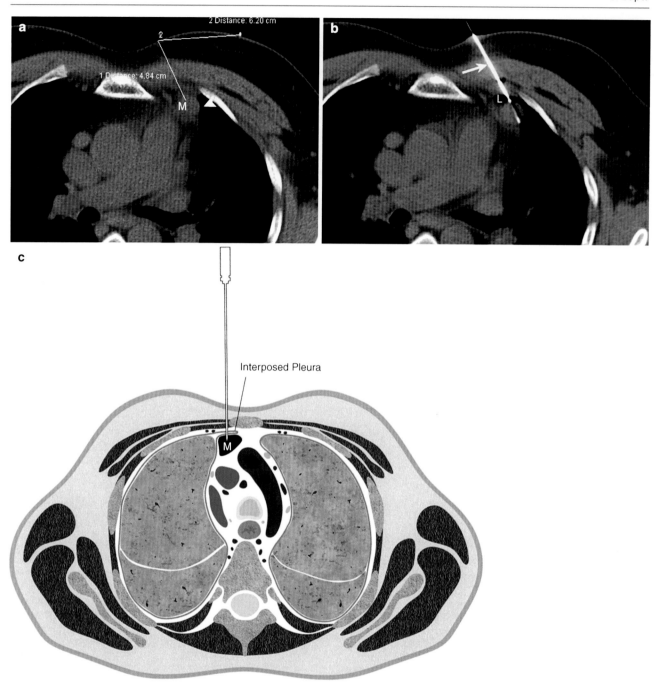

Fig. 10.4 Inadvertent pulmonary traversal during parasternal biopsy. (**a**) A CT scan shows an anterior mediastinal mass (*M*) in contact with the anterior chest wall. Note the extent of mediastinal fat (*arrowhead*) and the planned needle trajectory. (**b**) A CT scan shows lung (*L*) in the path of the needle causing separation of the mediastinal fat from the anterior chest wall. (**c**) A drawing illustrates how interposition of the parietal pleura into the needle's path can result in inadvertent traversal of the pleural space during a parasternal biopsy

The transsternal approach is used for biopsy of lesions that are not safely accessible by the parasternal approach. The transsternal approach is usually used for biopsy of anterior mediastinal masses (Fig. 10.13) [6, 13] but also allows access to middle or posterior mediastinal masses (Fig. 10.14) [8]. Traversal of a brachiocephalic vein with 22-gauge needles for biopsy of middle or posterior mediastinal masses has been shown to be safe (Fig. 10.15)

[8]. A curved 22-gauge Chiba needle can also be used to compensate for minor discrepancies in the trajectory of the guide needle (Fig. 10.16) [8]. Saline administration can be used to increase the contact between the mediastinum and the sternum to avoid pleural traversal as in the parasternal technique (Fig. 10.16).

The transsternal approach has some limitations. Mediastinal movements from patient respiration and

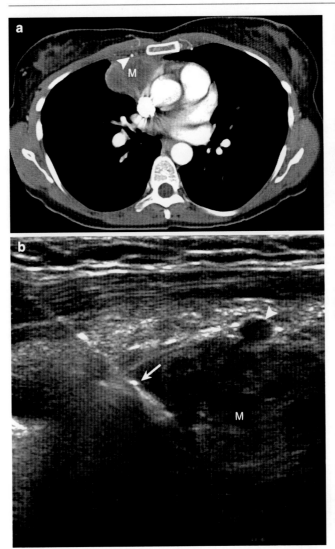

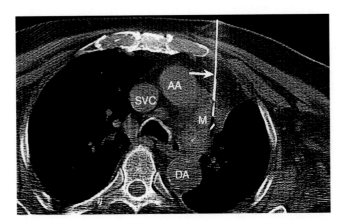

Fig. 10.5 US-guided parasternal biopsy. (**a**) A CT scan shows an anterior mediastinal mass (*M*). Note the position of the internal mammary vessels (*arrowhead*). (**b**) An ultrasonogram shows the biopsy needle (*arrow*) inserted via a parasternal approach and advanced lateral to the internal mammary artery (*arrowhead*) into the mass (*M*)

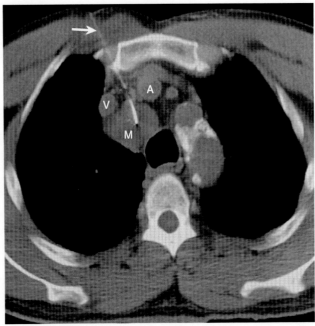

Fig. 10.7 Parasternal approach. A CT scan shows a biopsy needle (*arrow*) advanced between the right brachiocephalic vein (*V*) and artery (*A*) for biopsy of a pretracheal mass (*M*)

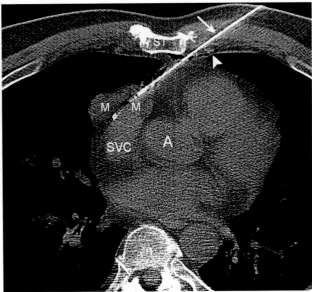

Fig. 10.6 Parasternal approach. A CT scan shows a biopsy needle (*arrow*) advanced through the mediastinal fat into an aortopulmonary window mass (*m*). Note the relationship of the mass to the aortic arch (*AA*), descending thoracic aorta (*DA*), and superior vena cava (*SVC*)

Fig. 10.8 Parasternal approach. A CT scan shows a biopsy needle (*arrow*) advanced between the sternum (*ST*) and internal mammary vessels (*arrowhead*) on the left side for biopsy of an anterior mediastinal mass (*m*) on the right side. Note the position of the superior vena cava (*SVC*) and aortic root (*A*)

cardiac or aortic pulsation can result in the lesion moving in and out of the biopsy plane, particularly in cases of small masses located close to the aortic arch. Also, once the needle has penetrated the sternum, the needle's trajectory cannot be altered without totally withdrawing the needle from the sternum. The degree of contact between the mediastinum and the sternum may sometimes change

Fig. 10.9 Schematic of the extrapleural paravertebral approach for needle biopsy of a posterior mediastinal mass (*M*) after widening of the mediastinal space by injection of saline solution

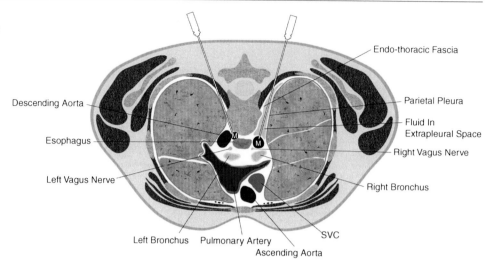

Fig. 10.10 Paravertebral approach for subcarinal mass. (**a**) A CT scan obtained with the patient prone shows a subcarinal mass (*M*); an 18-gauge needle (*arrow*) has been advanced to the edge of the paraver-

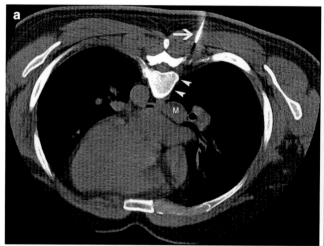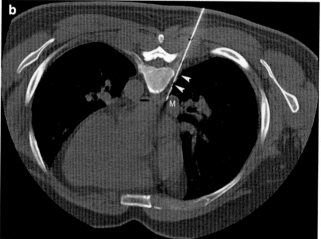

tebral space (*arrowheads*). (**b**) A CT scan obtained with the patient prone shows how the injection of saline solution has widened the mediastinum (*arrowheads*), creating a safe extrapleural path to the mass (*M*)

during the biopsy, resulting in inadvertent traversal of the pleural space.

Suprasternal Approach

In the suprasternal approach, the needle is inserted through the suprasternal fossa and advanced in a caudal direction toward the target lesion (Fig. 10.17). Two techniques can be used for CT-guided mediastinal biopsies by the suprasternal approach. One method involves placing the patient in a semierect position supported by pillows, with the patient's head turned to the side. Tilting the CT gantry craniocaudally allows imaging in a semicoronal plane and thus visualization of the projected needle path between the skin and the lesion (Fig. 10.18) [5]. The needle is inserted along the plane of the angled CT gantry using the gantry light for guidance. CT scans obtained with the gantry in the tilted position allow visualization of the entire length of the needle.

In the second method, the patient is placed in the supine position with pillows under the shoulders to allow hyperextension of the neck. Contiguous axial CT scans are obtained from the suprasternal level to the level of the target lesion. Using a triangulation method, the lesion depth from the skin entry site, the angle of incidence, and the anteroposterior and mediolateral inclination of the needle are estimated [20]. The needle path corresponds to the hypotenuse of a right triangle with the other two sides represented by the lesion depth and the craniocaudal distance between the axial level of the lesion and that of the skin entry site (Fig. 10.19a). The needle is advanced with CT guidance [4], and axial CT scans are obtained to check the needle-tip position (Fig. 10.19).

For US-guided procedures, a small-footprint transducer is used as it permits easy needle placement in the suprasternal notch and leaves enough room for simultaneous placement of a second needle. A 3.5-MHz or higher-frequency (5- to 7.5-MHz) transducer may be used, depending on the depth of the target lesion from the suprasternal notch [7, 11]. The patient is placed supine with pillows under the shoulder to keep the neck hyperextended. Because of limited space, a freehand technique is preferred over needle-attachment guides.

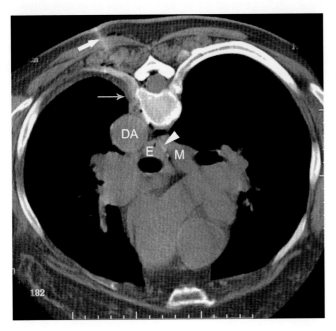

Fig. 10.11 Paravertebral retroaortic approach. A CT scan shows an 18-gauge guide needle (*thick arrow*) inserted into the paravertebral space (*thin arrow*) and advanced between the descending aorta (*DA*) and vertebral body after widening of these spaces by saline injection. A 22-gauge needle (*arrowhead*) was advanced through the guide needle to obtain aspirates from the subcarinal mass (*M*). *E* esophagus

Anterior mediastinal lesions that are large enough to extend above the cranial edge of the manubrium can be directly accessed by a US-guided suprasternal approach (Fig. 10.20). However, in most patients, these lesions are hidden behind the sternum. In these cases, the US transducer is positioned in the notch and angled downward to locate the lesion and identify a safe, avascular needle path. The soft tissues around the trachea and great blood vessels provide an adequate acoustic window, and the large arteries and veins act as anatomic guides for orientation of the needle in the superior mediastinum (Fig. 10.21). For pre- or paratracheal lesions, the needle is advanced between the blood vessels to reach the lesion. As with other approaches, traversal of the brachiocephalic vein with thin (22-gauge) needles is generally considered safe [7]. Occasionally, a small-caliber needle may be advanced through the thyroid gland to sample a retrotracheal lesion [19].

The suprasternal fossa offers an extrapleural window for access to superior mediastinal masses located above the level of the aortic arch. This approach can be used for biopsy of prevascular, pretracheal, and paratracheal lesions and lesions in the aortopulmonary window [4, 5, 7, 11, 12].

Angled suprasternal approaches with CT guidance using a gantry tilt or semicoronal route require excellent patient cooperation. The triangulation method involves contiguous localization scans to measure the distance between the lesion and the entry site, complex calculations of the degree of incline needed to direct the needle into the lesion, and multiple-level scanning to check the position of the needle tip during its advancement and before aspiration, all of which can be time-consuming and cumbersome. An inadequate acoustic window is a frequent problem with US

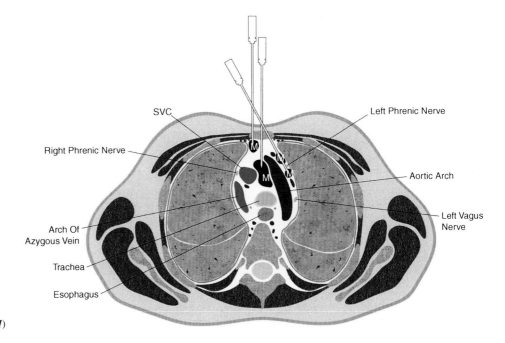

Fig. 10.12 Schematic of the transsternal approach showing needles traversing the sternum for biopsy of anterior mediastinal, preaortic, or pretracheal masses (*M*)

guidance of a suprasternal approach, limiting its use to biopsy of large anterior or middle mediastinal lesions located above the level of the aortic arch. US detection of small lesions situated immediately posterior to the sternum is also restricted.

Subxiphoid Approach

A subxiphoid approach is occasionally used for biopsy of mediastinal masses. With this approach, the needle is inserted below the xiphoid process of the sternum and is angled cranially. This approach allows biopsy of anterior pericardial lymph nodes and other pericardial masses. This approach can also be used for biopsy of posterior mediastinal masses by advancing the needle through the liver in a cranial direction (Fig. 10.22).

Approach Through the Pleural Space

For biopsy of anterior, middle, or posterior mediastinal lesions, the needle can sometimes be advanced through the pleural space created by an existing pleural effusion or an iatrogenic pneumothorax (Fig. 10.23). In patients with a free-flowing pleural effusion ipsilateral to the mediastinal mass, placing the patient in the contralateral decubitus position allows the fluid to move into the medial pleural recess [2, 5], thereby creating a "pleural window" for needle placement between the parietal and visceral layers of the pleura (Fig. 10.24). Patients with a loculated pleural effusion in the medial pleural recess do not require this positional maneuver [19]. The presence of pleural fluid provides an acoustic window for US visualization of mediastinal lesions, thus permitting US guidance of needle placement. US guidance is especially useful in patients with dyspnea who cannot tolerate a supine or prone position [19].

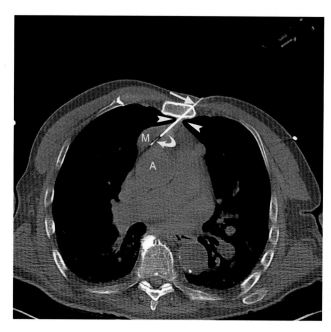

Fig. 10.13 Transsternal approach. A CT scan shows an 18-gauge needle (*arrow*) traversing the sternum and anterior mediastinal soft tissues and a 20-gauge core-biopsy needle (*curved arrow*) advanced through the 18-gauge needle into an anterior mediastinal mass (*M*) located anterior to the ascending aorta (*A*). Note that the anterior mediastinal soft tissues (*arrowheads*) do not extend laterally to allow parasternal extrapleural access

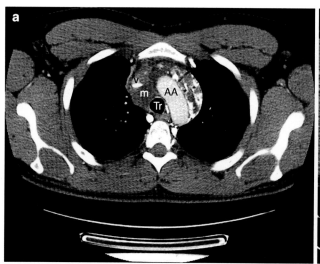
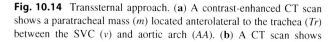
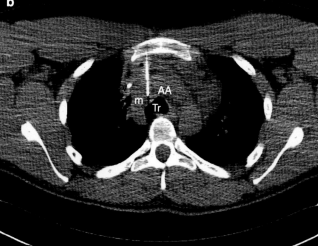

Fig. 10.14 Transsternal approach. (**a**) A contrast-enhanced CT scan shows a paratracheal mass (*m*) located anterolateral to the trachea (*Tr*) between the SVC (*v*) and aortic arch (*AA*). (**b**) A CT scan shows transsternal biopsy of the mass (*m*) with the biopsy needle passing between the superior vena cava (*v*) and the aortic arch (*AA*)

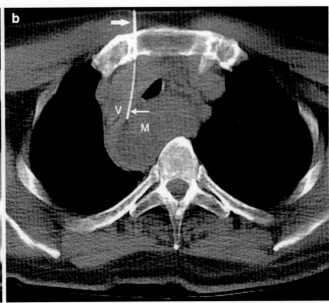

Fig. 10.15 Transsternal approach. (**a**) A contrast-enhanced CT scan shows a retrotracheal mass (*M*) posterior to the right and left brachiocephalic veins (*V*). (**b**) A CT scan shows a 22-gauge biopsy needle (*thin arrow*) coaxially introduced through an 18-gauge transsternal needle (*thick arrow*) and transgressing the left brachiocephalic vein (*V*) to obtain a sample of the mass (*M*)

A preexisting iatrogenic pneumothorax or intentionally injected intrapleural air can also create extrapulmonary access (Fig. 10.25) [2, 5]. In the latter procedure, an 18-gauge needle is advanced to the parietal pleura. The blunt needle cannula itself (from which the sharp stylet has been removed) or the needle with a blunt stylet is advanced through the parietal pleura and displaces the visceral pleura. Air is then injected into the pleural space to collapse the lung; the air is aspirated at the end of the biopsy procedure to reinflate the lung. This approach avoids puncture of visceral pleura and hence is useful in patients who have severe emphysema and are thus at a risk of developing persistent air leaks if a transpulmonary approach is used.

It may not always be possible to interpose pleural fluid between the skin and the target lesion, especially in the presence of pleural thickening and septations. The visceral pleura may be inadvertently punctured when using an approach through the pleural space during attempts to create an iatrogenic pneumothorax, resulting in air leakage. Moreover, inaccurate placement of the blunt needle outside the parietal pleura may result in dispersion of injected air into the extrapleural soft tissues [19].

Transpulmonary Approach

The transpulmonary approach to mediastinal biopsy allows access to masses in various anterior, middle, and posterior mediastinal locations [2, 5] (Fig. 10.26). This approach is generally used for biopsies of lesions that are not accessible by an extrapleural approach. The patient is placed in the appropriate position for easiest access to the mediastinal lesion. The needle passes through the lung parenchyma and two layers of visceral pleura. Attempts should be made to avoid fissures, emphysematous bullae, and major intrapulmonary vessels.

Complications

The most common complication of a mediastinal biopsy that involves needle traversal of the pleura and lung is pneumothorax. A transpulmonary approach for mediastinal biopsy is associated with an increased risk of pneumothorax because the needle traverses the lung and two layers of visceral pleura. Placement of the biopsy needle through the lung also creates a risk of alveolar hemorrhage and hemoptysis. Even during extrapleural approaches, inadvertent pleural or pulmonary traversal can result in pneumothorax.

Hemorrhage, a potential complication of any mediastinal biopsy, can be prevented by careful planning of the biopsy needle's path to avoid major blood vessels that are in proximity to the lesion. Small mediastinal hematomas are occasionally seen after transsternal biopsies; they are usually asymptomatic and self-limited and do not require treatment [19]. The parasternal approach carries the risk of accidental puncture of the internal mammary blood vessels, which

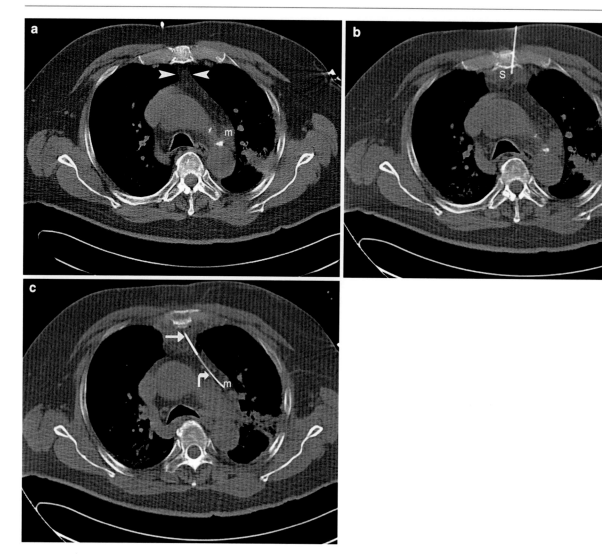

Fig. 10.16 Transsternal approach. (**a**) A CT scan shows an aortopulmonary window mass (*m*) and a narrow mediastinal window (*arrowheads*). (**b**) A CT scan shows placement of a needle and saline injections (*S*) to widen the degree of contact between the mediastinal soft tissues and the sternum. (**c**) A CT scan shows the transsternal placement of a guide needle (*arrow*) through the widened mediastinum. A curved 22-gauge Chiba needle (*curved arrow*) advances through the guide needle into the mass (*m*)

occasionally results in substantial extrapleural and pleural hemorrhage (Fig. 10.27). Similarly, the intercostal artery, paravertebral vessels, and azygos vein may be injured during a paravertebral approach, causing hemorrhage.

Rarely reported complications include vasovagal episodes, most likely secondary to apprehension, pain, or innervation of the pleura by the pulmonary plexus; intercostal neuritis caused by injury to the intercostal nerve; and transient Horner syndrome caused by irritation or injury to the ganglia of the sympathetic nervous system. The paravertebral approach carries the risk of injury to the intercostal nerves, spinal nerves, vagus nerve, and esophagus.

Other Invasive Methods for Obtaining Tissue Samples for Diagnosis of Mediastinal Lesions

Alternatives to percutaneous needle biopsy methods for obtaining tissue samples for cytologic or histologic evaluation of mediastinal lesions include other needle biopsy techniques such as transbronchial or endobronchial ultrasound (EBUS)-guided needle biopsy and endoscopic US-guided (EUS) transesophageal needle biopsy as well as surgical techniques, such as thoracoscopy, cervical mediastinoscopy, and anterior mediastinotomy [2, 21–23].

Fig. 10.17 Suprasternal approach. (**a**) A drawing illustrates suprasternal imaging in the sagittal oblique plane for biopsy of a superior mediastinal mass (*M*). (**b**) A drawing illustrates suprasternal imaging in the coronal oblique plane for biopsy of a mediastinal mass (*M*)

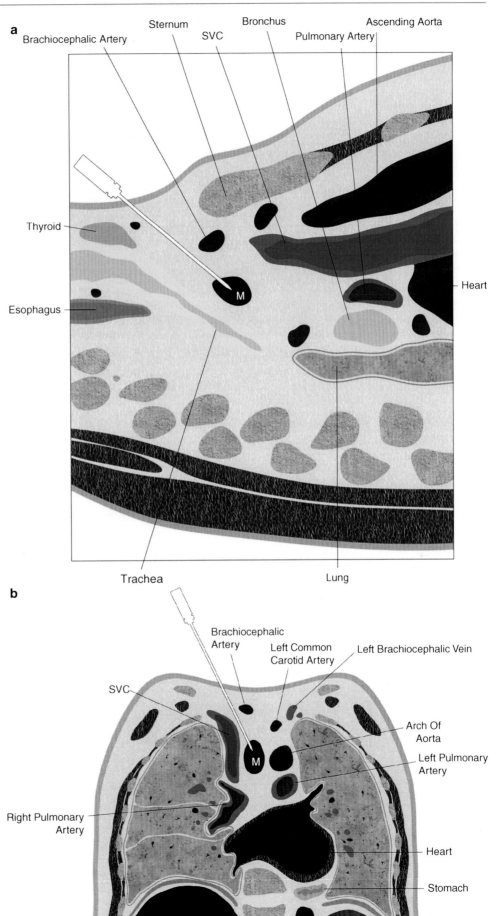

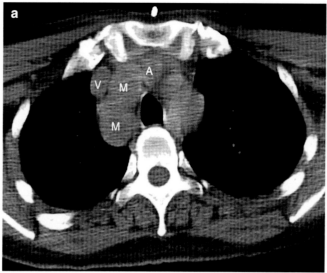 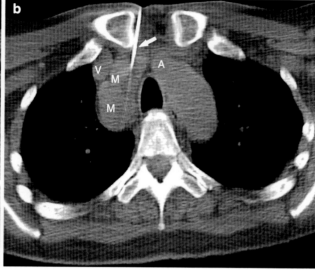

Fig. 10.18 Suprasternal approach using semicoronal CT scanning. (**a**) A transverse CT scan shows a bilobular retrosternal mediastinal mass (*M*) between the right brachiocephalic vein (*V*) and artery (*A*). (**b**) A semicoronal CT scan obtained after placing a pillow under the patient's shoulders and tilting the CT gantry craniocaudally shows a direct suprasternal access window, allowing safe placement of a biopsy needle (*arrow*) into the mass (*M*). *V* right brachiocephalic vein, *A* brachiocephalic artery

Fig. 10.19 Suprasternal approach using triangulation. (**a**) A schematic of the triangulation method. *Z* represents the point on the skin in the same transaxial plane as the target lesion. C, or the depth of needle insertion, is calculated by the Pythagorean theorem ($A^2 + B^2 = C^2$). The angle of needle insertion, *a*, equals the angle θ, which is calculated by the tangent of *B/A*. (**b**) A transverse contrast-enhanced CT scan shows an anterior mediastinal mass (*m*) located behind the sternum and between the aortic arch vessels (*v*). (**c**) A transverse CT scan shows the insertion site of the biopsy needle (*arrow*) in the suprasternal notch. The needle is angled caudally. (**d**) Transverse CT scan shows the tip of the biopsy needle (*arrow*) in the mass (*m*)

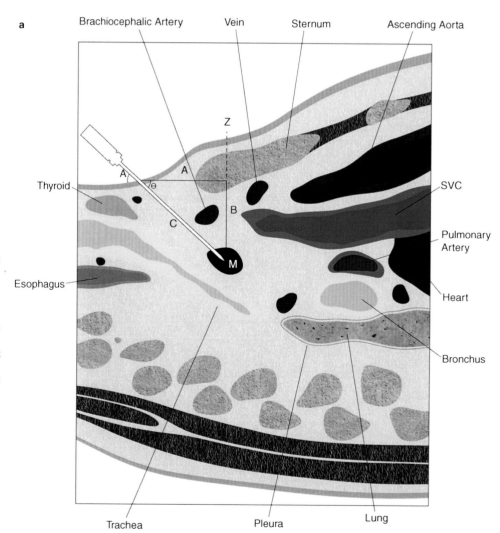

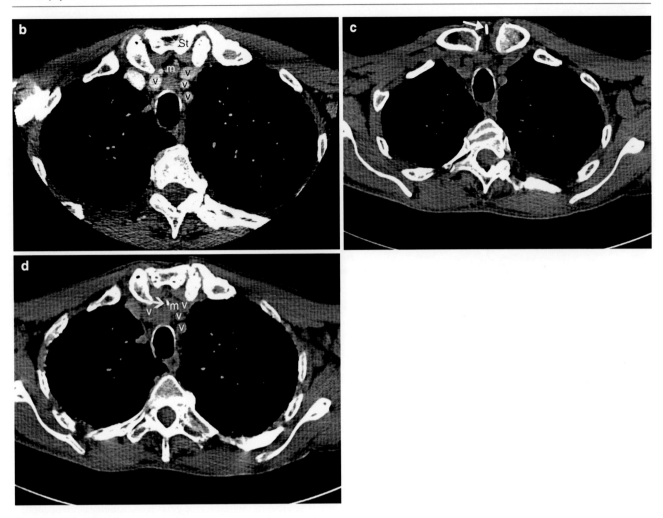

Fig. 10.19   (continued)

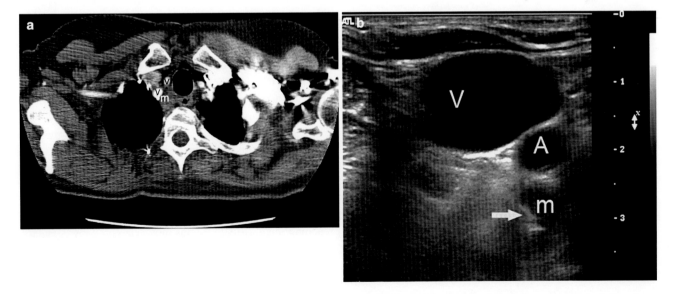

Fig. 10.20   US-guided suprasternal approach. (**a**) A CT scan shows a right paratracheal mass (*m*), which extends above the level of the manubrium. Note the presence of arch vessels (*v*) anterior to the mass. (**b**) A sagittal oblique ultrasonogram through the suprasternal window shows the needle (*arrow*) in the mass (*m*). *V* internal jugular vein, *A* brachiocephalic artery

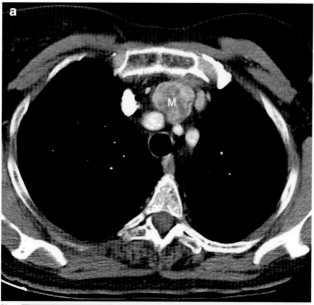

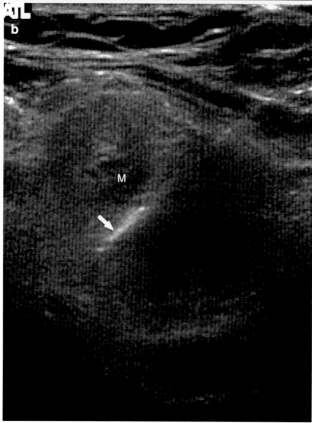

Fig. 10.21 US-guided suprasternal approach. (**a**) A CT scan shows an anterior mediastinal mass (*M*) that is located behind the sternum and anterior to the arteries arising from the aorta. (**b**) A suprasternal ultrasonogram in the semicoronal plane shows the biopsy needle (*arrow*) advanced into the mass (*M*) under US guidance

The transbronchial needle biopsy technique, which is performed during a flexible bronchoscopy, can be used to obtain FNABs or small core samples from subcarinal and paratracheal lymph nodes. A major limitation of this approach is the inability to visualize the target lesion and the needle tip during the biopsy. The sensitivity of transbronchial mediastinal biopsy for staging non-small-cell lung cancer is between 25 and 81 % [21]. Although the use of CT guidance may improve the yield of transbronchial needle biopsy, experience combining CT with this technique is still limited [24, 25]. EBUS-guided biopsy has been increasingly used for sampling mediastinal lymph nodes and has been shown to improve the diagnostic yield over that of transbronchial biopsies [21–24]. Real-time visualization of the needle during biopsy of the lymph nodes provides for a high diagnostic yield with EBUS-guided needle biopsy. However, mediastinal lymph nodes not in contact with the trachea or bronchus, e.g., prevascular nodes, aortopulmonary nodes, and posterior mediastinal nodes below the carina, are not accessible with this approach.

EUS-guided transesophageal needle biopsy allows access to the lower paratracheal, subcarinal, aortopulmonary, and paraesophageal regions. The advantages of EUS-guided biopsy include the ability to monitor the biopsy in real time, the decreased risk of pneumothoraces, and a high diagnostic yield. The reported sensitivity of EUS-guided biopsy in the mediastinum is 82–96 % [21, 22]. However, the interposition of the air-filled trachea prevents access to the anterior lymph nodes, including those in the pretracheal and upper right paratracheal regions.

Cervical mediastinoscopy has traditionally been accepted as the gold standard in preoperative disease staging involving the mediastinum in patients with non-small cell lung cancer and is especially useful in patients in whom multiple mediastinal nodes must be sampled for accurate staging. This method allows direct visualization and sampling of pretracheal, paratracheal, and anterior subcarinal lymph nodes and yields a diagnosis in 83–89 % of patients with lung cancer [2, 21, 22]. However, mediastinoscopy cannot provide access to the aortopulmonary, retrotracheal, posterior subcarinal, and inferior mediastinal lymph nodes. Also, mediastinoscopy requires general anesthesia and results in complications in 1–3 % of patients [2, 21, 22]. Potential complications include vascular, tracheobronchial, or phrenic nerve injury; esophageal perforation; mediastinitis; chylothorax; pericardial rupture; pneumothorax; arrhythmias; and death from stroke. Surgical techniques for reaching mediastinal regions not accessible by standard mediastinoscopy include extended cervical mediastinoscopy, anterior mediastinotomy, and thoracoscopy.

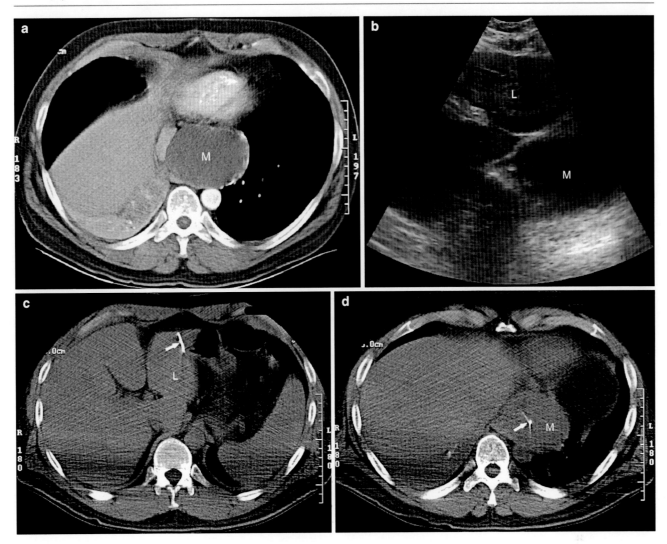

Fig. 10.22 Subxiphoid approach. (**a**) A CT scan shows a large posterior mediastinal mass (*M*). (**b**) An ultrasonogram from the subxiphoid approach with the transducer angled upward shows the mass (*M*) posterosuperior to the left lobe of the liver (*L*). The biopsy needle (not shown) was advanced under US guidance. (**c** and **d**) CT scans obtained to verify needle trajectory show the needle (*arrow*) passing through liver (*L*) (**c**) and the needle tip (*arrow*) in the mass (*M*) (**d**)

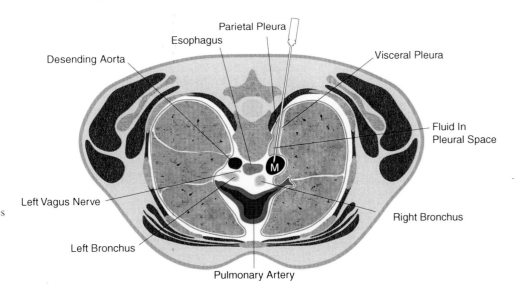

Fig. 10.23 Schematic illustrates needle advancement through the pleural space created by pleural fluid or an iatrogenic pneumothorax during biopsy of a posterior mediastinal mass

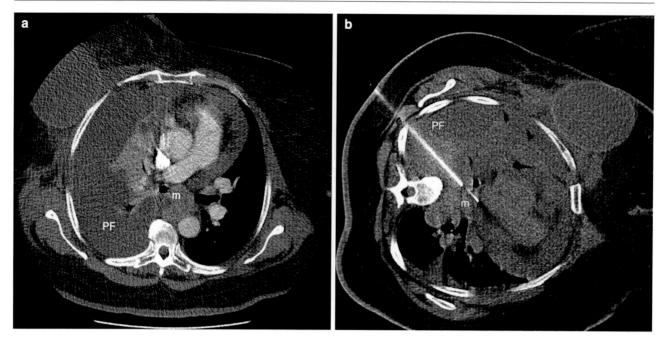

Fig. 10.24 Pleural space approach. (**a**) A CT scan shows a subcarinal mass (*m*) and right pleural fluid (*PF*). (**b**) A CT scan with the patient in the left lateral decubitus position shows placement of the biopsy needle into the subcarinal mass (*m*) through the pleural effusion (*PF*)

Image-guided percutaneous needle biopsy allows access to virtually all mediastinal regions, including those inaccessible by mediastinoscopy and transbronchial or EUS-guided needle biopsy. The accuracy of transthoracic biopsy in the diagnosis of mediastinal lesions ranges from 75 to 90 % [2, 21, 22]. Image-guided percutaneous needle biopsy is less invasive than mediastinoscopy and requires only local anesthesia and conscious sedation. A major limitation of this technique is that pneumothoraces occur in 10–60 % of cases. Various protective measures, such as saline administration, careful patient positioning, induction of iatrogenic pneumothorax, and the use of transsternal or suprasternal approaches can substantially decrease the rate of pneumothoraces.

Summary

This article summarizes the various approaches used for image-guided percutaneous mediastinal needle biopsy and discusses the anatomic and technical aspects, advantages, limitations, and potential complications of each technique as well as briefly describing several alternative methods for accessing mediastinal lesions. Familiarity with the mediastinal anatomy on cross-sectional images facilitates the planning of safe access routes for biopsies of deep-seated lesions. Various techniques, such as injection of physiologic saline solution and careful patient positioning, may help avoid puncture of the lung and visceral pleura, thus decreasing the risk of pneumothorax.

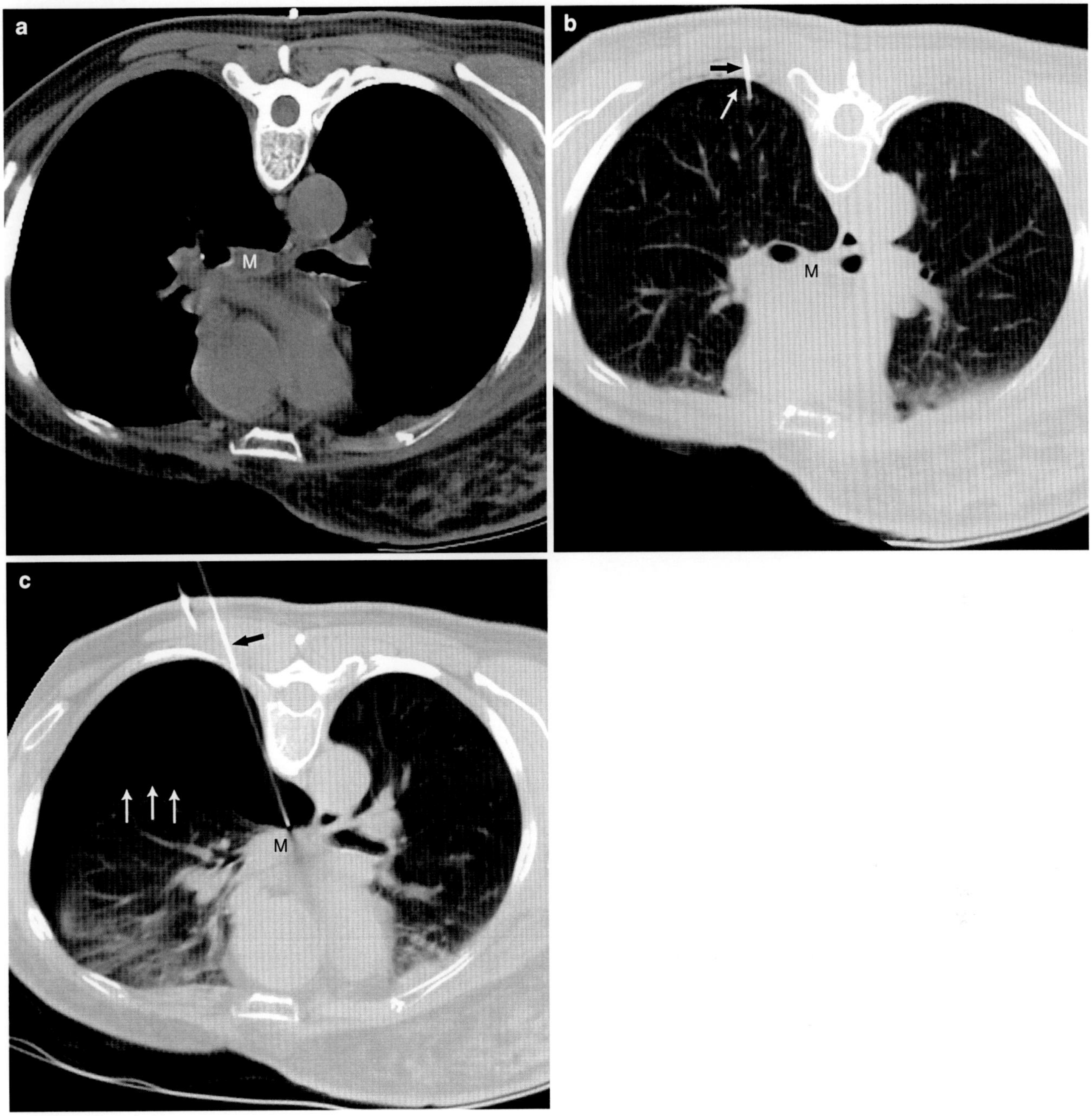

Fig. 10.25 Pleural space approach. (**a**) A CT scan shows a subcarinal mass. (**b**) A CT scan shows an 18-gauge blunt-tip needle (*black arrow*) advanced through the parietal pleura, displacing the visceral pleura (*white arrow*). (**c**) A CT scan shows lung collapse (*white arrows*) caused by the introduction of air into the pleural space. This has allowed advancement of the biopsy needle (*black arrow*) through the pleural space. The air was evacuated at the end of the biopsy procedure. *M* mass

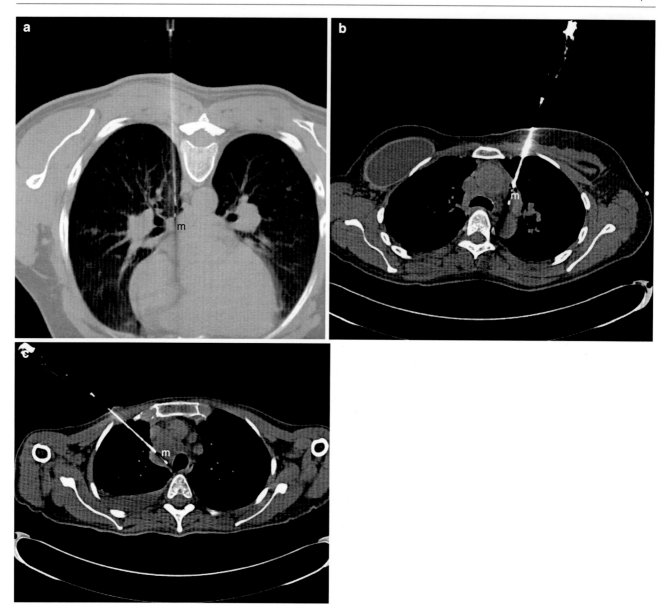

Fig. 10.26 Transpulmonary approach in three different patients. (**a**) A CT scan shows needle placement during transpulmonary biopsy of a subcarinal mass (*m*). (**b**) A CT scan shows needle placement during transpulmonary biopsy of an aortopulmonary mass (*m*). (**c**) A CT scan shows needle placement during transpulmonary biopsy of a right paratracheal mass (*m*)

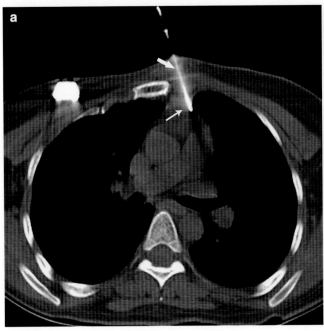 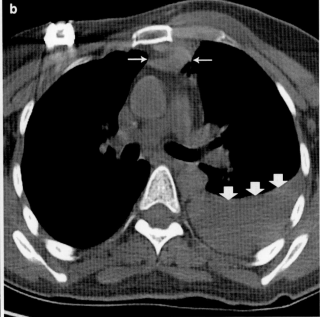

Fig. 10.27 Inadvertent internal mammary artery injury. (**a**) A CT scan shows a biopsy needle (*thick arrow*) advanced parasternally and causing a mediastinal hematoma (*thin arrow*) secondary to injury to the internal mammary vessels. (**b**) A postprocedural CT scan shows an enlarging mediastinal hematoma (*thin arrows*) and a left hemothorax (*short thick arrows*)

References

1. Morrissey B, Adams H, Gibbs AR, Crane MD. Percutaneous needle biopsy of the mediastinum: review of 94 procedures. Thorax. 1993;48:632–7.
2. Protopapas Z, Westcott JL. Transthoracic hilar and mediastinal biopsy. Radiol Clin North Am. 2000;38:281–91.
3. Westcott JL. Transthoracic needle biopsy of the hilum and mediastinum. J Thorac Imaging. 1987;2:41–8.
4. Belfiore G, Camera L, Moggio G, Vetrani A, Fraioli G, Salvatore M. Middle mediastinum lesions: preliminary experience with CT-guided fine-needle aspiration biopsy with a suprasternal approach. Radiology. 1997;202:870–3.
5. Bressler EL, Kirkham JA. Mediastinal masses: alternative approaches to CT-guided needle biopsy. Radiology. 1994;191:391–6.
6. D'Agostino HB, Sanchez RB, Laoide RM, et al. Anterior mediastinal lesions: transsternal biopsy with CT guidance. Work in progress. Radiology. 1993;189:703–5.
7. Gupta S, Gulati M, Rajwanshi A, Gupta D, Suri S. Sonographically guided fine-needle aspiration biopsy of superior mediastinal lesions by the suprasternal route. AJR Am J Roentgenol. 1998;171:1303–6.
8. Gupta S, Wallace MJ, Morello Jr FA, Ahrar K, Hicks ME. CT-guided percutaneous needle biopsy of intrathoracic lesions by using the transsternal approach: experience in 37 patients. Radiology. 2002;222:57–62.
9. Langen HJ, Klose KC, Keulers P, Adam G, Jochims M, Gunther RW. Artificial widening of the mediastinum to gain access for extrapleural biopsy: clinical results. Radiology. 1995;196:703–6.
10. vanSonnenberg E, Casola G, Ho M, et al. Difficult thoracic lesions: CT-guided biopsy experience in 150 cases. Radiology. 1988; 167:457–61.
11. Rubens DJ, Strang JG, Fultz PJ, Gottlieb RH. Sonographic guidance of mediastinal biopsy: an effective alternative to CT guidance. AJR Am J Roentgenol. 1997;169:1605–10.
12. Yang PC, Chang DB, Lee YC, Yu CJ, Kuo SH, Luh KT. Mediastinal malignancy: ultrasound guided biopsy through the supraclavicular approach. Thorax. 1992;47:377–80.
13. Astrom KG, Ahlstrom KH, Magnusson A. CT-guided transsternal core biopsy of anterior mediastinal masses. Radiology. 1996; 199:564–7.
14. Protopapas Z, Westcott JL. Transthoracic needle biopsy of mediastinal lymph nodes for staging lung and other cancers. Radiology. 1996;199:489–96.
15. Moulton JS, Moore PT. Coaxial percutaneous biopsy technique with automated biopsy devices: value in improving accuracy and negative predictive value. Radiology. 1993;186:515–22.
16. Sawhney S, Jain R, Berry M. Tru-Cut biopsy of mediastinal masses guided by real-time sonography. Clin Radiol. 1991;44:16–9.
17. Glassberg RM, Sussman SK, Glickstein MF. CT anatomy of the internal mammary vessels: importance in planning percutaneous transthoracic procedures. AJR Am J Roentgenol. 1990;155:397–400.
18. Grant TH, Stull MA, Kandallu K, Chambliss JF. Percutaneous needle biopsy of mediastinal masses using a computed tomography-guided extrapleural approach. J Thorac Imaging. 1998;13:14–9.
19. Gupta S, Seaberg K, Wallace MJ, et al. Imaging-guided percutaneous biopsy of mediastinal lesions: different approaches and anatomic considerations. Radiographics. 2005;25:763–86; discussion 786-768.
20. vanSonnenberg E, Wittenberg J, Ferrucci Jr JT, Mueller PR, Simeone JF. Triangulation method for percutaneous needle guidance: the angled approach to upper abdominal masses. AJR Am J Roentgenol. 1981;137:757–61.
21. Wiersema MJ, Vazquez-Sequeiros E, Wiersema LM. Evaluation of mediastinal lymphadenopathy with endoscopic US-guided fine-needle aspiration biopsy. Radiology. 2001;219:252–7.
22. Toloza EM, Harpole L, Detterbeck F, McCrory DC. Invasive staging of non-small cell lung cancer: a review of the current evidence. Chest. 2003;123:157S–66.
23. Lloyd C, Silvestri GA. Mediastinal staging of non-small-cell lung cancer. Cancer Control. 2001;8:311–17.
24. Shannon JJ, Bude RO, Orens JB, et al. Endobronchial ultrasound-guided needle aspiration of mediastinal adenopathy. Am J Respir Crit Care Med. 1996;153:1424–30.
25. Rong F, Cui B. CT scan directed transbronchial needle aspiration biopsy for mediastinal nodes. Chest. 1998;114:36–9.

Percutaneous Transthoracic Lung Biopsy

Antonio Gutierrez, Fereidoun Abtin, and Robert D. Suh

Background

Percutaneous transthoracic needle biopsy (TNB) has emerged as a viable and minimally invasive procedure for the diagnosis of indeterminate pulmonary nodules, masses, and consolidations. Lesions previously inaccessible can now be biopsied using cross-sectional imaging providing tissue samples for accurate histologic diagnosis. To date the most commonly used and widely studied technique for TNB is fine-needle aspiration with or without a coaxial system. Over the past two decades with continued improvements in small gauge coaxial core needle systems and biopsy technique, coaxial core biopsy is now a preferred technique for pulmonary lesions as it can obtain larger specimens for diagnosis and molecular analysis [1, 2]. Core needle samples are becoming increasingly important as recent advances in molecular profiling require adequate tumor tissue to identify specific mutations allowing for targeted cancer therapy, such as in primary lung adenocarcinomas; EGFR mutations are treated with tyrosine kinase inhibitors [2, 3]. In addition to targeted cancer therapy, molecular analysis can identify cancer-specific genetic profiles allowing for accurate prognosis [2, 4]. This major trend in molecular profiling highlights the importance for being proficient in obtaining adequate core samples in a reliable and safe manner [1–4]. With continued improvements in imaging technology, needle design, biopsy technique, and strategies for preventing and managing potential complications, TNB, or perhaps more appropriately, transthoracic core needle biopsy (TCNB) will continue to flourish as a minimally invasive diagnostic procedure for pulmonary lesions [5–7].

Indications and Patient Selection

The most common indication for TNB is an indeterminate solitary pulmonary nodule [5]. TNB is performed in cases where the nodule in question is almost certainly malignant but unsuitable for resection and is of equivocal or likely benign nature. In these cases, the TNB diagnosis will dictate management while avoiding thoracotomy (Fig. 11.1). Additionally, TNB is frequently performed for solitary or multiple pulmonary nodules, masses, or consolidations when tissue is required to diagnose and further characterize potentially malignant lesions (Fig. 11.2) [8]. TNB allows for the diagnosis of primary bronchogenic carcinoma and metastatic and/or pulmonary lymphoproliferative disease allowing for disease-specific management and in the era of molecular profiling, allowing for therapy targeting specific mutations and accurate prognosis [1–4, 8].

An increasingly common indication for TNB, particularly in the immunocompromised population, is a focal area of consolidation or suspected lung abscess in which bronchoscopy, or sputum cytology and culture have not yielded a diagnosis [9, 10]. Additional indications for TNB include enlarging ground glass opacities (Fig. 11.3) [11, 12] and evaluating for local recurrence following therapy (Fig. 11.4) [7].

A. Gutierrez, MD (✉)
Department of Radiological Sciences,
David Geffen School of Medicine at UCLA Medical Center,
Ronald Reagan UCLA Medical Center, 757 Westwood Plaza,
Suite 1638, Los Angeles, CA 90095-7437, USA
e-mail: angutierrez@mednet.ucla.edu

F. Abtin, MD
Department of Radiological Sciences,
Ronald Reagan UCLA Medical Center,
757 Westwood Plaza, Suite 1638,
Los Angeles, CA 90095-7437, USA
e-mail: fabtin@mednet.ucla.edu

R.D. Suh, MD
Department of Radiological Sciences,
David Geffen School of Medicine at UCLA Medical Center,
757 Westwood Plaza, Suite 1638,
Los Angeles, CA 90095-7437, USA

Thoracic Imaging and Intervention, Department of Radiology,
Ronald Reagan UCLA Medical Center, 757 Westwood Plaza,
Suite 1638, Los Angeles, CA 90095-7437, USA
e-mail: rsuh@mednet.ucla.edu

K. Ahrar, S. Gupta (eds.), *Percutaneous Image-Guided Biopsy*,
DOI 10.1007/978-1-4614-8217-8_11, © Springer Science+Business Media New York 2014

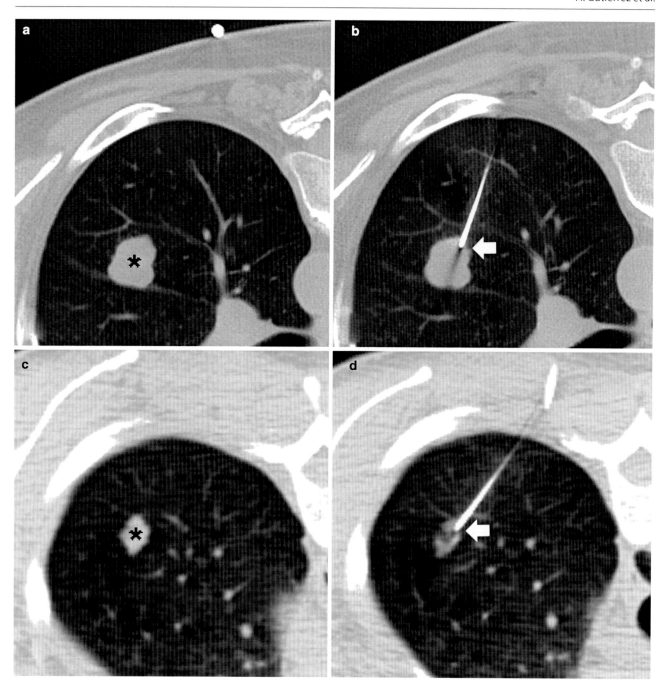

Fig. 11.1 Solitary pulmonary nodule: two different patients (**a**–**b** and **c**–**d**) undergoing TCNB for an indeterminate pulmonary nodule. (**a**) Pre-biopsy image demonstrates a 20 mm lobulated nodule (*) within the left lower lobe in close proximity to the oblique fissure with surrounding centrilobular emphysema. (**b**) A 19-gauge coaxial needle is placed into the nodule (*arrow*). Biopsy results demonstrated poorly differentiated adenocarcinoma. (**c**) Pre-biopsy CT image demonstrates a 13 mm lobulated nodule (*) within the left upper lobe with surrounding centrilobular emphysema. (**d**) A 19-gauge coaxial needle is placed into the nodule (*arrow*). Biopsy results demonstrated a hamartoma

The position of the lesion and its appearance on computed tomography (CT) continue to determine whether bronchoscopic biopsy or TNB is the more appropriate technique for establishing a diagnosis. In general, large central lesions with an endobronchial component are likely to be accurately diagnosed with flexible bronchoscopy, whereas peripheral tumors, especially those smaller than 3 cm in diameter, without a bronchus entering the proximal portion of the lesion are best suited for TNB [5, 7]. With improvements in technology and technique, TNB is an accurate method of diagnosing lesions regardless of their size or location where nodules less than 1 cm in diameter can be safely and accurately sampled [13]. This then provides new diagnostic options for patient populations requiring evaluation of an

Fig. 11.2 Biopsy indications: three different patients undergoing TCNB. (**a**) Pre-biopsy CT image demonstrates multiple pulmonary nodules (*arrows*). A 19-gauge coaxial needle (*arrowheads*) is positioned in the lateral left upper lobe nodule (*arrow*) via a parasternal approach. Biopsy results demonstrated colorectal adenocarcinoma. (**b**) Pre-biopsy CT image demonstrates a persistent left lower consolidation (*arrows*). A 19-gauge coaxial needle (*arrowheads*) is positioned in the consolidation via a posterior approach. Biopsy results demonstrated bronchoalveolar carcinoma. (**c**) Pre-biopsy CT image demonstrates a lobulated left lower lobe nodule (*) in a patient with Hodgkin's lymphoma. A 19-gauge coaxial needle (*arrowheads*) is positioned in the nodule via a posterior paraspinal approach. Biopsy results demonstrated treated lymphoproliferative disease

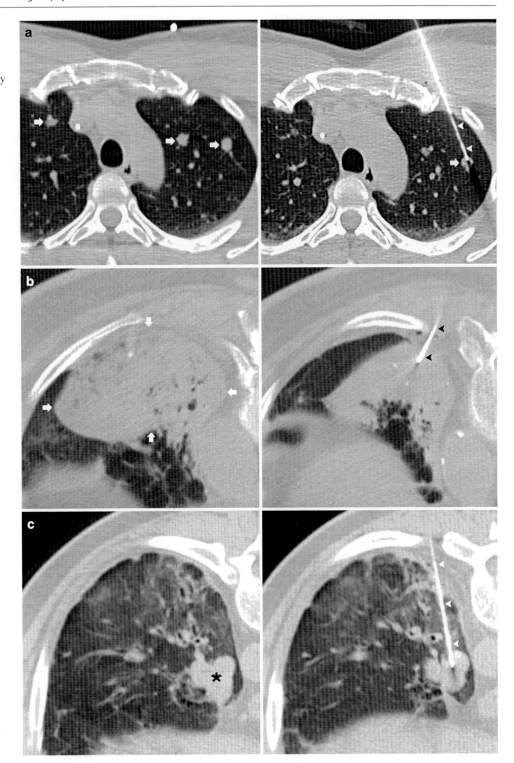

indeterminate nodule including patients undergoing staging and transplant evaluation (Fig. 11.5).

Regardless of the indication, the guiding principle used in all cases of TNB is that the potential benefits of a tissue diagnosis will affect patient management in such a manner that outweighs the risks of the procedure [5, 6, 14].

Contraindications

Although some authors claim that any case of an anatomic or functional single lung or severe pulmonary arterial hypertension (>40 mmHg) are absolute contraindications to TNB [2, 5], others insist that there are no absolute contraindications to the

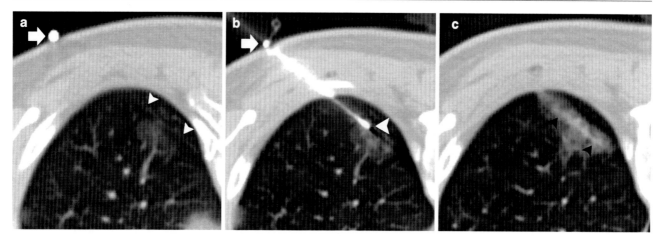

Fig. 11.3 Ground glass nodule. (**a**) Pre-biopsy CT image demonstrates a 23 mm ground glass nodule within the left lower lobe in close proximity to the oblique fissure (*arrowheads*). A radiopaque marker (*arrow*) is placed on the skin indicating a posterolateral approach to avoid transgression of the oblique fissure (*arrowheads*). (**b**) A 19-gauge coaxial needle is advanced via a perifissural route with confirmation of the needle tip (*arrowhead*) within the target lesion. Prior to obtaining specimens, the attachable depth marker (*arrow*) is positioned to prevent inadvertent advancement of the coaxial needle. (**c**) Post-biopsy images demonstrate a small amount of perinodular hemorrhage and autologous blood along the parenchymal needle tract (*arrowheads*). Biopsy results demonstrated bronchoalveolar cell carcinoma

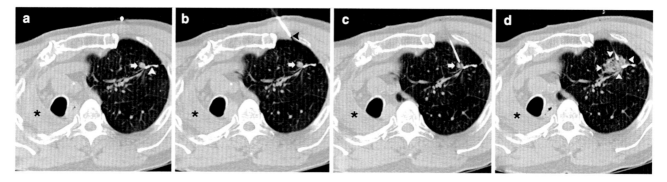

Fig. 11.4 Suture recurrence: 66-year-old man status post right pneumonectomy for primary bronchogenic adenocarcinoma and left upper lobe wedge resection of a metachronous primary bronchogenic carcinoma. (**a**) Pre-biopsy CT image demonstrates postoperative changes of a right pneumonectomy (*) and an 8 mm nodule (*arrow*) within the left upper lobe adjacent to the microsuture line (*arrowhead*). (**b**) A 19-gauge coaxial needle is placed in the left anterior chest wall with the tip in the extrapleural space (*arrowhead*) in the expected path to the target lesion (*arrow*). (**c**) The 19-gauge coaxial needle is advanced into the lung with the tip adjacent to the nodule (*arrow*). (**d**) Following needle tip confirmation, multiple 20-gauge core needle samples were obtained with development of perinodule hemorrhage (*arrowheads*). Biopsy results demonstrated recurrent adenocarcinoma

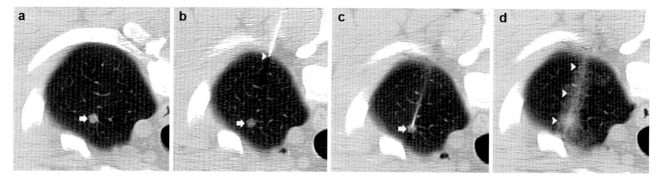

Fig. 11.5 4 mm nodule: 50-year-old man with hepatocellular carcinoma undergoing transplant evaluation with an indeterminate solitary pulmonary nodule. (**a**) Pre-biopsy CT image demonstrates a 4 mm nodule within the left upper lobe (*arrow*). (**b**) A 19-gauge coaxial needle is placed in the left anterior chest wall with the tip in the extrapleural space (*arrowhead*) in the expected path to the target lesion (*arrow*). (**c**) The 19-gauge coaxial needle is advanced into the lung with confirmation of the tip within the nodule (*arrow*). (**d**) Post-biopsy images demonstrate a small amount of perinodular hemorrhage and autologous blood along the parenchymal needle tract (*arrowheads*). Biopsy results demonstrated a necrotizing granuloma

procedure [7]. Overall, there are few relative contraindications to TNB, most authors agreeing that several preexisting conditions significantly increase the complication rate of TNB or render any complication more significant and therefore constitute relative contraindications to TNB. Relative contraindications include the inability to cooperate (lie flat and breath hold), although rectified with general anesthesia and deep sedation; coagulation disorders (international normalized ratio >1.3 or platelets <50,000) and anticoagulation medications; bulla or severe emphysema; relatively prominent airways or vasculature within the anticipated biopsy path; cardiac insufficiency; and pneumonectomy, although some authors believe that TNB can be safely performed even in this population if the proper preparations are made for rapid chest tube insertion (Fig. 11.4) [15]. Above all, TNB should be limited to cases that are truly indicated, technically feasible, and for which the anticipated benefits outweigh the risks.

Technique

Approach and Relevant Anatomy

Multiple anatomic factors should be taken into account when developing an approach for a TNB. The site of entry, adequate pleural anesthesia, and awareness of the bronchovascular planes, the fissures, and the hilar and mediastinal structures are critical in maximizing patient comfort to potentiate the success of the biopsy while minimizing the risk for significant complications.

Initial adequate placement of the coaxial needle is essential for achieving pleural anesthesia and optimal trajectory for needle placement into the target lesion. Adequate pleural anesthesia is the cornerstone of a successful biopsy, as patient comfort and cooperation are of the utmost importance. The parietal pleural is the second most sensitive structure aside from the skin in the path of the needle. The costal and diaphragmatic parietal pleura are innervated by the overlying intercostal nerve, where inadequate anesthesia is characterized by significant pain and discomfort along the dermatome or referred pain to the ipsilateral shoulder. Effective anesthesia of the parietal pleura requires the precise placement of the anesthesia needle tip in an extrapleural location immediately adjacent to and superficial to the parietal pleura (Fig. 11.6), while avoiding both the underlying parietal and visceral pleura, which if violated increases the risk of an early pneumothorax. Proper needle tip placement requires the combination of exact measurements obtained from localization scans and operator needle control. As the needle penetrates the different layers of the chest wall, the operator will feel many "pops," representing the needle traversing the different chest wall structures, the most important of which is the endothoracic fascia as its passages signify the exact location of the extrapleural fat space immediately superficial to the parietal pleura, where a few millimeters can mean the difference between a straightforward biopsy and one complicated by an early pneumothorax (Fig. 11.7).

An understanding of the central bronchovascular computed tomography (CT) anatomy allows the development of a safe transthoracic route to a central lesion. The pulmonary hila are composed of the major bronchi with accompanying pulmonary arteries and pulmonary veins that extend radially into the lobes, segments, and subsegments of the lungs. It is often difficult to avoid the vessels and airways in the periphery of the lung, but fortunately, such disturbances result in minimal to no significant complications. For central lesions, when developing a percutaneous transthoracic route, the radial nature of the bronchovascular structures from the hila to the periphery of the lung typically provides an abronchovascular route to the central portions of the lung and thus allowing safe access to a centrally located lesion (Fig. 11.8). By exploiting this abronchovascular plane, the risk of a threatening pulmonary hemorrhage with or without hemoptysis, and in a worst-case scenario, air embolism can be significantly reduced. In addition to conventional axial images, sagittal and coronal reformations can better delineate the relationship of the target lesion with the surrounding bronchovascular structures and may be beneficial in developing a safe transthoracic route. Of particular interest is the pulmonary venous anatomy as transgression should be avoided at all costs to minimize the risk of hemorrhage, bronchovenous fistula, and air embolism.

Awareness of the interlobar and accessory fissures is important, as these fissures should be avoided to reduce the risk of a pneumothorax, which may result in a problematic or persistent air leak. The relevant fissures are comprised of the major, minor, and accessory fissures. These fissures are best visualized on thin, less than 3 mm, CT sections; they appear as a white line that typically can be avoided when developing a path to the target lesion. However, if thin sections are not available, fissural position can be inferred from the location of a 1–2 cm thick avascular plane of lung. The minor fissure is usually difficult to visualize, as it parallels the plane of the scan, but it can be readily visualized on coronal and sagittal reconstructions. The fissures are not always complete and are often partial. Aziz et al. [16] catalogued in a large study population the incidence of partial or absent fissures and found centrally absent right major, left major, and right minor fissures in 48 %, 43 %, and 63 % of patients, respectively. Once recognized, incomplete fissure anatomic variation can be taken advantage of while planning a translobar approach to a central lung target (Fig. 11.9). Accessory fissures, seen in up to 30 % of individuals [17], should also be considered while planning an approach; common accessory fissures include the inferior accessory fissure that separates the medial basal segment from the remaining

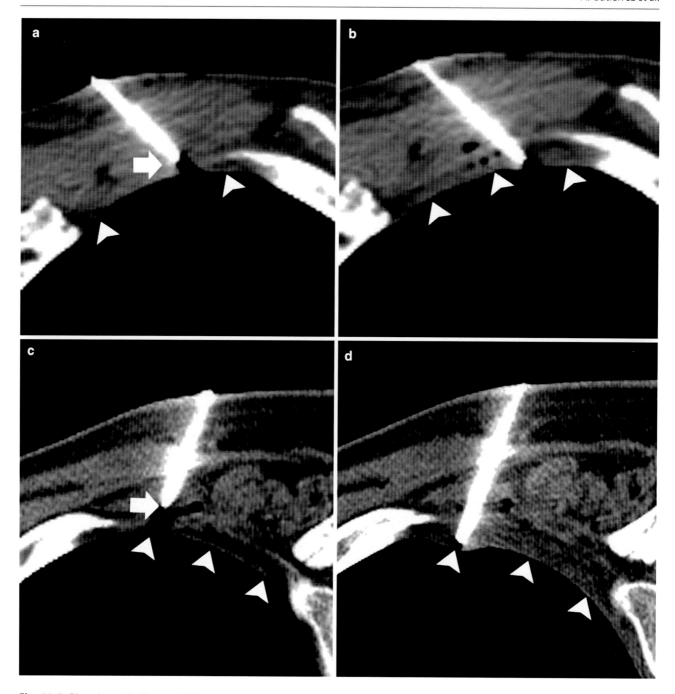

Fig. 11.6 Pleural anesthesia: two different patients (**a–b** and **c–d**) undergoing TCNB. (**a** and **c**) Preanesthesia: 19-gauge coaxial needle with the tip (*arrows*) superficial to the extrapleural fat (*arrowheads*). (**b** and **d**). Postanesthesia: 19-gauge coaxial needle has been advanced with the tip in the extrapleural fat status post administration of 1 % lidocaine in the extrapleural space (*arrowheads*)

basal segments, the azygos fissure (composed of four layers of pleura: two visceral and two parietal) that represents an invagination of the right apical pleura by the azygos vein, the superior accessory fissure that separates the superior segment from the basal segments of the lower lobe, and the left minor fissure that separates the lingula from the remaining portions of the upper lobe.

When planning a percutaneous transthoracic needle biopsy, lesions in a paramediastinal location must be approached and biopsied with caution, as they pose significant risk of injury to the cardiomediastinal structures. Those structures where the needle should preferably have a parallel course include the heart, the aorta and its branches and superior and inferior vena cava (Fig. 11.10) [2].

Preprocedure Evaluation

Evaluation of a potential candidate for TNB is preferably performed in an outpatient setting. Directed patient history

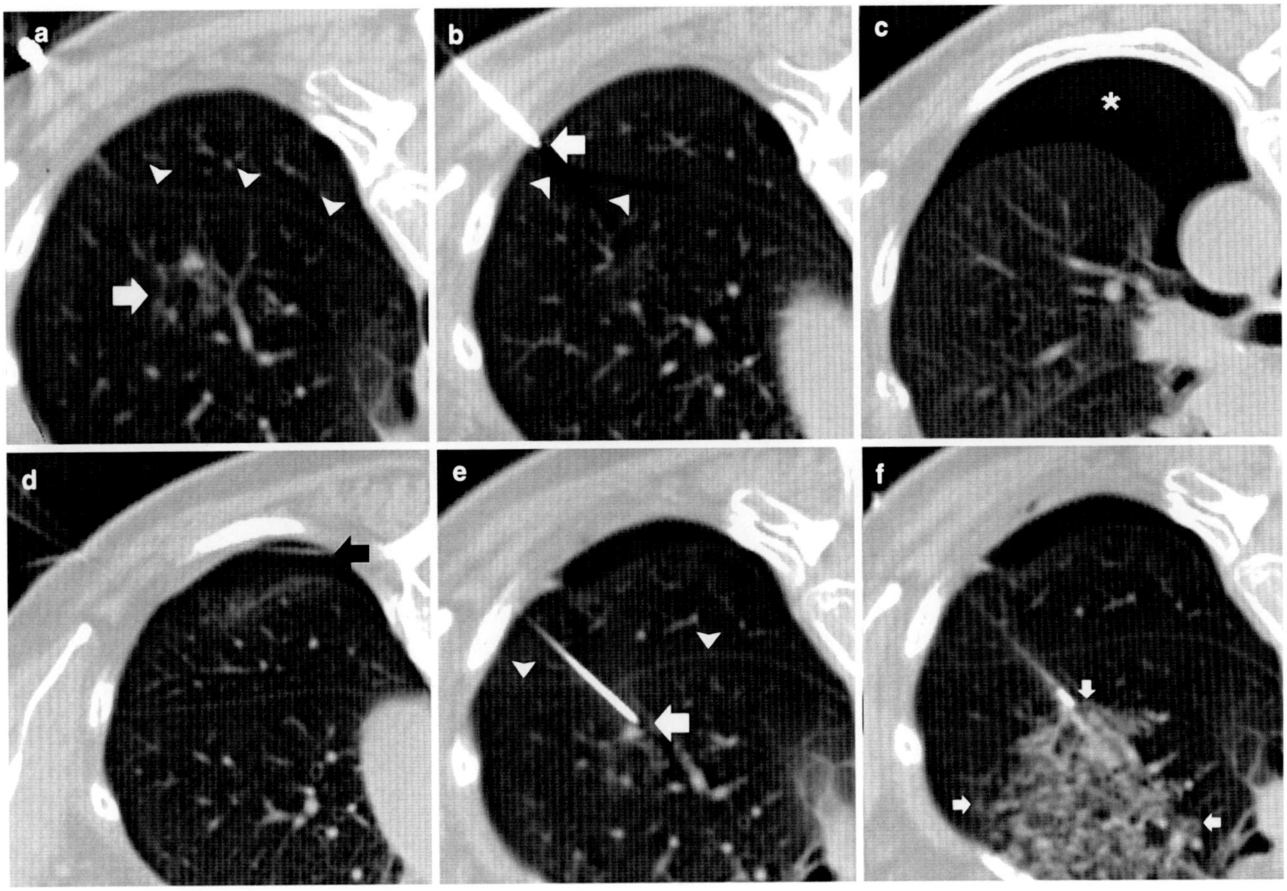

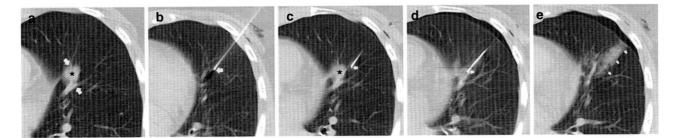

Fig. 11.7 Early pneumothorax. (**a**) Pre-biopsy CT image demonstrates an 8 mm ground glass nodule (*arrow*) within the left upper lobe in close proximity to the oblique fissure (*arrowheads*). (**b**) Following placement of a 19-gauge coaxial needle, the tip (*arrow*) is seen 3 mm into the thoracic cavity resulting in a premature pneumothorax with air tracking into the oblique fissure (*arrowheads*). (**c**) Repeat imaging demonstrates an enlarging pneumothorax (*) consistent with a persistent air leak. (**d**) Interval placement of a small angiocatheter (*black arrow*) with interval decrease in size of the pneumothorax status post aspiration. (**e**) A second 19-gauge coaxial needle is advanced into the target lesion via a transfissural route (*arrowheads*) to complete the procedure despite the air leak. (**f**) Following needle tip confirmation within the nodule, multiple 20-gauge core needle samples were obtained with development of perinodule hemorrhage (*arrows*). Biopsy results demonstrated invasive adenocarcinoma with bronchoalveolar cell features

Fig. 11.8 Abronchovascular route. (**a**) Pre-biopsy CT image demonstrates a spiculated 15 mm nodule (*) within the lingula intimately associated with the pulmonary vasculature (*arrows*). (**b**) A 19-gauge coaxial needle (*arrow*) is carefully advanced towards the target lesion. (**c**) Utilizing the abronchovascular plane, the needle (*arrow*) is slowly advanced into the centrally located target lesion (*). (**d**) Following needle tip confirmation, multiple 20-gauge core needle samples were carefully obtained with development of perinodule hemorrhage. (**e**) Upon removal of the coaxial needle, the patient's blood is injected into the needle tract (*arrows*) with a small but stable pneumothorax. Biopsy results demonstrated invasive adenocarcinoma with bronchoalveolar cell features

and physical examination are necessary, with special attention given to the patient's cardiopulmonary status and ability to cooperate, including the ability to perform adequate breath hold and the ability to lie still for an extended period of time.

A thorough evaluation of the patient's medication history is important, with attention paid to anticoagulant and antiplatelet medications, as these need to be discontinued prior to the procedure. Patients on warfarin require conversion to

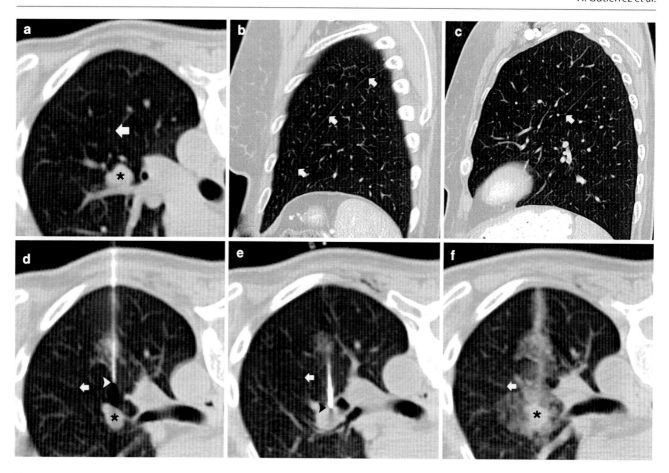

Fig. 11.9 Incomplete fissure. (**a**) Baseline axial CT image shows a centrally located 15 mm nodule (*) in the left upper lobe with an incomplete oblique fissure (*arrow*) seen posterior and lateral to the pulmonary nodule. (**b**) Sagittal multiplanar reformats demonstrates a complete left oblique fissure (*arrows*) laterally. (**c**) Sagittal multiplanar reformats medial to that in (**b**) confirms that the left oblique fissure is incomplete (*arrow*) medially. (**d**) and (**e**) The incomplete fissure is again seen (*arrows*) allowing the 19-gauge coaxial needle to approach the left upper lobe nodule (*) via the preferred posterior approach through the left lower lobe. (**f**) Following needle tip confirmation within the nodule, multiple 20-gauge core needle samples were carefully obtained with development of mild hemorrhage surrounding the nodule (*). Biopsy results demonstrated metastatic melanoma within an intrapulmonary lymph node

subcutaneous or low molecular weight heparin, which is then stopped at least 24 h before the procedure. Aspirin and clopidogrel bisulfate should be discontinued for at least 7 days. Increasingly, patients may require biopsy while on or immediately after non-chemotherapeutic systemic therapy, such as bevacizumab, and in these situations, additional precautions should be undertaken. Review of a recent electrocardiogram (ECG) and pulmonary function tests (PFTs) is particularly important in patients with comorbid heart and/or lung disease or prior resection. Many patients undergoing TNB are or have been smokers, and PFTs may be obtained to establish adequacy of oxygenation, pulmonary reserve, and flow-volume spirometry. Recent CT, magnetic resonance (MR), and computed tomography-positron emission tomography (CT-PET) scans should be available to ensure amenability of biopsy and to preliminary map out a safe needle path. In addition, the preprocedure CT demonstrates comorbid disease in the lung and the location and relationship of the lesion to vital structures, emphysema, and bulla.

Day of the Procedure

An informed consent for the procedure and other specific interventions should be obtained, detailing the benefits, risks, and alternatives. Laboratory data, including prothrombin time (PT), partial thromboplastin time (PTT), international normalized ratio (INR), and on minor occasion, bleeding time (BT) are required the day of the procedure or at least within the past 7 days, especially if the patient is on anticoagulation. A complete blood count (CBC), including hemoglobin and hematocrit, white count, and, most importantly, platelets, is recommended. Creatinine should be obtained if the administration of iodinated contrast is required to delineate vascular

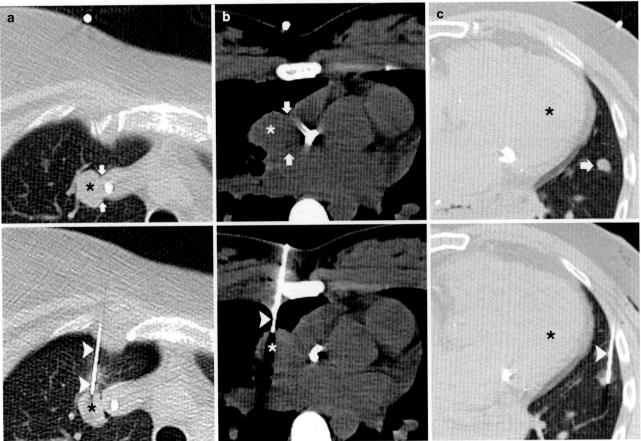

Fig. 11.10 Parallel approach: three different patients undergoing TCNB. (**a**) Pre-biopsy CT image demonstrates a right upper lobe nodule (*) adjacent to the superior vena cava (*arrows*). A 19-gauge coaxial needle (*arrowheads*) is advanced into the lung parallel to the mediastinum with the tip in the target lesion (*). Biopsy results demonstrated metastatic synovial sarcoma. (**b**) Pre-biopsy CT image demonstrates a right upper lobe nodule (*) adjacent to the right atrium (*arrows*). A 19-gauge coaxial needle (*arrowhead*) is advanced into the lung parallel to the heart with the tip in the target lesion (*). Biopsy results demonstrated lymphoma. (**c**) Pre-biopsy CT image demonstrates a lingula nodule (*arrow*) in close proximity to the left ventricle (*). A 19-gauge coaxial needle (*arrowhead*) is advanced into the lung parallel to the heart with the tip in the nodule. Biopsy results demonstrated dense fibrous tissue with chronic lymphoplasmacytic inflammation

structures and non-necrotic tumor margins. Every patient should have adequate peripheral intravenous access.

Breathing Instructions

Different techniques are used with regard to patient breath holding during the procedure and needle insertion, specifically consistent or constant volume breath holds versus continuous shallow breathing. When performing a TNB in a fully cooperative patient, constant volume breath holds allow for a relatively predictable nodule position resulting in shorter procedure times. The patient is instructed to take a small and comfortable breath that can be reproduced and held for 10–15 s. This is particularly helpful when biopsying small nodules near the diaphragm, cardiomediastinal structures, lingula, and right middle lobe, where any degree of respiratory motion can result in a significant change in the relative position of the needle, lesion, and surrounding vital nontarget structures [1, 2, 18].

Alternatively, for those patients who cannot hold their breath in a consistent fashion, allowing them to perform continuous shallow breathing takes the unpredictable changes in lung volume out of the equation. This requires an understanding of the nodule, needle, and entry site relationship throughout the respiratory cycle based on available imaging (fluoroscopy, CT, and CT fluoroscopy). Depending on the phase of the respiratory cycle, adjustments are made based on the relative position of the nodule and the needle, and additional adjustments are made accordingly as the patient is breathing [1, 18].

In addition, breathing instruction can be altered during the procedure to aid in nodule localization. Understanding the effect that breathing has on a nodule based on the volume can aid in instructing the patient to take a shallower or deeper breath depending on the relative needle and lesion position.

As a general rule, inspiration resulting in deeper volumes has the effect of moving the nodule in a caudal direction, and expiration resulting in shallower volumes has the effect of moving the nodule in a cranial direction. Thus, if attempts have failed to steer the needle to the nodule, intra-procedural breathing instructions may be altered to bring the nodule in line with the needle. Note is made that a lesion closer to the diaphragm demonstrates a greater degree of movement with variation in lung volume [1].

Sedation

Transthoracic needle biopsy is performed primarily as an outpatient procedure with preferably no or minimal conscious sedation as the patient is required to maintain an appropriate level of consciousness for cooperation and monitoring. If conscious sedation is required, a typical conscious sedation protocol includes midazolam and/or morphine sulfate titrated slowly to achieve the appropriate level of comfort. In addition, the antitussive effect of morphine is an added benefit to help decrease the incidence of significant coughing episodes. In certain circumstances, operators have used deep conscious sedation and even general anesthesia [19], in patients who are unable to lay still, breath hold, and in children. The advantages of deep conscious sedation and general anesthesia include a controlled patient environment, greater degree of intra-procedural patient comfort, better control of the airway, and the presence of an expert in cardiopulmonary management in case of a complication. The disadvantages of general anesthesia include higher cost, logistical challenges requiring a second participating service, longer procedure times related to anesthesia setup and availability, higher potential for pneumothorax due to positive pressure ventilation, and the risks specific to deep sedation and general anesthesia.

Imaging

Percutaneous TNB can be performed under fluoroscopy, CT, CT fluoroscopy, or ultrasonography; the choice of image guidance modality is dependent upon the size and location of the lesion, the availability of imaging systems, and operator expertise. Localization of the lesion by chest radiography and CT is necessary to determine the method of biopsy. The depth of the lesion and its relation to the major airways and vasculature, fissures, mediastinum, and ribs are used to plan the biopsy route.

Traditionally, percutaneous TNB was performed under fluoroscopic guidance. This technique has the advantages of real-time visualization, short procedure duration, and low cost. However, because of its limited ability to localize small

lesions, to guide access to central lesions, and to avoid bullae and vascular structures in the needle track, fluoroscopy is now reserved for large, peripheral lesions [5, 6].

In most centers, CT is now the standard imaging modality for TNB. CT enables selection of a biopsy route with the shortest distance between pleura and lesion and allows access to central lesions, while avoiding airways and vessels, fissures, bullae, and pronounced emphysema (Fig. 11.11). In addition, CT aids in distinguishing necrotic from solid portions of the lesions and allows unequivocal documentation of the needle tip within the lesion (paramount in the interpretation of absence of malignant cells) [20]. Procedure duration, one of the most commonly cited drawbacks of CT guidance, has significantly decreased with the advent of CT fluoroscopy [21]. This is of particular importance in less cooperative patients. In addition, CT fluoroscopy offers the advantage of near real-time visualization of needle placement. Real-time imaging is important within the lung, where extensive respiratory movement is present, causing small target lesions to shift and even disappear from the scan plane during needle advancement. Lack of real-time imaging has been cited as one of the most considerable reasons why CT-guided biopsies are unsuccessful or need to be repeated [22]. CT fluoroscopy has been shown to facilitate biopsy of smaller lesions as well as lesions situated in less favorable locations such as those in the costophrenic recess or close to the mediastinum. One of the major concerns regarding CT fluoroscopy remains the increased operator-related radiation exposure (although patient-related radiation exposure is essentially unchanged) [21].

In some instances, TNB can be performed under ultrasound guidance. Major advantages of ultrasound include real-time visualization of needle placement, portability, ability to target nonvascular, non-necrotic portions of a mass for sampling, and lack of exposure to ionizing radiation. Like CT, ultrasound also increases the likelihood of a positive biopsy in cavitating lesions. Ultrasound-guided TNB is limited to regions that provide an adequate acoustic window to the lesion and is best suited for peripheral pulmonary or mediastinal masses that abut the pleura (Fig. 11.12) [5, 7].

Devices

A variety of needle sizes, tip designs, and sampling mechanisms are used in TNB. Ideally, a biopsy needle should maximize specimen yield while minimizing bleeding complications. Bleeding complications are avoided today by using needles smaller than 18 gauge. Both single- and multiple-pass coaxial needles have been used in percutaneous TNB. The coaxial technique, which involves inserting a thin inner needle through a larger outer needle positioned within the lesion, has several advantages over the

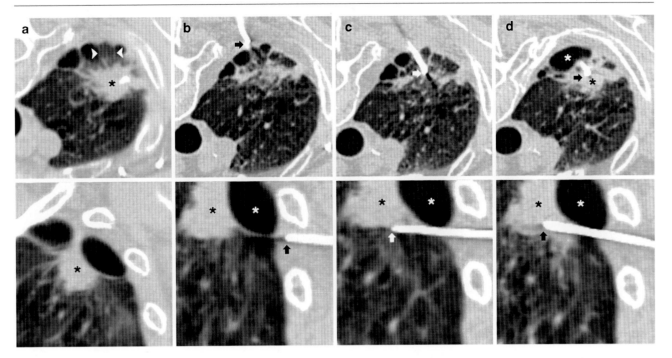

Fig. 11.11 Multiplanar reformats. (**a**) Axial (*top*) and sagittal (*bottom*) CT images demonstrates an irregular right apical nodule (*black* *) with surrounding emphysema and peripheral bullae. An intact secondary pulmonary lobule (*arrowheads*) is seen peripheral to the nodule and surrounded by bullae. (**b**) Axial (*top*) image demonstrates placement of a 19-gauge coaxial needle in the posterior chest wall with the tip in the extrapleural space (*arrow*) in the expected path to the target lesion. Sagittal (*bottom*) reformat images demonstrates the exact relationship of the target nodule (*black* *), bulla (*white* *), and needle tip (*arrow*).

(**c**) Axial (*top*) image demonstrates advancement of 19-gauge coaxial needle into the lung via the intact secondary pulmonary lobule. The sagittal (*bottom*) reformat image demonstrates the needle tip (*arrow*) inferior to the bulla (white *) and target lesion (*black* *). (**d**) Axial (*top*) image demonstrates repositioning of the 19-gauge coaxial needle into the target lesion (*black* *). The sagittal (*bottom*) reformat image confirms needle tip (*arrow*) placement into the nodule (*black* *) while avoiding the bulla (*white* *). Biopsy results demonstrated a fibroelastic scar with apical fibrous cap

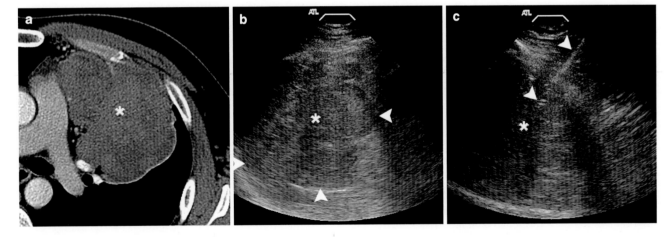

Fig. 11.12 Ultrasound biopsy. (**a**) Contrast-enhanced axial CT image demonstrates a large enhancing mass (*) within the left hemithorax abutting the chest wall providing an adequate acoustic window. (**b**) Grey-scale ultrasound image demonstrates a heterogenous predominantly hypoechoic mass (*) with the lung-mass interface clearly delineated (*arrowheads*). (**c**) Utilizing ultrasound guidance, a 19-gauge coaxial needle (*arrowheads*) is advanced into the mass (*). Biopsy results demonstrated a poorly differentiated carcinoma

single-needle technique, including limitation of the number of pleural punctures, easy repositioning of the needle, and the possible use of techniques to prevent leakage of air [18].

The biopsy needles currently used in TNB can be divided into two broad categories: aspirating and cutting needles

[7]. Commonly used aspirating needles include the Chiba, spinal, Westcott, and Greene needles, most ranging in size from 20 to 22 gauge [6]. Aspirating needles, when accurately placed within the lesion of interest, can provide high-quality cellular material for the diagnosis of malignancy [7]. When

TNB is used to isolate causative organisms in pneumonia or lung abscess, a 22-gauge Chiba or spinal needle usually provides an adequate specimen [7]. Cutting or core needles are generally larger than aspirating needles (usually 18–20 gauge) and are designed to provide histologic material using a circumferential cutting tip (e.g., Greene or Turner needles), a receptacle slot proximal to the tip (e.g., Westcott needle), an automated spring-loaded end cut or side-notched device (e.g., ASAP or Temno, Angiotech needles), or a drill bit stylet contained within a guiding cannula [7]. Core biopsy is best suited for large (>3 cm) peripheral lesions that abut the pleura; however, its use in the diagnosis of smaller (<3 cm) lesions has been reported [23] and increasingly more common. Coaxial models with small diameters have become available, allowing multiple core specimens to be obtained with a single pleural puncture [24]. Debate exists in the literature as to whether cutting needles offer any advantage over fine-needle aspiration in the diagnosis of malignancy [25, 26], but with the advent of molecular profiling, the importance in obtaining core samples is well established [1–4]. In addition, cutting needles are felt to be more accurate in the specific diagnosis of benign lesions, lymphoma, and in the setting where expert cytopathology is unavailable [24, 27, 28]. The two techniques are often used in complementary fashion, with cutting needles proposed when the diagnosis of malignancy is not made with fine-needle aspiration [29]. The initial choice between fine-needle aspiration and core needle biopsy depends on several factors, including operator expertise, the risk of complication, and the availability of an on-site cytopathologist. The use of core biopsy is now preferred in the current era of molecular profiling, in the absence of an on-site pathologist, and when the diagnosis of benign lesion or lymphoma is suspected [1–4, 24, 27, 28].

Biopsy Technique

The goal in performing TNB is to obtain sufficient material for diagnosis and characterization while minimizing potential complications. Special techniques may be utilized in TNB to maximize diagnostic yield and to avoid and/or minimize significant complications. These techniques are especially important when performing TNB in high-risk patients with significant cardiopulmonary disease as the potential impact of having to repeat a false-negative biopsy or experiencing a complication in these patients is much greater [15]. The following section outlines the biopsy process while focusing on various techniques that have been described to maximize success and to minimize potential complications. These include patient positioning, needle advancement, enhanced targeting, and procurement and evaluation of the specimen.

Patient positioning on the CT table warrants special attention as proper positioning is crucial for maximizing patient comfort and procedural success while minimizing potential complications. In general, the patient should be positioned so that the skin entry site allows the shortest, most vertical path to the lesion while avoiding fissures, bullae, major airways, and prominent vasculature. The shortest distance from skin to the tumor is optimal, although a lateral approach is less favorable due to the increased and opposite motion of ribs to the lungs during breathing, making needle placement difficult while increasing the risk of an air leak (Fig. 11.13). When equivocal, a posterior approach with the patient in the prone position is preferable to an anterior approach with the patient in the supine position, because the posterior ribs are less subject to respiratory variation and maintain a more consistent intercostal window with less need to rely upon breathing techniques (Fig. 11.14) [30]. In addition, since it is preferable for the patient to lie with the biopsy site dependent after completion of the procedure, lying supine postprocedure for an extended period of time is generally easier for the patient. If a supine position is required, an anterior parasternal approach is the next preferred route.

Once the patient is adequately positioned, an initial CT is performed that allows confirmation and final planning of a careful needle path. In general, access should pass over the superior margin of the rib to minimize the probability of intercostal artery or vein injury (Fig. 11.15), should avoid traversing bullae or interlobar fissures, and should avoid injury of essential nontarget structures. This often involves maneuvering around obstacles, including the osseous structures, blood vessels, and visceral pleura. Whenever possible, a needle path through abnormal lung and/or pleura including consolidation, postsurgical, or radiation scar should be chosen to minimize potential complications, e.g., pneumothorax [31]. In the prone position, the scapula is often the most difficult osseous structure around which to navigate. The scapula can be rotated out of the way by the following mechanism first described by Yankelevitz; the patient is positioned so that the arm of the ipsilateral side of the nodule is by his or her side and is then externally rotated (Fig. 11.16). This usually rotates the scapula out of the way; however, if the scapula remains an obstacle, the patient is rotated so that the side with the nodule is in a less dependent position. A pillow or towel roll may be placed under the side with the nodule, allowing more space for the scapula to move laterally when the arm is externally rotated [30].

The ribs may also block direct access to a lesion. One approach uses basic geometric principles to choose a plane that starts superior or inferior to the rib. The needle is placed above or below the obstructing rib and angulated inferiorly or superiorly, respectively, toward the nodule. Using several contiguous axial images, the craniocaudal needle angle can be estimated and the needle appropriately advanced (Fig. 11.14). This can be done with or without angling of the CT gantry [32]. When angling the gantry, once the plane

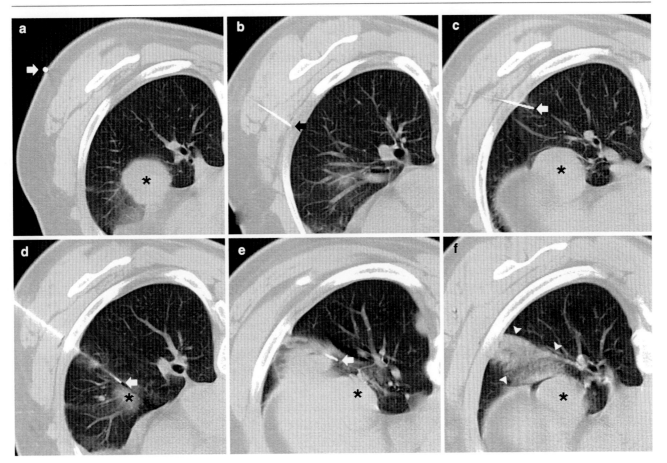

Fig. 11.13 Lateral approach. (**a**) Pre-biopsy CT image demonstrates a 3 cm mass (*) within the left lower lobe with a radiopaque marker on the lateral chest wall (*arrow*) indicating a lateral approach. (**b**) A 19-gauge coaxial needle is placed in the left lateral chest wall with the tip (*arrow*) located superior to the plane of the target lesion (not seen). (**c**) The 19-gauge coaxial needle is repositioned and advanced into the lung with the tip (*arrow*) now in plane with the target lesion (*). However, given increased motion of the lateral ribs, the tip is now displaced posteriorly (*arrow*). (**d**) The 19-gauge coaxial needle is repositioned and advanced further into the lung with the tip (*arrow*) now directed towards the target (*), but given marked increased motion of the lateral ribs, the tip is now displaced superiorly (*arrow*). (**e**) The increased and opposite motion of the ribs to the lungs during breathing and multiple attempts to position the needle tip (*arrow*) within the lesion (*) were unsuccessful with interval development of pulmonary hemorrhage. (**f**) Due to increasing pulmonary hemorrhage (*arrowheads*), the procedure was terminated without obtaining an adequate specimen

has been selected, the needle is inserted parallel to this new plane, allowing direct visualization of the needle as it avoids the rib, crosses the intercostal space and pleura, and enters the lesion. Using these techniques, TNB can be performed with relative ease, even for small nodules adjacent to an obstructing rib [33]. In addition to the osseous structures, it is sometimes necessary to maneuver around prominent or pertinent vasculature. Positioning the patient's arm either up or down can alter vascular anatomy, allowing vessels to be avoided. For instance, raising the patient's arms moves the axillary artery and vein superiorly, facilitating biopsy of an upper lobe lesion [34].

To minimize the risk of a pneumothorax, various techniques can be employed to avoid transgression of the visceral pleura adjacent to aerated lung. For example, extrapleural infusion of normal saline has been described as a technique for improving the safety of large-bore biopsies of subpleural

pulmonary lesions (Fig. 11.17) [35]. Other techniques for avoiding pleural transgression include a pleural space approach through a preexisting or iatrogenically induced pleural effusion and lateral decubitus positioning [34].

Following patient positioning and route selection, needle selection and advancement must be planned. The site of entry is marked using a radiopaque grid or radiopaque marker, like a lead ball (Fig. 11.18a). Once the skin entry site is confirmed with repeat imaging, it is prepped with antiseptic solution and draped with sterile towels. Consider a wider area of preparation to allow for possible chest tube placement especially in high-risk patients [15]. After cutaneous anesthesia is achieved, a coaxial needle is directed to the pleural surface (Fig. 11.6), where liberal local anesthetic is deposited to achieve pleural anesthesia, as previously described (see Anatomic Considerations, above). In addition to careful positioning within the extrapleural space, the

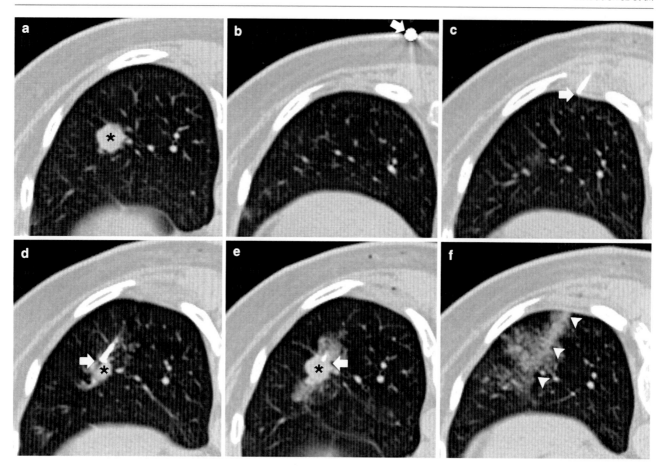

Fig. 11.14 Angulated approach. (**a**) Pre-biopsy CT image demonstrates a 20 mm nodule within the left lower lobe (*). (**b**) Given proximity to the diaphragm and spleen, an angulated inferior to superior approach was planned with the radiopaque marker (*arrow*) placed inferior to the target nodule. (**c**) A 19-gauge coaxial needle tip (*arrow*) is placed in the extrapleural space with subsequent administration of pleural anesthesia. Note that only the tip of the needle is seen at this level indicating the angulated inferior to superior approach. (**d**) The 19-gauge coaxial needle is advanced into the lung with only the tip now seen adjacent to the nodule (*) again indicating the angulated inferior to superior approach. (**e**) Following needle tip confirmation (*arrow*) within the nodule (*), multiple core needle samples were obtained with minimal hemorrhage anterior to the nodule indicating the throw of the biopsy gun. (**f**) Post-biopsy images demonstrate a small amount of perinodular hemorrhage and autologous blood along the parenchymal needle tract (*arrowheads*). Biopsy results demonstrated a metastatic colorectal adenocarcinoma

needle must be directed in such a manner where all major adjustments are performed in the chest wall so that the needle is directed along the appropriate path to the target lesion. By positioning the needle in an appropriate trajectory within the chest wall, only minor intrapulmonary adjustments will be required and thus further minimizing potential complications (Fig. 11.18).

Since even a slight misalignment can cause the needle tip to miss its target, meticulous planning and needle control are crucial. In patients with a thin body habitus or if a lateral approach is required, there may not be sufficient soft tissue to anchor the needle in the chest wall along the appropriate needle path. This can be corrected by using sterile towels or a needle holder to position the needle in the chest wall prior to entering the lung (Fig. 11.18) [1]. In addition, the use of bevel steering can further compensate for potential needle misalignment allowing for more precise needle control

[36, 37]. Bevel steering relies on the principle that the needle travels in the direction opposite to the bevel. If the needle is found to be off course, it is partially withdrawn, rotated so that the bevel faces in a direction opposite to the intended direction change, and then readvanced. Lastly, for deep lesions and in patients with a thick chest wall, performing a major adjustment at the skin level will be translated as a minor adjustment at the needle tip. By moving the needle, surrounding skin, and underlying muscles in unison in the intended direction (Fig. 11.19), the needle tip can be steered to the target lesion when prior attempts have failed.

For fluoroscopic or ultrasound-guided biopsies, the position of the needle can be checked and appropriately readjusted during advancement. Although a vertical approach to the lesion is usually preferred, an alternative approach is sometime necessary. For instance, subpleural lesions situated along the anterolateral or posterolateral lung are best

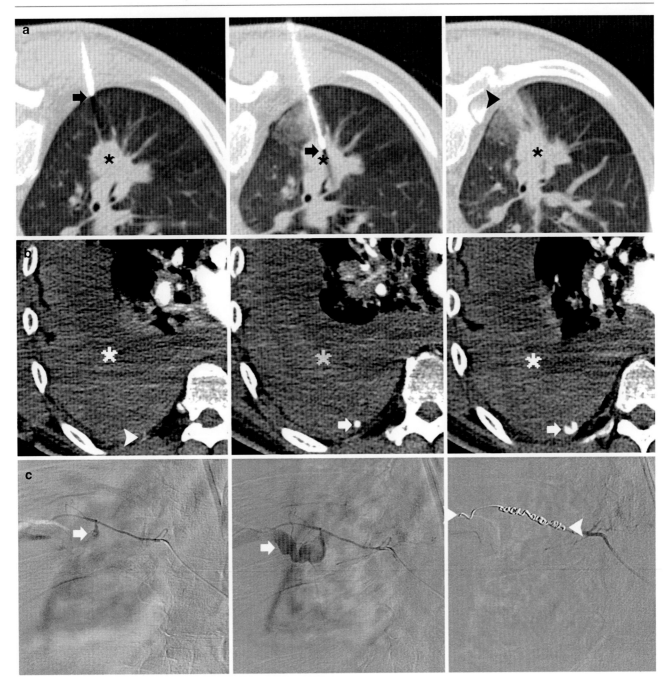

Fig. 11.15 Intercostal artery injury. (**a**) CT-guided biopsy of an irregular right lower lobe mass (*) with adequate placement of a 19-gauge coaxial needle (*arrows*). Post-biopsy image demonstrates a small amount of perinodular hemorrhage and autologous blood along the parenchymal needle tract without evidence of a chest wall hematoma (*arrowhead*). Biopsy results demonstrated a moderately differentiated adenocarcinoma. (**b**) Following hemodialysis and patient decompensation, a CT angiogram of the chest demonstrated a large hematoma (*) in the extrapleural space with opacification of a small intercostal artery (*arrowhead*) in the location of the needle path. Sequential images inferiorly demonstrated an area of active contrast extravasation (*arrows*). (**c**) Conventional angiogram demonstrating active extravasation (*arrows*) from an intercostal artery with the final image demonstrating coil embolization (*arrowheads*) with cessation of the extravasation

approached obliquely through the anterior or posterior intercostal space via a tangential approach (Fig. 11.19) [7]. This continuously situates the needle tip at the intended biopsy site, prevents respiratory misregistration (the needle tip and lesion move together), and ensures that the needle remains in the lung in case of a pneumothorax.

As the needle approaches the target lesion, enhanced targeting with correlation to prior contrast-enhanced/metabolic imaging, the use of intra-procedural contrast administration and the use of intra-procedural thin slice and reformatted images allow for accurate placement of the needle tip within the lesion allowing for accurate specimen

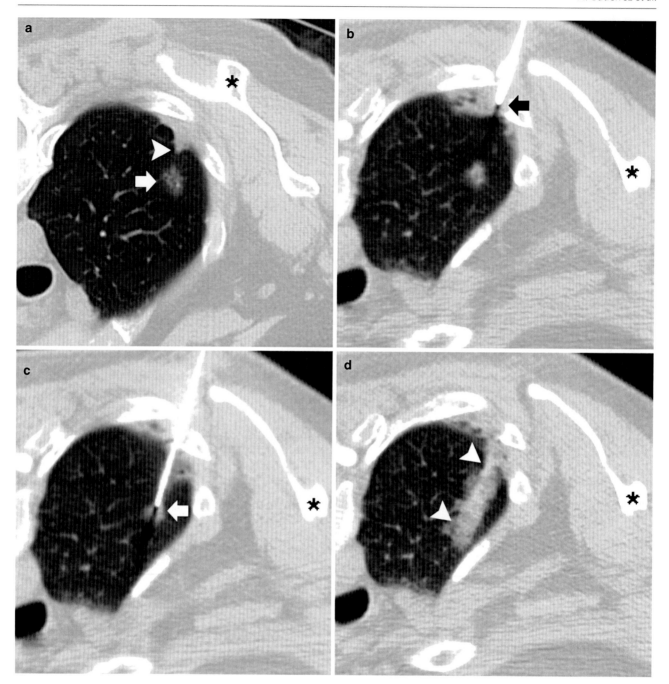

Fig. 11.16 Scapula maneuvers. (**a**) Pre-biopsy CT image demonstrates a 10 mm nodule within the right upper lobe (*arrow*) with an adjacent pleural-parenchymal scar (*arrowhead*). Note the scapula (*) obscuring the preferred route through the pleural-parenchymal scar. (**b**) Following repositioning of the arm by the patient's side and in external rotation, the scapula (*) is rotated laterally. A 19-gauge needle (*arrow*) is placed in the extrapleural space with administration of pleural anesthesia. (**c**) A 19-gauge coaxial needle is advanced into the lung with confirmation of the tip within the nodule (*arrow*). (**d**) Post-biopsy images demonstrate a small amount of perinodular hemorrhage and autologous blood along the parenchymal needle tract (*arrowheads*). Biopsy results demonstrated a bronchoalveolar cell carcinoma

yield. Correlation to prior contrast-enhanced CT/MR or CT-PET examinations allows for enhanced targeting by directing the needle tip to viable, metabolically active tumor allowing for improved specimen yield (Fig. 11.20). This is particularly important in cases where the target lesion is necrotic and/or surrounded by consolidated or atelectatic

lung (Fig. 11.20). Similarly intra-procedural contrast administration can help further differentiate viable tumor versus necrotic tumor and/or consolidated or atelectatic lung. In addition, intra-procedural contrast administration is useful in distinguishing the target lesion from surrounding vascular structures, especially for hilar lesions when

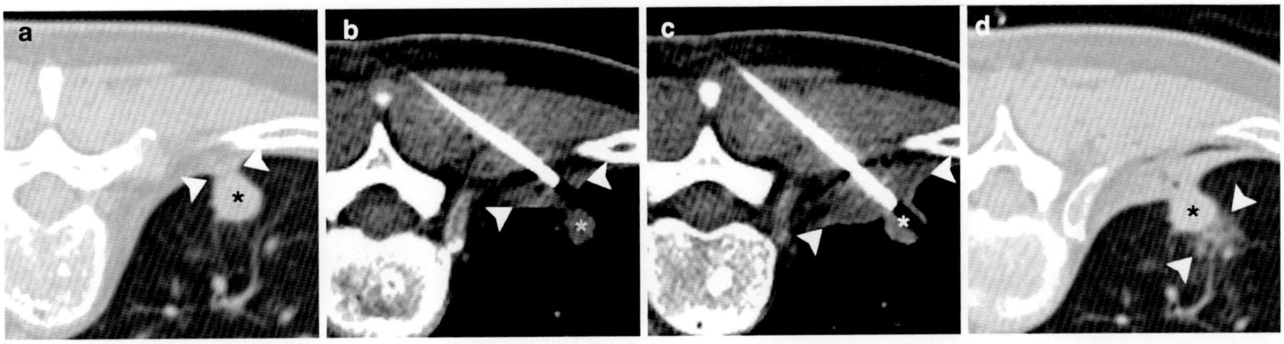

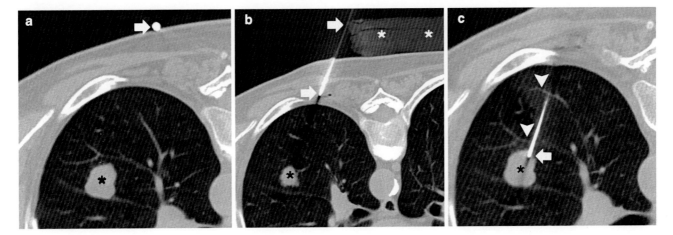

Fig. 11.17 Subpleural nodule: extrapleural infusion of normal saline. (**a**) Pre-biopsy CT image demonstrates a 14 mm nodule (*) within the right upper lobe with tethering of the adjacent pleura (*arrowheads*). (**b**) A 19-gauge coaxial needle is positioned with the tip in the extrapleural space with administration of pleural anesthesia (*arrowheads*) adjacent to the subpleural nodule (*). (**c**) Following the extrapleural infusion of normal saline (*arrowheads*), the coaxial needle is advanced through the enlarged extrapleural space toward the subpleural nodule (*). (**d**) Post-biopsy image demonstrates a small amount of perinodular hemorrhage (*arrowheads*) anterior to the nodule with air in the extrapleural space. Biopsy results demonstrated an adenocarcinoma with bronchoalveolar cell features

Fig. 11.18 Biopsy technique. (**a**) Pre-biopsy image demonstrates a 20 mm lobulated nodule (*) within the right lower lobe in close proximity to the oblique fissure with placement of a radiopaque marker (*arrow*) indicating the expected skin entry site. (**b**) A 19-gauge coaxial needle is placed in the right posterior chest wall with sterile towels (*) supporting the needle (*arrows*) in the expected path to the target lesion (*arrows*). (**c**) A 19-gauge coaxial needle tip (*arrow*) is placed into the nodule (*) while avoiding the larger vessels (*arrowheads*) in the biopsy path. Biopsy results demonstrated poorly differentiated adenocarcinoma

differentiation of the lesion from the surrounding hilar vessels is of utmost importance (Fig. 11.21).

Enhanced targeting for smaller lesions is important as partial volume averaging on CT can make the needle tip appear to be within the lesion when it is actually directly above or below. Misplacement of the needle tip can be avoided with the use of contiguous thin slices (1 mm). These images should be obtained in at least a group of three, using a slice thickness less than one half the diameter of the nodule. In this manner, the portion of the nodule not containing the needle tip can be seen above and below the slice that shows the needle tip within the lesion. In addition, volumetric acquisition of imaging data allows for computer reconstruction of three-dimensional (3D) volume data sets for pre-, intra-, and post-procedural analysis. Multiplanar reformatted (MPR) display of images both parallel to (long-axis views) and perpendicular to (short-axis views) the axis of the needle

can provide valuable information regarding depth of needle penetration, the exact position of the needle relative to the target lesion, and the relationship to essential and nontargeted structures (Fig. 11.22) [38].

New technologies have continued to improve enhanced targeting allowing for improved accuracy and safety. The development and refinement of navigation and image fusion technology has allowed the use of multiple modalities to create 3D maps of patient anatomy displaying needle position, orientation, and trajectory as well as anatomical landmarks. This will help guide needle tip placement to the target even if the lesion is small and hard to visualize, difficult to access, or close to vital nontarget structure [39]. Although these technologies have proven useful in other organ systems, multiple challenges still exist for their use in the lung, primarily lack of real-time imaging to evaluate for intra-procedural complications, such a pneumothorax.

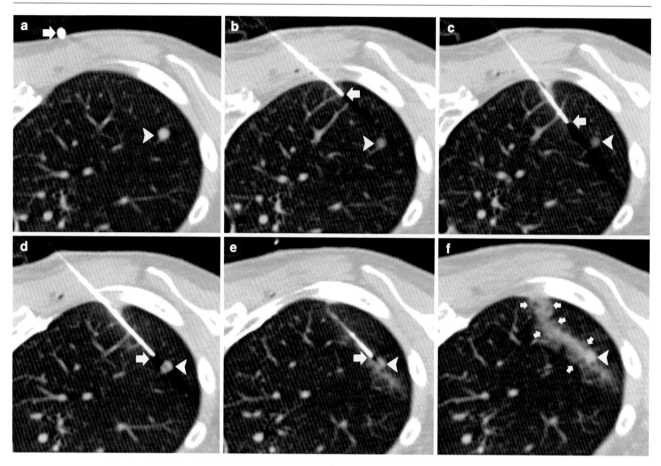

Fig. 11.19 Biopsy technique. (**a**) Pre-biopsy CT image demonstrates a 9 mm nodule (*arrowhead*) within the left upper lobe with placement of a radiopaque marker (*arrow*) indicating the expected skin entry site. (**b**) A 19-gauge coaxial needle tip (*arrow*) is carefully advanced into the lung (*arrow*) toward the target nodule (*arrowhead*) while avoiding the pulmonary vessels. (**c**) The 19-gauge coaxial needle is advanced in small increments while avoiding the vessels resulting in medial displacement of the needle tip (*arrow*) relative to the target nodule (*arrowhead*). (**d**) By moving the needle, surrounding skin, and underlying muscles in unison in a medial direction at the skin level and then advancing the needle, the needle tip (*arrow*) is steered in a lateral direction back in line with the nodule (*arrowhead*). (**e**) Following needle tip confirmation (*arrow*) within the nodule (*arrowhead*), multiple core needle samples were obtained with minimal hemorrhage anterior to the nodule indicating the throw of the biopsy gun. (**f**) Post-biopsy image demonstrates the autologous blood along the parenchymal needle tract (*arrowheads*) with note made of the abrupt turn near the pleural surface indicating the effect of steering. Biopsy results demonstrated a necrotizing granuloma with coccidioidomycosis

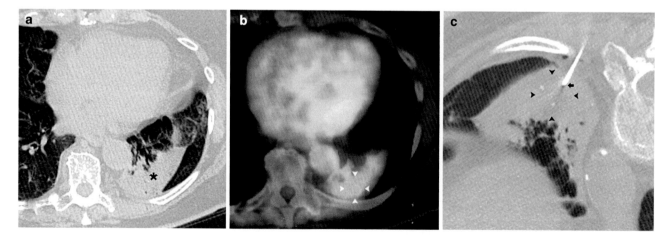

Fig. 11.20 Enhanced targeting: CT-PET correlation. (**a**) Supine axial CT image demonstrates a persistent left lower consolidation (*). B. Supine axial fused PET-CT image demonstrated focally intense hypermetabolic activity (*arrowheads*) within the central portion of the left lower lobe consolidation. (**c**) Prone axial CT image demonstrates placement of a 19-gauge coaxial needle (*arrow*) in the central portion of the left lower lobe consolidation that corresponds to the area of the focally intense hypermetabolic activity (*arrowheads*). Biopsy results demonstrated bronchoalveolar carcinoma

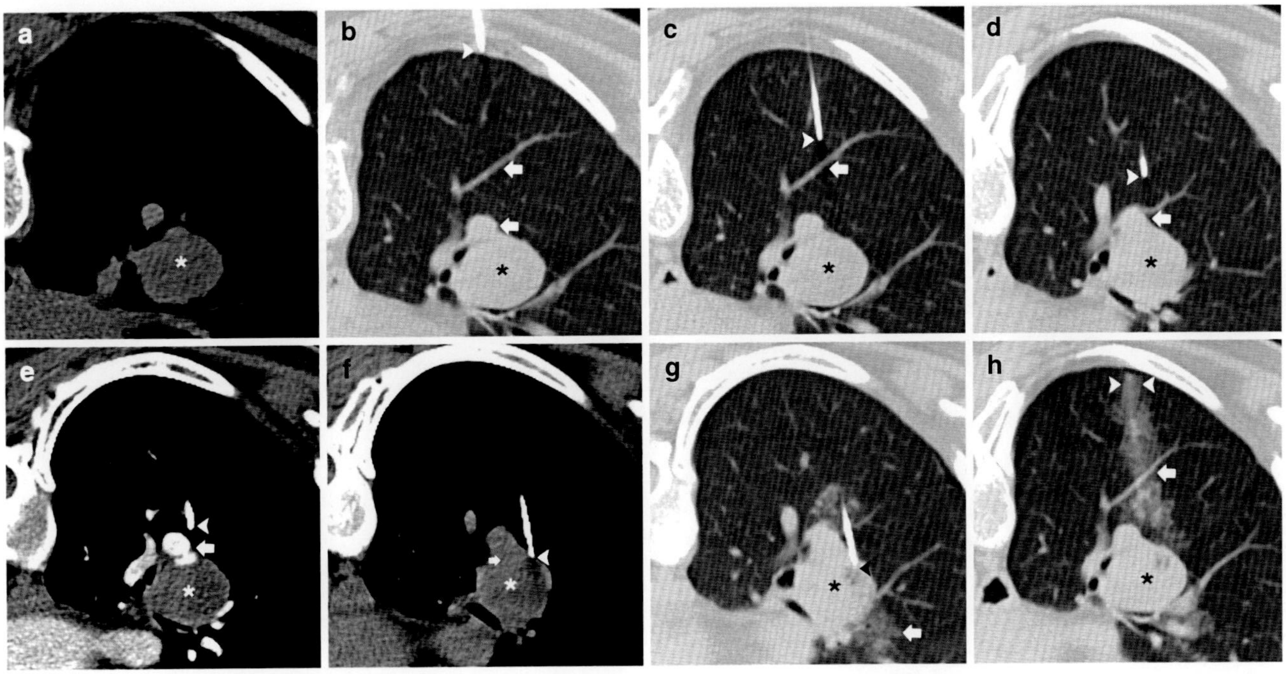

Fig. 11.21 Enhanced targeting: intra-procedural intravenous contrast. (a) Pre-biopsy CT image demonstrates a 3 cm right lower lobe perihilar mass (*). (b) A 19-gauge coaxial needle is positioned with the tip (*arrowhead*) in the extrapleural space with administration of pleural anesthesia with note made of pulmonary vessels (*arrows*) in close proximity to the expected needle path to the mass (*). (c) The 19-gauge coaxial needle tip (*arrowhead*) is carefully advanced into the lung toward the target mass (*) while stopping short of the pulmonary vessel (*arrow*). (d) The 19-gauge coaxial needle is steered superiorly and advanced a short distance with the tip (*arrowhead*) avoiding the vessel. (e) The 19-gauge coaxial needle is steered inferiorly and advanced a short distance with the tip (*arrowhead*) stopping short of the large hilar vessels (*arrow*). Following the administration of intravenous contrast, the hilar vessels are clearly delineated in relation to the needle path. (f) By moving the needle, surrounding skin, and underlying muscles in unison in a medial direction at the skin level and then advancing the needle, the needle tip (*arrowhead*) is steered in a lateral direction avoiding the hilar vessels (*arrow*) and into the mass (*). (g) Following needle tip confirmation (*arrowhead*) within the mass (*), multiple core needle samples were obtained with minimal hemorrhage (*arrow*) anterior to the mass indicating the throw of the biopsy gun. (h) Post-biopsy image demonstrates the autologous blood along the parenchymal needle tract extending to the pleural surface (*arrowheads*) without evidence of significant pulmonary hemorrhage with an intact pulmonary vessel (*arrow*). Biopsy results demonstrated metastatic melanoma

Following needle tip confirmation, an adequate specimen must be obtained. This can involve application of suction to the needle and withdrawal of the sample, as with aspiration techniques, or mechanical retrieval of the sample, as with automated devices. When TNB is performed on small lesions, even slight displacement of the needle can cause the tip to lie outside its intended position. Therefore, it has been recommended that needles with gridlines on their shafts or ones with attachable depth markers be used to control the depth of needle advancement (Fig. 11.3b). With aspiration techniques utilizing a coaxial system, the smaller aspirating needle needs to be longer than the coaxial needle to allow sampling of the lesion from multiple locations. The syringe should be large enough to achieve maximal suction while being easy to handle (usually either a 10- or 20-mL syringe). One study showed that the majority of carcinomas contain a reactive zone of variable thickness, representing approximately 10 % of the total tumor diameter [40], reinforcing the idea that multiple samples should be taken from several parts of a lesion. The wall of a necrotic or cavitary lesion should be carefully sampled. Because malignant cells tend to desquamate (especially in squamous cell carcinoma), aspiration of necrosis is also suggested [5]. When the specimen has been obtained, the pathologist must advise the radiologist as to whether an adequate specimen has been attained. The presence of an on-site expert cytopathologist is extremely valuable as it enables rapid assessment of the sample so that repeated aspirations or cutting needle biopsy can be performed immediately if necessary.

Post-procedure and Disposition

Following TNB, patients are placed in the puncture-site-down position and observed for potential complications from the procedure. Instructions are given for the patient to lie in the puncture-site-down position for at least 2 h post-procedure while minimizing any activities that will increase intrathoracic pressures including coughing, excessive talking, sitting up in bed without assistance, deep breathing, lifting, and straining [7, 18]. Patients should be observed and monitored in the postanesthesia care unit with regular vital signs (initially every 15 min

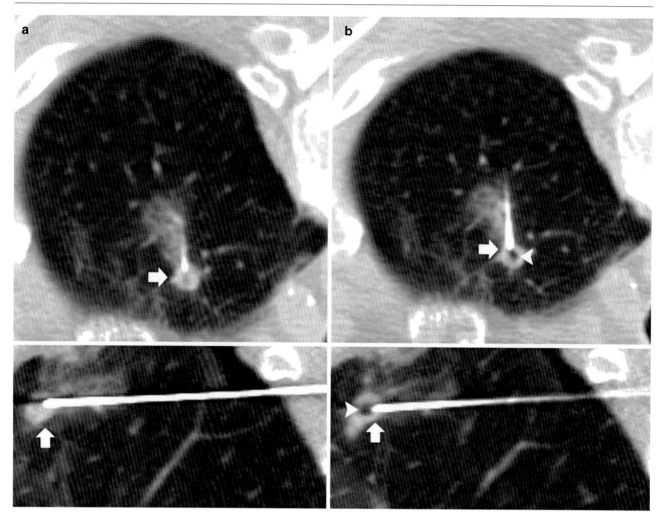

Fig. 11.22 Multiplanar reformats: needle tip confirmation. (**a**) Axial (*top*) image demonstrates an 8 mm left upper lobe with placement of a 19-gauge coaxial needle tip in the nodule (*arrow*) as confirmed by the sagittal (*bottom*) image (*arrow*). (**b**) Axial (*top*) and sagittal (*bottom*) CT images again demonstrates the coaxial needle tip (*arrows*) within the nodule status post core needle biopsy with interval development of air within the nodule (*arrowheads*) demonstrating adequate positioning. Biopsy results demonstrated an infectious granuloma

for 1 h) and continuous pulse oximetry. An upright expiratory chest radiograph should be obtained within 1–2 h of the procedure, and a second upright expiratory chest radiograph should be obtained 3–4 h post-procedure. Chest radiographs are obtained to exclude or follow-up immediate complications, such as a pneumothorax, hemothorax, and pulmonary hemorrhage. If pleural air is present, serial chest x-rays are required to determine if an air leak is present and to determine if further intervention is required. Some authors advocate allowing the patient to sit up or act as if they were at home prior to the final chest x-ray to ensure that a delayed pneumothorax does not develop with daily activities [18]. Post-procedure pain control if required is usually controlled with oral analgesics.

Depending on the patient's clinical course and assessment, most patients are routinely discharged on the same day within 3–4 h of the procedure. Admitting a patient for observation or further therapy is dependent on multiple factors including the size of a pneumothorax and the presence or absence of an air leak. In addition, the patient's home situation and location is

just as important when deciding to admit or discharge. Patients who can tolerate a pneumothorax with or without a chest tube, who have a responsible caretaker at home and/or live in close proximity to a hospital, may be discharged home with strict instructions and close follow-up. Patients and caregivers are instructed to monitor for symptoms or signs related to a delayed complication including shortness of breath, inability to catch their breath, dull or pleuritic chest pain, and hemoptysis (more than a teaspoon of pure fresh blood). If any of these develop, they are instructed to go to the nearest emergency department. Patients are instructed to avoid physical activities, particularly those that abruptly increase intrathoracic pressures, i.e., those that result in a Valsalva maneuver. Most medical guidelines recommend delaying air travel for up to 3 weeks following resolution of pleural air (aviation guidelines) [41]. Airplane cabins are not fully pressurized to sea level, and exposure to this environment could potentially exacerbate a known or an occult pneumothorax. However, many operators allow post lung biopsy patients to travel by air following a

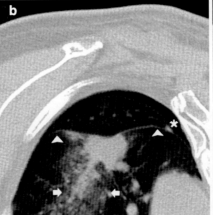
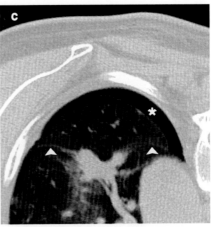

Fig. 11.23 Transfissural biopsy. (**a**) CT image demonstrates placement of a 19-gauge coaxial needle (*arrow*) within a 20 mm left upper lobe juxtafissural nodule through an intact oblique fissure (*arrowheads*). (**b**) Post-biopsy image demonstrates hemorrhage (*arrows*) anterior to the nodule indicating the throw of the biopsy gun with interval development of a small pneumothorax (***). (**c**) Delayed post-biopsy image demonstrated enlargement of the small pneumothorax (***), stressing the importance of avoiding fissures (*arrowheads*) as they result in transgression of four pleural surfaces rather than two. Biopsy results demonstrated invasive adenocarcinoma

24-h post-biopsy period if there was no pleural air or a small stable pneumothorax without a significant adverse event.

Written instructions and information detailing the above information is typically helpful for patients and family members and can also include the lung and lobe that was biopsied, whether a pneumothorax was present at discharge and if so the width in centimeters from the apex, this is particularly important if the patient returns to a different medical facility with post-procedure symptoms.

Potential Complications and Management

The most common complications of percutaneous lung biopsy are pneumothorax and bleeding [5]. Although most patients can tolerate a small pneumothorax or mild hemorrhage, when performing TNB in high-risk patients with significant cardiopulmonary disease or single functional or anatomic lung, even a small pneumothorax or mild hemorrhage may cause significant respiratory compromise. Thus, special techniques for preventing and managing complications as they occur are of paramount importance, particularly in high-risk patients.

Pneumothorax

Pneumothorax is the most common complication of TNB. The reported incidence of pneumothorax ranges from 0 to 61 %, 20 % in most large series, with 04–17 % (average 7 %) of patients requiring chest tube drainage [7]. Factors reported to be associated with a higher incidence of pneumothorax and chest tube insertion include obstructive airways disease, increased lesion depth, decreased lesion size, a small angle of the needle with the thoracic pleura, multiple pleural punctures, fissure and bulla transgression, small and deeply situated lesions, longer procedure duration, operator inexperience, and AIDS patients [31, 42–44].

Each of the factors implicated in producing pneumothorax should be minimized to the extent possible. Although there is generally not much that can be done about the status of the underlying lung parenchyma, it may be possible to choose a route for needle placement that minimizes that amount of disease lung transgressed. When possible, large bullae should be avoided (Fig. 11.11). The number of pleural punctures and the degree of needle manipulation within the lung should be minimized, and fissures should be avoided whenever possible, as they result in transgression of four pleural surfaces rather than two (Fig. 11.23). The time needed to perform the procedure must also be minimized. CT fluoroscopy, by shortening the length of the procedure and limiting the number of pleural punctures necessary to ensure accurate needle placement, may ultimately prove to decrease the incidence of a pneumothorax and subsequent chest tube placement, although this has yet to be proved.

Aspiration of air through indwelling biopsy needle or an angiocatheter has been reported to decrease the need for chest tube placement (Fig. 11.7) [45, 46]. Another technique that has been reported as both useful and effective in reducing chest tube placement following TNB is the use of a blood patch (Fig. 11.19) [47, 48]. With this technique, a small amount of the patient's clotted blood is injected into the needle tract, as the needle is withdrawn [47], most importantly the blood should be deposited in the peripheral 2 cm of the needle path. Lang et al. reported a significantly decreased incidence of chest tube placement with the use of a blood clot seal in 100 randomly assigned patients

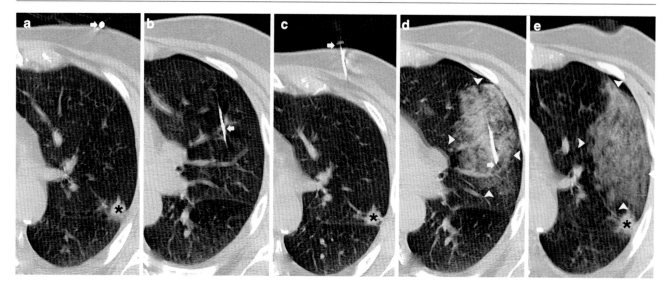

Fig. 11.24 Pulmonary hemorrhage. (**a**) Pre-biopsy CT image demonstrates an 18 mm nodule (*) within the juxtafissural left upper lobe with a radiopaque marker on the anterior chest wall (*arrow*). (**b**) A 19-gauge coaxial needle is advanced into the lung with the tip (*arrow*) in close proximity to a pulmonary artery. (**c**) The 19-gauge coaxial needle is advanced into the lung with the tip not seen in the same plane of the target nodule (*). Note is made of the coaxial needle hub (*arrow*) near the skin stressing the importance of selecting a needle with an appropriate length. (**d**) The 19-gauge coaxial needle tip (*arrow*) is repositioned and advanced further into the lung with interval development of significant pulmonary hemorrhage (*arrowheads*). (**e**) Due to increasing pulmonary hemorrhage (*arrowheads*), the procedure was terminated without obtaining an adequate specimen

undergoing TNB [47]. Alternatively, other investigators have reported a decreased incidence of pneumothorax with insertion of a collagen plug following needle withdrawal [49]. Positioning of the patient with the biopsy site dependent for at least 2 h following TNB has been shown to reduce post-biopsy pneumothorax [7]. In addition, supplemental nasal oxygen may be used to promote resorption of pleural air [45].

Most pneumothoraces are detected within the first hour after the procedure, do not require drainage, and can be managed conservatively with supplemental nasal oxygen [7]. If an air leak develops during follow-up, the patient should be placed in the puncture-side-down position, and repeat imaging is required to document stability of pleural air with a follow-up film following an hour of upright position. If an air leak returns, an additional cycle of puncture-side-dependent positioning and follow-up imaging may be attempted. However, radiologists performing lung biopsy should have a low threshold for chest tube insertion in high-risk patients, as even a small pneumothorax may cause significant ventilatory compromise [15, 18]. Long-term pleural drainage may be required for a persistent air leak despite conservative management, or for a large (>20–30 %) or symptomatic pneumothorax. A small-gauge drainage catheter (<16-French) can be placed in a relative quick and safe manner using either a direct trocar method versus guide wire approach. Once in place, the catheter can be connected to Pleur-evac suction or to a Heimlich valve depending on the rate of air leak (techniques) [15, 18].

Hemoptysis and Pulmonary Hemorrhage

Hemorrhage, with or without hemoptysis, is the second most common complication of TNB. Although most bleeding is self-limited, hemorrhage is considered by most to be the most dangerous potential complication of percutaneous lung biopsy [5]. Major intrathoracic hemorrhage causing cardiac tamponade and death has been reported [50, 51].

The risk of hemorrhage is reportedly increased with the use of cutting needles, in biopsy of mediastinal and paracardiomediastinal lesions, vascular lesions such as metastatic renal cell carcinoma, from enlarged bronchial artery branches associated with chronic cavities or bronchiectasis, and in patients with clotting disorders or pulmonary hypertension [2, 6, 52]. The use of fine needles for aspiration and biopsy has reduced the incidence of significant bleeding to 0–10 % with most series reporting an incidence of less than 5 % [40]. In addition, small-gauge (18–20 gauge) automated cutting needles are now widely available and do not appear to be associated with a significantly increased risk of hemorrhage compared with aspirating needles, particularly when their use is confined to lesions in the peripheral third of the lung [52]. Hemorrhage is characterized by the development of peri-lesional airspace and ground glass opacities on CT (Fig. 11.24).

If hemoptysis occurs, the patient should be placed with the biopsy site dependent to prevent transbronchial aspiration of blood. This maneuver usually suffices, and the hemoptysis usually resolves within minutes. If the hemorrhage continues or is more severe, bronchoscopic tamponade, arterial embolization, or surgery may be required. In addition, hemoptysis is often associated with coughing secondary to airway irritation. Severe coughing can result in pleural laceration and increases the risk of a pneumothorax. If pulmonary venous damage has occurred, the swings from negative (inspiration) to positive (coughing) intrathoracic pressure increases the risk for air embolism and Trendelenburg positioning may be added to facilitate clearance of blood and reduce the risk of an air embolus reaching the cerebral circulation [15].

Other Complications

Rare complications of TNB include systemic arterial air embolism, malignant seeding of the biopsy track, and vasovagal reaction. Systemic air embolism usually presents as sudden deterioration in the patient's neurologic status or with coronary ischemia or arrhythmia. The mechanism is thought to be either air entry through the needle directly into a pulmonary vein or the iatrogenic creation of a bronchovenous or alveolovenous fistula along the biopsy needle. Predisposing factors cited include coughing, biopsy of consolidated lung, cavitary or vascular masses, and an associated vasculitis [6]. To minimize the risk of air embolism, TNB should never be performed with the patient in an upright position, and the patient should be instructed not to cough, move, or talk during the procedure [53]. A styleted needle should be used to minimize exposure to the atmosphere [6]. In the event of suspected air embolism, patients should be placed in either the left lateral decubitus position or the Trendelenburg position to prevent residual air within the left atrium from systemically embolizing. Oxygen should be administered by face mask to promote resorption of air, and blood pressure and ventilator support should be provided. A whole body CT may be performed to evaluate the extent of air embolization and determine need for definitive therapy (Fig. 11.25). If possible, patients should be transferred immediately to a hyperbaric decompression chamber [54].

Malignant seeding of the biopsy track is another rare complication of TNB. An early report of two cases of pleural seeding following TNB led authors to recommend that TNB be reserved for inoperable lesion; however, subsequent large series have shown that this complication is extremely uncommon [55, 56]. A survey of the Society of Thoracic Radiology and literature review found an incidence of needle track metastasis of 0.012 %. Additional rare complications of TNB include vasovagal reaction and lung torsion [7].

Outcomes and Results

TNB is highly accurate for the diagnosis of intrathoracic malignancy, with most series reporting an overall sensitivity of 70–100 % [5, 7]. A large study involving 12,000 transthoracic needle aspirations reported a sensitivity of 89 %, specificity of 95 %, positive predictive value of 99 %, and negative predictive value of 70 % [57]. Even small lesions may be accurately evaluated, with Westcott et al. reporting a sensitivity of 93 % when sampling nodules <15 mm [58]. The most common causes for a false-negative biopsy are sampling error and inaccurate needle placement [5].

Another study showed TNB to be highly accurate in the diagnosis of hilar lymph node metastases [59]. This high success rate allows TNB to be offered as an alternative to transbronchial biopsy, mediastinoscopy, or thoracotomy in the nodal staging of lung cancer and confirmation of nodal metastases. With the use of cutting needles, TNB has a yield of cytology approximately 60–75 % in the diagnosis of lymphoma [7]. This technique provides material sufficient to guide therapy in 83–95 % of cases [7].

Perhaps the greatest limitation of TNB is in its ability to diagnose benign disease. Several large studies report an overall yield for benign disease of 88–97 %; however, a specific benign diagnosis was detected in only 16–68 % of cases [7]. This is a major drawback as a "negative" biopsy cannot reliably exclude malignancy (and thereby prevent a thoracotomy) unless a specific benign diagnosis can be made. Nonetheless, with sampling of multiple portions of a lesion, the use of cutting needles when repeated aspirations fail to show definitive evidence of malignancy, and expert cytopathology, the yield for benign lesions is increased [7]. Improvements in the design of cutting needles permit good samples to be obtained for histologic evaluation without significantly increasing patients' mortality [6].

TNB has long been used to diagnose pulmonary infection, particularly when other methods fail to isolate a causative organism. Castellino and Blank reported a diagnostic yield of 73 % from 108 biopsies in 82 immunocompromised patients suspected to have focal infection [9]. Conces et al. identified the causative organism in 35 of 46 patients ultimately found to have infection [10]. More recently, Grinan et al. described fluoroscopically guided needle aspiration in 49 patients with lung abscess, with a diagnostic yield of 82 % [60]. The results of TNB led to a change in antibiotic therapy in 47 % of these patients. TNB has also been shown to be of use in patients with acquired immunodeficiency syndrome (AIDS) and focal chest lesions that may be secondary to Kaposi's sarcoma, tuberculosis, and rarely pneumocystis pneumonia [61, 62]. Gruden et al. determined the cause of a focal lesion by TNB in 27 of 32 patients with AIDS [61]. Careful preparation of samples for microbiology is of utmost importance when TNB is performed in these patients.

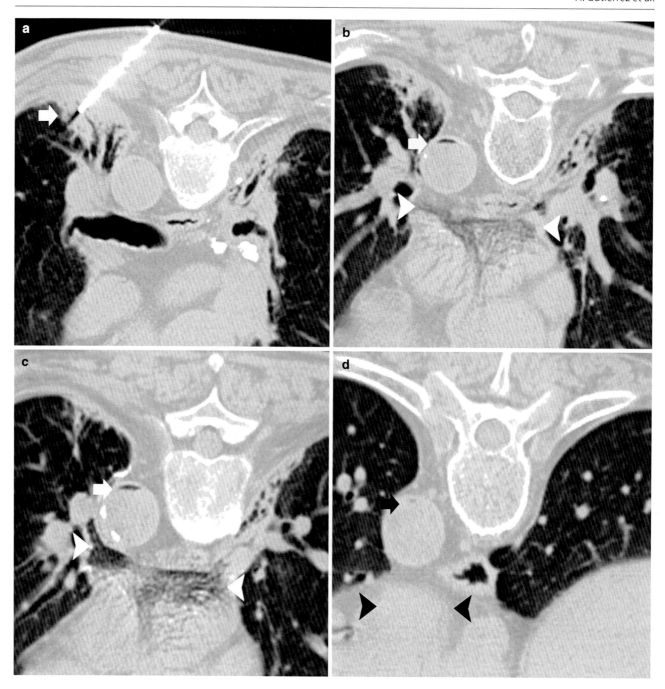

Fig. 11.25 Air embolism. (**a**) Axial CT image demonstrates placement of a 19-gauge coaxial needle (*arrow*) in the right lower lobe consolidation. Biopsy results demonstrated a dense fibroelastic scar. (**b** and **c**) Post-biopsy images demonstrated air within the descending aorta (*arrow*) and within the left atrium and right inferior pulmonary vein (*arrowheads*) consistent with an air embolism. (**d**) The patient was positioned in Trendelenburg with 100 % oxygen administered via face mask with repeat imaging of the entire body demonstrating resolution of air in the aorta (*arrow*) and left atrium (*arrowhead*) without new foci of systemic arterial air. Patient was admitted to ICU for 24-h observation without adverse events

Summary

Transthoracic needle biopsy is a widely used, reliable, and minimally invasive procedure for the diagnosis and characterization of indeterminate pulmonary lesions. With the continued improvement in imaging technology, needle design, biopsy technique, enhanced targeting, and strategies for preventing and managing potential complications, previously inaccessible pulmonary lesions can be biopsied in a safe and reliable manner. With the increasing role in diagnosing benign disease and with continued advances in molecular profiling and targeted therapy, transthoracic core needle biopsy will continue to flourish as a minimally invasive diagnostic procedure for pulmonary lesions.

References

1. Cham MD, Lane ME, Henschke CI, Yankelevitz DF. Lung biopsy: special techniques. Semin Respir Crit Care Med. 2008;29(4):335–49.

2. Moore EH. Percutaneous lung biopsy: an ordering clinician's guide to current practice. Semin Respir Crit Care Med. 2008;29(4):323–34.

3. Maemondo M, Inoue A, Kobayashi K, et al. Gefitinib or chemotherapy for non-small-cell lung cancer with mutated EGFR. N Engl J Med. 2010;362(25):2380–8.

4. Borczuk AC, Shah L, Pearson GD, et al. Molecular signatures in biopsy specimens of lung cancer. Am J Respir Crit Care Med. 2004;170(2):167–74.

5. Laurent F, Montaudon M, Latrabe V, et al. Percutaneous biopsy in lung cancer. Eur J Radiol. 2003;45:60–8.

6. Murphy JM, Gleeson FV, Flower CD. Percutaneous needle biopsy of the lung and its impact on patient management. World J Surg. 2001;25:373–80.

7. Klein JS, Zarka MA. Transthoracic needle biopsy. Radiol Clin North Am. 2000;38:235–66.

8. Manhire A, Charig M, Clelland C, et al. Guidelines for radiologically guided lung biopsy. Thorax. 2003;58(11):920–36.

9. Castellino RA, Blank N. Etiologic diagnosis of focal pulmonary infection in immunocompromised patients by fluoroscopically guided percutaneous needle aspiration. Radiology. 1979;132:563–7.

10. Conces DJ, Clark SA, Tarver RD, et al. Transthoracic aspiration needle biopsy: value in the diagnosis of pulmonary infections. AJR Am J Roentgenol. 1989;152:31–4.

11. Hur J, Lee HJ, Nam JE, et al. Diagnostic accuracy of CT fluoroscopy-guided needle aspiration biopsy of ground-glass opacity pulmonary lesions. AJR Am J Roentgenol. 2009;192(3):629–34.

12. Kim TJ, Lee JH, Lee CT, et al. Diagnostic accuracy of CT-guided core biopsy of ground-glass opacity pulmonary lesions. AJR Am J Roentgenol. 2008;190:234–9.

13. Wallace MJ, Krishnamurthy S, Broemeling LD, et al. CT guided percutaneous fine-needle aspiration biopsy of small (< or ¼1-cm) pulmonary lesions. Radiology. 2002;225:823–8.

14. Charig MJ, Stutley JE, Padley SPG, et al. The value of negative needle biopsy in suspected operable lung cancer. Clin Radiol. 1991;44(3):147–9.

15. Wallace AB, Suh RD. Percutaneous transthoracic needle biopsy: special considerations and techniques used in lung transplant recipients. Semin Intervent Radiol. 2004;21(4):247–58; https://www.thieme-connect.com/ejournals/abstract/sir/doi/10.1055/s-2004-861559.

16. Aziz A, Ashizawa K, Nagaoki K, Hayashi K. High resolution CT anatomy of the pulmonary fissures. J Thorac Imaging. 2004;19:186–91.

17. Yildiz A, Gölpinar F, Calikoğlu M, Duce MN, Ozer C, Apaydin FD. HRCT evaluation of the accessory fissures of the lung. Eur J Radiol. 2004;49(3):245–9.

18. Moore EH. Technical aspects of needle aspiration lung biopsy: a personal perspective. Radiology. 1998;208:303–18.

19. Cahill AM, Baskin KM, Kaye RD, Fitz CR, Towbin RB. CT-guided percutaneous lung biopsy in children. J Vasc Interv Radiol. 2004;15(9):955–60.

20. Yankelevitz DF, Henschke CI, Koizumi JH, et al. CT-guided transthoracic needle biopsy of small solitary pulmonary nodules. Clin Imaging. 1997;21:107–10. (alternative – Ng YL CT-Guided percut 2008).

21. Froelich JJ, Ishaque N, Regn J, et al. Guidance of percutaneous pulmonary biopsies with real-time CT fluoroscopy. Eur J Radiol. 2002;42:74–9.

22. Katada K, Kato R, Anno H, et al. Guidance with real-time CT fluoroscopy: early clinical experience. Radiology. 1996;200:851–6.

23. Li H, Boiselle PM, Shepard JO. Diagnostic accuracy and safety of CT-guided percutaneous needle aspiration biopsy of the lung: comparison of small and large pulmonary nodules. AJR Am J Roentgenol. 1996;167:105–9.

24. Haramati LB. CT-guided automated needle biopsy of the chest. AJR Am J Roentgenol. 1995;165:53–5.

25. Greif J, Marmur S, Schwarz Y, et al. Percutaneous core cutting needle biopsy compared with fine-needle aspiration in the diagnosis of peripheral lung malignant lesions: results in 156 patients. Cancer. 1998;84:144–7.

26. Klein JS, Schultz S. Interventional chest radiology. Curr Probl Diagn Radiol. 1992;21:219–77.

27. Klein JS, Salomon G, Stewart EA. Transthoracic needle biopsy with a coaxially placed 20-gauge automated cutting needle: results in 122 patients. Radiology. 1996;198:715–20.

28. Greif J, Marmur S, Schwarz Y, et al. Percutaneous core needle biopsy vs. fine-needle aspiration in diagnosing benign lung lesions. Acta Cytol. 1999;43:756–60.

29. Staroselsky AN, Schwarz Y, Man A, et al. Additional information from percutaneous cutting needle biopsy following fine-needle aspiration in the diagnosis of chest lesions. Chest. 1998;113:1522–5.

30. Yankelevitz DF, Vazquez M, Henschke CI. Special techniques in transthoracic needle biopsy of pulmonary nodules. Radiol Clin North Am. 2000;38:267–79.

31. Haramati LB, Austin JHM. Complications after CT-guided needle biopsy through aerated versus nonaerated lung. Radiology. 1991;181:778.

32. Stern EJ, Webb WR, Gamsu G. CT gantry tilt: utility in transthoracic fine-needle aspiration biopsy. Radiology. 1993;187:873–4.

33. Yankelevitz DF, Henschke CI, Davis SD. Percutaneous CT biopsy of chest lesions: an in vitro analysis of the effect of partial volume averaging on needle positioning. AJR Am J Roentgenol. 1993;161:273–8.

34. Sandhu J, Meglin AJ, Trerotola SO. Thoracic and visceral nonvascular interventions. Fairfax: The Society of Cardiovascular and Interventional Radiology; 1997. p. 159–70.

35. Klose KC. CT-guided large-bore biopsy: extrapleural injection of saline for safe transpleural access to pulmonary lesions. Cardiovasc Intervent Radiol. 1993;16:259–61.

36. Horton JA, Bank WO, Kerber CW. Guiding the thin spinal needle. AJR Am J Roentgenol. 1980;134:845–84.

37. Yankelevitz DF, Davis SD, Chiarella D, et al. Needle-tip repositioning during computed-tomography-guided transthoracic needle aspiration biopsy of small deep pulmonary lesions: minor adjustments make a big difference. J Thorac Imaging. 1996;11:279–82.

38. Ohno Y, Hatabu H, Takenaka D, Imai M, Ohbayashi C, Sugimura K. Transthoracic CT-guided biopsy with multiplanar reconstruction image improves diagnostic accuracy of solitary pulmonary nodules. Eur J Radiol. 2004;51(2):160–8.

39. Santos RS, Gupta A, Ebright MI. Electromagnetic navigation to aid radiofrequency ablation and biopsy of lung tumors. Ann Thorac Surg. 2010;89(1):265–8.

40. Layfield LJ, Liu K, Erasmus JJ. Radiologically determined diameter, pathologic diameter, and reactive zone surrounding pulmonary neoplasms: implications for transthoracic fine needle aspiration of pulmonary neoplasms. Diagn Cytopathol. 1999;21:250–2.

41. Aerospace Medical Association Medical Guidelines Task Force. Medical guidelines for airline travel, 2nd ed. Aviat Space Environ Med. 2003;74(5 Suppl):A1–19.

42. Moore EH, Shepard JO, McLoud TC, et al. Positional precautions in needle aspiration lung biopsy. Radiology. 1990;175:733–5.

43. Berquist TH, Bailey PB, Cortese DA, et al. Transthoracic needle biopsy: accuracy and complications in relation to location and type of lesion. Mayo Clin Proc. 1980;55:475–81.

44. Fish GD, Stanley JH, Miller S, et al. Postbiopsy pneumothorax: estimating the risk by chest radiography and pulmonary function tests. AJR Am J Roentgenol. 1988;150:71–4.

45. Yankelevitz DF, Davis SD, Henschke CI. Aspiration of a large pneumothorax resulting from transthoracic needle biopsy. Radiology. 1996;200:695–7.

46. Yamagami T, Nakamura T, Iida S, et al. Management of pneumothorax after percutaneous CT-guided lung biopsy. Chest. 2002;121:1159–64.

47. Lang EK, Ghavami R, Schreiner VC, et al. Autologous blood clot seal to prevent pneumothorax at CT-guided lung biopsy. Radiology. 2000;216:93–6.

48. Herman SJ, Weisbrod GL. Usefulness of the blood patch technique after transthoracic needle aspiration biopsy. Radiology. 1990; 176:395–7.

49. Engeler CE, Hunter DW, Castaneda-Zuniga W, et al. Pneumothorax after lung biopsy: prevention with transpleural placement of compressed collagen foam plugs. Radiology. 1992;184:787–9.

50. Man A, Schwarz Y, Greif J. Case report: cardiac tamponade following fine needle aspiration (FNA) of a mediastinal mass. Clin Radiol. 1998;53:151–2.

51. Milner LB, Ryan K, Gullo J. Fatal intrathoracic hemorrhage after percutaneous aspiration lung biopsy. AJR Am J Roentgenol. 1979;132:280–1.

52. Arakawa H, Nakajima Y, Kurihara H, et al. CT-guided transthoracic needle biopsy: a comparison between automated biopsy gun and fine needle aspiration. Clin Radiol. 1996;51:503–6.

53. Aberle DR, Gamsu G, Golden JA. Fatal systemic arterial air embolism following lung needle aspiration. Radiology. 1987;165:351–3.

54. Murphy BP, Harford FJ, Cramer FS. Cerebral air embolism resulting from invasive medical procedures: treatment and hyperbaric oxygen. Ann Surg. 1985;201:242–5.

55. Berger RL, Dargan EL, Huang BL. Dissemination of cancer cells by needle biopsy of the lung. J Thorac Cardiovasc Surg. 1972;63:430–2.

56. Khouri NF, Stitik FP, Erozan YS, et al. Transthoracic needle aspiration biopsy of benign and malignant lung lesions. AJR Am J Roentgenol. 1985;144:281–8.

57. Zarbo RJ, Fenoglio-Presier CM. Inter-institutional database for comparison of performance in lung fine-needle aspiration cytology: a College of American Pathologists Q-probe study of 5264 cases with histologic correlation. Arch Pathol Lab Med. 1992; 116:463–70.

58. Westcott JL, Najmussaqib R, Colley DP. Transthoracic needle biopsy of small pulmonary nodules. Radiology. 1997;202: 97–103.

59. Protopapas Z, Westcott JL. Transthoracic needle biopsy of mediastinal lymph nodes for staging lung and other cancers. Radiology. 1996;199:489–96.

60. Grinan NP, Lucena FM, Romero JV, et al. Yield of percutaneous needle lung aspiration in lung abscess. Chest. 1990;97: 69–74.

61. Gruden JF, Klein JS, Webb WR. Percutaneous transthoracic needle biopsy in AIDS: analysis in 32 patients. Radiology. 1993;189:567–71.

62. Scott WW, Kuhlman JE. Focal pulmonary lesions in patients with AIDS: percutaneous transthoracic needle biopsy. Radiology. 1991;180:419–21.

Pleural Biopsy

12

Kamran Ahrar and Sanaz Javadi

Background

Pleural disease may present with focal nodules or patchy or diffuse pleural thickening. Effusion is often an early sign of pleural disease and may be detected before any nodules or thickening of the pleura has developed. Aspiration of pleural fluid is accepted as the first diagnostic test in the detection of pleural disease [1, 2]. However, cytological evaluation of pleural fluid is diagnostic in only 60 % of patients with malignant effusion and in only 30 % of cases associated with malignant pleural mesothelioma (MPM) [3, 4]. Evaluation of pleural fluid against a panel of monoclonal antibodies or tumor markers used in conjunction with cytological analysis may improve the sensitivity for diagnosing malignant pleural effusion [5, 6]. Some patients with pleural disease may have no effusion. Thus, pleural biopsy is an important diagnostic tool for evaluating pleural disease with or without effusion. This chapter will cover the indications, contraindications, patient selection for pleural biopsy, the technique, complications and their management, and outcomes and results.

K. Ahrar, MD, FSIR (✉)
Department of Interventional Radiology,
Department of Thoracic and Cardiovascular Surgery,
The University of Texas MD Anderson Cancer Center,
1515 Holcombe Boulevard, Unit 1471, Houston, TX, USA
e-mail: kahrar@mdanderson.org

S. Javadi, MD
Department of Radiology, Baylor College of Medicine,
One Baylor Plaza, Unit 360, Houston, TX, USA
e-mail: sjavadi@bcm.edu

Indications and Patient Selection for Pleural Biopsy

When evaluation of the pleural effusion does not reveal the underlying pathology or when no effusion is present, pleural histology is required to establish a diagnosis. The vast majority of pleural biopsies are performed to evaluate for malignant diseases of the pleura, including MPM, metastatic disease from a nonpleural primary, and lymphoma. However, many benign conditions may also involve the pleura. The most common benign pleural disease evaluated via biopsy is pleural tuberculosis [7–9]. Benign asbestos-related pleural thickening is usually diagnosed on the basis of clinical and radiological features [10]. When imaging studies demonstrate atypical findings or progression of pleural thickening, a biopsy is warranted to exclude malignant disease. For other benign diseases of pleura, specific histological findings occasionally point to a specific diagnosis (e.g., amyloidosis) [11]. But more often, histological findings of fibrosis or chronic inflammation are nonspecific and do not suggest a clear diagnosis. In these cases, a prolonged period of follow-up is recommended. In a study at the Mayo Clinic, 25 % of patients with negative histological findings on open surgical pleural biopsy went on to develop malignant disease [12].

Patients with focal pleural nodules (Fig. 12.1) or patchy or diffuse pleural thickening (Fig. 12.2) are good candidates for image-guided biopsy [14]. When multiple nodules or areas of pleural thickening are present, a positron-emission tomography (PET) scan can help identify metabolically active areas of disease (Fig. 12.3). For patients with pleural thickening, image-guided biopsy can be performed even when pleural thickening is minimal (i.e., <5 mm) [15].

Contraindications

The only contraindication for image-guided pleural biopsy is the presence of uncorrectable coagulopathy. Some researchers have suggested that pleural biopsy is contraindicated in

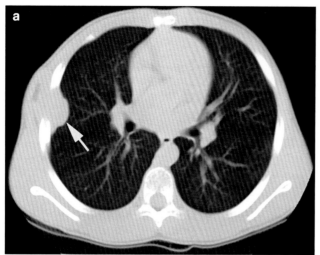

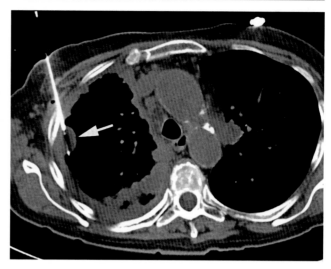

Fig. 12.2 CT-guided pleural biopsy. Axial CT image shows diffuse right pleural thickening with a focal nodular mass (*arrow*). A core biopsy needle is placed within the pleural mass (Ahrar et al. [13])

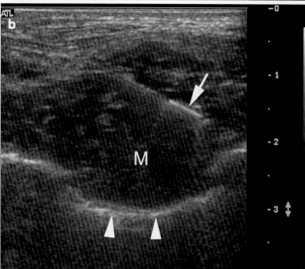

Fig. 12.1 US-guided pleural biopsy. Axial CT image of the chest (**a**) shows a focal pleural mass (*arrow*). Grayscale ultrasound image (**b**) during the biopsy shows the echogenic biopsy needle (*arrow*) within the mass (*M*). The thin echogenic band (*arrowheads*) signifies the interface of the mass (*M*) and the underlying lung tissue (Ahrar et al. [13])

patients who cannot control their breathing or who cannot cooperate during the biopsy [16]. In our experience, most patients under moderate sedation take regular, shallow breaths that help target even small pleural nodules.

Pleural Biopsy Technique

Overview

Surgical pleural biopsy, also referred to as "open" pleural biopsy, is the "gold standard" for diagnosis of pleural diseases, but thoracotomy is associated with substantial morbidity [17–20]. Minimally invasive surgical approaches

to pleural biopsy, including video-assisted thoracoscopic surgery (VATS) and physician-based thoracoscopy, have also demonstrated a high diagnostic yield (>90 %) [21–26]. However, VATS and thoracoscopy require a safe separation of the visceral and parietal pleura, and medical thoracoscopy requires the presence of a moderate effusion [27], whereas image-guided pleural biopsy is not limited by these factors.

Nonsurgical percutaneous pleural biopsy, also known as "blind" or "closed" pleural biopsy, was first described in patients with pleural effusion in the 1950s by Abrams and Cope [28, 29]. In this technique, a reverse-beveled needle is advanced into the pleural cavity and pulled back to "hook" the pleura and obtain a biopsy sample (Fig. 12.4). Four to six passes are usually necessary to obtain an adequate diagnostic specimen [8]. Although blind pleural biopsy can be performed at the bedside and is relatively simple, the diagnostic yield is suboptimal and the complication rates are higher than those for image-guided biopsy [30]. Simultaneous fluid analysis with blind pleural biopsy has demonstrated better diagnostic value than blind biopsy alone [31].

Over the last two decades, the trend has been away from blind pleural biopsy and toward image-guided pleural biopsy, using either ultrasonography or computed tomography (CT) [32].

Imaging

Both CT and ultrasonography can be used to guide pleural biopsies. Initially, a diagnostic imaging study, usually a CT (Fig. 12.5) scan or a PET-CT (Fig. 12.3) scan, identifies

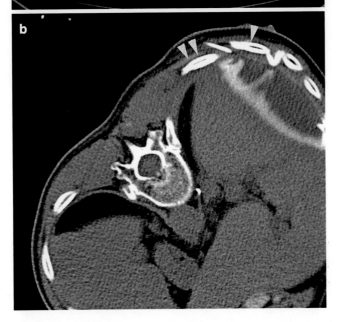

Fig. 12.3 CT-guided pleural biopsy with minimal pleural thickening. A 53-year-old man with history of epithelioid malignant mesothelioma and extrapleural pneumonectomy underwent PET-CT imaging for surveillance. Fused axial PET-CT image (**a**) showed a focal area of FDG uptake in the posterolateral chest wall between the *right* 10th (*arrowhead*) and the 11th (*double arrowhead*) ribs. Minimal pleural thickening was targeted in that particular interspace under CT guidance (**b**). Pathology confirmed recurrent malignant mesothelioma

areas of nodular, patchy, or diffuse pleural thickening. Subsequently, the choice between CT and ultrasound depends on personal preference, local expertise, and equipment availability. Ultrasonography provides real-time imaging, is widely available, and is relatively inexpensive. However, pleural lesions near or behind the ribs or along the paravertebral or medial surfaces may be difficult to image with ultrasound, and small pleural nodules in the absence of pleural effusion may be challenging to localize with ultrasound (Fig. 12.6). CT can help identify and target virtually any nodule or area of pleural thickening in the thoracic cavity.

Devices

For blind pleural biopsy, Abrams or Cope needles are used. These needles range in size from 11 to 8 gauge (up to 4 mm in diameter). Each needle is fitted with a "cutting window" to trap and extract a sample of the pleura. Safe application of these devices requires the presence of a moderate-sized pleural effusion (Fig. 12.4).

For image-guided biopsies, both fine-needle aspiration (FNA) biopsy (Fig. 12.7) and automated tissue-cutting biopsy guns (Fig. 12.2) have been used. Cutting-needle biopsy has been shown to be more sensitive than FNA biopsy in diagnosing pleural malignancies [14, 33]. The size of the needle (14 vs. 18 gauge) used in cutting-needle biopsy does not influence diagnostic sensitivity [14, 34]. The use of FNA biopsy and core biopsy together may help increase the diagnostic yield for malignant disease [14, 35].

Approaches and Relevant Anatomy

In ultrasonography, patients can be positioned in a sitting or a recumbent position. A sitting position is advantageous in patients with large pleural effusions to avoid worsening of respiratory symptoms such as shortness of breath, which is frequently encountered in these patients. Positioning of the patient for CT-guided biopsy depends on the location of the target tissue. Patients can be placed in a supine, prone, lateral decubitus, or oblique position. Tilting the CT gantry helps target lesions located behind a rib. To biopsy areas of minimal pleural thickening, the needle should be aligned almost parallel to the pleural surface that is to be biopsied to allow the longest interface of the needle with the area of abnormality (Fig. 12.2). This is important for both FNA and tissue-cutting biopsies.

Potential Complications

Potential complications of pleural biopsies include pneumothorax, hemothorax, hemoptysis, subcutaneous hematoma, damage to the diaphragm or abdominal viscera, and tract seeding. For image-guided biopsies, the complication rate is less than 5 %. For blind pleural biopsies, the complication rate is higher, with 15 % of patients developing pneumothorax and 5 % of patients developing hemothorax or vasovagal reactions (Table 12.1) [14, 34–41].

It is generally believed that MPM has a tendency to seed the biopsy tract [42]. In one study, the rate of tract seeding was directly proportional to the size of the biopsy tract and has been reported to be as high as 24 % for thoracotomy, 16 % for thoracoscopy, and 5 % for image-guided

Fig. 12.4 Artist rendition of bilateral diffuse pleural thickening. With the patient in prone position, the right pleura can be sampled by blind biopsy (e.g., with Abrams needle) due to presence of large pleural effusion. On the *left side*, the lack of pleural effusion precludes blind pleural biopsy. A core biopsy needle is shown in the pleural thickening on the *left*

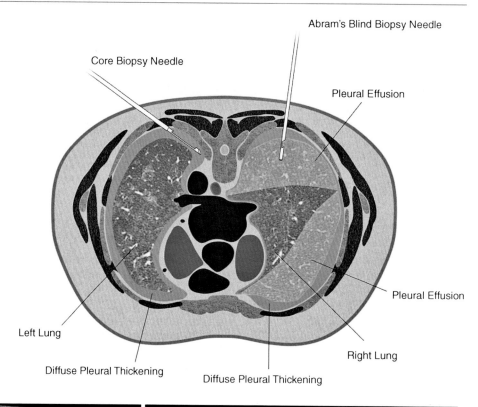

Fig. 12.5 Ultrasound-guided biopsy of pleural mass extending into the chest wall. An 84-year-old man with new onset of pain underwent CT imaging which showed multiple pleural masses involving the left hemithorax (**a**). The largest mass (*) was found in the anterolateral aspect of the left lower chest wall. Grayscale ultrasound image of the chest wall (**b**) shows the hypoechoic pleural mass (*). Biopsy was carried out under ultrasound guidance (**c**). *Arrowheads* indicate the cutting tip of a core biopsy needle. Pathology showed high-grade carcinoma of unknown primary

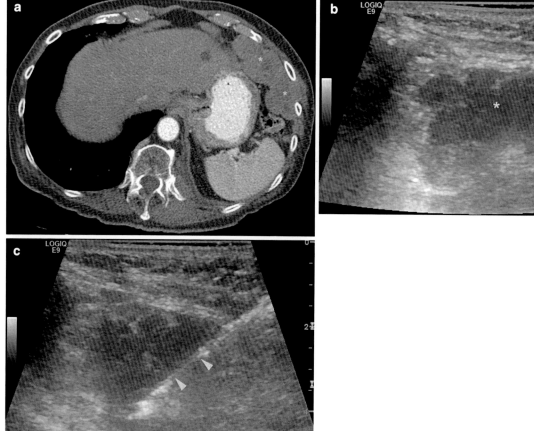

Fig. 12.6 Artist rendition of focal pleural nodules along the superior-lateral aspect of the right pleural cavity (**a**) and along the inferior-medial aspect of the left pleural cavity (**b**). CT guidance is preferred for targeting these small nodules that are difficult to visualize with ultrasound

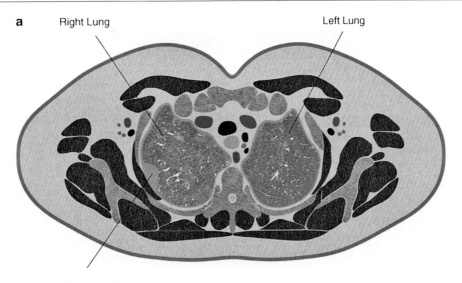

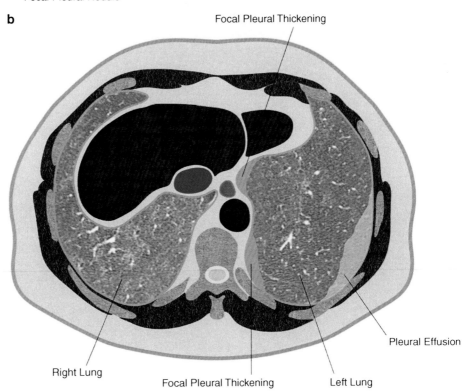

biopsy [36]. In other studies, no correlation between biopsy tract invasion and size of the biopsy tract was reported [42–44].

Management of Complications

Small iatrogenic pneumothorax often resolves spontaneously (Fig. 12.7) [45–47]. Simple aspiration may obviate the need for placement of a thoracostomy tube [48, 49]. An aspiration volume greater than 600 mL may indicate the need for a chest drain insertion [49]. Thoracostomy tube can be placed under CT or fluoroscopic guidance. Most patients do not

require admission to the hospital and can be managed as outpatients [50].

Traditionally, patients with intrathoracic hemorrhage owing to intercostal artery injury have been managed by exploratory thoracotomy. Thoracotomy has limited success in identifying and blocking the bleeding artery and has substantial morbidity [51]. Transcatheter arterial embolization is a safe and effective therapeutic option for these patients [51–57].

A randomized trial of local radiotherapy for prevention of malignant seeding after invasive diagnostic procedures in patients with MPM showed a benefit from radiation therapy [42]. On the contrary, two recent randomized trials have

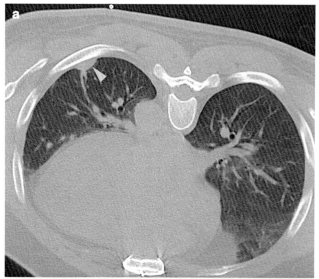

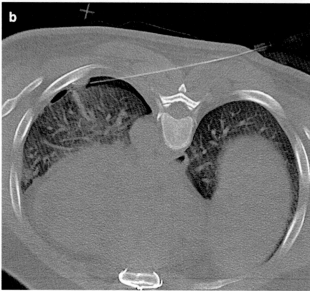

Fig. 12.7 A 46-year-old man with history of thymoma returns after definitive therapy with a focal pleural nodule. Axial CT image of the chest in prone position (**a**) shows a small focal area of pleural thickening covered by the left 7th rib. Initial attempts at accessing the nodule led to development of a small pneumothorax, but the biopsy was ultimately completed (**b**). Small pneumothorax remained stable and did not require any further intervention. Pathology confirmed recurrent thymoma

shown a lack of therapeutic benefit from prophylactic radiation therapy in these patients [43, 44].

Outcomes and Results

In patients with tuberculosis, the pleura is often diffusely involved. Under these circumstances, the diagnostic yield of blind pleural biopsy can reach as high as 79 % [7], although for the same group of patients, image-guided biopsy and thoracoscopy can achieve 86 % and 100 % sensitivity, respectively [7, 38].

Accurate diagnosis of malignant pleural disease is essential for treatment planning. Malignant pleural involvement seen on imaging studies or at thoracoscopy is often patchy and not uniformly confluent. As such, blind pleural biopsy is not an appropriate technique for diagnosing malignant pleural disease. The highest diagnostic sensitivity rates reported for this technique are about 50 % [58], and the sensitivity of blind pleural biopsy is even lower in patients with MPM [39, 41, 59, 60].

On the other hand, CT can help target any focal pleural nodule or thickening regardless of its anatomic location. Several case series of image-guided pleural biopsy have reported high diagnostic yield [14, 34–39], with overall diagnostic sensitivities of 70–88 % (Table 12.1). Even for patients with MPM, sensitivity of 86 % and specificity of 100 % have been reported [33]. In a prospective randomized trial, the sensitivity of CT-guided biopsy and blind pleural biopsy were 87 % and 47 %, respectively [39].

To date, no studies have directly compared the diagnostic yield of pleural biopsy under CT with that using ultrasound guidance. Some studies have reported equally high and comparative diagnostic yield for both techniques [14, 33]. While in other studies, higher diagnostic sensitivity was achieved with CT than with ultrasound [61].

In summary, image-guided biopsy is superior to blind pleural biopsy allowing biopsy of diffuse pleural thickening or focal pleural nodules. Even minimal pleural thickening without associated pleural effusion can be targeted under CT guidance.

Table 12.1 Image-guided pleural biopsy outcomes and complications

| | | | | Outcome | | | |
References	Patients/biopsies	Imaging	Needle	Sensitivity	Specificity	Accuracy or adequacy	Complications
Adams and Gleeson [14]	33/33	CT 24 US 9	Core needle 18 and 14 G	88 %	100 %	91 %	1 chest wall hematoma
Heilo et al. [34]	70[a]/70	US	Core needle 18 and 14 G	77 %	88 %	80 %	1 hemoptysis 1 chest pain
Scott et al. [35]	42/45	CT	Core 18 G	83 %	100 %	92 %	1 hemoptysis 1 stroke
Agrawal et al. [36]	22[a]/23	CT 10 US 1 Fluoroscopy 12	Core needle 20 to 14 G	86 %	NR	87 %	1 seeding
Benamore et al. [37]	82/85	CT 80 US 5	Core needle 21, 18, and 14 G	76 %	100 %	88 %	4.7 % pneumothorax No chest tube
Chang [38]	25/25	US	Tru-cut 16 G	70 %[b] to 86 %[c]	100 %	84 %	0
Maskell et al. [39]	23	CT	Core 18 G	87 %	100 %	91 %	0

CT computed tomography, *US* ultrasonography, *G* gauge, *NR* not reported
[a]Patients with malignant pleural mesothelioma
[b]Sensitivity for detection of malignancy
[c]Sensitivity for detection of tuberculosis

References

1. Antunes G, Neville E, Duffy J, Ali N. BTS guidelines for the management of malignant pleural effusions. Thorax. 2003;58 Suppl 2:ii29–38.
2. American Thoracic Society. Management of malignant pleural effusions. Am J Respir Crit Care Med. 2000;162:1987–2001.
3. Renshaw AA, Dean BR, Antman KH, Sugarbaker DJ, Cibas ES. The role of cytologic evaluation of pleural fluid in the diagnosis of malignant mesothelioma. Chest. 1997;111:106–9.
4. Fenton KN, Richardson JD. Diagnosis and management of malignant pleural effusions. Am J Surg. 1995;170:69–74.
5. Aerts JG, Delahaye M, van der Kwast TH, Davidson B, Hoogsteden HC, van Meerbeeck JP. The high post-test probability of a cytological examination renders further investigations to establish a diagnosis of epithelial malignant pleural mesothelioma redundant. Diagn Cytopathol. 2006;34:523–7.
6. Porcel JM, Vives M, Esquerda A, Salud A, Perez B, Rodriguez-Panadero F. Use of a panel of tumor markers (carcinoembryonic antigen, cancer antigen 125, carbohydrate antigen 15-3, and cytokeratin 19 fragments) in pleural fluid for the differential diagnosis of benign and malignant effusions. Chest. 2004;126:1757–63.
7. Diacon AH, Van de Wal BW, Wyser C, et al. Diagnostic tools in tuberculous pleurisy: a direct comparative study. Eur Respir J. 2003;22:589–91.
8. Khadadah ME, Muqim AT, Al-Mutairi AD, et al. Closed percutaneous pleural biopsy. A lost art in the new era. Saudi Med J. 2009;30:793–7.
9. Chakrabarti B, Davies PD. Pleural tuberculosis. Monaldi Arch Chest Dis. 2006;65:26–33.
10. Chapman SJ, Cookson WO, Musk AW, Lee YC. Benign asbestos pleural diseases. Curr Opin Pulm Med. 2003;9:266–71.
11. Schwarz D, Jue C, Sikov W. Primary systemic amyloidosis and persistent pleural effusions. Amyloid. 2009;16:239–42.
12. Ryan CJ, Rodgers RF, Unni KK, Hepper NG. The outcome of patients with pleural effusion of indeterminate cause at thoracotomy. Mayo Clin Proc. 1981;56:145–9.
13. Ahrar K, Wallace M, Javadi S, Gupta S. Mediastinal, Hilar, and Pleural Image-Guided Biopsy: Current Practice and Techniques. Seminars in Respiratory and Critical Care Medicine. 2008;29(4). Thieme Publishers.
14. Adams RF, Gleeson FV. Percutaneous image-guided cutting-needle biopsy of the pleura in the presence of a suspected malignant effusion. Radiology. 2001;219:510–14.
15. Mueller PR, Saini S, Simeone JF, et al. Image-guided pleural biopsies: indications, technique, and results in 23 patients. Radiology. 1988;169:1–4.
16. Duncan M, Wijesekera N, Padley S. Interventional radiology of the thorax. Respirology. 2010;15:401–12.
17. Dajczman E, Gordon A, Kreisman H, Wolkove N. Long-term post-thoracotomy pain. Chest. 1991;99:270–4.
18. Gaeta RR, Macario A, Brodsky JB, Brock-Utne JG, Mark JB. Pain outcomes after thoracotomy: lumbar epidural hydromorphone versus intrapleural bupivacaine. J Cardiothorac Vasc Anesth. 1995;9:534–7.
19. Kalso E, Perttunen K, Kaasinen S. Pain after thoracic surgery. Acta Anaesthesiol Scand. 1992;36:96–100.
20. Perttunen K, Tasmuth T, Kalso E. Chronic pain after thoracic surgery: a follow-up study. Acta Anaesthesiol Scand. 1999;43:563–7.
21. Harris RJ, Kavuru MS, Rice TW, Kirby TJ. The diagnostic and therapeutic utility of thoracoscopy. A review. Chest. 1995;108:828–41.
22. Harris RJ, Kavuru MS, Mehta AC, et al. The impact of thoracoscopy on the management of pleural disease. Chest. 1995;107:845–52.
23. de Groot M, Walther G. Thoracoscopy in undiagnosed pleural effusions. S Afr Med J. 1998;88:706–11.
24. Blanc FX, Atassi K, Bignon J, Housset B. Diagnostic value of medical thoracoscopy in pleural disease: a 6-year retrospective study. Chest. 2002;121:1677–83.
25. Hansen M, Faurschou P, Clementsen P. Medical thoracoscopy, results and complications in 146 patients: a retrospective study. Respir Med. 1998;92:228–32.
26. Menzies R, Charbonneau M. Thoracoscopy for the diagnosis of pleural disease. Ann Intern Med. 1991;114:271–6.

27. Rahman NM, Gleeson FV. Image-guided pleural biopsy. Curr Opin Pulm Med. 2008;14:331–6.

28. Abrams LD. A pleural-biopsy punch. Lancet. 1958;1:30–1.

29. Cope C. New pleural biopsy needle; preliminary study. J Am Med Assoc. 1958;167:1107–8.

30. Von Hoff DD, LiVolsi V. Diagnostic reliability of needle biopsy of the parietal pleura. A review of 272 biopsies. Am J Clin Pathol. 1975;64:200–3.

31. Poe RH, Israel RH, Utell MJ, Hall WJ, Greenblatt DW, Kallay MC. Sensitivity, specificity, and predictive values of closed pleural biopsy. Arch Intern Med. 1984;144:325–8.

32. Gopal M, Romero AB, Baillargeon J, Sharma G. Trends in pleural biopsies between 1996 and 2006 at a tertiary medical center. Am J Med Sci. 2010;339:345–9.

33. Adams RF, Gray W, Davies RJ, Gleeson FV. Percutaneous image-guided cutting needle biopsy of the pleura in the diagnosis of malignant mesothelioma. Chest. 2001;120:1798–802.

34. Heilo A, Stenwig AE, Solheim OP. Malignant pleural mesothelioma: US-guided histologic core-needle biopsy. Radiology. 1999;211:657–9.

35. Scott EM, Marshall TJ, Flower CD, Stewart S. Diffuse pleural thickening: percutaneous CT-guided cutting needle biopsy. Radiology. 1995;194:867–70.

36. Agarwal PP, Seely JM, Matzinger FR, et al. Pleural mesothelioma: sensitivity and incidence of needle track seeding after image-guided biopsy versus surgical biopsy. Radiology. 2006;241: 589–94.

37. Benamore RE, Scott K, Richards CJ, Entwisle JJ. Image-guided pleural biopsy: diagnostic yield and complications. Clin Radiol. 2006;61:700–5.

38. Chang DB, Yang PC, Luh KT, Kuo SH, Yu CJ. Ultrasound-guided pleural biopsy with Tru-Cut needle. Chest. 1991;100:1328–33.

39. Maskell NA, Gleeson FV, Davies RJ. Standard pleural biopsy versus CT-guided cutting-needle biopsy for diagnosis of malignant disease in pleural effusions: a randomised controlled trial. Lancet. 2003;361:1326–30.

40. Maskell NA, Butland RJ. BTS guidelines for the investigation of a unilateral pleural effusion in adults. Thorax. 2003;58 Suppl 2: ii8–17.

41. Prakash UB, Reiman HM. Comparison of needle biopsy with cytologic analysis for the evaluation of pleural effusion: analysis of 414 cases. Mayo Clin Proc. 1985;60:158–64.

42. Boutin C, Rey F, Viallat JR. Prevention of malignant seeding after invasive diagnostic procedures in patients with pleural mesothelioma. A randomized trial of local radiotherapy. Chest. 1995;108:754–8.

43. Bydder S, Phillips M, Joseph DJ, et al. A randomised trial of single-dose radiotherapy to prevent procedure tract metastasis by malignant mesothelioma. Br J Cancer. 2004;91:9–10.

44. O'Rourke N, Garcia JC, Paul J, Lawless C, McMenemin R, Hill J. A randomised controlled trial of intervention site radiotherapy in malignant pleural mesothelioma. Radiother Oncol. 2007;84: 18–22.

45. Kazerooni EA, Lim FT, Mikhail A, Martinez FJ. Risk of pneumothorax in CT-guided transthoracic needle aspiration biopsy of the lung. Radiology. 1996;198:371–5.

46. Anderson JM, Murchison J, Patel D. CT-guided lung biopsy: factors influencing diagnostic yield and complication rate. Clin Radiol. 2003;58:791–7.

47. Gupta S, Krishnamurthy S, Broemeling LD, et al. Small (</=2-cm) subpleural pulmonary lesions: short- versus long-needle-path CT-guided Biopsy–comparison of diagnostic yields and complications. Radiology. 2005;234:631–7.

48. Delius RE, Obeid FN, Horst HM, Sorensen VJ, Fath JJ, Bivins BA. Catheter aspiration for simple pneumothorax. Experience with 114 patients. Arch Surg. 1989;124:833–6.

49. Yamagami T, Kato T, Hirota T, Yoshimatsu R, Matsumoto T, Nishimura T. Usefulness and limitation of manual aspiration immediately after pneumothorax complicating interventional radiological procedures with the transthoracic approach. Cardiovasc Intervent Radiol. 2006;29:1027–33.

50. Gupta S, Hicks ME, Wallace MJ, Ahrar K, Madoff DC, Murthy R. Outpatient management of postbiopsy pneumothorax with small-caliber chest tubes: factors affecting the need for prolonged drainage and additional interventions. Cardiovasc Intervent Radiol. 2008;31:342–8.

51. Carrillo EH, Heniford BT, Senler SO, Dykes JR, Maniscalco SP, Richardson JD. Embolization therapy as an alternative to thoracotomy in vascular injuries of the chest wall. Am Surg. 1998;64:1142–8.

52. Barbaric ZL, Luka NL. Angiographic demonstration and transcatheter embolic control of post-traumatic intercostal arterial hemorrhage. Surgery. 1977;81:409–12.

53. Hagiwara A, Iwamoto S. Usefulness of transcatheter arterial embolization for intercostal arterial bleeding in a patient with burst fractures of the thoracic vertebrae. Emerg Radiol. 2009;16:489–91.

54. Kessel B, Alfici R, Ashkenazi I, et al. Massive hemothorax caused by intercostal artery bleeding: selective embolization may be an alternative to thoracotomy in selected patients. Thorac Cardiovasc Surg. 2004;52:234–6.

55. Muthuswamy P, Samuel J, Mizock B, Dunne P. Recurrent massive bleeding from an intercostal artery aneurysm through an empyema chest tube. Chest. 1993;104:637–9.

56. Yu WY, Wang CP, Ng KC, Chen WK, Tzeng IH. Successful embolization of a ruptured intercostal artery after violent coughing. Am J Emerg Med. 2006;24:247–9.

57. Chemelli AP, Thauerer M, Wiedermann F, Strasak A, Klocker J, Chemelli-Steingruber IE. Transcatheter arterial embolization for the management of iatrogenic and blunt traumatic intercostal artery injuries. J Vasc Surg. 2009;49:1505–13.

58. Chakrabarti B, Ryland I, Sheard J, Warburton CJ, Earis JE. The role of Abrams percutaneous pleural biopsy in the investigation of exudative pleural effusions. Chest. 2006;129:1549–55.

59. Escudero Bueno C, Garcia Clemente M, Cuesta Castro B, et al. Cytologic and bacteriologic analysis of fluid and pleural biopsy specimens with Cope's needle. Study of 414 patients. Arch Intern Med. 1990;150:1190–4.

60. Salyer WR, Eggleston JC, Erozan YS. Efficacy of pleural needle biopsy and pleural fluid cytopathology in the diagnosis of malignant neoplasm involving the pleura. Chest. 1975;67:536–9.

61. Qureshi NR, Gleeson FV. Imaging of pleural disease. Clin Chest Med. 2006;27:193–213.

Liver Biopsy

Ashraf Thabet and Debra A. Gervais

Background

The liver is the most commonly biopsied organ by the interventional radiologist [1]. Not only is image-guided biopsy the gold standard for the staging of diffuse parenchymal liver disease such as viral hepatitis [2], it is the most commonly employed means for evaluating focal hepatic lesions that do not demonstrate definite benign features on ultrasound (US), computed tomography (CT), or magnetic resonance imaging (MRI). It may also be an effective means of obtaining specimen for microbiologic analysis.

Image-guided liver biopsy may be performed via direct percutaneous or transjugular approaches. The choice of approach is dependent on whether a non-focal or focal biopsy is desired; whether the patient's clinical status raises the risk of percutaneous biopsy (e.g., coagulation disorders), the presence of ascites; and whether hepatic venous pressure gradient measurements are desired. With regard to non-focal percutaneous liver biopsy, consensus is evolving that image guidance improves the quality of the biopsy specimen, reduces complications, and is cost-effective compared to when no imaging is used [2–5]. The safety of direct percutaneous and transjugular biopsy has also been established in children [4, 6].

Endobiliary biopsy is an important tool in the evaluation of benign and malignant biliary strictures. With the advent of endoscopic retrograde cholangiopancreatography (ERCP), the majority of endobiliary work is performed by gastroenterologists in the endoscopy suite. However, percutaneous transhepatic cholangiography is a means to secure access to the biliary system when the endoscopic approach is impossible or has failed. As such, endobiliary biopsy can be a valuable service provided by the interventional radiologist.

Indications and Patient Selection

Safe and successful liver biopsy is predicated on appropriate pre-procedure planning. The three major facets of pre-procedure planning are clinical history, laboratory work-up, and pre-procedure imaging.

When considering a request for a liver biopsy, the patient's clinical history is evaluated to determine whether biopsy is indicated and to identify and potentially modify factors that may increase the risk of the procedure. Non-focal percutaneous liver biopsy is performed in patients with suspected or known diffuse parenchymal disease and is useful in establishing diagnosis as well as evaluating prognosis, staging, and/or response to treatment (Table 13.1). In patients with coagulation disorders or when hepatic venous pressure gradient measurements are needed, transjugular liver biopsy may provide a safer or more appropriate alternative to a direct percutaneous technique [6–9].

Focal hepatic lesions without definite benign features on imaging may prompt a focal image-guided biopsy. History of malignancy may raise the suspicion for metastatic disease; alternatively, factors predisposing to malignancy such as cirrhosis may raise suspicion for hepatocellular carcinoma. Image-guided biopsy of portal vein thrombus may be performed to evaluate tumor thrombus [10, 11]. In patients with

Table 13.1 Etiologies of diffuse parenchymal liver disease for which biopsy may be useful

Viral hepatitis
Hemochromatosis
Wilson's disease
Glycogen storage disease
Autoimmune hepatitis
Primary biliary cirrhosis
Nonalcoholic steatohepatitis
Amyloidosis
Sarcoidosis
Diffuse metastatic disease

A. Thabet, MD • D.A. Gervais, MD (✉)
Division of Abdominal Imaging and Intervention,
Department of Radiology, Massachusetts General Hospital,
55 Fruit Street, White-270, Boston, MA 02114, USA
e-mail: athabet@partners.org; dgervais@partners.org

K. Ahrar, S. Gupta (eds.), *Percutaneous Image-Guided Biopsy*,
DOI 10.1007/978-1-4614-8217-8_13, © Springer Science+Business Media New York 2014

Table 13.2 Factors which may increase the risk of complication

Bleeding diathesis
Anticoagulation or antiplatelet therapy
Ascites
Congestive heart failure
Oxygen-dependent chronic obstructive pulmonary disease
Allergy to latex, medications used in sedation, intravenous iodinated contrast

history of lymphoma, specimens are typically submitted for flow cytometry. Immunosuppression (e.g., chemotherapy) may be an indication to submit specimens for microbiologic analysis.

Factors in the patient's clinical history that may increase the risk of the procedure are also assessed (Table 13.2). For example, history of bleeding diathesis or easy bruising should prompt laboratory evaluation of coagulation and platelet function. Patients with severe cardiac or pulmonary disease may not be candidates for procedural sedation; the assistance of an anesthesiologist may be indicated. Pre-procedure antibiotics are typically given in liver transplant patients and prior to biliary procedures. A determination may also be made from the patient's clinical history as to whether the patient is able to give informed consent for the procedure.

The liver is a vascular organ, and hence, patients need to be optimized to reduce the risk of post-procedure bleeding. Along with review of the clinical history, laboratory work-up is important. A coagulation profile is often necessary, particularly in patients with history of liver dysfunction, in whom synthesis of coagulation factors may be compromised. Patients may also need to be screened for thrombocytopenia. Practices vary in the threshold levels that prompt action such as blood product transfusion. Given the risk of post-procedure bleeding, some physicians will require a pre-procedure hematocrit level to be checked and blood bank sample to be submitted.

The importance of pre-procedure imaging will depend on whether a focal or non-focal biopsy is to be performed. For non-focal liver biopsy, pre-procedure imaging is not routinely requested, although, if available, may be reviewed to assess for the presence of ascites as well as anatomical variants (e.g., course of colon relative to liver).

Pre-procedure imaging is mandatory, however, for focal hepatic biopsies for at least four reasons. First, cross-sectional imaging may be useful to exclude patients with lesions that demonstrate definite benign imaging features (e.g., hemangioma). Second, imaging will demonstrate location of the mass and help assess for distant disease. Third, pre-procedure imaging is crucial to planning a safe access route for the biopsy. Fourth, pre-procedure imaging may help the interventionalist select the best imaging modality to guide the biopsy, i.e., ultrasound, CT, or MRI.

As with other interventional radiologic procedures, pre-procedure preparation also includes withholding anticoagulants and antiplatelet agents. If sedation is to be administered, patients are generally made NPO for solid foods 8 h and for clear liquids 2 h prior to the procedure, although practices vary slightly in this regard.

Some practices routinely perform non-focal liver biopsies without procedural sedation. In such circumstances, indications for procedural sedation may include patient anxiety and pediatric age. The assistance of an anesthesiologist is rarely indicated but may be required in pediatric patients or in patients with hemodynamic or respiratory instability.

When a non-focal liver biopsy is desired, an alternative to the direct percutaneous approach is the transjugular liver biopsy. Specimens obtained by way of transjugular approach may be inferior compared to those obtained by direct percutaneous biopsy [8, 12–15]; hence, transjugular liver biopsy is generally performed in specific circumstances. Transjugular biopsy is appropriate if hepatic vein pressure gradient measurements are desired for the assessment of portal hypertension [7, 8]. It may be preferred in patients with severe coagulopathy or congenital clotting disorder, in which the risk of intraperitoneal hemorrhage is reduced by using the transjugular route [7]. Massive ascites has also been described as an indication [6, 8, 9]; however, whether ascites increases the risk of bleeding after direct percutaneous approach is controversial [16, 17]. Transjugular liver biopsy may also be used in children [6].

Contraindications

In most instances, when an image-guided liver biopsy is indicated, factors that may increase the risk of the procedure may be modified to an acceptable level. Rarely do circumstances arise in which a biopsy cannot be performed. These include uncorrectable coagulopathy, hemodynamic or respiratory instability, and lack of safe access to a hepatic lesion. In patients in need of a non-focal biopsy and who present with coagulopathy or massive ascites, a transjugular liver biopsy may be preferred [8]. Massive ascites may restrict the ability to secure safe access to a lesion or liver; pre-procedure paracentesis may be helpful.

Percutaneous Liver Biopsy

Technique (Table 13.3)

Imaging

Non-focal liver biopsies are generally performed using sonography. Focal liver biopsies may be guided using ultrasound, CT, or rarely, MRI.

Table 13.3 General technique for percutaneous liver biopsy

1. Clinical history is reviewed for indications, contraindications, and risk factors that may need to be modified prior to biopsy
2. Laboratory values are reviewed, particularly coagulation profile and platelet count; estimated glomerular filtration rate is calculated if intravenous contrast is to be administered
3. Prior imaging is reviewed, which is mandatory for focal liver biopsy. Putative needle entry site and trajectory are planned
4. Informed consent is obtained. If a hepatic dome lesion is being biopsied, discussion of pneumothorax and chest tube placement may be important
5. Based on review of prior imaging, patient is positioned on the table or stretcher to facilitate the biopsy, e.g., supine, prone, or left lateral oblique or decubitus position
6. Procedural sedation or anesthesia is administered if applicable. Patient is generally made NPO as per institutional guidelines
7. Preliminary images are obtained. The application of a skin grid may be helpful for CT- or MRI-guided focal liver biopsy (see text)
8. Needle entry site, angle of entry, and distance to lesion, if applicable, are assessed
9. Clean and sterilize skin using standard technique
10. Apply local anesthetic, such as 1 % lidocaine. Local anesthesia is optimally administered if given along the planned needle trajectory from the skin to the liver capsule. Allow one to two minutes for anesthetic to take effect
11. A 5-mm skin incision is made with a scalpel blade to facilitate introduction of the introducer (coaxial technique) or biopsy needle
12. With US, needle is advanced into the liver under real-time imaging guidance. Using CT or MRI, a stepwise approach may be used (see text). CT or MRI fluoroscopy may enable real-time visualization
13. Coaxial-, tandem-, or single-needle technique is performed as described in the text

Ultrasound

Ultrasound is the preferred modality for non-focal (Fig. 13.1) and focal (Fig. 13.2) percutaneous liver biopsy for several reasons. US offers real-time visualization and multiplanar capability, is relatively inexpensive, and is readily accessible. The lack of radiation is another advantage, particularly in younger patients. However, sonography is limited in its ability to identify the pleural space, which may increase the risk of post-procedure pneumothorax. Additionally, collapsed bowel may be difficult to discern.

Preliminary sonography is performed to evaluate the liver as well as the position of the gallbladder, if present. Doppler sonography is useful for the identification of intervening vessels [10, 18]. The most common practice is use of freehand technique. In general, one hand controls the transducer, whereas the other controls the biopsy needle. Some physicians prefer to use a biopsy needle guide, which attaches to the transducer. In either case, the needle can be visualized as an echogenic complex; visualization of the needle may be improved with a jiggling "in-and-out"

motion [18]. Echogenic needle-tip enhancers are also commercially available.

CT

CT guidance is associated with longer procedure times, higher cost, and radiation compared to US. In addition, the needle trajectory is generally restricted to the axial plane. CT guidance is indicated in cases where the target lesion is not well demonstrated on sonography (e.g., cirrhosis) or if there is a concern for intervening structures such as bowel based on pre-procedure imaging. CT guidance may also be helpful in obese patients or patients who had a nondiagnostic result from a prior US-guided biopsy. New practitioners may also find that CT-guided biopsy is generally easier to perform than US guidance, with a shorter learning curve.

Pre-procedure images are reviewed, and a grid with radiopaque lines is placed on the patient's skin in the area of the expected needle entry site. A preliminary CT is performed and the biopsy trajectory is confirmed (Fig. 13.3). The needle entry position on the grid is selected; the angle of entry and distance to the lesion are also assessed on the images. The skin is then marked. If an entry site is chosen that is outside the field demarcated by the grid, the skin entry site may be marked by measuring the transverse and/or craniocaudal distances of the entry site from a selected point on the grid. For example, in an anterior approach, if the planned entry site is located medial to the most medial radiopaque grid line, the distance between that line and the entry site can be measured on the images and translated on the skin. A craniocaudal component can also be assessed by counting the number of axial images above or below the CT image in which the grid is last seen and multiplying that number by the slice thickness. Alternatively, the grid position can be modified and repeat CT images obtained. After a sterile preparation and the application of local anesthetic, a needle is inserted at the marked entry site and advanced in step-by-step fashion, with intermittent CT imaging to confirm needle position. If a coaxial needle is used, the stylet may be removed prior to each CT scan to reduce needle artifact that may obscure the lesion (Fig. 13.4).

Although many practitioners use a stepwise approach as outlined above, CT fluoroscopy (CTF) may be useful as it may reduce procedure duration [19, 20]. Although reduction in needle placement time has been documented, CTF has not proven to provide a statistically significant increase in procedure success [19]. In CTF, images may be reconstructed at a rate of up to 8 images per second and may be utilized in either continuous fluoroscopy mode or as a quick-check technique [19, 21]. With the former, the use of CT is analogous to conventional fluoroscopy, as needle manipulation is visualized in real time. The quick-check technique involves the use of single CT fluoroscopic spot images to intermittently check needle position. The quick-check

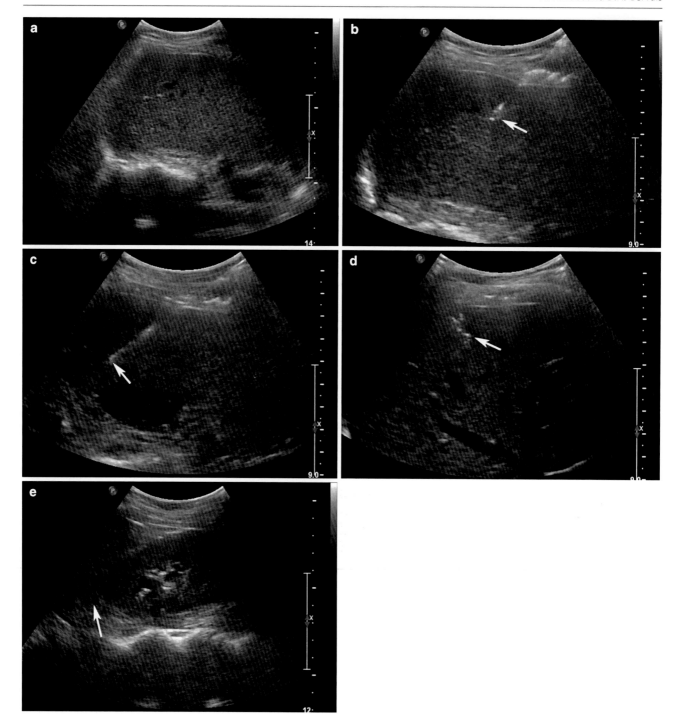

Fig. 13.1 Ultrasound-guided non-focal liver biopsy in a 51-year-old man with hepatitis C. Preliminary sonogram of the liver (**a**) is used to determine a clear needle trajectory to the liver. (**b**) A 17-gauge introducer needle (*arrow*), part of a coaxial needle kit, is advanced into the liver under real-time US guidance. (**c**) An 18-gauge core biopsy gun (*arrow*) is advanced into the liver (*arrow*) through the introducer needle. Post-biopsy sonogram of the liver at the level of the biopsy (**d**, *arrow*) and Morrison's pouch (**e**, *arrow*) demonstrate no hemorrhage

technique is analogous to the conventional step-by-step CT technique but improves upon it in that the operator has use of a "floating table," enabling quick movement of the table and the aid of a laser light to demarcate the axial slice, as well as hand and foot controls. Although the quick-check technique does not fully utilize the real-time capability of

CTF, it improves on procedure time compared to conventional CT technique and significantly lowers radiation to patient and operator compared with the continuous fluoroscopy technique [19].

The success of any image-guided procedure is predicated on visibility of the lesion. CT-guided biopsy may be

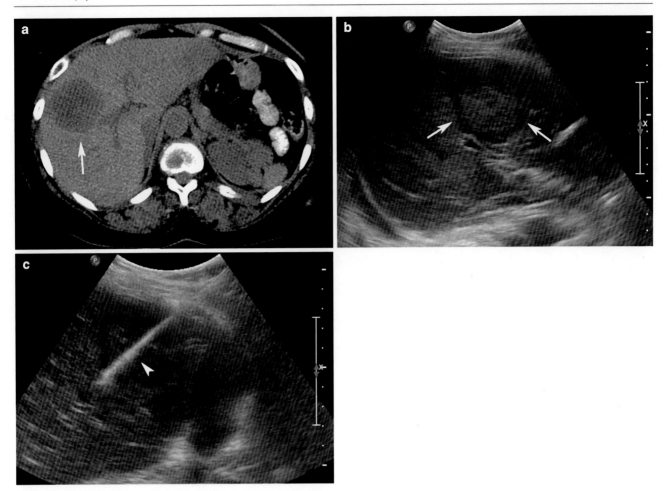

Fig. 13.2 Ultrasound-guided focal liver biopsy in a 62-year-old man with metastases of unknown primary. (**a**) CT scan of the abdomen and pelvis performed with intravenous contrast demonstrates a 5-cm hypodense mass (*arrow*) within the right lobe of the liver. (**b**) Preliminary sonogram demonstrates an echogenic mass with hypoechoic rim (*arrows*). (**c**) Core biopsy needle (*arrowhead*) is advanced into the mass through an introducer needle. Pathology demonstrated metastatic non-small cell lung adenocarcinoma

challenging when the targeted lesion is isodense to surrounding liver parenchyma on non-contrast images. In such cases, prior cross-sectional imaging that best demonstrates the lesion should be reviewed and the position of the lesion on preliminary CT images located based on anatomic landmarks. A reference needle (e.g., 20-gauge Chiba) may be advanced to this position using CT guidance (Fig. 13.4). Contrast-enhanced images can then be obtained and the location of the lesion relative to the reference needle assessed. A second needle entry site may be selected and the biopsy needle advanced to the lesion; although the lesion may no longer be enhancing while the second needle is inserted, the first needle continues to serve as a reference. Lesions identified on MRI images are occasionally not visible on US and contrast-enhanced CT. If MR guidance is unavailable, then CT guidance may be considered with the sole use of anatomic landmarks.

Another limitation of CT guidance is the lack of multiplanar capability. Hepatic dome lesions, for instance, may be better suited for US guidance if visible sonographically

or MRI guidance, if available. If CT is to be used, gantry angulation may be helpful to avoid pleural or pulmonary transgression, although this may be time-consuming. A transpleural or transpulmonary trajectory may be unavoidable (22). The need for such a trajectory may be anticipated on prior imaging, in which case informed consent of the patient may include a discussion of pneumothorax and chest tube placement. The decision to pursue a transpleural or transpulmonary route depends on the clinical scenario; it may be performed safely although the operator should be prepared for a pneumothorax if one is detected on CT images (Fig. 13.5). A transpleural or transpulmonary route may be a relative contraindication in patients with tenuous clinical status who may not be able to tolerate a pneumothorax with chest tube placement. The risk of pneumothorax increases with the number of pleural transgressions; hence, the risk of pneumothorax with a transpulmonary approach is generally considered higher than with a transpleural approach as two pleural surfaces need to be traversed [22–25].

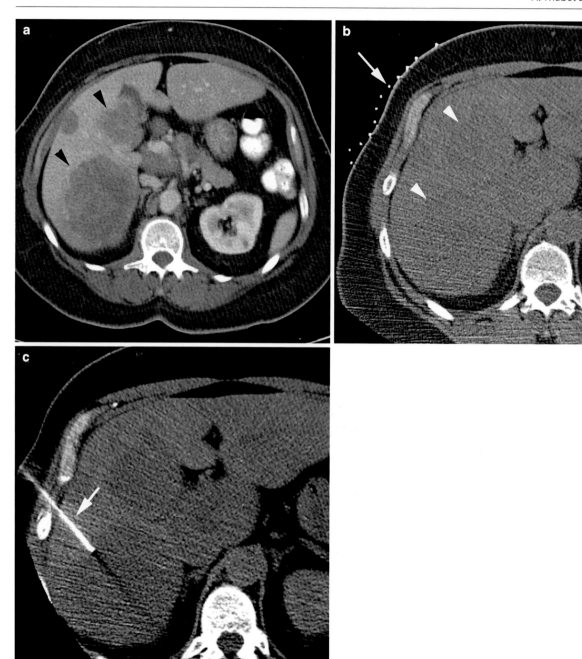

Fig. 13.3 CT-guided focal liver biopsy in a 54-year-old woman. Intravenous contrast-enhanced CT scan (**a**) performed to evaluate abdominal pain demonstrated multiple hypodense hepatic masses (*arrowheads*). Review of this scan at liver biopsy was necessary to plan grid placement (**b**, *arrow*). The hypodense masses (**b**, *arrowheads*) are visible on the non-contrast-enhanced preliminary scan. (**c**) A 17-gauge introducer needle (*arrow*) is advanced into the lesion. Subsequently, fine needle aspiration and core biopsy were performed using coaxial technique (not shown); pathology demonstrated metastatic small cell lung cancer

MRI

MR guidance offers multiplanar imaging capability and excellent soft tissue contrast and lacks radiation [26]. However, its use is limited by procedure duration, cost, and limited availability compared to US and CT [27]. MR guidance is rarely indicated and may be helpful when encountering lesions within the hepatic dome, lesions which are poorly visible on US or CT, or when a nondiagnostic result is obtained after an US- or CT-guided biopsy.

The technique varies with the available equipment, and as such, a complete description of the available MR-guided techniques is beyond the scope of this chapter; the reader is referred to several excellent papers [26, 27]. In general, open- and closed-bore systems are available for interventional

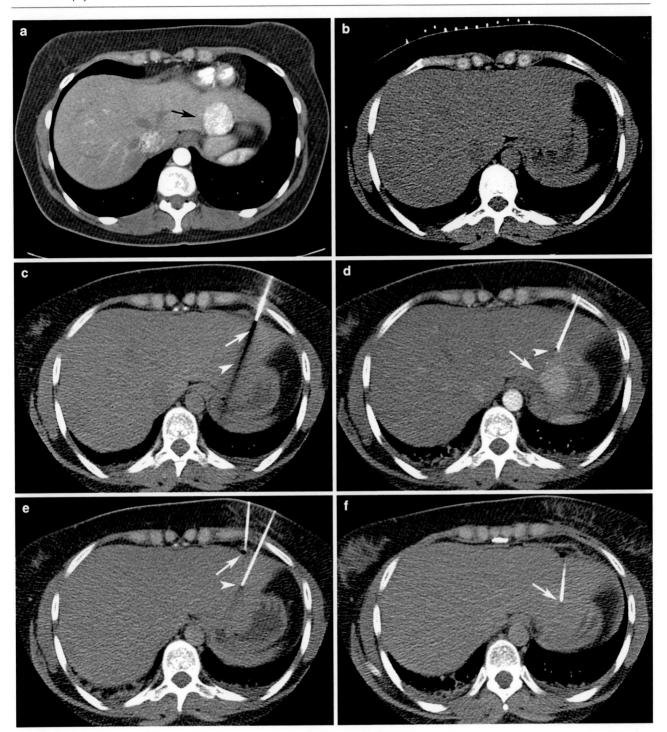

Fig. 13.4 CT-guided focal liver biopsy in a 33-year-old woman with history of melanoma. (**a**) Intravenous contrast-enhanced CT scan of the abdomen and pelvis demonstrates a 3.5-cm arterially enhancing mass (*arrow*) in segment 2 of the liver. (**b**) Preliminary CT performed at liver biopsy demonstrates the lesion is isodense to normal unenhanced liver parenchyma. (**c**) A 17-gauge introducer needle (*arrow*) is advanced into segment 2 based on anatomic landmarks. Needle artifact (*arrowhead*) is prominent as the stylet is present within the needle. (**d**) Contrast-enhanced scan at biopsy demonstrates that the trajectory of the needle is not optimally aligned with the mass (*arrow*). Note, with the stylet removed, needle artifact is absent (*arrowhead*). (**e**) A second 17-gauge introducer needle (*arrow*) is advanced into the liver, using the first needle as a reference (*arrowhead*). (**f**) The second needle (*arrow*) is optimally aligned for biopsy of the mass. Pathology demonstrated focal nodular hyperplasia

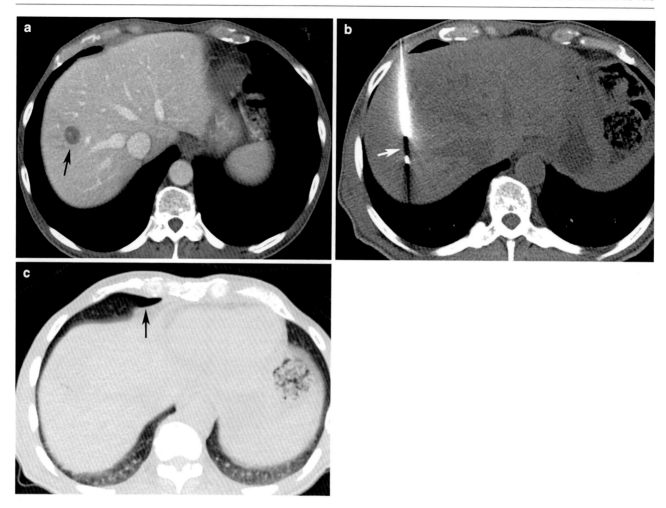

Fig. 13.5 Pneumothorax after CT-guided focal liver biopsy using a transpleural route in a 65-year-old man with history of pancreatic cancer. (**a**) Intravenous contrast-enhanced CT scan of the abdomen demonstrates a 1.8 cm hypodense mass (*arrow*) in segment 8 of the liver. (**b**) A core biopsy needle placed by coaxial technique encompasses the mass (*arrow*). (**c**) CT scan after removal of the needle demonstrates a small right anterior pneumothorax (*arrow*). The patient was asymptomatic and was discharged after a 2-h follow-up chest radiograph (not shown) demonstrated no pneumothorax. Pathology demonstrated metastatic pancreatic adenocarcinoma

procedures. Open-bore designs offer improved patient access compared to closed-bore systems. C-shaped open-bore designs enable improved horizontal but poor vertical access; hence, some patients may need to be positioned in a decubitus position for anterior or posterior approaches [21]. Double-doughnut configuration open-bore systems enable excellent vertical and horizontal access [21]. These systems typically operate in the 0.2-T–0.5-T range, and hence, the quality of imaging is poorer compared to closed-bore systems that operate in the 1-T–1.5-T range but nevertheless may be sufficient for biopsy [26, 28]. Although a closed-bore design may offer better signal-to-noise and contrast-to-noise ratio, patient access is restricted, particularly in obese patients; instrument manipulations are thus often performed with the patient outside of the magnet as with conventional CT guidance. However, the availability of closed-, short-, wide-bore 1.5-T systems may offer improved access for interventions allowing needle manipulations when the patient is in the magnet while maintaining excellent imaging quality [27].

A step-by-step technique similar to CT has been described with both systems, although MR fluoroscopy may also be performed [27]. In general, preliminary non-contrast MRI images are obtained with a three-plane localizer sequence as well as fast T2-weighted spin-echo sequences; gradient-echo sequences can also be employed before and after gadolinium administration [26]. If a step-by-step technique is employed, as is commonly with conventional closed-bore systems, an MR-compatible grid visible on either T1- or T2-weighted sequences is applied to the skin. The technique is similar to CT, with the exception that the needle trajectory is not restricted to the axial plane [26]. T1- or T2-weighted sequences are obtained depending on the type of grid used. Software specific to the MR scanner is used to select the needle entry site, plan the angle of the needle trajectory, and measure the distance

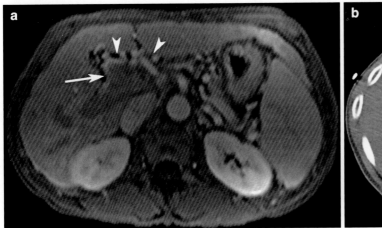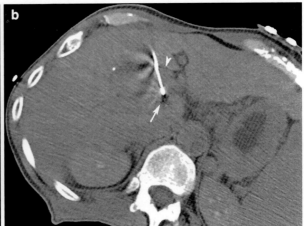

Fig. 13.6 CT-guided liver biopsy in a 53-year-old man with a liver mass and portal thrombus. (**a**) T1-weighted fat-saturated post-gadolinium MRI image of the liver demonstrates enhancing thrombus within the portal vein (*arrow*) with cavernous transformation. A 4-cm segment 7 mass was also seen (not shown). (**b**) At liver biopsy, the 2-cm notch of the core biopsy gun (*arrow*) is well seated within the portal vein mass (*arrowhead*). Biopsy of the segment 7 mass was also performed (not shown) during the same session. Pathology demonstrated hepatocellular carcinoma and tumor thrombus

to the lesion. The needle is inserted at the entry site and is advanced using a stepwise technique, with each manipulation performed while the patient is outside the magnet.

Open-bore as well as closed-, short-, wide-bore systems may enable real-time guidance. By repeating fast imaging sequences, the operator's palpating finger rather than a grid may be use to mark the needle entry site [26, 27]. Confirmatory images in two orthogonal planes may be obtained when the needle tip is at the edge of the lesion to detect any significant deviation of the needle [27]. If there is difficulty correcting needle deviation after several attempts using MR fluoroscopy (e.g., firm liver due to cirrhosis that restricts manipulation of soft MR-compatible needles), the stylet can be inserted into the needle while the patient is outside the magnet and the needle redirected, with intermittent imaging used as in a conventional step-by-step approach [27].

In general, the needle appears hypointense with a hyperintense rim on MR [26]. Many variables affect the degree of artifact induced by the needle. Distortion is worse with smaller needles, increased needle angle relative to B0, higher-field MR scanners, and gradient-echo versus spin-echo sequences [26].

Devices

Cytologists and pathologists may require multiple biopsy specimens in order to make an accurate and confident diagnosis. Biopsy techniques have evolved to facilitate obtaining multiple specimens while reducing the risk of complication. The most established method is the coaxial technique [21], although tandem- and single-needle techniques may also be performed.

The coaxial technique enables multiple tissue samples to be obtained with a single pass through overlying tissues and liver capsule, reducing patient discomfort, procedure duration, number of images required, and risk of complication [21]. This is of particular benefit in deep-seated lesions, in which single- or tandem-needle technique may be cumbersome [21]. In general, an introducer needle is advanced into the lesion under imaging guidance. Introducer needles are available from 11 G to 19 G, depending on the biopsy system to be used, although 17 G to 19 G is usually sufficient. Once the introducer needle is within the lesion, core biopsy and/or fine needle aspiration may be performed through the indwelling introducer needle.

Fine needle aspirates may be obtained with the use of a 20-G to 22-G hollow (e.g., Chiba) needle. The aspiration needle is advanced through the introducer needle. A "to-and-fro" motion is performed such that cells are acquired by capillary action. A 10-mL syringe may also be attached to the needle with a small degree of aspiration (1–3 mL) applied to improve cytologic yield, although suction is not applied while withdrawing the needle to reduce the amount of blood within the specimen.

Core biopsy guns are available in multiple designs and sizes. It is important to be familiarized with operation of the biopsy system available prior to use. The most commonly used is an automated, spring-activated side-cutting biopsy gun, available from 14 to 20 G. Automated devices generally provide more diagnostic specimens than their manual counterparts [21, 29, 30]. For hepatic lesions, 18-G to 20-G systems are most commonly used. Use of larger systems may be associated with a higher complication rate, although randomized trials are lacking [21, 31–33]. The core biopsy gun is advanced through the introducer needle while the inner trochar is retracted into the gun's outer cannula. Subsequently, the inner trochar may be

Table 13.4 Summary of preparation of biopsy specimens (these are representative; consultation with individual pathology departments is suggested as practices vary)

General histopathology	Two or three 2-cm non-fragmented core biopsy specimens in saline (or possibly formalin if pathology processing cannot be performed same day), additional samples if fragmented specimens encountered
General cytopathology	At least two sets of fine needle aspirates smeared on glass slides. These should be placed in 95 % ethanol quickly after smears are made to minimize dry air contact time. Additional samples in sterile saline or methanol–water solution for cell block
Lymphoma	Separate fine needle aspirates in sterile saline for flow cytometry
Breast cancer	Hormone receptor/Her2 staining
Prostate cancer	PSA staining
Microbiology	Gram stain, culture, sensitivity, AFB, mycobacterial culture, fungal stain, and culture
Research	As per protocol

advanced into the lesion prior to firing the system; if desired, this allows the use of imaging to confirm that the side-cutting portion of the needle is well seated within the lesion prior to firing the system (Figs. 13.5 and 13.6). Typically, two or three 2-cm non-fragmented samples are sufficient for histopathology, although additional specimens may be needed if fragmented specimens are obtained. Representative methods of specimen preparation are summarized in Table 13.4.

Because the coaxial technique involves the placement of a single introducer needle into the lesion, multiple samples may be obtained within a specific portion of the lesion. Hence, as additional samples are obtained, the diagnostic yield may diminish as the same area is biopsied. It is generally possible to rotate the core biopsy needle with each pass such that the notch faces a different orientation with respect to the lesion. If the lesion is sufficiently large and the introducer needle tip is in the proximal portion of the needle, the stylet may be reinserted into the introducer needle and the system advanced further into the lesion. If this is performed, note should be made of the sample size of the notch within the side-cutting needle, typically measuring 2 cm, such that any further core biopsy samples are performed within the lesion. Occasionally, necrotic lesions are encountered. Biopsy of the periphery of such lesions may improve diagnostic yield, and this may be taken into account when planning placement of the introducer needle.

Although the coaxial technique is well established, a tandem-needle technique is also possible for focal liver biopsy. The principal disadvantage of this technique is the multiple passes through overlying tissues and liver capsule required. In general, a 20 G reference needle is advanced into the needle using imaging guidance. A 22-G needle may also be used, although such needles may deflect more easily in firm, cirrhotic livers or when traversing long distances. Along and parallel to this needle, a 20- to 22-G hollow needle may be advanced into the lesion to obtain fine needle aspirations. A core biopsy gun may also be advanced alongside the reference needle. This technique requires imaging for every pass, as opposed to coaxial technique, thereby prolonging the procedure. In addition, multiple passes through the liver capsule may result in more patient discomfort and increase the risk of procedure complication [21].

A single-needle approach to non-focal hepatic biopsy may also be performed [34]. The principal advantage of this technique is that several areas of the liver may be biopsied [34], although the clinical significance of this is uncertain. Another advantage is that the larger introducer needle is not required; instead, a core biopsy gun is used directly, although this advantage should be weighed against the need for multiple punctures of the liver capsule with the single-needle technique. Hatfield et al. found no difference in the complication rate between coaxial and noncoaxial techniques [34].

Practices vary in the need for core biopsy specimens for focal hepatic lesions. Fine needle aspiration is limited by the expertise of the cytopathologist and its ability to specifically diagnose benign lesions and subtype particular malignancies [21]. Some practices will use an on-site cytopathologist to determine if a specimen is adequate and obtain core biopsy specimens only if fine needle aspirates are insufficient. Other practices may routinely get both fine needle and core biopsy specimens without the assistance of a cytopathologist. In the absence of a cytologist, a predetermined number of three passes may be diagnostic in nearly 90 % of cases [35]. It appears that a combination of core biopsy and fine needle specimens may improve the diagnostic yield of the procedure [21, 36].

Approach and Relevant Anatomy

Ideally, any needle advanced into the liver courses through no other structures other than the skin, fat, muscle, and liver capsule. Other structures that may be encountered include gallbladder, pleura, lung, bowel, and vessels.

The liver is divided into two lobes, with the left lobe separated from the right by the middle hepatic vein and gallbladder fossa. If present, it is important to document the position of the gallbladder relative to the needle trajectory on preliminary images as inadvertent gallbladder puncture risks bile peritonitis. The normal anatomy of the pleura is also important: the inferior extent of the pleura increases when coursing from anterior to posterior in the axial plane. Hence, an intercostal approach may increase the risk of transpleural trajectory compared to a subcostal approach. In addition, the superior epigastric artery descends within the rectus sheath and is an important structure to be aware of when planning

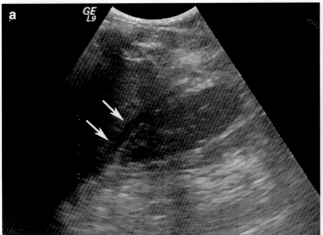 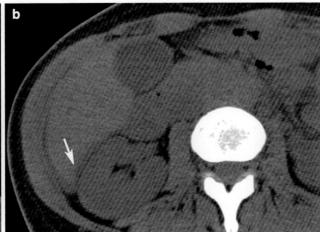

Fig. 13.7 Mild hemorrhage after US-guided non-focal liver biopsy in a 46-year-old woman with hemochromatosis. (**a**) Sonogram of Morrison's pouch after removal of the needle demonstrates a small amount of fluid (*arrows*). The patient had mild pain but was hemody- namically stable with an unchanged hematocrit. (**b**) Two-hour follow-up CT demonstrated a small hematoma in Morrison's pouch. Patient was admitted for observation and discharged the following day. No transfu- sion of blood products was required

an anterior approach. The colon may be interposed between the abdominal wall and the anterior and/or lateral aspects of the liver. The liver may also migrate cranially with dimin- ished respiratory excursion.

For non-focal liver biopsy and in some focal liver biop- sies, a subcostal, subxiphoid, or midaxillary intercostal approach may be available. Some interventionalists prefer a subcostal or subxiphoid approach to reduce the risk of pain. Increased pain with an intercostal approach may be due to the injury to intercostal muscles or nerves, transgression of the pleura, or larger tear of the liver capsule secondary to greater respiratory motion [37]. However, in a randomized trial comparing pain scores and complication rates between subcostal and intercostals, Tan et al. demonstrated no statis- tically significant difference in pain or complication rates [37]. An intercostal approach may be preferable in patients undergoing procedural sedation, where the liver may rise too cranially for a subcostal or subxiphoid approach. In addition, when a biopsy of the right lobe is performed under sonographic guidance, a medial-to-lateral needle trajec- tory may be preferable to avoid inadvertent injury to the gallbladder.

Planning the needle entry site and trajectory for a focal liver biopsy depends on lesion location and the presence of intervening structures. For hepatic dome lesions, US enables craniocaudal angulation of the needle trajectory. Occasionally, CT guidance may be required, in which case pleural transgression may be unavoidable, although angu- lation of the gantry may help to reduce this risk. When a lesion abuts the liver capsule, some interventional radiolo- gists prefer a needle trajectory that traverses through nor- mal liver parenchyma first, which may theoretically provide a tamponading effect to reduce the risk of intraperitoneal

hemorrhage [38]. Necrotic liver lesions may also be encoun- tered. As discussed previously, it may be helpful to place the needle within the periphery of such lesions to improve the chance of sampling viable tissue.

The presence of ascites may also be documented on prelimi- nary imaging. Ascites may displace the liver surface away from the abdominal wall, which may make obtaining needle purchase more difficult or may increase the risk of intraperitoneal hemor- rhage. In such cases, interventionalists may perform pre-proce- dure paracentesis or, alternatively, recommend a transjugular biopsy. However, some studies have reported that there is no increased risk of complication from liver biopsy in the presence of ascites [16, 17]. Although such data suggests that ascites should not be a contraindication to liver biopsy, pre-procedure paracentesis may be a prudent measure given its low risk.

Potential Complications

Percutaneous liver biopsy is generally a safe procedure [10, 18, 37–41]. As delineated by the Society of Interventional Radiology, a major complication is defined as one requiring hospital admission after an outpatient procedure, unplanned increase in care, prolonged hospital stay, or resulting in per- manent adverse event or death [42]. A minor complication is one that requires no or nominal care, including overnight hospital admission for observation [42]. Less than 5 % of outpatient liver biopsy patients require admission [10].

Major complications of percutaneous biopsy include hemorrhage requiring transfusion or other intervention, pneumothorax, malignant tract seeding, infection, gallbladder or bowel perforation, and death [10]. Minor complications include mild hemorrhage not requiring intervention (Fig. 13.7). The most common complications are pain and hemorrhage, the latter of which is found more commonly after biopsy of a malignant lesion than after a non-focal biopsy [10]. Both of these complications account for the majority of hospital admissions after biopsy [43]. Pain is an expected finding after liver biopsy. Most studies estimate the complication rate at less than 2 %, with mortality not exceeding 0.1 %. In one population-based study of 4275 focal and non-focal liver biopsies, the overall complication rate was 0.75 %, with pain found in 0.51 % and bleeding in 0.35 % of all biopsy patients [43].

Although such complications occur with both focal and non-focal biopsies, it is noteworthy that some physicians perform non-focal liver biopsy without US guidance [44]. Numerous studies have demonstrated that the use of US guidance results in a statistically significant decrease in the complication rate. In one study, the rate with and without US guidance was 0.53 % and 2.1 %, respectively [44, 45]. There is also a decreased rate of hospitalization for pain and bleeding [3, 44].

Management of Complications

Immediate post-procedure care after US-guided biopsy includes evaluation of the biopsy site and Morrison's pouch after removal of the needle to assess for hemorrhage. A chest radiograph may be obtained if there is suspicion for pneumothorax. Post-procedure CT images after needle removal are reviewed for hemorrhage and pneumothorax. Bowel or gallbladder perforation is rare and may manifest as a delayed complication such as abscess.

The most common symptom and sign of hemorrhage are abdominal/shoulder pain and tachycardia [10]. Postprocedure pain should be evaluated first by assessment of vital signs. If tachycardia is present, CT may be helpful to evaluate for hemorrhage. However, if hemodynamic instability ensues, intravenous hydration may be administered, serial hematocrit levels checked, and blood bank sample submitted. Of note, the normal tachycardiac response during hemorrhage may be blunted if the patient is on beta-blocker therapy. In general, a low threshold for non-contrast CT imaging of the abdomen is prudent. Angiography with embolization may be required in some cases (Fig. 13.8).

If coaxial technique was performed, some interventionalists choose to administer a slurry of absorbable gelatin sponge into the introducer needle routinely or after brisk back bleeding is noted, particularly after biopsy of hypervascular lesions. However, a study by Hatfield et al. demonstrated no statistically significant difference in complication rates among patients who underwent biopsy with or without gelatin sponge embolization of the tract [34]. Although this was a retrospective analysis, there is otherwise little evidence suggesting that gelatin sponge administration reduces hemorrhage after biopsy.

Outcomes and Results

The reported accuracy of liver biopsy ranges from 83 to 95 % [39]. With fine needle aspiration alone, the sensitivity and specificity of focal liver biopsy is approximately 94 % and 93 %, respectively [10, 46]. In general, fine needle aspiration alone in focal liver biopsy is limited by the expertise of the cytopathologist and is less accurate in providing specific benign diagnoses and subtyping malignancies [21]. A statistically significant increase in accuracy in establishing a specific benign or malignant diagnosis has been reported when histologic core biopsy specimens are combined with cytologic samples after focal liver biopsy [36].

Core biopsy is generally required in non-focal liver biopsy [44]. The quality of liver biopsy specimens for the evaluation of diffuse liver disease is determined by the number of complete portal tracts, with specimens of sufficient quality to stage and grade hepatic disease typically containing more than 11 [44]; specimens containing at least six complete portal tracts may be sufficient for diagnosis [8]. Automated core biopsy specimens appear to provide better quality tissue for the evaluation of liver parenchyma, particularly in hepatitis C and hepatic fibrosis, compared to aspiration techniques [44].

Transjugular Liver Biopsy

Technique
Imaging

Two necessary guidance tools for transjugular interventional work are sonography and fluoroscopy. Although needle access to the internal jugular vein may be performed using anatomic landmarks, the use of ultrasound guidance reduces the risk of puncture-related complications such as neck hematoma [8, 9]. Pre-procedure sonography of the liver and abdomen may be useful to assess for hepatic vein and IVC patency [9]. Fluoroscopy is utilized for manipulation of guidewires, catheters, and biopsy devices, as well as for venography [8].

Devices

The most commonly used biopsy device is an automated, spring-activated cutting needle. These typically measure 18–19 G and consist of a 2-cm notch which captures the specimen (Fig. 13.9). Fragmentation of specimens appears to be worse when devices larger than 18 G are used [8]. Older aspiration-type devices such as the 16-G Menghini needle are described in the literature; tissue specimens obtained with Menghini needles appear to be shorter and more fragmented, contain fewer complete portal tracts, and are less likely to be adequate for histologic diagnosis given the same number of passes than automated, cutting needles [8].

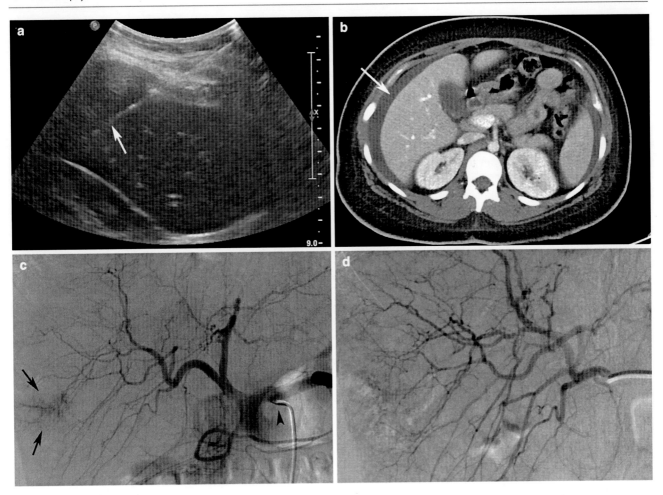

Fig. 13.8 Hemorrhage after US-guided non-focal liver biopsy in a 19-year-old woman who was admitted for new-onset jaundice. (**a**) Sonography of the liver during liver biopsy demonstrates an 18-gauge core biopsy needle (*arrow*) within the right lobe. After removal of the needle, sonography demonstrated no evidence of hemorrhage (not shown). Patient was transferred back to the inpatient ward. That evening, the patient complained of abdominal pain and became hypotensive. Hematocrit dropped from 41 to 22. (**b**) Unenhanced CT scan of the abdomen and pelvis demonstrates new intraperitoneal fluid measuring 30 Hounsfield units, consistent with hemorrhage. (**c**) Celiac arteriography (*arrowhead*) demonstrates active extravasation (*arrows*) from a branch of the right hepatic artery. Embolization of the branch was performed with 500 **μ**m polyvinyl alcohol particles. (**d**) Post-embolization arteriogram demonstrates no further extravasation. The patient's blood pressure and hematocrit stabilized; the patient was subsequently discharged 2 days later. Pathology demonstrated autoimmune hepatitis

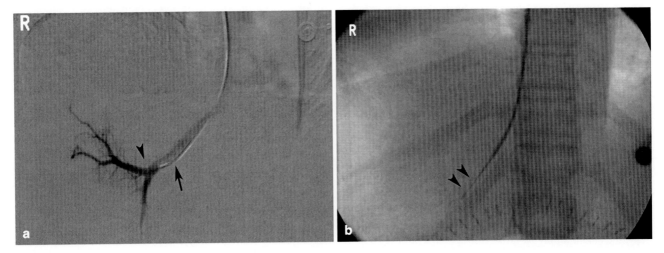

Fig. 13.9 Transjugular liver biopsy in a 38-year-old man with hepatocellular carcinoma, acute renal failure, and thrombocytopenia. (**a**) Hepatic venography after cannulation of the right hepatic vein with a 5-French angiographic catheter (*arrow*) demonstrates patency (*arrowhead*) of the right hepatic venous system. (**b**) Transjugular biopsy with a 19-gauge automated cutting needle (*arrowheads*) is guided with fluoroscopy

Approach and Relevant Anatomy

The right internal jugular vein (RIJV) approach is most commonly used [6, 8, 9]. The left internal jugular vein (LIJV) may be used when the RIJV is not available such as due to thrombosis, although technically more challenging to navigate given the course of the left brachiocephalic vein across the mediastinum [47]. The RIJV communicates with the subclavian and subsequently right brachiocephalic vein and the superior vena cava (SVC). From the SVC and through the right atrium, the intrahepatic inferior vena cava (IVC) is reached, where the orifices of the right, middle, and left hepatic veins may be found.

The right hepatic vein (RHV) generally courses laterally or posterolaterally. The middle (MHV) and left hepatic veins (LHV) course anterolaterally and anteriorly, respectively. In most patients, the right lobe of the liver is significantly larger than then the left lobe of liver; hence, biopsy via the right hepatic vein is generally preferred, as this may reduce the risk of perforation of the liver capsule.

While supine, the patient's head is turned to the side opposite the side of internal jugular vein puncture, usually to the left. The RIJV is identified with US, and after sterile preparation and the application of local anesthetic, the RIJV is accessed using standard Seldinger or micropuncture technique. Venous distention may be improved with Trendelenburg position and intravenous hydration [8]. A 0.035-in. guidewire (e.g., J-wire) is advanced into the venous system followed by a vascular sheath. Over the wire, an angled 5-French catheter can be navigated through the right atrium into the IVC; continuous electrocardiographic and hemodynamic monitoring is important to assess for possible arrhythmia [8]. A multipurpose catheter and guidewire can then be used to cannulate the hepatic vein, preferably the right. The left hepatic vein may be cannulated if the left lobe is hypertrophied [9]. After cannulation of the RHV, hepatic venography may be performed to confirm patency and selection of correct hepatic vein. If indicated, hepatic venous pressure gradients may be evaluated with the use of an occlusion-balloon catheter.

A curved 9-French cannula is advanced through into the vein. If a LIJV approach is used, a 0.035-in. super-stiff Amplatz wire may facilitate negotiation of the cannula across the mediastinum [9]. Over a guidewire, the biopsy device is advanced into the hepatic vein, approximately 1 cm distal to the cannula. Peripheral positioning of the cannula/needle assembly in the hepatic vein is avoided to reduce the risk of capsular perforation [8, 9]. In the right hepatic vein, the cannula is typically turned counterclockwise, directing the needle anteriorly into the liver [7, 9]. In the MHV, the cannula may be turned clockwise to direct the needle laterally. In the LHV, the cannula may be turned clockwise as well.

Once the needle is advanced into the liver parenchyma and the system is fired, the needle is withdrawn out of the patient and the specimen inspected and collected. After a sufficient number of specimens are obtained (generally, two to three specimens), hepatic venography may be performed to assess for capsular perforation. After removal of the sheath, manual compression at the neck venipuncture site is generally applied for 5 min until hemostasis is achieved.

Potential Complications

Transjugular liver biopsy is generally a safe procedure. The rate of major complications is 0.5 % [8]. Approximately half of these are related to intraperitoneal hemorrhage. Ventricular arrhythmia represents another major complication. Caroticojugular fistula is very rarely encountered [8]. Minor complications occur in approximately 6.5 % of patients [8]. Those related to neck puncture include hematoma, carotid artery puncture, and pneumothorax, which occur less frequently with ultrasound guidance [8]. Reported mortality rate is under 0.1 % [8]. A major factor associated with increased frequency of complication is pediatric age, possibly due to smaller size of the liver [8].

Management of Complications

Complications may be subdivided among those related to neck puncture, liver puncture, and cardiac arrhythmias. Neck hematomas may respond to manual compression and compression bandage [9]. Symptomatic or large pneumothoraces may require chest tube placement; otherwise, observation with serial chest radiographs is reasonable. Caroticojugular fistula may be treated with surgery or stent graft [9]. Hemoperitoneum due to capsular perforation may be followed with serial hematocrit levels and hemodynamic monitoring. In refractory cases, transfusion of packed red blood cells, correction of abnormal coagulation profile and/or thrombocytopenia, or possibly embolization or surgery may be required. Some physicians may perform hepatic venography after the biopsy is complete to assess for extravasation; if perforation is detected, coil embolization may be performed or the patient may be observed for hemoperitoneum as described [6, 8]. Treatment of cardiac arrhythmias depends on the rhythm type but may respond to carotid massage and removal of the catheter and guidewire [9].

Outcomes and Results

Transjugular liver biopsy is technically successful in 95–98 % of cases [8, 9]. The most common reason for technical failure is inability to cannulate the hepatic vein. Given the smaller mean number of complete portal triads obtained with each pass from transjugular biopsy, specimens are generally adequate for histologic diagnosis, but may not be as sufficient for staging and grading of diffuse liver disease when compared to direct percutaneous liver biopsy unless multiple specimens are provided [8, 9]. The use of automated cutting needles has been advocated as these may provide longer, better quality specimens than Menghini needles [8, 9].

Endobiliary

Technique
Imaging
Endobiliary sampling by interventional radiologists is performed through percutaneous transhepatic biliary tracts. Hence, guidance of most devices requires fluoroscopy. Fluoroscopy is also effective in establishing access for a choledochoscope, if forceps biopsy under direct visualization is desired.

Devices
Masses which produce biliary obstruction may be best evaluated by fine needle aspiration and/or core biopsy techniques using US, CT, or endoscopic US guidance [48]. However, some biliary lesions are too small for US- or CT- guided biopsy. Such strictures may be good candidates for endobiliary sampling. Methods of sampling include bile cytology, fluoroscopically guided endobiliary brush biopsy, or fluoroscopic- or choledochoscopic-guided clamshell forceps biopsy [48].

Malignant biliary tumors may shed cells into the biliary system. Because it is simple, requires minimal effort, and is inexpensive, submission of a 10–15-mL sample of bile after catheter decompression of the biliary system is generally performed when malignancy is suspected [48–51].

Other endobiliary tools are available. Endobiliary brush biopsy via percutaneous transhepatic tracts involves placement of a peel-away sheath through the percutaneous tract (Fig. 13.10). After securing a safety guidewire, a 3-mm brush may be advanced into the tract through the sheath and placed distal to the stricture [48]. The brush is brought back and forth across the lesion and removed. The brush may be clipped, placed in normal saline, and sent to cytology, or, a smear may be made on glass slides, which are placed into 95 % ethanol, and the procedure repeated [48, 52].

Fluoroscopic- or choledochoscopic-guided clamshell forceps biopsy may also be performed. When using fluoroscopic guidance, a peel-away sheath is advanced just proximal to the stricture; a 5.2- or 7-French clamshell bioptome forceps is advanced through a peel-away sheath and exposed just proximal to the stricture [48]. The clamshell-shaped head of the forceps device is in apposition to the duct wall and a specimen obtained and placed in formalin [48]. When choledochoscopy is used, a 3–5-French flexible forceps may be advanced through the working channel of a choledochoscope and a specimen obtained under direct visualization [48]. Of note, the tract may need to be dilated to 16–18 French to allow use of the choledochoscope [48]. Progressive dilatation of the tract may be performed over 2–3 weeks [48].

Approach and Relevant Anatomy
Endobiliary sampling requires a percutaneous transhepatic biliary access or endoscopic approach. Once access is established, a bile fluid sample may be sent for exfoliative cytology. Brush or clamshell forceps biopsy may be performed at initial percutaneous drainage, although if there is concern for cholangitis, sepsis, or significant hemobilia, biopsy may be delayed until the patient's clinical status is stabilized [48]. Biopsy of lesions involving the left and right hepatic ducts, duct confluence, common hepatic and bile duct, ampullary segment, or biliary-enteric anastomosis is generally possible once a tract is established [48].

Potential Complications
Complications after endobiliary sampling procedures include cholangitis and sepsis, as well as bile extravasation with biloma formation, and hemobilia. The overall reported complication rate from endobiliary biopsy ranges from 0 to 6 % [48, 53]. A majority of these complications are minor and include biloma or self-limiting hemobilia. It may be difficult to ascertain whether such complications are a result of the biopsy or secondary to the percutaneous drainage procedure when performed at the same setting [53].

Management of Complications
Biloma formation may require percutaneous drainage [53]. Hemobilia is usually self-limiting. Refractory hemorrhage may require arteriography and embolization, although such a major complication has not been reported in the literature after biopsy [53]. Cholangitis and sepsis are other potential complications; broad-spectrum antibiotics are generally administered prior to any biliary intervention [48].

Outcomes and Results
The sensitivity of exfoliative cytology ranges from 15 to 34 %, with a specificity of up to 100 %. Although the sensitivity for the detection of malignant disease may be low, it is simple to perform and inexpensive. Brush biopsy has shown to be a safe technique; reported sensitivity ranges from 26 to 67 % with specificity as high as 96 % [48, 53]. Forceps biopsy may prove to be more sensitive than brush biopsy or cytology in the diagnosis of malignant stricture, with sensitivity, specificity, and accuracy reported as high as 78 %, 100 %, and 79.2 %, respectively [53]. Endobiliary sampling may be more effective in diagnosis of cholangiocarcinoma than in extrahepatic tumors that result in biliary stricture (e.g., metastases to portal lymph nodes); this is presumably due to the relatively superficial tissue penetration by the biopsy technique [48, 53]. False-positive diagnoses are rare but may be seen particularly in the setting of sclerosing cholangitis, where fibrosis may mimic pancreatic carcinoma [48]. Choledochoscopic-guided forceps biopsy may offer higher sensitivity in the detection of malignancy, although it

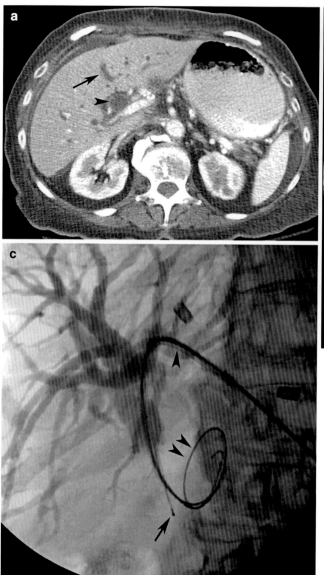

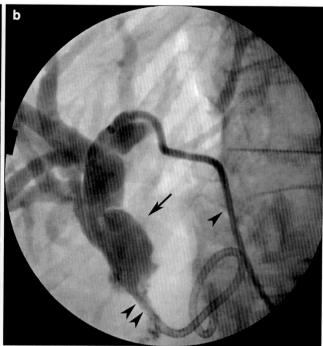

Fig. 13.10 Endobiliary brush biopsy in an 88-year-old woman with history of Klatskin tumor. (**a**) Intravenous contrast-enhanced CT scan 1 year after surgical resection of the primary tumor demonstrates intrahepatic (*arrow*) and extrahepatic (*arrowhead*) biliary duct dilatation. (**b**) Percutaneous biliary drainage was performed after failed endoscopic retrograde pancreatography. Contrast injection of the biliary drain (*sin-* *gle arrowhead*) demonstrates severe biliary duct dilatation (*arrow*) which abruptly terminates (*double arrowhead*) at the biliary-enteric anastomosis. (**c**) 2 days after drainage, the drain is exchanged over a wire (*double arrowheads*) for a peel-away sheath (*single arrowhead*). Brush biopsy device is advanced (*arrow*) into the level of the stricture. Cytology demonstrated no malignant cells

is generally more expensive and challenging to employ, with larger percutaneous tracts required [48, 53].

Summary

Image-guided liver biopsy is among the most valuable tools offered by interventional radiology. It represents the gold standard in evaluation of diffuse parenchymal liver disease and may be invaluable when assessing focal hepatic lesions which do not demonstrate benign imaging features. Endobiliary biopsy, whether using a brush or clamshell forceps device, can serve as an important tool for the interventionalist when ERCP is not readily available. The safety and efficacy of these procedures are well documented; very rarely is an absolute contraindication encountered. Proficiency with US-, CT-, and MR-guidance tools will offer the interventionalist maximum flexibility when encountering a challenging case.

References

1. Hahn PF, Gervais DA, O'Neill MJ, Mueller PR. Nonvascular interventional procedures: analysis of a 10-year database containing more than 10,000 cases. Radiology. 2001;220:730–6.

2. Flemming JA, Hurlbut DJ, Mussari B, Hookey LC. Liver biopsies for chronic hepatitis C: should nonultrasound-guided biopsies be abandoned? Can J Gastroenterol. 2009;23:425–30.

3. Lindor KD, Bru C, Jorgensen RA, et al. The role of ultrasonography and automatic-needle biopsy in outpatient percutaneous liver biopsy. Hepatology. 1996;23:1079–83.

4. Farrell RJ, Smiddy PF, Pilkington RM, et al. Guided versus blind liver biopsy for chronic hepatitis C: clinical benefits and costs. J Hepatol. 1999;30:580–7.

5. Pasha T, Gabriel S, Therneau T, Dickson ER, Lindor KD. Cost effectiveness of ultrasound-guided liver biopsy. Hepatology. 1998;27:1220–6.

6. Kaye R, Sane S, Towbin RB. Pediatric intervention: an update—Part II. J Vasc Interv Radiol. 2000;11:807–22.

7. Bromley PJ, Kaufman JA. In: Kaufman JA, Lee MJ, editors. Vascular and interventional radiology: the requisites. Philadelphia: Mosby; 2004. p. 377–406.

8. Kalambokis G, Manousou P, Vibhakorn S, et al. Transjugular liver biopsy—indications, adequacy, quality of specimens, and complications—a systematic review. J Hepatol. 2007;47:284–94.

9. Mammen T, Keshava SN, Eapen CE, et al. Transjugular liver biopsy: a retrospective analysis of 601 cases. J Vasc Interv Radiol. 2008;19:351–8.

10. Kinney TB. Percutaneous biopsy. In: Valji K, editor. Vascular and interventional radiology. 2nd ed. Philadelphia: Saunders Elsevier; 2006. p. 495–515.

11. Withers CE, Casola G, Herba MJ, et al. Intravascular tumors: transvenous biopsy. Radiology. 1988;167:713–15.

12. Bravo AA, Sheth SG, Chopra S. Liver biopsy. N Engl J Med. 2001;344:495–500.

13. Dotter CT. Catheter biopsy. Experimental technique for transvenous liver biopsy. Radiology. 1964;82:312–14.

14. Guido M, Rugge M. Liver biopsy sampling in chronic viral hepatitis. Semin Liver Dis. 2004;24:89–97.

15. Sheela H, Seela S, Caldwell C, Boyer JL, Jain D. Liver biopsy: evolving role in the new millennium. J Clin Gastroenterol. 2005;39:603–10.

16. Little AF, Ferris JV, Dodd III GD, Baron RL. Image-guided percutaneous hepatic biopsy: effect of ascites on the complication rate. Radiology. 1996;199:79–83.

17. Murphy FB, Barefield KP, Steinberg HV, Bernardino ME. CT- or sonographically-guided biopsy of the liver in the presence of ascites: frequency of complications. Am J Roentgenol. 1988;151:485–6.

18. Lee MJ. Image-guided percutaneous biopsy. In: Kaufman JA, Lee MJ, editors. Vascular and interventional radiology: the requisites. Philadelphia: Mosby; 2004. p. 469–88.

19. Paulson EK, Sheafor DH, Enterline DS, McAdams HP, Yoshizumi TT. CT fluoroscopy-guided interventional procedures: techniques and radiation dose to radiologists. Radiology. 2001;220:161–7.

20. Silverman SG, Tuncali K, Adams DF, Nawfel RD, Zou KH, Judy PF. CT fluoroscopy-guided abdominal interventions: techniques, results, and radiation exposure. Radiology. 1999;212:673–81.

21. Gupta S. New techniques in image-guided percutaneous biopsy. Cardiovasc Intervent Radiol. 2004;27:91–104.

22. Gervais DA, Gazelle GS, Lu DSK, Hahn PF, Mueller PR. Percutaneous transpulmonary CT-guided liver biopsy: a safe and technically easy approach for lesions located near the diaphragm. Am J Roentgenol. 1996;167:482–3.

23. Westcott J. Percutaneous transthoracic needle biopsy. Radiology. 1988;169:593–601.

24. Sinner W. Complications of percutaneous transthoracic needle aspiration biopsy. Acta Radiol. 1976;17:813–28.

25. Berquist T, Bailey P, Cortese D, Miller W. Transthoracic needle biopsy: accuracy and complications in relation to location and type of lesion. Mayo Clin Proc. 1980;55:475–81.

26. Adam G, Bucker A, Nolte-Ernsting C, Tacke J, Gunther RW. Interventional MR imaging: percutaneous abdominal and skeletal biopsies and drainages of the abdomen. Eur Radiol. 1999; 9:1471–8.

27. Stattaus J, Maderwald S, Baba HA, et al. MR-guided liver biopsy within a short, wide-bore 1.5 Tesla MR system. Eur Radiol. 2008;18:2865–73.

28. Durek JL, Lewin JS, Wendt M, Petersilge C. Remember true-FISP? A high SNR, near 1 second imaging method for T2-like contrast interventional MRI at 0.2 T. J Magn Reson Imaging. 1999;8:203–8.

29. Hopper KD, Abendroth CS, Sturtz KW, Matthews KW, Stevens LA, Shirk SJ. Automated biopsy devices: a blinded evaluation. Radiology. 1993;187:653–60.

30. Hopper KD, Abendroth CS, Sturtz KW, Matthews YL, Shirk SJ, Stevens LA. Blinded comparison of biopsy needles and automated devices in vitro. 1. Biopsy of diffuse hepatic disease. Am J Roentgenol. 1993;161:1293–7.

31. Haaga JR, LiPuma JP, Bryan PJ, Balsara VJ, Cohen AM. Clinical comparison of small- and large- caliber cutting needles for biopsy. Radiology. 1983;146:665–7.

32. Erwin BC, Brynes RK, Chan WC, et al. Percutaneous needle biopsy in the diagnosis and classification of lymphoma. Cancer. 1986;57:1074–8.

33. Welch TJ, Sheedy 2nd PF, Johnson CD, Johnson CM, Stephens DH. CT-guided biopsy: prospective analysis of 1,000 procedures. Radiology. 1989;171:493–6.

34. Hatfield MK, Beres RA, Sane SS, Zaleski GX. Percutaneous imaging-guided solid organ core needle biopsy: coaxial versus noncoaxial method. Am J Roentgenol. 2008;190:413–17.

35. Appelbaum L, Kane RA, Kruskal JB, Romero J, Sosna J. Focal hepatic lesions: US-guided biopsy—lesions from review of cytologic and pathologic examination. Radiology. 2008;250:453–8.

36. Moulton JS, Moore PT. Coaxial percutaneous biopsy technique with automated biopsy devices: value in improving accuracy and negative predictive value. Radiology. 1993;186:515–22.

37. Tan KT, Rajan DK, Kachura JR, et al. Pain after percutaneous liver biopsy for diffuse hepatic disease: a randomized trial comparing subcostal and intercostals approaches. J Vasc Interv Radiol. 2005;16:1215–19.

38. Smith EH. Complications of percutaneous abdominal fine-needle biopsy. Radiology. 1991;178:253–8.

39. Silverman SG. Percutaneous image-guided abdominal biopsy. In: Kandarpa K, Aruny JE, editors. Handbook of interventional radiologic procedures. 3rd ed. Philadelphia: Lippincott Williams & Wilkins; 2002. p. 342–53.

40. Pietrobattista A, Fruwirth R, Natali G, et al. Is juvenile liver biopsy unsafe? Putting an end to a common misapprehension. Pediatr Radiol. 2009. Published online ahead of print.

41. Brown DB, Gonsalves CF. Percutaneous biopsy before interventional oncologic therapy: current status. J Vasc Interv Radiol. 2008;19:973–9.

42. Cardella JF, Bakal CW, Bertino RE, et al. Quality improvement guidelines for image-guided percutaneous biopsy in adults. J Vasc Interv Radiol. 2003;14:S227–30.

43. Myers RP, Fong A, Shahee AAM. Utilization rates, complications and costs of percutaneous liver biopsy: a population-based study including 4275 biopsies. Liver Int. 2008;28:705–12.

44. Al Knawy B, Shiffman M. Percutaneous liver biopsy in clinical practice. Liver Int. 2007;27:1166–73.

45. Caturelli E, Giacobbe A, Facciorusso D, et al. Percutaneous biopsy in diffuse liver disease: increasing diagnostic yield and decreasing

complication rate by routine ultrasound assessment of puncture site. Am J Gastroenterol. 1996;91:1318–21.

46. Luning M, Schroder K, Woldd H, et al. Percutaneous biopsy of the liver. Cardiovasc Intervent Radiol. 1991;14:40–2.

47. Yavuz K, Geyik S, Petersen B, Lakin P, Keller FS, Kaufman JA. Transjugular liver biopsy via the left jugular vein. J Vasc Interv Radiol. 2007;18:237–41.

48. Savader SJ, Prescott CA, Lund GB, Osterman FA. Intraductal biliary biopsy: comparison of three techniques. J Vasc Interv Radiol. 1996;7:743–50.

49. Savader SJ, Lynch FC, Radvany MG, et al. Single-specimen bile cytology: a prospective study of 80 patients with obstructive jaundice. J Vasc Interv Radiol. 1998;9:817–21.

50. Harell GS, Anderson MF, Berry PF. Cytologic bile examination in the diagnosis of biliary duct strictures. Am J Roentgenol. 1981;137:1123–6.

51. Muro A, Mueller PR, Ferrucci Jr JT, Taft PD. Bile cytology: a routine addition to percutaneous biliary drainage. Radiology. 1983;149:846–7.

52. Lee MJ. Biliary intervention. In: Kaufman JA, Lee MJ, editors. Vascular and interventional radiology: the requisites. Philadelphia: Mosby; 2004. p. 558–87.

53. Jung GS, Huh JD, Lee SU, Han BH, Chang HK, Cho YD. Bile duct: analysis of percutaneous transluminal forceps biopsy in 130 patients suspected of having malignant biliary obstruction. Radiology. 2002;224:725–30.

Percutaneous Biopsy of the Pancreas

Sanjay Gupta

Background

A focal pancreatic mass identified on imaging may represent pancreatic adenocarcinoma; other malignant lesions such as islet cell tumors, lymphomas, or metastases or benign conditions such as focal chronic pancreatitis. These lesions are not always distinguishable by standard imaging studies and laboratory tests alone. Pathologic evaluation of tissue samples is generally required to differentiate between benign and malignant lesions and to differentiate among various types of malignancies in patients presenting with pancreatic lesions.

Before the 1970s, tissue acquisition was possible only via open surgery [1]. Since the introduction of image-guided percutaneous needle biopsy in the 1970s, percutaneous needle biopsy has become the preferred technique. Percutaneous needle biopsy with computed tomographic (CT) or ultrasound guidance is less invasive than surgery and allows access to nearly all pancreatic lesions. Both fine-needle aspiration biopsy (FNAB) and core-needle biopsy (CNB), and the safety and accuracy of these techniques, have been well documented in the medical literature [2–8].

Indications

Image-guided percutaneous biopsy of the pancreas is generally performed to obtain a pathologic diagnosis in patients who present with a pancreatic mass. The results of pancreatic biopsy play a crucial role in determining treatment options [9]. For example, histologic examination of biopsy tissue can help protect patients with pseudotumors or benign lesions from inappropriate and aggressive therapeutic regimens. Pathologic examination of biopsy specimens also

allows diagnosis of the specific malignancy type. The various malignant pancreatic lesions, including adenocarcinomas, islet cell carcinomas, and lymphomas, carry very different prognoses and are treated differently [10, 11], and for those who are surgical candidates, the surgical approach is often quite different. Likewise, in patients with a pancreatic mass that is considered unresectable based on imaging findings, it is important to verify the diagnosis before neoadjuvant or palliative therapy is initiated.

Although the diagnosis of cystic pancreatic lesions can often be made with imaging findings alone, needle biopsy may be required to obtain a definitive diagnosis in some patients who present with atypical clinical and imaging findings [12–19]. Accurate differentiation of serous and mucinous cystic neoplasms is essential for appropriate disease management. Whereas serous tumors are considered benign and can likely be managed with observation alone; mucinous tumors have malignant potential and require resection, if possible.

Technique

Image Guidance

Percutaneous needle biopsy of the pancreas is generally performed with ultrasound or CT guidance [2, 3]. The real-time monitoring capability of ultrasonography allows continuous monitoring of the needle placement and biopsy procedure [20]. Other advantages of ultrasound guidance include speed, ease of availability, and low cost. In addition, ultrasound's multiplanar imaging capability allows free selection of needle entry points and oblique needle paths, yet so that important structures such as the gallbladder and hepatic and gastroduodenal arteries can be avoided. Furthermore, Doppler ultrasonography can help identify and avoid perilesional vessels. However, the presence of gas-containing bowel loops and obesity occasionally hinders visualization of small pancreatic lesions

S. Gupta, MD, DNB
Department of Interventional Radiology, Department of Diagnostic Radiology, The University of Texas MD Anderson Cancer Center, 1515 Holcombe Blvd., Unit 1471, Houston, TX 77030, USA
e-mail: sgupta@mdanderson.org

K. Ahrar, S. Gupta (eds.), *Percutaneous Image-Guided Biopsy*,
DOI 10.1007/978-1-4614-8217-8_14, © Springer Science+Business Media New York 2014

with ultrasonography. During ultrasound-guided biopsy, abdominal compression with the transducer will displace the intervening bowel loops, improve the depiction of deep lesions, and shorten the needle path. Although inadvertent transgression of bowel loops with the biopsy needle may occur, such transgression with small-caliber needles is generally considered safe.

CT, with its high spatial resolution and ability to clearly visualize intervening structures, such as bowel loops and blood vessels, is the most common imaging modality for guiding percutaneous pancreatic biopsies. CT visualization of pancreatic lesions is unhindered by intestinal gas. Unlike ultrasound guidance, which allows only an anterior biopsy approach to pancreatic lesions, CT guidance allows anterior, posterior, or lateral biopsy approaches. Administration of a contrast medium is occasionally required to identify vessels in the needle path.

Pancreatic malignancies often initiate an intense desmoplastic reaction around the tumor or obstruct the major pancreatic duct, causing acute or chronic pancreatitis. Hence, on CT scans, a pancreatic mass may appear larger than the actual tumor itself, thereby increasing the chances of sampling error [4, 7, 21]. Tumor necrosis or bleeding can also lead to insufficient recovery of tumor cells. Therefore, administration of a contrast medium may help differentiate viable portions of the pancreatic tumor from surrounding areas of fibrosis and necrosis; this allows for more accurate needle positioning, thus potentially increasing the diagnostic yield. In a study by Brandt et al. [2], researchers administered contrast medium for 92 % of CT-guided biopsies. Intermittent CT fluoroscopy can be used to avoid injury to major intervening structures [22, 23].

Patients with early pancreatic cancer may present with a ductal stricture without any identifiable mass. Obtaining a pathologic diagnosis in such patients can be difficult, as washings from ductal strictures are positive in only 30 % of patients. In five patients who had a ductal stricture but no demonstrable mass and in whom cytologic brushings were atypical but not diagnostic for malignancy, Pelsang et al. [24] successfully performed CT-guided percutaneous biopsies by targeting the biopsy needles at the ductal stents that had been inserted during endoscopic retrograde cholangiopancreatography (ERCPs). Use of a stent as a target for percutaneous biopsies under ultrasound, CT, or fluoroscopic guidance has also been reported by other authors [7, 25, 26]. When percutaneous biopsies are being performed in patients with plastic biliary stents, the needle should be aimed directly at the stent so that the operator may feel the contact of the needle with the stent. Some groups advocate the use of a power-cutting needle to obtain samples of the stent along with the tissue biopsy [25]. However, caution is advised when biopsying a mass around a metal stent, because of the risk of snagging the wires of the stent in the enclosed notch of the cutting needle and the possibility of

difficulty in retrieving the needle and tissue [25]. Fluoroscopy and pancreatography can also be used to guide percutaneous biopsy in such patients. Gagnon et al. [27] used biplane fluoroscopy during pancreatography to guide percutaneous biopsies in 14 patients with pancreatic strictures but without identifiable masses and reported a sensitivity of 90 % and a specificity of 100 %. There were no complications in any of these patients.

Needles and Pathologic Considerations

A variety of needles of different calibers, lengths, and needle tip configurations and a variety of mechanisms for sample acquisition have been used for percutaneous biopsies of pancreatic masses [5, 23, 28, 29]. Small-caliber (20- to 25-gauge) aspiration needles are generally used for FNABs. These needles provide specimens suitable for cytologic evaluation. FNAB is the most commonly used technique for biopsy of pancreatic masses because it combines a high diagnostic yield and a low complication rate. CNBs yield tissue specimens suitable for histologic evaluation. Although 14- to 16-gauge cutting needles have been used for pancreatic CNB, their use has not been associated with any improvement in overall diagnostic accuracy rates over smaller-gauge needles [23]. The small-caliber (18- to 20-gauge) cutting needles now available consistently provide high-quality histopathologic specimens, reduce the number of passes needed to obtain adequate tissue for diagnosis, and decrease the durations of the procedures without increasing the complication rate [28]. Various studies have shown that image-guided percutaneous CNB can be an effective and safe procedure in the evaluation of pancreatic masses [23, 28]. The main advantages of CNB over FNAB include the preservation of the tissue architecture and the relative ease of obtaining a sufficient amount of tissue for immunohistochemical analysis, both of which may be important in distinguishing well-differentiated adenocarcinomas from chronic inflammation and in subtyping some tumors.

The presence of an on-site cytopathologist during biopsy allows for optimal handling of the tissue and immediate assessment of the adequacy of the specimen. Immediate cytologic evaluation permits the cytopathologist and the radiologist to determine whether subsequent needle passes are required to obtain additional specimens or to perform ancillary studies. An immediate cytologic result also allows the radiologist to decide whether to attempt a biopsy of a different area of the lesion (e.g., if the initial aspirate shows only necrotic material, fibrotic tissue, or nonspecific inflammatory cells). This is especially important in pancreatic biopsies because pancreatic tumors are associated with extensive fibrosis and inflammation in the surrounding tumor-free pancreatic tissue [7, 21].

Approaches and Techniques

As mentioned earlier, pancreatic lesions can be accessed percutaneously via anterior, posterior, or lateral approaches (Fig. 14.1). The selection of approach depends on the location of the lesion within the pancreas and of the surrounding structures. Most interventional radiologists prefer an anterior approach to avoid the large retroperitoneal blood vessels

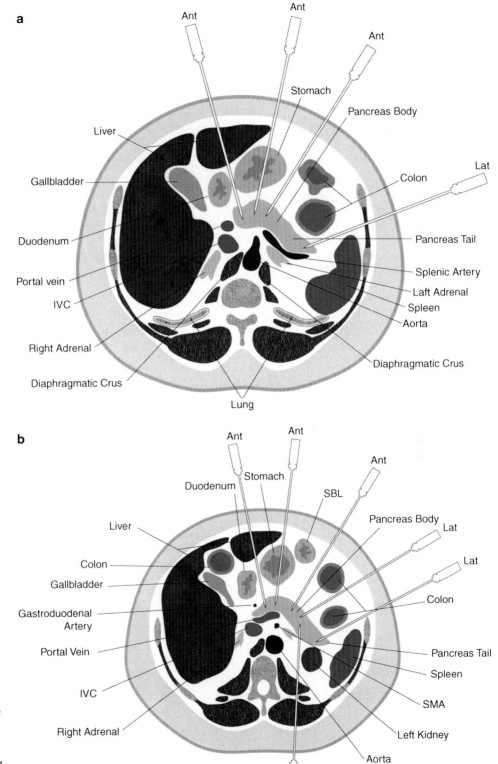

Fig. 14.1 Schematic drawings showing the relevant anatomy and needle trajectories for anterior (*Ant*), posterior (*Post*), and lateral (*Lat*) approaches for percutaneous pancreatic biopsy at various levels: upper pancreatic body and tail (**a**), lower pancreatic body and tail (**b**), pancreatic head (**c**), and uncinate process (**d**). The needle has been advanced via a posterior approach and traverses the IVC in **c**. *IVC* inferior vena cava, *SMA* superior mesenteric artery, *SMV* superior mesenteric vein, *SBL* small bowel loops

Fig. 14.1 (continued)

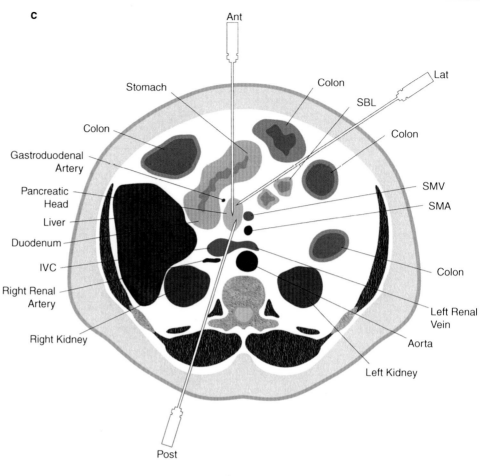

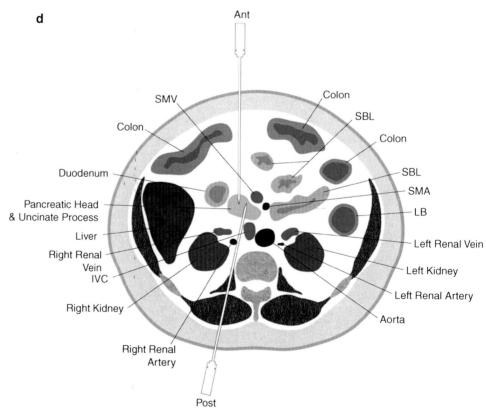

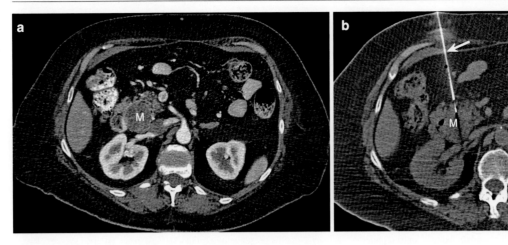

Fig. 14.2 Direct anterior approach. (**a**) Contrast-enhanced transverse CT scan obtained with the patient in a supine position shows a hypoenhancing mass (*M*) in the head of the pancreas. (**b**) Transverse CT scan during the biopsy procedure shows the biopsy needle (*arrow*) advanced via an anterior approach into the pancreatic mass (*M*)

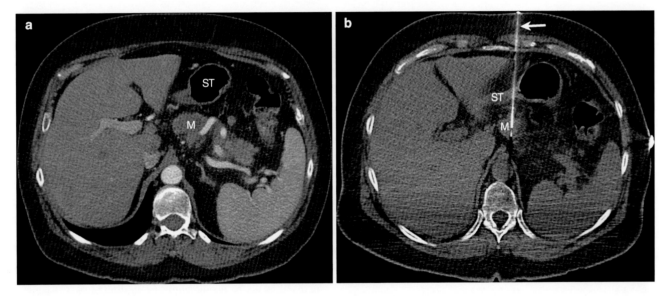

Fig. 14.3 Transgastric approach. (**a**) Contrast-enhanced transverse CT scan obtained with the patient in a supine position shows a pancreatic mass (*M*) posterior to the stomach (*ST*). (**b**) Transverse CT scan during the biopsy procedure shows the biopsy needle (*arrow*) advanced through the collapsed stomach (*ST*) into the pancreatic mass (*M*)

(Fig. 14.2). Generally, a direct path to the mass that does not traverse any organs or major vessels is preferred. However, masses within or around the head of the pancreas are often shielded by the stomach, duodenum, transverse colon, liver, and mesenteric vessels, precluding direct access to the lesion by an anterior approach. In a retrospective review of pancreatic biopsies performed with CT (*n*=195) or ultrasound (*n*=56) guidance, Brandt et al. [2] found that the biopsy needle had to traverse other organs in 24 % of the ultrasound-guided and in 40 % of the CT-guided biopsy procedures. The needle was passed through the liver in 27 cases, through the gastrointestinal tract in 66 cases (through the stomach, small bowel, or colon in 41, 18, and 7 cases, respectively), and through the spleen in 1 case. Multiple organs were traversed in 4 patients.

The incidence of bowel traversal during ultrasound-guided biopsies reported by Brandt et al. [2] may be an underestimation, because the inadvertent traversal of bowel loops while they are being compressed by the ultrasound probe (a maneuver commonly used during ultrasound-guided biopsy procedures to improve the visualization of lesions in deep abdominal structures) is not uncommon. It is generally acceptable to traverse the gastrointestinal tract in an immunocompetent patient when performing FNABs of abdominal masses [2, 30]. In the study by Brandt et al. [2], none of the patients had complications related to biopsy route. Many other studies have also shown that traversal of the stomach (Fig. 14.3) or small bowel (Fig. 14.4) during percutaneous pancreatic biopsy is unlikely to result in substantial

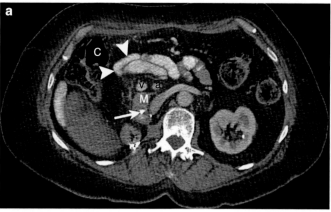

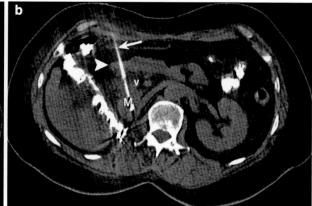

Fig. 14.4 Needle traversing small bowel loops. (**a**) Contrast-enhanced transverse CT scan obtained with the patient in a supine position shows a mass (*M*) in the head of pancreas. A direct anterior approach is precluded by the presence of the hepatic flexure of the colon (*C*), small bowel loops (*arrowheads*), and superior mesenteric vein (*v*) and artery

(*a*). Note the presence of a biliary stent (*arrow*). (**b**) Transverse CT scan during the biopsy procedure shows the biopsy needle (*arrow*) advanced through the small bowel loops (*arrowheads*) and medial to the superior mesenteric vein (*v*) into the pancreatic mass (*M*)

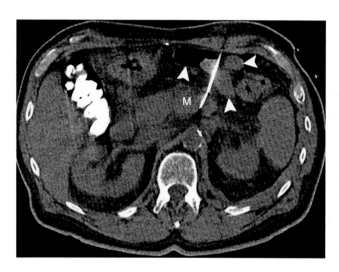

Fig. 14.5 Use of a Hawkins needle. Transverse CT scan during the biopsy procedure shows a Hawkins biopsy needle advanced in between multiple bowel loops (*arrowheads*) into a pancreatic mass (*M*)

complications [2, 30–32]. Although some authors state that traversing the colon is acceptable during pancreatic biopsies, others avoid the colon, especially when using large-bore needles [5]. Injection of physiologic saline solution through the guide needle can help displace the colon or small bowel loops from the intended needle path and thereby decrease the risks associated with the procedure [33, 34]. Alternatively, using a Hawkins-Akins (Meditech, Westwood, MS) needle with a blunt trocar may also reduce the risk of injury to the bowel and/or major vessels in the needle path [31] (Fig. 14.5). When necessary, an out-of-plane route can be taken to avoid injury to the stomach or bowel.

A transhepatic approach can be used for needle biopsies of lesions in the pancreatic head. Occasionally, an anterior approach to lesions of the pancreatic body may require

needle placement through the left lobe of the liver (Fig. 14.6). Needle biopsy through the liver is generally considered safe; however, there is a small risk of needle-track seeding with malignant cells [31].

If a safe anterior approach is not available, a posterior approach can be used. In our experience, a posterior approach is less painful to the patient because it avoids a transperitoneal puncture. A direct posterior approach from the left side can occasionally be used for lesions involving the distal body or tail of the pancreas (Fig. 14.7). With this approach, care should be taken to avoid injury to the splenic artery and vein, left adrenal gland, upper pole of the left kidney, and spleen. This approach may be precluded by the presence of interposed lung and pleura. The triangulation method, which involves a caudal-skin entry and uses the Pythagorean theorem to calculate the needle angle, or angling of the CT gantry can be used to allow an angled posterior approach that avoids pleural transgression in biopsy of pancreatic tail lesions [35]. Electromagnetic navigation systems can also be used to assist in such out-of-plane approaches [36, 37] (Fig. 14.8). Alternatively, placing the patient in the ipsilateral decubitus position may cause the diaphragm to move superiorly, allowing for a direct posterior approach (Fig. 14.9).

While one is using a posterior approach to lesions involving the pancreatic head and uncinate process, the needle is inserted through the right paraspinal muscles and is advanced lateral to the inferior vena cava (IVC); between the IVC and the vertebra (Fig. 14.10); or, if neither route is feasible, through the IVC itself (Fig. 14.11). For the transcaval approach, an 18-gauge guide needle is positioned posterior to the cava IVC, and an inner 22-gauge Chiba needle traverses the vena cava IVC to biopsy the target lesion [7, 38]. Studies have shown that the transgression of vascular structures, especially low-pressure veins, with small-caliber needles

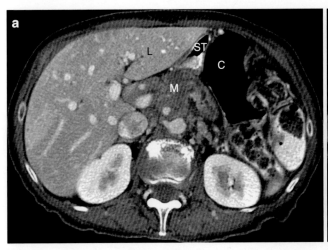
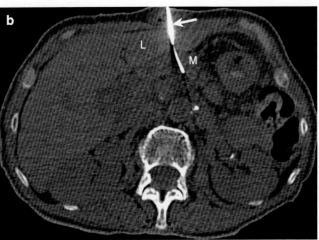

Fig. 14.6 Transhepatic approach. (**a**) Contrast-enhanced transverse CT scan obtained with the patient in a supine position shows a mass (*M*) in the pancreatic body. A direct anterior approach is precluded by the inter- posed liver (*L*), stomach (*ST*), and colon (*C*). (**b**) Transverse CT scan during the biopsy procedure shows the biopsy needle (*arrow*) advanced through the left lobe of the liver (*L*) into a pancreatic mass (*M*)

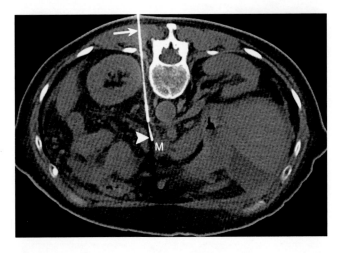

Fig. 14.7 Direct posterior approach. Transverse CT scan with the patient in a prone position shows an 18-gauge guide needle (*arrow*) advanced through the paravertebral space. A 22-gauge needle (*arrowhead*) was advanced through the guide needle to sample a mass (*M*) involving the distal body of the pancreas

does not increase the complication rates of needle biopsy procedures [7, 39]. Two studies describing the use of the transcaval approach for pancreatic biopsies did not report any major hemorrhagic complications [7, 38]. However, when the transcaval approach is used, it is important to identify and avoid the right renal artery, which courses posterior to the IVC.

A direct lateral or anterolateral approach can also be used for needle biopsy of lesions involving the distal body and tail of the pancreas (Fig. 14.1). The structures that may be present in the needle path with this approach include the small and large bowel, spleen, and mesenteric vessels. Saline injection to displace bowel loops or use of a blunt-tip Hawkins-Akins (Meditech) needle can help avoid injury to the bowel.

When pancreatic cancer presents as an isolated cuff of tumor surrounding the superior mesenteric artery or celiac trunk, without an identifiable mass [40], a posterior needle biopsy approach under CT guidance can be used. Administration of a contrast medium may be required to identify and avoid major blood vessels [41]. Particular attention must be used to identify and avoid the superior mesenteric artery; the celiac trunk; and the splenic, superior mesenteric, and portal veins. The needle is inserted and advanced via a posterior-oblique approach lateral to these vessels. Some authors have described the use of an anterior approach with real-time ultrasound guidance for biopsying such lesions; a combination of gray-scale ultrasonography and color-Doppler imaging helps to avoid inadvertent transgression of the artery [41].

Most ultrasound-guided pancreatic biopsies are performed using a single-needle technique that involves using a new needle for each pass. On the other hand, CT-guided pancreatic biopsies generally involve the use of a coaxial technique that requires initial placement of a thin-walled guide needle in or close to the target lesion followed by advancement of the biopsy needle through the guide needle to obtain tissue samples. The coaxial technique allows multiple samples of tissue to be obtained without the need for additional passes through overlying tissues, thus decreasing the risk of complications and patient discomfort. Unlike the single-needle technique, the coaxial technique requires the precise placement of only the guide needle, thus substantially decreasing the duration of the procedure and the number of images required, especially for deep lesions with difficult access routes. Also, the coaxial technique allows for small-caliber CNBs to be performed through the same guide needle. One potential problem with the coaxial technique is that after the

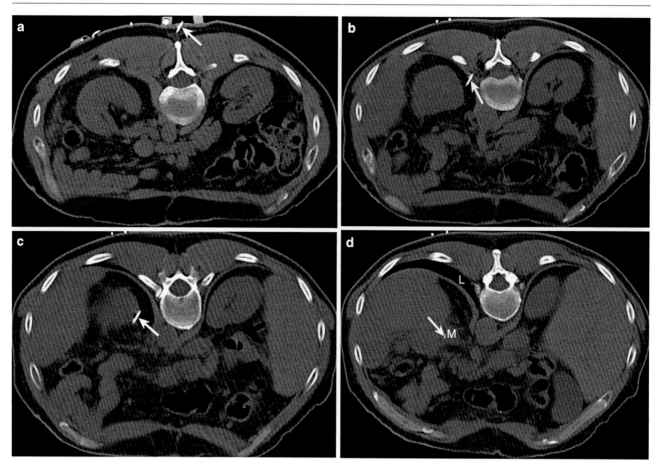

Fig. 14.8 Use of electromagnetic navigation system for an angled caudo-cranial approach. Transverse CT scans from caudal to cranial levels with the patient in a prone position show an 18-gauge guide needle (*arrow*) inserted at a level caudal to the mass (**a**) and directed cranially (**b–d**) to sample a mass (*M*) involving the tail of the pancreas. A direct approach would have involved a needle passing through the interposed lung (*L*). The needle was advanced to the lesion in a single pass using virtual real-time multiplanar reconstructions to guide the needle trajectory

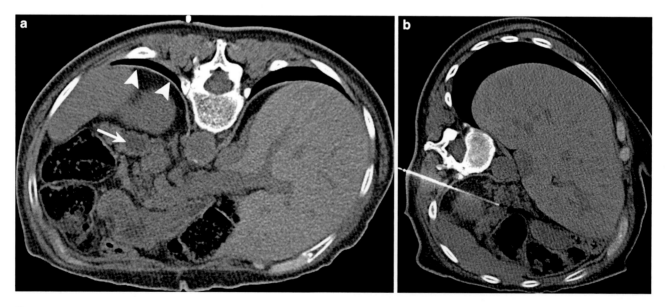

Fig. 14.9 Use of an ipsilateral decubitus position to avoid the interposed lung. (**a**) Transverse CT scan with the patient in a prone position shows the interposed lung (*arrowheads*) obstructing the direct path to a pancreatic tail lesion (*arrow*). (**b**) CT scan with the patient in an ipsilateral decubitus position causes the diaphragm to move superiorly, allowing for a direct posterior approach

first-needle pass, subsequent passes tend to follow the same path and may yield little additional tissue. This problem can be overcome by the use of a custom-made curved 22-gauge needle, which is advanced through a straight 18-gauge guide needle to sample different parts of the lesion, potentially increasing the diagnostic yield [26]. The needle is customized by grasping its tip with a forceps and gently bending the needle so that the distal part of its shaft curves. The curved-needle technique can also help avoid intervening structures or correct for an inaccurately positioned guide needle.

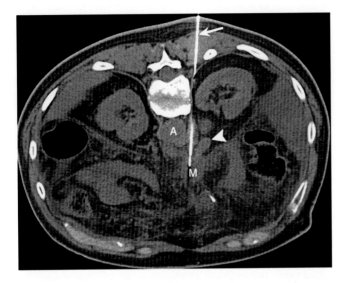

Fig. 14.10 Direct posterior approach. Transverse CT scan with the patient in a prone position shows the biopsy needle (*arrow*) advanced through the paravertebral space to sample a mass (*M*) involving the head of the pancreas. The needle passes between the inferior vena cava (*arrowhead*) and the aorta (*A*)

Results

The reported accuracy of image-guided percutaneous biopsy for assessing pancreatic lesions ranges from 45 to 100 % (2). The reported accuracy of CT-guided pancreatic biopsy ranges from 50 to 94 % [2, 42], whereas that of ultrasound-guided biopsy ranges from 67 to 97 % [2, 3, 8, 43]. The wide variability in accuracy reported in the literature may be related to a variety of factors, such as lesion size and location, needle size, biopsy device, and the experience level of the individual performing the biopsy.

The literature comparing the diagnostic efficacies of FNAB and CNB also shows variable results [3, 5, 29, 44]. While some authors favor FNAB to obtain cytologic specimens [45, 46], others suggest that better results can be achieved with CNB using cutting-type needles, which allow for histologic examination [5, 23, 44, 47]. The accuracy of FNAB is dependent on the expertise of the cytopathologist. The high false-negative rates reported for FNAB in some series may be related in part to the difficulty in distinguishing between well-differentiated adenocarcinomas and reactive conditions such as pancreatitis in cytologic specimens. Because CNB yields large solid-tissue specimens, which are suitable for both histologic evaluation and immunohistochemical analysis, it has been suggested that CNB may be more appropriate than FNAB for diagnosing some types of malignant pancreatic tumors (e.g., well-differentiated adenocarcinomas) [23].

Another reason for false-negative results with percutaneous biopsy is that pancreatic carcinoma is often associated with a strong desmoplastic reaction, which increases the probability of sampling nonmalignant cells by inadvertently placing the biopsy needle in an area where the tumor consists

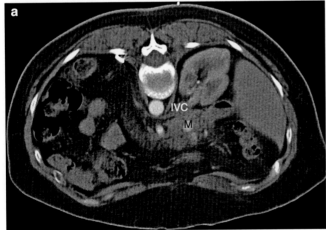
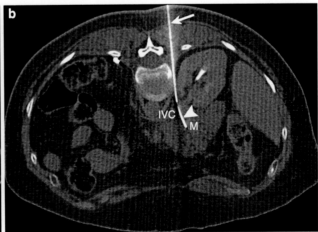

Fig. 14.11 Posterior transcaval approach. (**a**) Contrast-enhanced transverse CT scan obtained with the patient in a prone position shows a mass (*M*) in the head of the pancreas. Note the presence of the inferior vena cava (*IVC*) posterior to the mass. (**b**) Transverse CT scan during the biopsy procedure with the patient in a prone position shows the 18-gauge needle (*arrow*) posterior to the IVC and the curved 22-gauge needle (*arrowhead*) traversing the IVC to sample the mass (*M*)

mostly of fibrous tissue. Various methods can be used to increase the diagnostic yield, including obtaining CNB specimens or multiple samples and sampling different portions of the visible mass.

In general, lesion size is an important factor affecting the diagnostic accuracy of percutaneous pancreatic biopsy, with such accuracy being higher in larger masses [2, 23]. Correct needle placement is particularly difficult if the lesion is small, which may lead to sampling errors. In the study by Brandt et al. [2], percutaneous needle biopsy had an accuracy of 92 % for pancreatic lesions larger than 3 cm and 81 % for smaller lesions. In the same study, greater accuracy was achieved for masses in the pancreatic body or tail (93 %) than for those in the head (84 %), which may be related to the larger size of masses in the pancreatic body or tail.

Biopsy After Pancreas Transplantation

After pancreatic transplantation, percutaneous needle biopsy may be needed to determine the cause of graft dysfunction. Rejection of a pancreas graft by the body's immune system must be detected early so that appropriate antirejection therapy can be initiated to prevent destruction of pancreatic tissue and prolong graft survival. However, clinical signs and symptoms, laboratory tests, and imaging findings lack specificity and cannot reliably differentiate between various causes of graft dysfunction, such as pancreas graft rejection, cyclosporine toxicity, decreased oral intake, graft anastomotic leak, necrosis, pancreatitis, and ischemia [48]. A histologic diagnosis is needed to differentiate among these causes of graft dysfunction prior to the initiation of therapy.

Biopsy of a pancreas graft can be performed by open surgery (for enteric-drained grafts) or a cystoscopic approach (for bladder-drained grafts) [49–51]. Unfortunately, both these time-consuming and invasive procedures usually require general anesthesia and an operating room. On the other hand, percutaneous needle biopsy of pancreatic grafts using ultrasound or CT guidance has been shown to be safe and reliable, with an excellent tissue yield [52, 53]. Generally, the portion of the pancreatic graft that is most accessible is sampled. This requires an anterior, anterolateral, or direct lateral approach [52, 53]. It is important to avoid the vessels supplying the graft, which are usually located medial to the graft and can be visualized easily in most patients. Percutaneous biopsy offers significant advantages over cystoscopic biopsy in that percutaneous biopsies are performed with local anesthesia and allow biopsy of multiple sites. Results of some studies suggest that simultaneous biopsy of multiple sites within the graft can increase the diagnostic yield [53].

Complications

The reported complication rate for image-guided percutaneous biopsy of the pancreas is remarkably low – between 0.5 and 3 % – with the most frequent complication being acute pancreatitis [54–57]. Furthermore, only six cases of biopsy-related deaths have been reported in the literature; five were attributed to acute pancreatitis and one to sepsis [54–57]. The type of needle used does not seem to affect complication rates; various published series on percutaneous pancreatic biopsies suggest that CNBs have a complication rate similar to that of FNABs. Levin et al. [48] reported a case of hemorrhagic pancreatitis that led to the death of a patient after CT-guided percutaneous FNAB of a pseudolesion of the uncinate process. Pancreatitis after percutaneous biopsy is more likely to occur when normal pancreatic tissue has been traversed or when there has been a puncture of the pancreatic duct or its branches; this increased risk may be due to the release of pancreatic enzymes each time the biopsy needle passes through the pancreatic tissue or dilated pancreatic ducts. Hence, care should be taken to place the needle directly into the mass and minimize traversal of normal pancreatic tissue or dilated pancreatic ducts [58].

Because of the deep location of the pancreas within the body and the presence of mesenteric vessels in the needle path, it is not uncommon to see small hemorrhages along the needle path after percutaneous CT-guided biopsies (Fig. 14.12); however, most are asymptomatic and do not require any treatment. It is important to avoid the superior mesenteric artery, the celiac trunk, and the splenic, superior mesenteric, and portal veins. Inadvertent puncture of these vessels has the potential to cause hemorrhage, pseudoaneurysm formation, or thrombosis.

Whether percutaneous needle biopsy can lead to peritoneal dissemination of malignant cells remains controversial. Warshaw et al. [59] reported that the frequency of malignant peritoneal cytology findings was higher in patients with pancreatic cancer who had undergone CT or ultrasound-guided biopsy than in those who had not. However, others have reported no differences in the rates of malignant peritoneal cytology findings (approximately 10–20 %) in patients who had undergone FNABs compared with those who had not [60, 61]. Although there are a few anecdotal reports of tumor seeding along the needle track, most authors believe that the risk of needle-track seeding is extremely low [2, 21, 62, 63].

Bowel traversal can potentially contaminate a sterile biopsy procedure; maintaining sterility is especially important during biopsy of cystic masses. Ferrucci et al. [30] reported a case of gram-negative sepsis after pancreatic biopsy, presumably resulting from bowel transgression and resultant needle implantation of intestinal flora in the lesion.

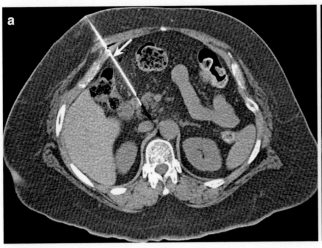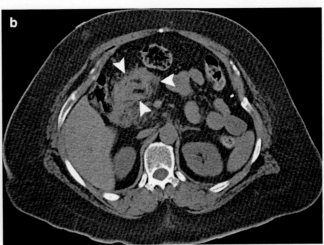

Fig. 14.12 Biopsy-related bleeding. (**a**) Transverse CT scan with the patient in a supine position shows the biopsy needle (*arrow*) advanced via an anterior approach to sample a mass involving the head of the pancreas. (**b**) Transverse CT scan obtained after removal of the needle shows a hematoma (*arrowheads*) in the needle path

Comparison with Endoscopic Ultrasonography and Biopsy

Endoscopic ultrasonography (EUS) is an alternative technique that is increasingly used to guide biopsies of pancreatic masses. Placement of a high-frequency ultrasound probe close to the pancreas through an endoscope positioned in the stomach or duodenum allows for high-resolution imaging of the head and proximal body of the pancreas and helps in visualization of small intra- and peripancreatic lesions. EUS-guided FNAB is performed through the endoscope, which avoids the percutaneous punctures necessary with external ultrasound- or CT-guided biopsy. Another important advantage of EUS-guided biopsy is its ability to target small intrapancreatic lesions not detectable by CT or external ultrasonography. However, lesions located in the distal body and tail of the pancreas are not amenable to EUS-guided procedures [64]. An important limitation of EUS-guided biopsy is that only FNAB is possible, which may lower the diagnostic yield for lesions that require large-caliber cores for accurate pathologic diagnosis. Recently, a 19-gauge Tru-Cut needle was introduced for EUS use, but experience with this needle is limited and its stiffness precludes adequate sampling of small or difficult-to-reach lesions, especially those located in the head and uncinate process of the pancreas. The accuracy of EUS-guided FNAB is similar to that of CT-guided FNAB: up to 100 % for CT and 96 % for EUS [64–67].

Summary

CT- or ultrasound-guided percutaneous needle biopsies are common, safe, and highly effective diagnostic techniques for patients who present with pancreatic masses. Pancreatic lesions can be percutaneously accessed via anterior, posterior, or lateral approaches, with the choice of approach depending on the lesion location and the presence or absence of intervening structures. The results of pancreatic biopsy play a crucial role in determining treatment options.

References

1. Hancke S, Holm HH, Koch F. Ultrasonically guided percutaneous fine needle biopsy of the pancreas. Surg Gynecol Obstet. 1975;140:361–4.
2. Brandt KR, Charboneau JW, Stephens DH, Welch TJ, Goellner JR. CT- and US-guided biopsy of the pancreas. Radiology. 1993;187:99–104.
3. Di Stasi M, Lencioni R, Solmi L, et al. Ultrasound-guided fine needle biopsy of pancreatic masses: results of a multicenter study. Am J Gastroenterol. 1998;93:1329–33.
4. Dodd LG, Mooney EE, Layfield LJ, Nelson RC. Fine-needle aspiration of the liver and pancreas: a cytology primer for radiologists. Radiology. 1997;203:1–9.
5. Elvin A, Andersson T, Scheibenpflug L, Lindgren PG. Biopsy of the pancreas with a biopsy gun. Radiology. 1990;176:677–9.
6. Goldstein HM, Zornoza J. Percutaneous transperitoneal aspiration biopsy of pancreatic masses. Am J Dig Dis. 1978;23:840–3.
7. Gupta S, Ahrar K, Morello Jr FA, Wallace MJ, Hicks ME. Masses in or around the pancreatic head: CT-guided coaxial fine-needle aspiration biopsy with a posterior transcaval approach. Radiology. 2002;222:63–9.
8. Hajdu EO, Kumari-Subaiya S, Phillips G. Ultrasonically guided percutaneous aspiration biopsy of the pancreas. Semin Diagn Pathol. 1986;3:166–75.
9. Edoute Y, Lemberg S, Malberger E. Preoperative and intraoperative fine needle aspiration cytology of pancreatic lesions. Am J Gastroenterol. 1991;86:1015–19.
10. Di Stasi M, Cavanna L, Fornari F, et al. Obstructive jaundice secondary to non-Hodgkin's lymphoma: usefulness of ultrasound-guided fine-needle aspiration biopsy (UG-FNAB). Eur J Haematol. 1990;44:265–6.
11. Webb TH, Lillemoe KD, Pitt HA, Jones RJ, Cameron JL. Pancreatic lymphoma. Is surgery mandatory for diagnosis or treatment? Ann Surg. 1989;209:25–30.

12. Carlson SK, Johnson CD, Brandt KR, Batts KP, Salomao DR. Pancreatic cystic neoplasms: the role and sensitivity of needle aspiration and biopsy. Abdom Imaging. 1998;23:387–93.

13. Delatour NR, Policarpio-Nicolas ML, Yazdi H, Islam S. Fine needle aspiration biopsy for preoperative workup of pancreatic cystic neoplasms: report of 4 cases. Acta Cytol. 2007;51:925–33.

14. Attasaranya S, Pais S, LeBlanc J, McHenry L, Sherman S, DeWitt JM. Endoscopic ultrasound-guided fine needle aspiration and cyst fluid analysis for pancreatic cysts. JOP. 2007;8:553–63.

15. Khalid A, Zahid M, Finkelstein SD, et al. Pancreatic cyst fluid DNA analysis in evaluating pancreatic cysts: a report of the PANDA study. Gastrointest Endosc. 2009;69:1095–102.

16. Lewandrowski K, Lee J, Southern J, Centeno B, Warshaw A. Cyst fluid analysis in the differential diagnosis of pancreatic cysts: a new approach to the preoperative assessment of pancreatic cystic lesions. Am J Roentgenol. 1995;164:815–19.

17. Lewandrowski KB, Southern JF, Pins MR, Compton CC, Warshaw AL. Cyst fluid analysis in the differential diagnosis of pancreatic cysts. A comparison of pseudocysts, serous cystadenomas, mucinous cystic neoplasms, and mucinous cystadenocarcinoma. Ann Surg. 1993;217:41–7.

18. Ryu JK, Woo SM, Hwang JH, et al. Cyst fluid analysis for the differential diagnosis of pancreatic cysts. Diagn Cytopathol. 2004;31:100–5.

19. Sperti C, Pasquali C, Guolo P, et al. Evaluation of cyst fluid analysis in the diagnosis of pancreatic cysts. Ital J Gastroenterol. 1995;27:479–83.

20. D'Onofrio M, Malago R, Zamboni G, Manfrin E, Pozzi Mucelli R. Ultrasonography of the pancreas. 5. Interventional procedures. Abdom Imaging. 2007;32:182–90.

21. Robins DB, Katz RL, Evans DB, Atkinson EN, Green L. Fine needle aspiration of the pancreas. In quest of accuracy. Acta Cytol. 1995;39:1–10.

22. Carlson SK, Bender CE, Classic KL, et al. Benefits and safety of CT fluoroscopy in interventional radiologic procedures. Radiology. 2001;219:515–20.

23. Zech CJ, Helmberger T, Wichmann MW, Holzknecht N, Diebold J, Reiser MF. Large core biopsy of the pancreas under CT fluoroscopy control: results and complications. J Comput Assist Tomogr. 2002;26:743–9.

24. Pelsang RE, Johlin FC. A percutaneous biopsy technique for patients with suspected biliary or pancreatic cancer without a radiographic mass. Abdom Imaging. 1997;22:307–10.

25. Amin Z, Kessel D, Lees WR. Percutaneous biopsy of pancreatic masses in patients with biliary metal stents: the snags! Clin Radiol. 1995;50:276.

26. Gupta S, Ahrar K, Morello Jr FA, Wallace MJ, Madoff DC, Hicks ME. Using a coaxial technique with a curved inner needle for CT-guided fine-needle aspiration biopsy. Am J Roentgenol. 2002;179:109–12.

27. Gagnon P, Boustiere C, Ponchon T, Valette PJ, Genin G, Labadie M. Percutaneous fine-needle aspiration cytologic study of main pancreatic duct stenosis under pancreatographic guidance. Cancer. 1991;67:2395–400.

28. Li L, Liu LZ, Wu QL, et al. CT-guided core needle biopsy in the diagnosis of pancreatic diseases with an automated biopsy gun. J Vasc Interv Radiol. 2008;19:89–94.

29. Solmi L, Muratori R, Bacchini P, Primerano A, Gandolfi L. Comparison between echo-guided fine-needle aspiration cytology and microhistology in diagnosing pancreatic masses. Surg Endosc. 1992;6:222–4.

30. Ferrucci Jr JT, Wittenberg J, Mueller PR, et al. Diagnosis of abdominal malignancy by radiologic fine-needle aspiration biopsy. Am J Roentgenol. 1980;134:323–30.

31. Gupta S, Madoff DC. Image-guided percutaneous needle biopsy in cancer diagnosis and staging. Tech Vasc Interv Radiol. 2007;10:88–101.

32. Gupta S, Nguyen HL, Morello Jr FA, et al. Various approaches for CT-guided percutaneous biopsy of deep pelvic lesions: anatomic and technical considerations. Radiographics. 2004;24:175–89.

33. Haaga JR, Beale SM. Use of CO_2 to move structures as an aid to percutaneous procedures. Radiology. 1986;161:829–30.

34. Langen HJ, Jochims M, Gunther RW. Artificial displacement of kidneys, spleen, and colon by injection of physiologic saline and CO_2 as an aid to percutaneous procedures: experimental results. J Vasc Interv Radiol. 1995;6:411–16.

35. van Sonnenberg E, Wittenberg J, Ferrucci Jr JT, Mueller PR, Simeone JF. Triangulation method for percutaneous needle guidance: the angled approach to upper abdominal masses. Am J Roentgenol. 1981;137:757–61.

36. Gupta S. New techniques in image-guided percutaneous biopsy. Cardiovasc Intervent Radiol. 2004;27:91–104.

37. Wallace MJ, Gupta S, Hicks ME. Out-of-plane computed-tomography-guided biopsy using a magnetic-field-based navigation system. Cardiovasc Intervent Radiol. 2006;29:108–13.

38. Sofocleous CT, Schubert J, Brown KT, Brody LA, Covey AM, Getrajdman GI. CT-guided transvenous or transcaval needle biopsy of pancreatic and peripancreatic lesions. J Vasc Interv Radiol. 2004;15:1099–104.

39. Gupta S, Seaberg K, Wallace MJ, et al. Imaging-guided percutaneous biopsy of mediastinal lesions: different approaches and anatomic considerations. Radiographics. 2005;25:763–86; discussion 786–8.

40. Megibow AJ, Bosniak MA, Ambos MA, Beranbaum ER. Thickening of the celiac axis and/or superior mesenteric artery: a sign of pancreatic carcinoma on computed tomography. Radiology. 1981;141:449–53.

41. O'Connell MJ, Paulson EK, Jaffe TA, Ho LM. Percutaneous biopsy of periarterial soft tissue cuffs in the diagnosis of pancreatic carcinoma. Abdom Imaging. 2004;29:115–19.

42. Sperti C, Pasquali C, Di Prima F, et al. Percutaneous CT-guided fine needle aspiration cytology in the differential diagnosis of pancreatic lesions. Ital J Gastroenterol. 1994;26:126–31.

43. Hall-Craggs MA, Lees WR. Fine-needle aspiration biopsy: pancreatic and biliary tumors. Am J Roentgenol. 1986;147:399–403.

44. Mitchell CJ, Wai D, Jackson AM, MacFie J. Ultrasound guided percutaneous pancreatic biopsy. Br J Surg. 1989;76:706–7.

45. Wittenberg J, Mueller PR, Ferrucci Jr JT, et al. Percutaneous core biopsy of abdominal tumors using 22 gauge needles: further observations. Am J Roentgenol. 1982;139:75–80.

46. Pinto MM. CT-guided needle biopsy of the pancreas. Am J Gastroenterol. 1993;88:967–8.

47. Jennings PE, Donald JJ, Coral A, Rode J, Lees WR. Ultrasound-guided core biopsy. Lancet. 1989;1:1369–71.

48. Munn SR, Engen DE, Barr D, Carpenter HA, Perkins JD. Differential diagnosis of hypoamylasuria in pancreas allograft recipients with urinary exocrine drainage. Transplantation. 1990;49:359–62.

49. Sibley RK, Sutherland DE. Pancreas transplantation. An immunohistologic and histopathologic examination of 100 grafts. Am J Pathol. 1987;128:151–70.

50. Carpenter HA, Engen DE, Munn SR, et al. Histologic diagnosis of rejection by using cystoscopically directed needle biopsy specimens from dysfunctional pancreatoduodenal allografts with exocrine drainage into the bladder. Am J Surg Pathol. 1990;14:837–46.

51. Perkins JD, Munn SR, Marsh CL, Barr D, Engen DE, Carpenter HA. Safety and efficacy of cystoscopically directed biopsy in pancreas transplantation. Transplant Proc. 1990;22:665–6.

52. Aideyan OA, Schmidt AJ, Trenkner SW, Hakim NS, Gruessner RW, Walsh JW. CT-guided percutaneous biopsy of pancreas transplants. Radiology. 1996;201:825–8.

53. Bernardino M, Fernandez M, Neylan J, Hertzler G, Whelchel J, Olson R. Pancreatic transplants: CT-guided biopsy. Radiology. 1990;177:709–11.

54. Evans WK, Ho CS, McLoughlin MJ, Tao LC. Fatal necrotizing pancreatitis following fine-needle aspiration biopsy of the pancreas. Radiology. 1981;141:61–2.
55. Levin DP, Bret PM. Percutaneous fine-needle aspiration biopsy of the pancreas resulting in death. Gastrointest Radiol. 1991;16:67–9.
56. Mueller PR, Miketic LM, Simeone JF, et al. Severe acute pancreatitis after percutaneous biopsy of the pancreas. Am J Roentgenol. 1988;151:493–4.
57. Smith EH. Complications of percutaneous abdominal fine-needle biopsy. Review. Radiology. 1991;178:253–8.
58. Kane NM, Korobkin M, Francis IR, Quint LE, Cascade PN. Percutaneous biopsy of left adrenal masses: prevalence of pancreatitis after anterior approach. Am J Roentgenol. 1991;157:777–80.
59. Warshaw AL. Implications of peritoneal cytology for staging of early pancreatic cancer. Am J Surg. 1991;161:26–9; discussion 29–30.
60. Leach SD, Rose JA, Lowy AM, et al. Significance of peritoneal cytology in patients with potentially resectable adenocarcinoma of the pancreatic head. Surgery. 1995;118:472–8.
61. Johnson DE, Pendurthi TK, Balshem AM, et al. Implications of fine-needle aspiration in patients with resectable pancreatic cancer. Am Surg. 1997;63:675–9; discussion 679–80.
62. Smith FP, Macdonald JS, Schein PS, Ornitz RD. Cutaneous seeding of pancreatic cancer by skinny-needle aspiration biopsy. Arch Intern Med. 1980;140:855.
63. Rashleigh-Belcher HJ, Russell RC, Lees WR. Cutaneous seeding of pancreatic carcinoma by fine-needle aspiration biopsy. Br J Radiol. 1986;59:182–3.
64. Mallery JS, Centeno BA, Hahn PF, Chang Y, Warshaw AL, Brugge WR. Pancreatic tissue sampling guided by EUS, CT/US, and surgery: a comparison of sensitivity and specificity. Gastrointest Endosc. 2002;56:218–24.
65. Erickson RA, Sayage-Rabie L, Beissner RS. Factors predicting the number of EUS-guided fine-needle passes for diagnosis of pancreatic malignancies. Gastrointest Endosc. 2000;51: 184–90.
66. Rodriguez J, Kasberg C, Nipper M, Schoolar J, Riggs MW, Dyck WP. CT-guided needle biopsy of the pancreas: a retrospective analysis of diagnostic accuracy. Am J Gastroenterol. 1992;87: 1610–13.
67. Tillou A, Schwartz MR, Jordan Jr PH. Percutaneous needle biopsy of the pancreas: when should it be performed? World J Surg. 1996;20:283–6, discussion 287.

Spleen Biopsy

Alda Lui Tam

Background

In many parts of the world, image-guided biopsy of the spleen plays a useful role in diagnosing infectious and systemic diseases such as kala-azar, tuberculosis, sarcoidosis, and amyloidosis [1, 2]. In the United States, however, there has been some reluctance to routinely perform image-guided biopsy for focal splenic lesions or diffuse splenomegaly. This aversion could be related to several misconceptions, such as the perceived increased risk of hemorrhage; the assumption that isolated splenic lesions are uncommon; and the presumed increase in technical difficulty due to the spleen being surrounded by overlying lung, colon, or kidney [3–5]. When compared with other intra-abdominal organs, primary and isolated metastatic tumors of the spleen are relatively rare [6, 7]. However, advances in imaging technology and oncologic therapy have contributed to an increased incidence of reported cases of splenic metastases and a corresponding increased need for splenic biopsy [1, 6]. In addition, with the regular use of immunosuppressive drugs in therapy, which makes patients susceptible to infection, the differentiation between disease recurrence and benign lesions of the spleen can substantially alter treatment and prognosis. Percutaneous image-guided splenic biopsy is a minimally invasive, viable alternative to diagnostic splenectomy, which may be associated with a potentially fatal risk of sepsis [8]. Consensus from the most recent publications regarding percutaneous image-guided splenic biopsy is that the procedure is safe and accurate [3, 9–12].

A.L. Tam, MD, MBA, FRCPC
Department of Interventional Radiology,
Department of Diagnostic Radiology,
The University of Texas MD Anderson Cancer Center,
1515 Holcombe Boulevard, Unit 1471,
Houston, TX 77030-4009, USA
e-mail: alda.tam@mdanderson.org

Indications and Patient Selection

Splenic biopsy can be used to evaluate both focal lesions and splenomegaly of unknown significance [3, 5]. In the setting of a known diagnosis of a solid tumor, autopsy series have demonstrated that the rates of tumor involvement of the spleen range between 1.6 and 30 % [13, 14]. The most common solid tumors that metastasize to the spleen are breast and lung carcinomas, melanoma, and gynecologic malignancies [14]. In patients with a history of a solid tumor, biopsy is indicated to distinguish between metastases and a benign process.

Splenic involvement can occur in up to 40 % of patients with non-Hodgkin or Hodgkin lymphoma [7]. When the spleen is the only organ involved, biopsy may be indicated to establish a diagnosis of lymphoma. For patients with a prior history of lymphoma, new lesions in the spleen may require biopsy to differentiate residual disease from necrosis, infection, or transformation to a higher grade of lymphoma [1]. Nontarget biopsy of an enlarged spleen can be helpful in diagnosing systemic disorders, such as sarcoidosis, amyloidosis, storage diseases, or lymphoreticular disorders [1–3]. Splenic biopsy is also appropriate for pediatric patients, as the risk of sudden, fatal sepsis following splenectomy is particularly high in children [8].

Contraindications

There are no absolute contraindications to splenic biopsy; however, patients with infectious mononucleosis, polycythemia vera, or megakaryocytic myelosis with thrombocytosis have an increased risk of hemorrhagic complications, and it is recommended that biopsy not be performed in these patients [15]. While some authors feel that hilar lesions should be avoided because of the increased risk of

K. Ahrar, S. Gupta (eds.), *Percutaneous Image-Guided Biopsy*,
DOI 10.1007/978-1-4614-8217-8_15, © Springer Science+Business Media New York 2014

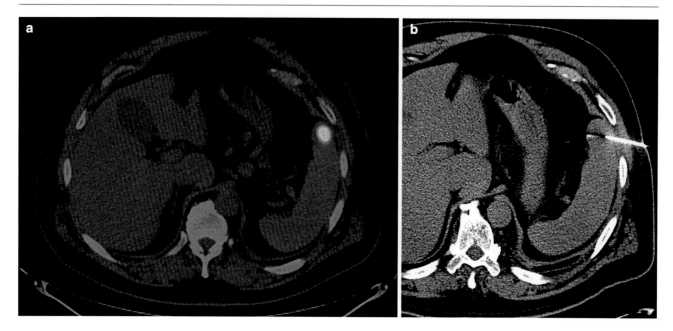

Fig. 15.1 CT-guided splenic biopsy targeting FDG-avid lesion. A 60-year-old man with a history of diffuse large B-cell lymphoma presents with a new FDG-avid lesion in the upper pole of the spleen (**a**). The specific area of FDG avidity was targeted during the CT-guided biopsy (**b**). A lateral approach was taken to traverse the least amount of splenic tissue during biopsy. A coaxial technique was used and the CT image demonstrates the core-biopsy needle within the hypodense lesion. Both fine-needle aspiration and core biopsy were performed and a pathologic diagnosis of B-cell lymphoma was made

hemorrhagic complication, others have found no difference in the complication rate based on the location of the lesion [4, 16].

Preprocedural Work-Up

Preparation for splenic biopsy involves a review of the patient's diagnostic imaging and procedural indications. Diagnostic images should be reviewed to confirm that biopsy is indicated, determine a trajectory for the biopsy needle, establish the modality for guidance, and anticipate patient positioning during the procedure. If positron emission tomography or positron emission tomography/computed tomography (PET/CT) was performed, the images obtained may aid in targeting a specific area of the lesion that is fluoro-2-deoxy-D-glucose (FDG) positive to improve diagnostic yield (Fig. 15.1).

Coagulation studies (platelet count, prothrombin time, international normalized ratio (INR), and partial thromboplastin time) should be examined and any coagulopathies should be corrected prior to biopsy. In general, an INR ≤1.5 and platelet count ≥50,000/L are acceptable parameters for solid-organ biopsy. Written informed consent must be obtained before each procedure. Splenic biopsy is well tolerated and can be performed either with local anesthesia alone or with monitored, conscious sedation using intravenous midazolam and fentanyl citrate. Preprocedural, prophylactic antibiotics are not routinely recommended.

Technique

Imaging

Either ultrasound guidance or non-contrast enhanced, CT guidance can be used for splenic biopsy. The imaging modality that best demonstrates the lesion within the spleen should be selected. The advantage of ultrasound guidance is that it provides real-time imaging in multiple planes and visualization of the needle during biopsy (Fig. 15.2). An advantage of CT guidance is the ability to accurately visualize adjacent organs, such as the colon, lung, and kidney, and their anatomic relationships to the spleen (Fig. 15.3). In some cases, the lesion cannot be seen with non-contrast-enhanced CT and the administration of intravenous contrast may be necessary for lesion localization. Another advantage of CT guidance is that a non-contrast-enhanced CT scan can be obtained immediately after the procedure to evaluate for potential complications, such as pneumothorax and hemorrhage.

Devices

Fine-needle aspiration of the spleen is usually performed using 20- to 22-gauge needles [3, 4, 7, 16]. Core-needle biopsies using 18- to 20-gauge needles have also been reported [17]. Biopsy with larger gauge needles (e.g., 14-gauge needles) has been reported, but the use of these larger needles is associated with an increased risk of hemorrhage [18].

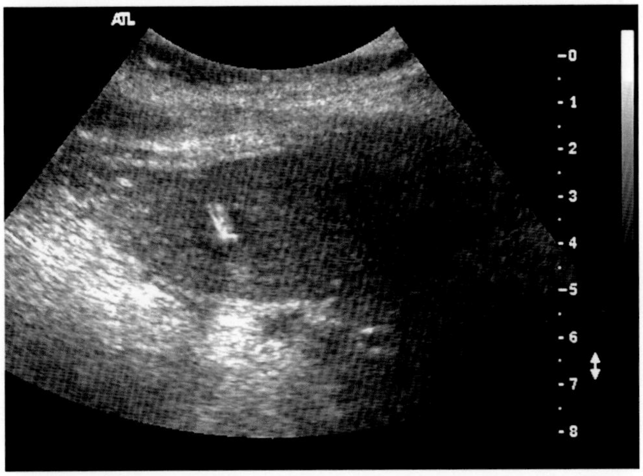

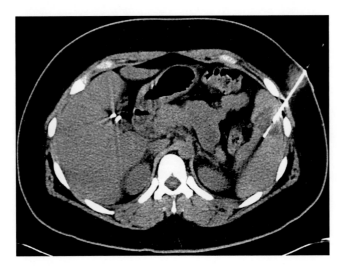

Fig. 15.2 Ultrasound-guided splenic biopsy. A 58-year-old woman with a history of mucinous cystadenoma of the ovary presented with an enlarging focal lesion within the spleen. Ultrasound image demonstrates the echogenic tip of the 22-gauge Chiba needle within the hypoechoic lesion in the inferior pole of the spleen. The biopsy tract was chosen to traverse the least amount of splenic tissue. The biopsy specimen yielded benign splenic tissue and the lesion is being followed clinically and by imaging

Fig. 15.3 CT-guided splenic biopsy. A 26-year-old woman with large cell lymphoma presents following chemotherapy with a residual lesion within the spleen. Biopsy was requested to evaluate for residual disease versus transformation to a higher grade of lymphoma. Axial non-contrast CT scan demonstrates use of the coaxial technique. A 19-gauge Chiba needle was inserted into the periphery of the splenic lesion using an anterolateral, intercostal approach. A 22-gauge Chiba needle was inserted coaxially and the tip lies within the center of the lesion. Both fine-needle aspiration and core biopsy were performed of this lesion. A pathologic diagnosis of atypical lymphohistiocytic infiltrate in a background of mild sclerosis and increased histiocytes, suspicious for lymphomatous involvement, was made on the examination of the 20-gauge core biopsy

Approaches and Relevant Anatomy

In contrast to liver biopsy, for which a biopsy tract through normal liver tissue is recommended to provide a tamponade effect, splenic biopsy should be performed on the most peripherally located lesion, thereby traversing the least amount of splenic tissue and minimizing the potential for hemorrhagic complications. The patient should be positioned so that the most direct path for biopsy of the lesion is accessible. Typically, when biopsy is performed under ultrasound guidance, the patient is in a supine or right lateral decubitus position [9, 17]. Several authors recommend that the patient be instructed to suspend respiration during needle insertion and biopsy to minimize needle movement and the resulting trauma to the splenic tissue [2, 8, 9, 19]. A subcostal approach is favored, although an intercostal approach may be necessary depending on the lesion's location. For splenic lesions in the upper pole, the triangulation method or angling of the CT gantry may be necessary to avoid traversal of the pleural reflection [20]. Most ultrasound-guided biopsies are performed using a free-hand technique, as most lesions are located in the periphery of the spleen [4]. For deeper lesions, a coaxial technique may be helpful and allows for both fine-needle aspiration and core biopsy to be performed with only one puncture of the spleen.

Potential Complications and Management of Complications

Splenic biopsies can be performed on an outpatient basis. Following the procedure, patients should be observed for potential complications. Postprocedural observation times vary between 2 and 4 h [9, 11, 19] and include monitoring of the patient's blood pressure, pulse, and oxygen saturation. Postprocedural chest radiography should be performed in patients in whom a pleural surface was traversed to evaluate for pneumothorax. Patients who remain stable following the observation period, with minimal or no discomfort, can be discharged home. Patients should be instructed to avoid heavy lifting and strenuous activity for at least 3 days, as delayed hemorrhagic complications have been reported [4, 11, 18, 19].

In 1976, Soderstrom reported no complications in a series of more than 1,000 "blind" splenic biopsies [2]. More recently, complication rates ranging from zero to 16.7 % have been reported for splenic biopsy (Table 15.1). Unfortunately, uniform criteria for reporting complications have not been applied across the studies, making direct comparisons difficult. Most postbiopsy complications are minor and self-limited, requiring no additional treatment. For example, postprocedural pain occurring in the left upper quadrant or radiating to the left shoulder has been described in up to 50 % of patients after percutaneous splenic biopsy [18]. Hemorrhage following splenic biopsy has been reported in zero to 8.3 % of patients [3, 5, 11, 16, 17, 21]. Most cases of hemorrhage are self-limited, perisplenic hematomas that do not require further intervention (Fig. 15.4); however, although rare, uncontrolled hemorrhage has been reported

Table 15.1 Comparison of results of percutaneous splenic biopsy

Study	No. of biopsies	Diagnostic yield (%)	Overall accuracy (%)	Complication rate (%)
Siniluoto et al. [23]	42	97.6	88.1	0
Caraway et al. [1]	50	88	NR	2
Venkataramu et al. [21]	35	62.8	NR	2.9
Keogan et al. [7]	20	88.9	NR	0
Civardi et al. [3]	398	90	91	5.3 (<1 % major)
Muraca et al. [8]	30	90	83	0
Lucey et al. [16]	39	91	NR	10.3
Lieberman et al. [17]	24	90	NR	8.3
Lal et al. [12]	56	90	100	16.3 (6 % major)
Kang et al. [9]	78	84	NR	1.1
Liang et al. [10]	43	97.6	85.7	2.3
Tam et al. [11]	156	92.3	84.7	16.7 (1.9 % major)

NR not reported

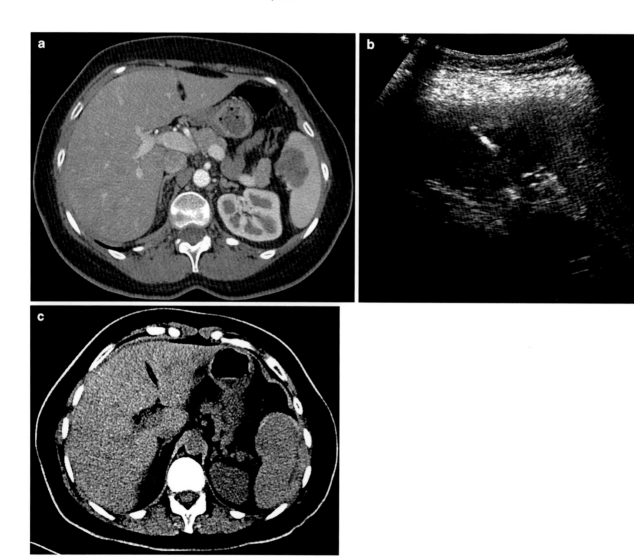

Fig. 15.4 Self-limited perisplenic hematoma following biopsy. A 48-year-old woman with a history of lung cancer and endometrial cancer presented with a focal splenic lesion. The axial image from the contrast-enhanced CT scan demonstrates a low-density lesion within the spleen, near the hilum (**a**). Ultrasound-guided splenic biopsy was performed from a lateral approach and the ultrasound image demonstrates the echogenic tip of the 22-gauge Chiba needle within the lesion (**b**). One hour following the procedure, the patient complained of left upper quadrant abdominal pain that radiated to her left shoulder. A limited, non-contrast-enhanced CT scan of the abdomen was obtained and showed a small, perisplenic hematoma (**c**). The patient was admitted overnight for monitoring and observation. She was discharged the next day without complication. A pathologic diagnosis of metastatic endometrial cancer was made based on the evaluation of the fine-needle aspiration

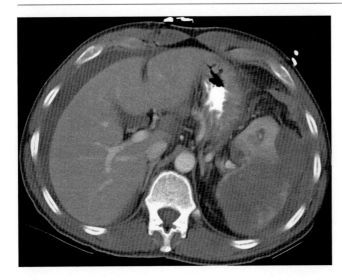

Fig. 15.5 Delayed postbiopsy splenic rupture. A 39-year-old man with a history of follicular lymphoma underwent a diagnostic ultrasound-guided fine-needle aspiration biopsy of a new focal splenic lesion. There were no immediate complications from the biopsy and the patient was discharged home following a 4-h observation period. Four days later, the patient presented to the emergency room with worsening left upper quadrant abdominal pain. The axial image from the contrast-enhanced CT scan demonstrates intraperitoneal hemorrhage and a large low-density defect within the inferior pole of the spleen with subcapsular fluid consistent with splenic rupture and hematoma. The patient underwent emergent splenectomy which confirmed lymphomatous involvement of the spleen

and can result in the need for blood transfusions, the need for emergent splenectomy, or death[1, 11, 16] (Fig. 15.5). Other complications such as pneumothorax, pleural effusion, and colonic injury have also been described [3, 5].

Outcome and Results

The reported diagnostic accuracy rates for splenic biopsy range from 83 to 100 % (Table 15.1) [1, 3, 5, 7, 11, 16, 21–23]. Civardi et al. demonstrated that operator experience and skill were factors in improved diagnostic accuracy [3]. The patient's underlying diagnosis can also affect the diagnostic accuracy rate. Fine-needle aspiration of focal splenic lesions is most effective for patients with malignancies other than lymphoma [11, 23]. In our series of 156 biopsies, the diagnostic yield and accuracy in patients with a history of solid tumor were 97 % and 93.8 %, respectively [11]. In contrast, in patients with lymphoma, the diagnostic yield and accuracy were 90.8 % and 84.1 %, respectively [11].

While several authors have demonstrated the efficacy of fine-needle aspiration of splenic lesions for diagnosing non-Hodgkin lymphoma [1, 21, 22], many have noted its limited role in diagnosing or staging Hodgkin lymphoma [1, 18]. Our results show that fine-needle aspiration is not particularly effective for diagnosing Hodgkin lymphoma, with a

sensitivity of only 50 %, negative predictive value of 33.3 %, accuracy of 60 %, and diagnostic yield of 83.3 % [11]. These findings are similar to those reported by Lindgren et al., who used a 14-gauge core-biopsy needle to obtain samples. In that series, only three of 15 patients with Hodgkin lymphoma had a positive splenic biopsy [18]. In another study of Hodgkin lymphoma patients, when laparoscopic excisional biopsy of the spleen was followed by splenectomy, splenic involvement was detected in only 30 % of patients [24]. In general, core biopsy is associated with greater accuracy rates in lymphoma patients. In a series of 183 lymphoma patients (out of a study population of 398), fine-needle aspiration was associated with an accuracy rate of 68.5 %, while core biopsy had an improved accuracy rate of 90.9 % [3]. However, the authors found that the best results for lymphoma patients were obtained after "double sampling," in which fine-needle aspiration and core biopsy were performed concurrently. The accuracy rate for patients with double sampling was 95.4 % [3]. Other studies have also concluded that core biopsy improves diagnostic accuracy and decreases the number of false-negative results [17, 18, 25]. Similarly, our results show that concurrent fine-needle aspiration and core biopsy of a lesion improves the accuracy to 91.7 % compared with 84.1 % for fine-needle aspiration alone [11]. As treatment regimens for lymphoma become increasingly targeted to specific lymphoma subtypes, the ability to subclassify a lymphoma takes on added importance. Double sampling would ensure sufficient material to send for flow cytometry analysis and provide material for morphologic analysis.

Summary

A number of benign and malignant disease processes can involve the spleen, resulting in focal or diffuse abnormalities. In oncology patients, it is particularly important to determine the etiology of splenic involvement as treatment can vary from observation only to active therapeutic intervention, with adverse consequences if the diagnosis is incorrect. Histopathologic yield from splenic biopsy is reliable, and the procedure is safe and effective for the evaluation of focal lesions or splenomegaly of unknown significance. In a patient who has or is suspected to have lymphoma, concurrent fine-needle aspiration and core biopsy should be performed to maximize diagnostic yield.

References

1. Caraway NP, Fanning CV. Use of fine-needle aspiration biopsy in the evaluation of splenic lesions in a cancer center. Diagn Cytopathol. 1997;16:312–16.
2. Soderstrom N. How to use cytodiagnostic spleen puncture. Acta Med Scand. 1976;199:1–5.

3. Civardi G, Vallisa D, Berte R, et al. Ultrasound-guided fine needle biopsy of the spleen: high clinical efficacy and low risk in a multicenter Italian study. Am J Hematol. 2001;67:93–9.

4. O'Malley ME, Wood BJ, Boland GW, et al. Percutaneous imaging-guided biopsy of the spleen. AJR Am J Roentgenol. 1999;172:661–5.

5. Quinn SF, vanSonnenberg E, Casola G, et al. Interventional radiology in the spleen. Radiology. 1986;161:289–91.

6. Comperat E, Bardier-Dupas A, Camparo P, et al. Splenic metastases: clinicopathologic presentation, differential diagnosis, and pathogenesis. Arch Pathol Lab Med. 2007;131:965–9.

7. Keogan MT, Freed KS, Paulson EK, et al. Imaging-guided percutaneous biopsy of focal splenic lesions: update on safety and effectiveness. AJR Am J Roentgenol. 1999;172:933–7.

8. Muraca S, Chait PG, Connolly BL, et al. US-guided core biopsy of the spleen in children. Radiology. 2001;218:200–6.

9. Kang M, Kalra N, Gulati M, et al. Image guided percutaneous splenic interventions. Eur J Radiol. 2007;64:140–6.

10. Liang P, Gao Y, Wang Y, et al. US-guided percutaneous needle biopsy of the spleen using 18-gauge versus 21-gauge needles. J Clin Ultrasound. 2007;35:477–82.

11. Tam A, Krishnamurthy S, Pillsbury EP, et al. Percutaneous image-guided splenic biopsy in the oncology patient: an audit of 156 consecutive cases. J Vasc Interv Radiol. 2008;19:80–7.

12. Lal A, Ariga R, Gattuso P, et al. Splenic fine needle aspiration and core biopsy. A review of 49 cases. Acta Cytol. 2003;47: 951–9.

13. Klein B, Stein M, Kuten A, et al. Splenomegaly and solitary spleen metastasis in solid tumors. Cancer. 1987;60:100–2.

14. Wolf B, Neiman R. Disorders of the spleen. In: Bennington JL, editor. Major problems in pathology. Philadelphia: WB Saunders; 1989. p. 5–204.

15. Linsk J, Franzen S. Disease of the lymph node and spleen. In: Linsk J, Franzen S, editors. Clinical aspiration cytology. 2nd ed. Philadelphia: JB Lippincott; 1989. p. 354–8.

16. Lucey BC, Boland GW, Maher MM, et al. Percutaneous nonvascular splenic intervention: a 10-year review. AJR Am J Roentgenol. 2002;179:1591–6.

17. Lieberman S, Libson E, Maly B, et al. Imaging-guided percutaneous splenic biopsy using a 20- or 22-gauge cutting-edge core biopsy needle for the diagnosis of malignant lymphoma. AJR Am J Roentgenol. 2003;181:1025–7.

18. Lindgren PG, Hagberg H, Eriksson B, et al. Excision biopsy of the spleen by ultrasonic guidance. Br J Radiol. 1985;58:853–7.

19. Lieberman S, Libson E, Sella T, et al. Percutaneous image-guided splenic procedures: update on indications, technique, complications, and outcomes. Semin Ultrasound CT MR. 2007;28:57–63.

20. van Sonnenberg E, Wittenberg J, Ferrucci Jr JT, et al. Triangulation method for percutaneous needle guidance: the angled approach to upper abdominal masses. AJR Am J Roentgenol. 1981;137:757–61.

21. Venkataramu NK, Gupta S, Sood BP, et al. Ultrasound guided fine needle aspiration biopsy of splenic lesions. Br J Radiol. 1999;72:953–6.

22. Silverman JF, Geisinger KR, Raab SS, et al. Fine needle aspiration biopsy of the spleen in the evaluation of neoplastic disorders. Acta Cytol. 1993;37:158–62.

23. Siniluoto T, Paivansalo M, Tikkakoski T, et al. Ultrasound-guided aspiration cytology of the spleen. Acta Radiol. 1992;33:137–9.

24. Veronesi U, Spinelli P, Bonadonna G, et al. Laparoscopy and laparotomy in staging Hodgkin's and non-Hodgkin's lymphoma. AJR Am J Roentgenol. 1976;127:501–3.

25. Suzuki T, Shibuya H, Yoshimatsu S, et al. Ultrasonically guided staging splenic tissue core biopsy in patients with non-Hodgkin's lymphoma. Cancer. 1987;60:879–82.

Adrenal Gland Biopsy

Alda Lui Tam

Background

Adrenal lesions are common. Autopsy series have found that adrenal masses can be found in up to 9 % of patients and 27 % of cancer patients [1–3]. The adrenal gland is the most common site of extranodal metastases in lung cancer [4–6]. Additionally, lymphoma, melanoma, and carcinomas (breast, gastric, pancreatic, renal, and colon) often metastasize to the adrenal gland [7]. With the increase in the use of cross-sectional imaging, incidental adrenal masses have been found in 4–6 % of the imaged population [8]. The most common adrenal masses found on cross-sectional imaging are nonfunctioning adenomas and metastases (Table 16.1), and determining the presence of malignant disease, either primary or secondary, is a priority when an adrenal mass is discovered [9, 10]. Advances in diagnostic imaging techniques, including lipid-sensitive computed tomography (CT), CT densitometry, and magnetic resonance imaging (MRI), have increased the ability to detect and characterize adrenal masses. The sensitivity and specificity for detecting adrenal adenoma is reported to be 95 % and 80 %, respectively, for MRI and 98 % and 92 %, respectively, for CT [11, 12]. This refinement of diagnostic imaging protocols has decreased the number of lesions referred for percutaneous biopsy and decreased the number of benign diagnoses in patients with known malignancies who undergo biopsy of an adrenal mass to less than 12 % [13]. Still, despite these imaging advances, percutaneous biopsy continues to be a useful tool for evaluating focal lesions of the adrenal gland.

Indications and Patient Selection

Adrenal biopsy can be performed to establish a diagnosis in an indeterminate lesion, stage a known malignancy, or establish a diagnosis of malignancy in diffuse disease [14]. The indication for biopsy of an adrenal lesion is clear in patients with known extra-adrenal malignancies or suspected infection; however, not all adrenal masses warrant tissue sampling, and the role of percutaneous biopsy in the evaluation of adrenal "incidentalomas" is less certain.

An adrenal incidentaloma is defined as an adrenal mass, ≥1 cm in diameter, that has been incidentally discovered during a radiologic examination performed for purposes other than the evaluation of adrenal disease [10]. Most adrenal incidentalomas are benign, nonfunctioning adenomas; however, other common diagnoses include cortisol-secreting adenomas, pheochromocytomas, adrenal cortical carcinomas, and metastatic disease [15, 16]. According to the 2003 National Institutes of Health State-of-the-Science statement on adrenal incidentalomas, all patients with an adrenal incidentaloma require evaluation with a complete history and physical examination and hormonal testing [17]. It is

Table 16.1 Differential diagnosis of adrenal lesions

	Differential diagnosis
Unilateral lesion	Adrenal adenomas (functional vs. nonfunctional)
	Myelolipoma
	Adrenal cyst
	Metastases
	Primary adenocarcinoma
	Pheochromocytoma
	Lymphoma
	Neuroblastoma
Bilateral lesions	Hyperplasia
	Hemorrhage
	Infection (histoplasmosis or tuberculosis)
	Metastases
	Bilateral pheochromocytoma
	Lymphoma

A.L. Tam, MD, MBA, FRCPC
Department of Interventional Radiology,
Department of Diagnostic Radiology,
The University of Texas MD Anderson Cancer Center,
1515 Holcombe Boulevard, Unit 1471,
Houston, TX 77030-4009, USA
e-mail: alda.tam@mdanderson.org

K. Ahrar, S. Gupta (eds.), *Percutaneous Image-Guided Biopsy*,
DOI 10.1007/978-1-4614-8217-8_16, © Springer Science+Business Media New York 2014

recommended that all patients undergo a 1-mg overnight dexamethasone suppression test and measurement of fractionated urinary or plasma metanephrines and catecholamines. In hypertensive patients, additional evaluations of the serum potassium levels and plasma aldosterone concentration-plasma renin activity ratio are needed to assess for primary aldosteronism. If the biochemical test results are consistent with a functional adrenal cortical tumor or pheochromocytoma, surgical management is recommended [10, 17]. If the biochemical test results are normal, the radiologic images should be reviewed for lesion morphology, as larger lesions are associated with an increased risk for malignancy. An incidentaloma >4 cm in size is associated with an increased risk of malignancy of approximately 70 % and the risk increases to 85 % if the incidentaloma is >6 cm; conversely, nearly all lesions <4 cm are benign [10, 15, 17]. Given the increased risk of malignancy, surgical management is usually recommended for lesions ≥4 cm [10, 18]. For lesions <4 cm, yearly biochemical testing and repeat imaging at 6, 12, and 24 months following the initial scan are suggested [10, 17]. Percutaneous biopsy may be considered in patients with an incidentaloma and a history of malignancy; however, there are few studies demonstrating the utility of percutaneous biopsy in patients with an incidentaloma who do not have a history of malignancy [10, 17].

Contraindications

There are no absolute contraindications to adrenal gland biopsy. Relative contraindications include uncorrectable coagulopathy, an uncooperative patient, and lesion inaccessibility. Generally, biopsy of a suspected pheochromocytoma is not indicated as it can precipitate a potentially life-threatening hypertensive crisis.

Preprocedural Workup

Preparation for adrenal biopsy involves a review of the patient's diagnostic imaging results, procedural indications, biochemical studies of adrenal function, and coagulation profile. Diagnostic images should be reviewed to confirm that biopsy is indicated, determine a trajectory for the biopsy needle, establish the modality for guidance, and anticipate patient positioning during the procedure. If positron emission tomography (PET) or PET/CT is available, the images may aid with targeting a specific area of the lesion that is fluoro-2-deoxy-D-glucose (FDG) positive to improve diagnostic yield.

It is essential to review all available biochemical studies, as they can affect the clinical management of adrenal masses: functional lesions do not require biopsy.

Additionally, adrenal biopsy should not be performed until a pheochromocytoma has been excluded biochemically [19–21]. If biopsy of a suspected pheochromocytoma is categorically required, pre-biopsy consultation with an endocrinologist, who can provide for prophylactic blockade of the adrenergic receptors prior to the procedure, and anesthesiology support during the procedure, are strongly recommended.

Coagulation studies (platelet count, prothrombin time, international normalized ratio (INR), and partial thromboplastin time) should be examined and coagulopathies should be corrected prior to biopsy. In general, an INR ≤ 1.5 and a platelet count ≥50,000/L are acceptable parameters for solid organ biopsy. Written informed consent must be obtained before each procedure. Adrenal biopsy is well tolerated and can be performed either with local anesthesia alone or with monitored, conscious sedation using intravenous midazolam and fentanyl citrate. Preprocedural, prophylactic antibiotics are not routinely recommended.

Technique

Imaging

Ultrasound guidance can be used for very large adrenal lesions and provides the advantage of real-time monitoring of the needle during biopsy; however, CT is usually the imaging guidance modality of choice for adrenal biopsy. CT clearly delineates the anatomic detail of the adrenal gland and adjacent structures. It also demonstrates the position of the biopsy needle within the lesion and can be used to detect procedure-related complications, such as intra-abdominal hemorrhage or pneumothorax, quickly. Non-contrast-enhanced CT is usually adequate for procedure planning and execution. Axial images acquired in 3- or 5-mm thick slices are obtained to confirm the location of the lesion and to plan needle trajectory.

Devices

Small-caliber needles (20–22 gauge) provide fine-needle aspirates for cytologic assessment, and cutting needles (18–20 gauge) provide core biopsy samples for histologic analysis. Coaxial technique using a 16–19-gauge guide needle is often used during adrenal biopsy to allow for the acquisition of both fine-needle aspirates and core biopsies. Thin-wall Chiba needles, with a beveled tip, are common guide needles. A Hawkins needle, with interchangeable blunt and sharp stylets, may be useful when the needle path lies in close proximity to major vessels or when artificial paravertebral widening with saline injection is planned.

Fig. 16.1 Anatomy of the upper abdomen. Schematic representation of the adrenal glands lying within the upper abdominal cavity and their anatomic relationships to other surrounding solid organs

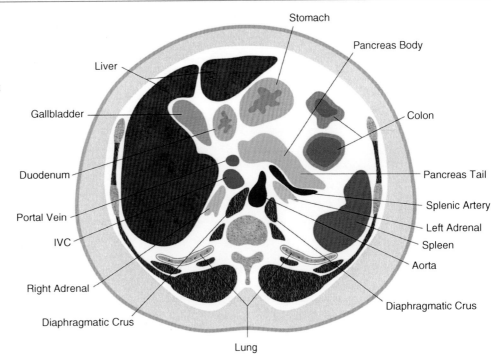

Approaches and Relevant Anatomy

The adrenal glands are located deep within the upper abdomen, surrounded by lung, liver, kidney, spleen, and pancreas (Fig. 16.1). The presence of these overlying structures can make adrenal gland biopsy technically challenging. Most image-guided adrenal biopsies are performed from a posterior approach. With the patient in the prone position, a direct, vertical approach to the adrenal gland is often not possible without transgressing the pleural space, which is associated with a risk of pneumothorax (Fig. 16.2). To avoid this potential complication, special techniques, such as angled approaches with or without CT gantry angulation, have been developed [22–24]. The triangulation method involves the construction of a right triangle and the use of the Pythagorean theorem and tangent ratios to calculate an extrapleural, extraperitoneal route to the lesion of interest with the patient in the prone position [23] (Fig. 16.3). The point on the skin directly overlying the lesion is marked (Z), and the depth from the skin surface to the center of the lesion is then calculated. This length (B) represents one side of the right triangle. A point on the skin surface, in the same parasagittal plane as point Z, is chosen for the needle entry site. The entry site should be below the posterior pleural reflection, either lower than the 12th rib or the transverse process of the first lumbar vertebra. The length (A) between the skin entry point and point Z represents the second side of the right triangle. The hypotenuse (C), representing the actual needle distance and an extrapleural, extraperitoneal path from the entry site to the center of the lesion, can now be calculated using the Pythagorean theorem for right triangles, $(A^2 + B^2 = C^2)$. The angle of needle insertion is determined from the tangent ratio of the two sides of the right triangle. Once the ratio is calculated, the angle can be extrapolated from a table of trigonometric ratios. It should be noted that with the angled approach, the entire needle length will not be visualized on a single transverse slice, and successive cephalad scans may be required to locate the needle tip (Fig. 16.4).

Alternatively, with the patient in the prone position, angulation of the CT gantry towards the patient's feet to create a caudocephalad beam direction can be used to avoid the posterior costophrenic sulcus during adrenal biopsy [22, 24]. With this technique, the biopsy needle is inserted along the plane of the angled CT gantry. Beam angulation then allows for visualization of a direct path to the adrenal lesion without having to perform geometric calculations. Another advantage of this technique is that the entire path of the needle can often be seen on a single transverse slice. Beam angulation between 15° and 25° has been shown to be sufficient for most adrenal lesions.

Other authors recommend a posterior approach to the adrenal gland while the patient is in an ipsilateral decubitus position, with the side of the gland of interest down [14, 25, 26]. In the decubitus position, the dependent diaphragm is elevated, removing the risk of costophrenic sulcus transgression, and allows for a more direct approach to the adrenal gland (Fig. 16.5).

Besides the presence of interposed lung, access to the adrenal gland in the prone position may be hampered by the kidney or vertebral body (Fig. 16.6). Artificial widening of the paravertebral space using the injection of saline is a well-known technique in the biopsy of mediastinal lesions; this technique can

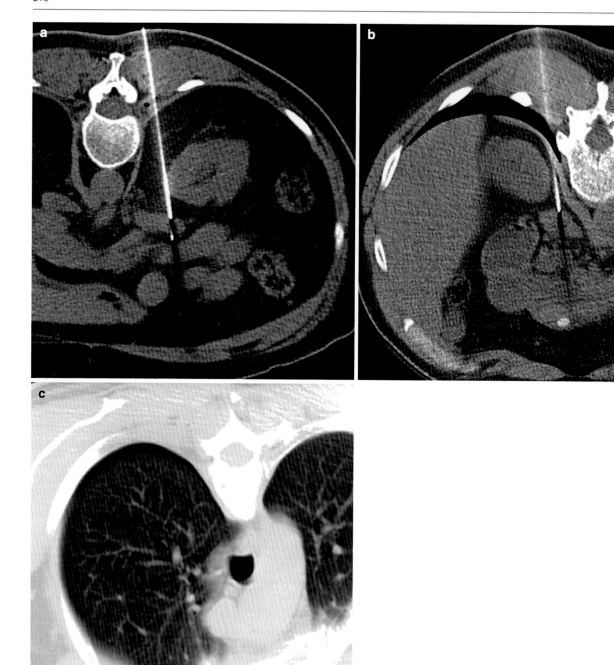

Fig. 16.2 Posterior approach for biopsy of adrenal gland. (**a**) Axial non-contrast-enhanced CT image demonstrates a direct, extrapleural, posterior approach to a left adrenal gland mass in a patient in the prone position. A coaxial biopsy technique was used where the 18-gauge Chiba guide needle has been positioned at the periphery of the left adrenal gland and a 22-gauge Chiba needle has been inserted coaxially into the left adrenal gland lesion. Both fine-needle aspiration and core biopsy were obtained and the pathologic diagnosis was metastatic non-small cell lung cancer. (**b**) Axial non-contrast-enhanced CT image shows a posterior approach, involving traversal of the pleural space, to a right adrenal gland lesion in a patient in the prone position. The pathologic diagnosis of metastatic colon cancer was made. Traversal of the pleural reflection resulted in a post biopsy pneumothorax as shown on the axial non-contrast-enhanced CT image in lung windows (**c**). The pneumothorax remained stable in size during the observation period and the patient was discharged home without a chest tube being placed

also be applied to the biopsy of the adrenal gland [27]. Injecting saline into the posterior paravertebral space results in lateral displacement of the parietal pleura, providing an extrapleural path to the adrenal lesion (Figs. 16.7 and 16.8). When no alternative access to the adrenal gland is available, transrenal adrenal biopsy can be performed [25] (Fig. 16.9).

Fig. 16.3 Triangulation method. Schematic representation of use of the Pythagorean theorem and tangent ratios to calculate an extrapleural, extraperitoneal route to the adrenal gland in a patient in the prone position

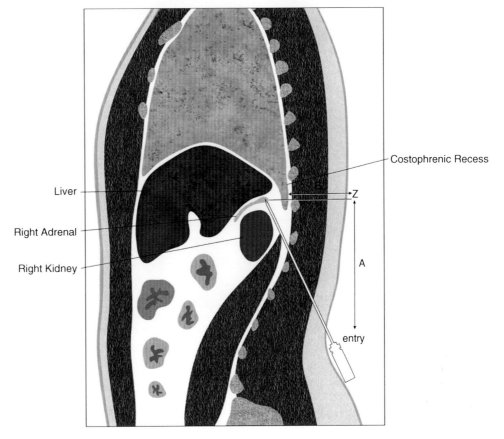

Various anterior approaches to the adrenal gland have been described but are rarely used, such as a transhepatic approach for the right adrenal gland and transgastric, transpancreatic, or transsplenic approaches for the left adrenal gland [28–30]. It has been argued that the liver parenchyma serves to tamponade the needle track when the transhepatic approach is used [30] (Fig. 16.10). Nevertheless, a posterior approach to the adrenal gland is generally preferred, as this approach usually represents the shortest distance to the adrenal gland and does not involve the traversal of another solid organ. Also, the potential complication associated with a posterior approach—pneumothorax—is easier to manage than the potential complications associated with an anterior approach.

Potential Complications and Management of Complications

Complication rates from adrenal biopsy range from 0 to 12 % [29, 31, 32]. The most common complications associated with adrenal gland biopsy are pneumothorax and hemorrhage [31, 33, 34]. Pancreatitis, adrenal abscess, bacteremia, needle-track seeding, and hypertensive crisis are uncommon complications that have also been described [19, 28, 29, 31, 35].

Following biopsy, patients are observed for 3 h to monitor hemodynamic stability and respiratory status. Hemorrhage following adrenal biopsy has been reported in 4–7 % of cases; hemorrhage can occur either in the abdomen or thorax, is usually self-limited, and typically resolves over time [25, 31, 32, 35] (Fig. 16.11). Rarely, transfusions may be indicated if hemorrhage occurs [29, 31] (Fig. 16.12). In a review of 83 cases, Mody et al. noted a higher overall complication rate when the transhepatic route was used than when the posterior approach was used. The transhepatic route-related complications (hepatic or subcapsular hematoma, needle-track seeding) were associated with significant morbidity. Similarly, anterior approaches to the left adrenal gland that traverse the pancreas are associated with a 6 % risk of acute pancreatitis, which can result in significant morbidity and mortality [28].

For biopsies during which a pleural surface was crossed, a chest radiograph should be performed immediately and 3 h following the biopsy to evaluate for pneumothorax. While the management of postprocedural pneumothorax varies across institutions, we and other authors have found that patients with small, stable, asymptomatic pneumothoraces may be discharged home without the need for additional intervention [25, 36]. Patients with enlarging or symptomatic pneumothoraces require chest tube placement. The placement of a small bore (8 French) chest tube may be accomplished either under fluoroscopic or under CT guidance. To allow for

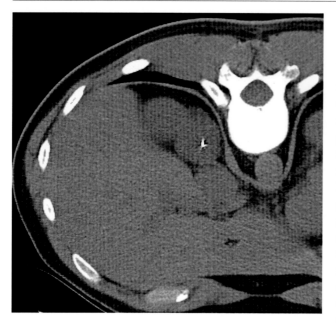

Fig. 16.4 CT-guided adrenal biopsy using triangulation method. The triangulation method was used to biopsy the right adrenal lesion, and an axial non-contrast-enhanced CT image demonstrates the tip of the biopsy needle within the adrenal lesion. The angled, subcostal approach avoids traversal of the pleural space by the biopsy needle; however, as is common with the angled approach, the entire needle length is not visualized on this single transverse image

outpatient management of the pneumothorax, the chest tube can be attached to a one-way Heimlich valve, and the patient can then be discharged home with instructions to return the next day for evaluation of chest tube removal. If required, the chest tube can be placed to Pleurovac, with or without suction, and the patient admitted for observation and more aggressive air-leak management.

One potentially life-threatening complication is the provocation of a hypertensive crisis during biopsy of a pheochromocytoma. At least 14 % of pheochromocytomas present with atypical clinical and/or biochemical features [19]; therefore, biopsy of an unsuspected pheochromocytoma does occasionally occur and the radiologist should be prepared to address pheochromocytoma reactions [19, 21, 37]. Reported complications of biopsy of pheochromocytoma include transient headaches, labile blood pressure, abdominal pain, hemodynamic instability, uncontrolled hemorrhage, and death [38]. An acute hypertensive crisis is treated with 1 mg of phentolamine given intravenously, followed by an intravenous phentolamine drip (20 mg in 500 mL of 5 % dextrose water) titrated to blood pressure. Intravenous nitroprusside (50 mg in 500 mL of 5 % dextrose water) can also be used to control hypertension. A beta-adrenergic blocking agent, such as propranolol, may be useful to treat cardiac arrhythmias (1 mg/min intravenously until a response is noted) or hypotension (1 mg/min intravenously for a total of 5–10 mg until hypotension resolves) [19].

Outcome and Results

In general, the accuracy rates of image-guided adrenal gland biopsy range from 90 to 96 % [31, 33, 34, 39, 40] and the sensitivity ranges from 81 to 93 % [6, 32, 33, 40, 41]. The utility of adrenal biopsy in distinguishing between benign and malignant adrenal cortical tumors has been debated, and despite some positive studies [42, 43], the pervasive opinion is that the differentiation and classification of primary adrenal cortical tumors remains unreliable [17, 18, 20]. However, results from a study by Saeger et al. suggest that core biopsy of the adrenal gland can provide sufficient sensitivity and specificity for the diagnosis of primary adrenocortical tumors if strict criteria for the diagnosis of adrenal cortical carcinoma in combination with immunohistochemistry are applied [44]. In 2003, Saeger et al. validated the high diagnostic accuracy rate of adrenal core biopsy in a prospective, multicenter study using an ex vivo approach. Core biopsies were obtained from 220 consecutive patients who underwent adrenalectomy. The biopsies were evaluated for pathohistologic diagnosis using paraffin sections, routine staining, and immunohistochemistry. The overall sensitivity and specificity for malignancy was 94.6 % and 95.3 %, respectively. The overall accuracy rate, where there was concordance with surgical pathology findings, was 90 %. The positive predictive value was 98.8 %, and the negative predictive value was 81.4 % [44].

In cancer patients, adrenal biopsy is believed to be associated with a 100 % positive predictive value [33]. Other studies have shown that the negative predictive value of adrenal biopsy is 90–100 %—in other words, when normal- or benign-appearing adrenal tissue is obtained at biopsy, even in patients with primary malignancy, it is predictive of a benign lesion [33, 45, 46]. However, these studies considered only biopsies in which normal or benign adrenal tissue was sampled and excluded nondiagnostic biopsies. In contrast, the negative predictive value of a nondiagnostic result was reported to be 82 %, and it is thus recommended that adrenal gland biopsies with insufficient tissue for diagnosis be repeated [33, 40, 46]. In the study by Silverman et al., 20 % (2/11) of the patients with nondiagnostic biopsies were subsequently proven to have a malignancy by surgery or autopsy [33].

Several authors have described factors that contribute to increased diagnostic yield [40, 46, 47]. Welch et al. noted that accuracy was improved when the right adrenal gland was biopsied and when larger needles (18 or 19 gauge) were used [40]. Biopsy of lesions ≥3 cm in size was associated with better accuracy (100 %) than biopsy of lesions <3 cm (90 %) [33]. In two series examining two institutions' experiences with adrenal biopsy over a ten-year period, an improvement in the accuracy rate was noted between the first 5 years and the last 5 years of the study. This was attributed to the increased experience of the radiologists performing biopsies, as well as the addition of on-site, immediate evaluation of the biopsy samples by a trained cytopathologist [40, 47].

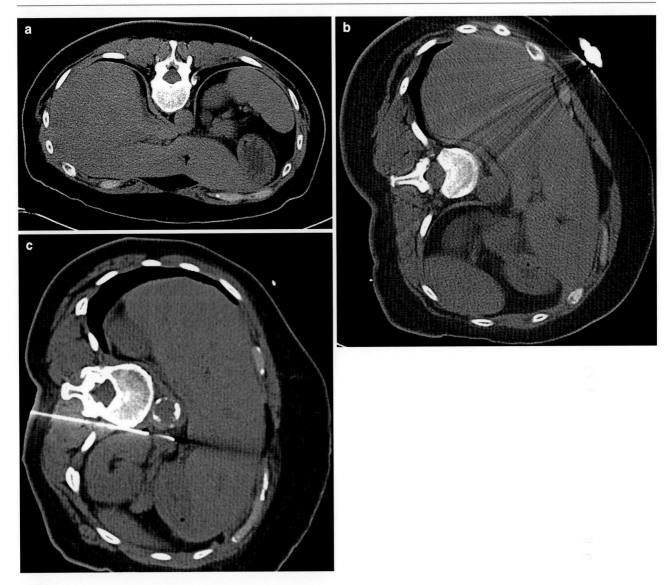

Fig. 16.5 Effects of position change on biopsy approach to adrenal gland. (**a**) A 39-year-old woman with lung cancer presented with a 1-cm left adrenal nodule. In the prone position, the left lower lobe of the lung is interposed between the skin and the left adrenal nodule. (**b**) Repositioning the patient into the ipsilateral decubitus position (*left side down*) elevates the dependent diaphragm, moves the lung out of the path of the biopsy needle, and provides a more direct approach to the adrenal lesion. (**c**) Axial non-contrast CT image depicts the coaxial technique using an 18-gauge Hawkins guide needle and a 22-gauge Chiba needle for biopsy of a different patient with a left adrenal lesion in the ipsilateral decubitus position

Summary

Adrenal gland biopsy is an important tool in diagnosing focal lesions of the adrenal gland. For cancer patients, a biopsy can contribute to accurate staging of disease and often differentiates those patients who are eligible for potentially curative surgical resection from those who are not. Review of the preprocedural, biochemical workup is particularly important, as functional adrenal lesions and pheochromocytomas should not be biopsied. Guidelines for the management of adrenal incidentalomas should be followed and all radiologists who perform adrenal biopsies should be familiar with the treatment of an acute hypertensive crisis.

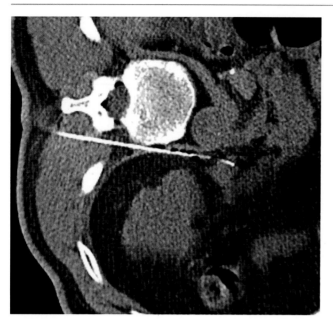

Fig. 16.6 Ipsilateral decubitus approach for biopsy of adrenal gland. Axial non-contrast-enhanced CT image demonstrates an extrapleural, paravertebral approach to a left adrenal gland lesion with the patient in the ipsilateral decubitus position. Note the slight curvature on the 22-gauge Chiba needle within the adrenal lesion. Putting a small curve on the 22-gauge biopsy needle can help to redirect the needle into the lesion. The pathologic diagnosis was metastatic renal cell carcinoma

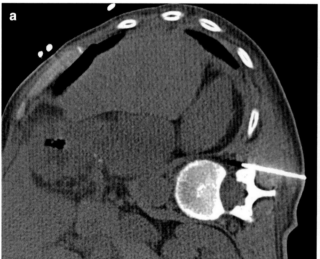
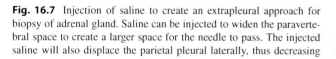
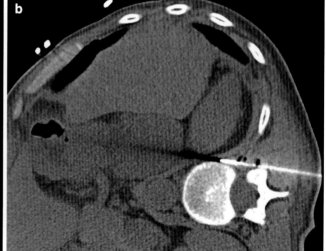

Fig. 16.7 Injection of saline to create an extrapleural approach for biopsy of adrenal gland. Saline can be injected to widen the paravertebral space to create a larger space for the needle to pass. The injected saline will also displace the parietal pleural laterally, thus decreasing the risk of pleural transgression (**a, b, c, d**). This patient was placed in the contralateral decubitus position because of the significant beam-hardening artifact from residual contrast in the colon (not shown). The pathologic diagnosis was metastatic non-small cell carcinoma

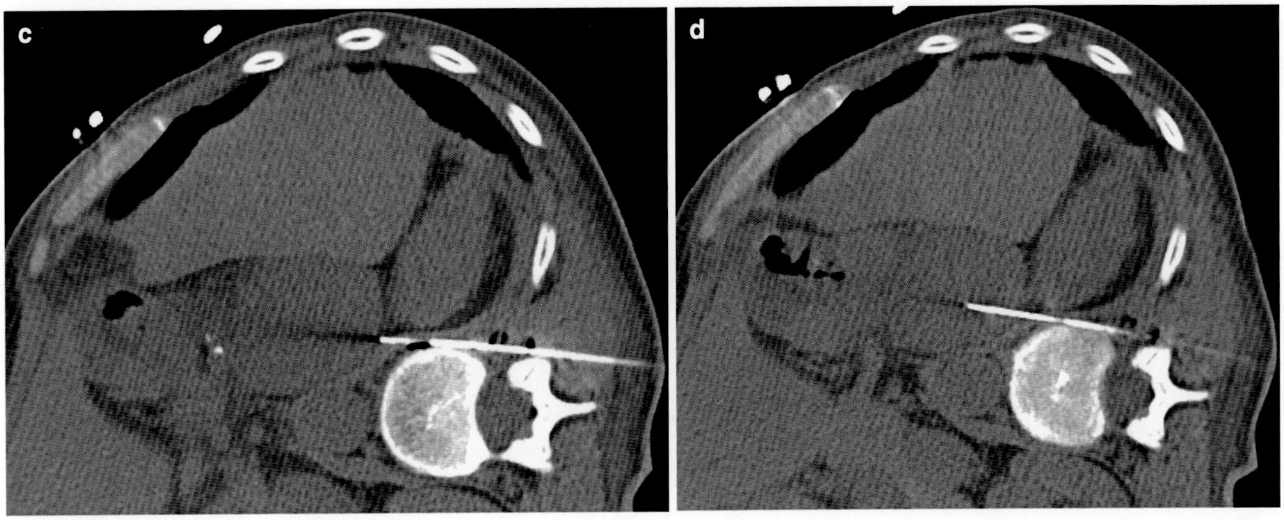

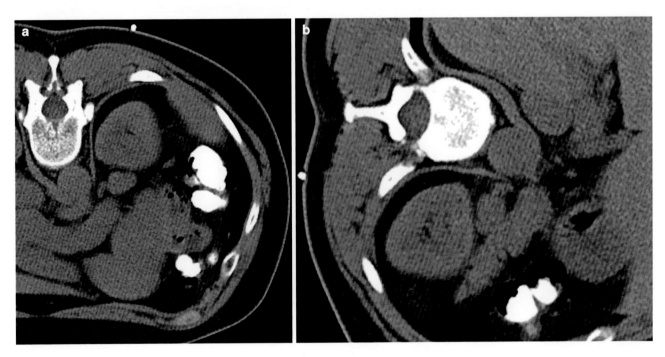

Fig. 16.7 (continued)

Fig. 16.8 Injection of saline to displace kidney during biopsy of adrenal gland. (**a**) A 43-year-old woman with squamous cell carcinoma of the right tonsil presented with a left adrenal mass. Axial non-contrast-enhanced CT image with the patient in the prone position demonstrates the left kidney directly overlying the left adrenal gland without a clear approach to the adrenal gland for the biopsy needle. (**b**) Repositioning the patient in the ipsilateral decubitus position was not particularly helpful as the left kidney still prevented direct access to the left adrenal gland. (**c**) The injection of saline during needle placement provided adequate displacement of the kidney laterally and to allow for left adrenal gland biopsy without traversing the left kidney (**c, d, e**). The low-density posterior and medial to the left kidney represents the injected saline. The pathologic diagnosis in this case was an adrenal cortical adenoma

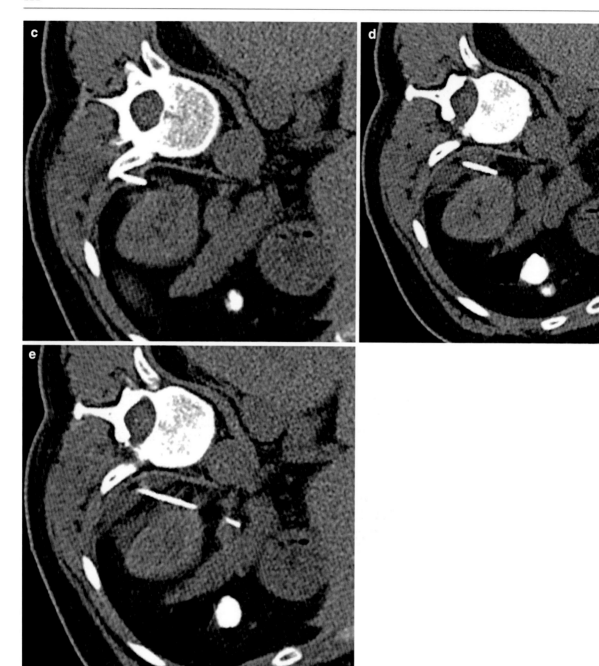

Fig. 16.8 (continued)

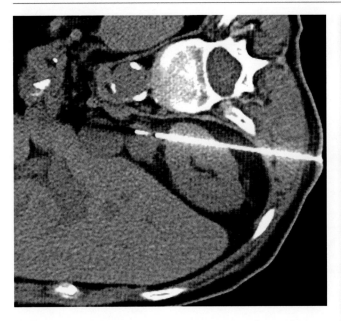

Fig. 16.9 Transrenal approach for biopsy of adrenal gland. A 56-year-old man with non-small cell lung cancer presented with an FDG-avid right adrenal lesion. With the patient in the ipsilateral decubitus position, the transrenal approach to the right adrenal lesion was the only available access. Coaxial biopsy technique was used, and both fine-needle aspiration and core biopsy were performed. The pathologic diagnosis was metastatic non-small cell carcinoma

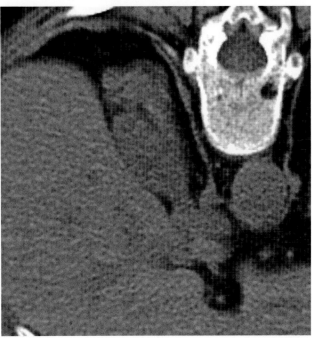

Fig. 16.11 Self-limited hemorrhage following biopsy of adrenal gland. A 66-year-old woman with a history of ovarian cancer and new bilateral adrenal lesions underwent CT-guided right adrenal gland biopsy in the prone position. Axial non-contrast-enhanced CT image obtained immediately following removal of the biopsy needle reveals a small amount of periadrenal hemorrhage posterior to the right adrenal gland. The patient was asymptomatic and discharged home following an uneventful 3-h observation period. The pathologic diagnosis was metastatic ovarian cancer

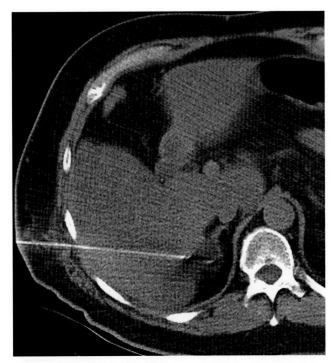

Fig. 16.10 Transhepatic approach for biopsy of adrenal gland. A 66-year-old man with transitional cell cancer of the bladder presented with a right adrenal nodule. Axial non-enhanced CT image demonstrates a transhepatic approach to the right adrenal gland using a coaxial biopsy technique. An 18-gauge Chiba needle was used as the guide needle and 22-gauge Chiba needles were inserted coaxially for fine-needle aspiration. A 20-gauge core biopsy needle was used to obtain histologic specimens. The pathologic diagnosis of adrenal cortical nodule was made on examination of the aspirates and core specimens

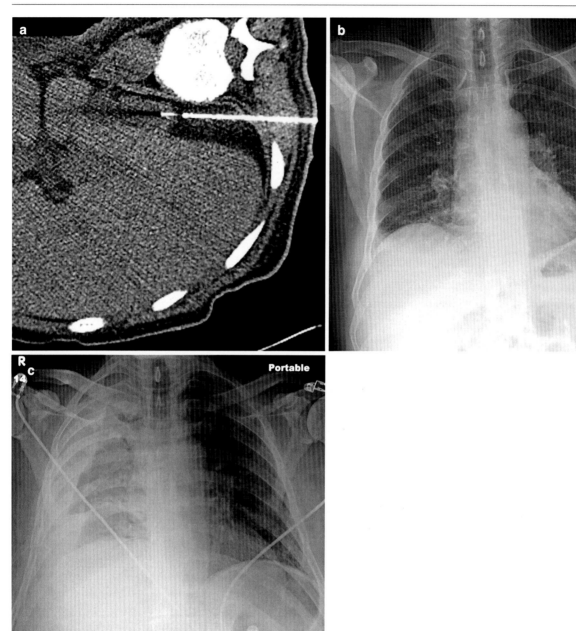

Fig. 16.12 Hemothorax following adrenal biopsy. A 70-year-old man with no known cancer history presented with nonfunctioning, bilateral adrenal masses. (**a**) Axial non-contrast-enhanced CT image demonstrates biopsy of the right adrenal gland via an ipsilateral decubitus approach. Coaxial biopsy technique was used, and fine-needle aspiration and core biopsy were performed. Samples were also sent for microbiological analysis to evaluate for infection. (**b**)The patient was asymptomatic after the biopsy, and an immediate postbiopsy chest radiograph was performed and demonstrated no pneumothorax. (**c**) Chest radiograph performed 24 h following the procedure demonstrated a significant right hemothorax and clinically the patient experienced a drop in hemoglobin. The patient required a red blood cell transfusion and the insertion of a large-bore chest tube (not shown) for the management of this delayed bleeding complication. The pathologic diagnosis was *Candida* infection

References

1. Abrams HL, Spiro R, Goldstein N. Metastases in carcinoma; analysis of 1000 autopsied cases. Cancer. 1950;3:74–85.
2. Barzon L, Sonino N, Fallo F, et al. Prevalence and natural history of adrenal incidentalomas. Eur J Endocrinol. 2003;149:273–85.
3. Kloos RT, Gross MD, Francis IR, et al. Incidentally discovered adrenal masses. Endocr Rev. 1995;16:460–84.
4. Arellano RS, Boland GW, Mueller PR. Adrenal biopsy in a patient with lung cancer: imaging algorithm and biopsy indications, technique, and complications. AJR. 2000;175:1613–17.
5. Berkman WA, Bernardino ME, Sewell CW, et al. The computed tomography-guided adrenal biopsy. An alternative to surgery in adrenal mass diagnosis. Cancer. 1984;53:2098–103.
6. Katz RL, Patel S, Mackay B, et al. Fine needle aspiration cytology of the adrenal gland. Acta Cytol. 1984;28:269–82.
7. Thomas JL, Barnes PA, Bernardino ME, et al. Diagnostic approaches to adrenal and renal metastases. Radiol Clin North Am. 1982;20:531–44.
8. Korobkin M. CT characterization of adrenal masses: the time has come. Radiology. 2000;217:629–32.
9. Dunnick NR, Korobkin M, Francis I. Adrenal radiology: distinguishing benign from malignant adrenal masses. AJR. 1996;167:861–7.
10. Young Jr WF. Clinical practice. The incidentally discovered adrenal mass. N Engl J Med. 2007;356:601–10.
11. Caoili EM, Korobkin M, Francis IR, et al. Adrenal masses: characterization with combined unenhanced and delayed enhanced CT. Radiology. 2002;222:629–33.
12. Korobkin M, Francis IR, Kloos RT, et al. The incidental adrenal mass. Radiol Clin North Am. 1996;34:1037–54.
13. Paulsen SD, Nghiem HV, Korobkin M, et al. Changing role of imaging-guided percutaneous biopsy of adrenal masses: evaluation of 50 adrenal biopsies. AJR. 2004;182:1033–7.
14. Uppot RN, Gervais DA, Mueller PR. Interventional uroradiology. Radiol Clin North Am. 2008;46:45–64.
15. Mansmann G, Lau J, Balk E, et al. The clinically inapparent adrenal mass: update in diagnosis and management. Endocr Rev. 2004;25:309–40.
16. Young Jr WF. Management approaches to adrenal incidentalomas. A view from Rochester, Minnesota. Endocrinol Metab Clin North Am. 2000;29:159–85.
17. Grumbach MM, Biller BM, Braunstein GD, et al. Management of the clinically inapparent adrenal mass ("incidentaloma"). Ann Intern Med. 2003;138:424–9.
18. Mazzaglia PJ, Monchik JM. Limited value of adrenal biopsy in the evaluation of adrenal neoplasm: a decade of experience. Arch Surg. 2009;144:465–70.
19. Casola G, Nicolet V, van Sonnenberg E, et al. Unsuspected pheochromocytoma: risk of blood-pressure alterations during percutaneous adrenal biopsy. Radiology. 1986;159:733–5.
20. Quayle FJ, Spitler JA, Pierce RA, et al. Needle biopsy of incidentally discovered adrenal masses is rarely informative and potentially hazardous. Surgery. 2007;142:497–502.
21. Sood SK, Balasubramanian SP, Harrison BJ. Percutaneous biopsy of adrenal and extra-adrenal retroperitoneal lesions: beware of catecholamine secreting tumours! Surgeon. 2007;5:279–81.
22. Hussain S. Gantry angulation in CT-guided percutaneous adrenal biopsy. AJR. 1996;166:537–9.
23. Van Sonnenberg E, Wittenberg J, Ferrucci Jr JT, et al. Triangulation method for percutaneous needle guidance: the angled approach to upper abdominal masses. AJR. 1981;137:757–61.
24. Yueh N, Halvorsen Jr RA, Letourneau JG, et al. Gantry tilt technique for CT-guided biopsy and drainage. J Comput Assist Tomogr. 1989;13:182–4.
25. Arellano RS, Harisinghani MG, Gervais DA, et al. Image-guided percutaneous biopsy of the adrenal gland: review of indications, technique, and complications. Curr Probl Diagn Radiol. 2003;32:3–10.
26. Heiberg E, Wolverson MK. Ipsilateral decubitus position for percutaneous CT-guided adrenal biopsy. J Comput Assist Tomogr. 1985;9:217–18.
27. Karampekios S, Hatjidakis AA, Drositis J, et al. Artificial paravertebral widening for percutaneous CT-guided adrenal biopsy. J Comput Assist Tomogr. 1998;22:308–10.
28. Kane NM, Korobkin M, Francis IR, et al. Percutaneous biopsy of left adrenal masses: prevalence of pancreatitis after anterior approach. AJR. 1991;157:777–80.
29. Mody MK, Kazerooni EA, Korobkin M. Percutaneous CT-guided biopsy of adrenal masses: immediate and delayed complications. J Comput Assist Tomogr. 1995;19:434–9.
30. Price RB, Bernardino ME, Berkman WA, et al. Biopsy of the right adrenal gland by the transhepatic approach. Radiology. 1983;148:566.
31. Bernardino ME, Walther MM, Phillips VM, et al. CT-guided adrenal biopsy: accuracy, safety, and indications. AJR. 1985;144:67–9.
32. Heaston DK, Handel DB, Ashton PR, et al. Narrow gauge needle aspiration of solid adrenal masses. AJR. 1982;138:1143–8.
33. Silverman SG, Mueller PR, Pinkney LP, et al. Predictive value of image-guided adrenal biopsy: analysis of results of 101 biopsies. Radiology. 1993;187:715–18.
34. Welch TJ, Sheedy 2nd PF, Johnson CD, et al. CT-guided biopsy: prospective analysis of 1,000 procedures. Radiology. 1989;171:493–6.
35. Masmiquel L, Hernandez-Pascual C, Simo R, et al. Adrenal abscess as a complication of adrenal fine-needle biopsy. Am J Med. 1993;95:244–5.
36. Gurley MB, Richli WR, Waugh KA. Outpatient management of pneumothorax after fine-needle aspiration: economic advantages for the hospital and patient. Radiology. 1998;209:717–22.
37. McCorkell SJ, Niles NL. Fine-needle aspiration of catecholamine-producing adrenal masses: a possibly fatal mistake. AJR. 1985;145:113–14.
38. Valji K. Vascular and interventional radiology. 2nd ed. Philadelphia: WB Saunders; 2006. p. 508.
39. Katz RL, Shirkhoda A. Diagnostic approach to incidental adrenal nodules in the cancer patient. Results of a clinical, radiologic, and fine-needle aspiration study. Cancer. 1985;55:1995–2000.
40. Welch TJ, Sheedy 2nd PF, Stephens DH, et al. Percutaneous adrenal biopsy: review of a 10-year experience. Radiology. 1994;193:341–4.
41. Saboorian MH, Katz RL, Charnsangavej C. Fine needle aspiration cytology of primary and metastatic lesions of the adrenal gland. A series of 188 biopsies with radiologic correlation. Acta Cytol. 1995;39:843–51.
42. Lumachi F, Borsato S, Brandes AA, et al. Fine-needle aspiration cytology of adrenal masses in noncancer patients: clinicoradiologic and histologic correlations in functioning and nonfunctioning tumors. Cancer. 2001;93:323–9.
43. Wu HH, Cramer HM, Kho J, et al. Fine needle aspiration cytology of benign adrenal cortical nodules. A comparison of cytologic findings with those of primary and metastatic adrenal malignancies. Acta Cytol. 1998;42:1352–8.
44. Saeger W, Fassnacht M, Chita R, et al. High diagnostic accuracy of adrenal core biopsy: results of the German and Austrian adrenal network multicenter trial in 220 consecutive patients. Hum Pathol. 2003;34:180–6.
45. Harisinghani MG, Maher MM, Hahn PF, et al. Predictive value of benign percutaneous adrenal biopsies in oncology patients. Clin Radiol. 2002;57:898–901.
46. Phillips MD, Silverman SG, Cibas ES, et al. Negative predictive value of imaging-guided abdominal biopsy results: cytologic classification and implications for patient management. AJR. 1998;171:693–6.
47. de Agustin P, Lopez-Rios F, Alberti N, et al. Fine-needle aspiration biopsy of the adrenal glands: a ten-year experience. Diagn Cytopathol. 1999;21:92–7.

Renal Mass Biopsy

17

Kamran Ahrar, Sanaz Javadi, and Judy U. Ahrar

Background

Presentation and treatment of renal masses have changed drastically over the years. The classic triad of groin pain, hematuria, or flank mass is rarely encountered anymore [1]. The trend has been toward incidental detection of small renal masses on cross-sectional imaging performed for non-urological complaints [2]. Advances in imaging technologies have made it possible to detect even subcentimeter renal masses and to distinguish between cystic and solid masses with ease. On the other hand, there is significant overlap in the radiological appearance between benign and malignant solid renal lesions. It is estimated that up to 30 % of small renal masses that are removed at surgery are histologically benign [3–5].

The differential diagnosis of renal masses includes primary renal tumors (malignant or benign), metastatic disease from an extrarenal malignancy, lymphoma, and infection [6–8]. The role of image-guided renal mass biopsy has been well established in evaluating metastatic disease, lymphoma, and infection [9, 10]. Patients with renal cell carcinoma (RCC) who are not suitable candidates for surgery should undergo biopsy to obtain an accurate diagnosis before systemic therapy is begun [11]. Historically, patients with small resectable tumors that were presumed to be RCCs did not undergo preoperative biopsy, but recently there is a trend toward performing image-guided biopsy in a subset of patients with small renal tumors [12]. This chapter will cover the indications, contraindications, and techniques for renal mass biopsy as well as outcomes and results.

K. Ahrar, MD, FSIR (✉)
Department of Interventional Radiology,
Department of Thoracic and Cardiovascular Surgery,
The University of Texas MD Anderson Cancer Center,
1515 Holcombe Boulevard, Unit 1471,
Houston, TX 77030, USA
e-mail: kahrar@mdanderson.org

S. Javadi, MD
Department of Radiology, Baylor College of Medicine,
One Baylor Plaza, Unit 360, Houston,
TX 77030, USA
e-mail: sjavadi@bcm.edu

J.U. Ahrar, MD
Department of Interventional Radiology,
The University of Texas MD Anderson Cancer Center,
1515 Holcombe Blvd., Unit 1471,
Houston, TX 77030, USA
e-mail: judy.ahrar@mdanderson.org

Indications for Renal Mass Biopsy

Patients with Known or Suspected Extrarenal Malignancy or Lymphoma

Nearly any type of cancer can metastasize to the kidney, but the most common extrarenal malignancies that metastasize to the kidney are lung, colon, and liver cancers and melanoma [10, 13]. It is estimated that 8–13 % of renal masses are metastatic foci from extrarenal primaries; however, a solitary enhancing renal mass in a patient with a history of extrarenal malignancy is most likely a primary renal tumor (Fig. 17.1) [14]. Similarly, in a patient with an extrarenal primary, a cystic renal mass is unlikely to represent a metastasis [14]. For example, in one study, half of the renal tumors were found to be RCCs despite a possibility of metastatic disease [14]. Image-guided biopsy can help differentiate metastatic disease from RCC, and this distinction has substantial clinical implications (Figs. 17.2 and 17.3). Virtually all metastatic disease to the kidney is treated by nonsurgical means, whereas RCC confined to the kidney is managed more aggressively with resection or percutaneous ablation.

In some reported autopsy series of patients with lymphoma, the kidneys were found to be involved in 34–60 % of cases [15]. However, renal lymphoma is detected on routine abdominal imaging in only 2.7–15 % of patients who undergo computed tomography (CT) scans during lymphoma staging investigation [16, 17]. The discrepancy between actual cases and imaging-detected cases of renal lymphoma during staging may be due to variations in the radiological appearance of renal lymphoma; on imaging, the

K. Ahrar, S. Gupta (eds.), *Percutaneous Image-Guided Biopsy*,
DOI 10.1007/978-1-4614-8217-8_17, © Springer Science+Business Media New York 2014

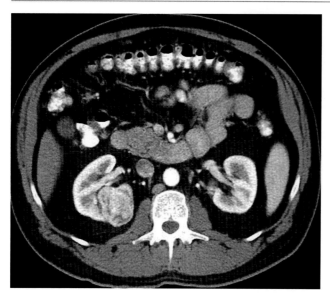

Fig. 17.1 A 48-year-old man with melanoma. An axial CT image of the abdomen reveals a hypervascular mass in the right kidney. A biopsy revealed renal cell carcinoma

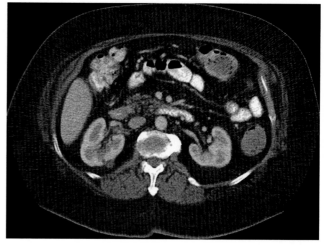

Fig. 17.3 A 64-year-old woman with primary peritoneal carcinoma. A CT image of the abdomen reveals a mass in the right kidney. A biopsy revealed metastatic disease

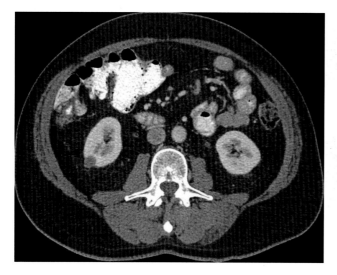

Fig. 17.2 A 64-year-old man with a history of prostate cancer. A CT image of the abdomen reveals a low-density mass in the right kidney. A biopsy revealed renal cell carcinoma

appearance of renal lymphoma can vary from a well-defined mass resembling primary renal tumors to diffuse involvement and enlargement of the kidney [18]. Image-guided biopsy can help differentiate renal lymphoma from epithelial tumors of the kidney (Fig. 17.4). Patients with renal lymphoma are treated with chemotherapy; surgery or ablation does not have a role in treating these patients.

Patients with Unresectable RCC

RCC is a heterogeneous malignancy and has several subtypes that exhibit distinct clinical and histological features [19, 20]. In patients who have an unresectable renal mass, who are

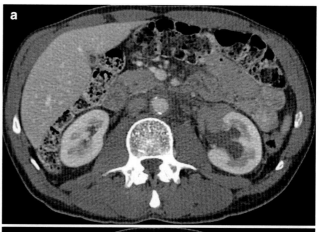

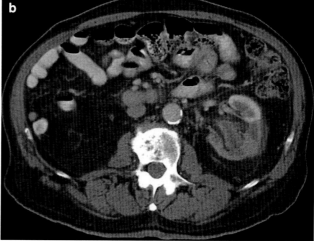

Fig. 17.4 (**a**) A 58-year-old man with a history of lymphoma was found to have a left renal mass. A biopsy revealed lymphoma. (**b**) A CT of the abdomen in an 86-year-old man with a history of lymphoma reveals an infiltrative left renal mass. A biopsy revealed urothelial carcinoma

poor surgical candidates, or who have metastatic RCC, renal mass biopsy can establish the diagnosis so that optimal treatment and/or treatment sequence can be determined [11]

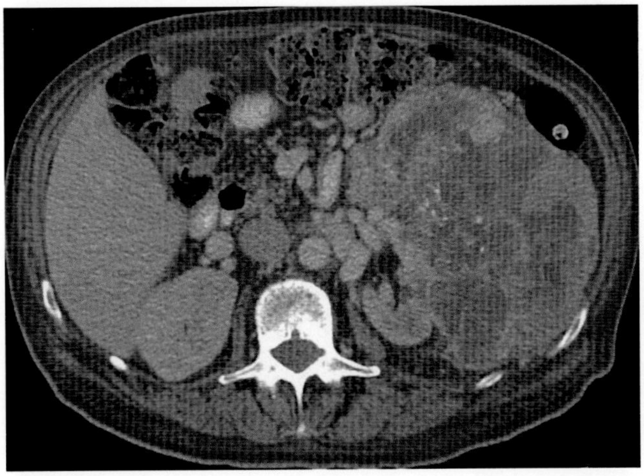

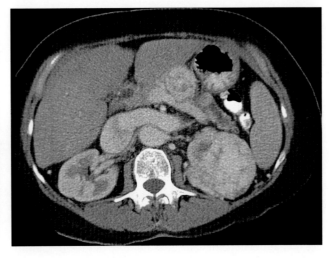

Fig. 17.5 A 67-year-old man with a large renal mass. A biopsy of the left renal tumor revealed renal cell carcinoma. He underwent cytore-ductive nephrectomy

Fig. 17.6 A 63-year-old woman with a left renal tumor underwent biopsy. A pathologic evaluation revealed renal cell carcinoma. She was treated with radical nephrectomy

(Figs. 17.5 and 17.6). This is particularly important in the current era of molecular targeted therapy, where several agents with distinct mechanisms of action are now available to treat patients with advanced RCC [21].

therapy and follow-up imaging may obviate biopsy; however, if the mass persists, image-guided biopsy is indicated to confirm an infectious process and to rule out renal cancer.

Patients with a Renal Mass and Febrile Urinary Tract Infection

Renal infections such as focal bacterial infections and xantho-granulomatous pyelonephritis can present as mass-like lesions on imaging studies [22–24], although ill-defined margins and perinephric stranding may suggest an infectious condition rather than a neoplastic process [25, 26]. In patients with clinical signs and symptoms of urinary tract infection and a focal mass-like lesion shown on imaging, appropriate antibiotic

Patients with an Indeterminate Cystic Renal Mass

Complex cystic masses present a diagnostic and management dilemma. Approximately 10–15 % of RCCs have cystic components on cross-sectional imaging [27]. The Bosniak renal cyst classification system categorizes cystic lesions of the kidney into one of five groups: categories I, II, IIF (F: follow-up), III, and IV (Table 17.1) [28]. According to this classification system, cystic lesions in categories I and II are benign and do not require further evaluation or intervention

Table 17.1 Bosniak renal cyst classification system

Category	Description
I	A benign simple cyst with a hairline thin wall that does not contain septa, calcifications, or solid components. It measures water density and does not enhance.
II	A benign cyst that may contain a few hairline thin septa in which "perceived" enhancement[a] may be present. Fine calcification or a short segment of slightly thickened calcification may be present in the wall or septa. Uniformly high-attenuation lesions <3 cm (so-called high-density cysts) that are well marginated and do not enhance are included in this group. Cysts in this category do not require further evaluation.
IIF	Cysts that may contain multiple hairline thin septa or minimal smooth thickening of their wall or septa. Perceived enhancement of their septa or wall may be present. Their wall or septa may contain calcification that may be thick and nodular, but no measurable contrast enhancement is present. These lesions are generally well marginated. Totally, intrarenal nonenhancing high-attenuation renal lesions >3 cm are also included in this category. These lesions require follow-up studies to prove benignity.
III	"Indeterminate" cystic masses that have thickened irregular or smooth walls or septa in which measurable enhancement is present. These are surgical lesions, although some will prove to be benign (e.g., hemorrhagic cysts, chronic infected cysts, and multiloculated cystic nephroma) and some will be malignant, such as cystic renal cell carcinoma and multiloculated cystic renal cell carcinoma.
IV	These are clearly malignant cystic masses that can have all the criteria of category III but also contain enhancing soft tissue components adjacent to, but independent of, the wall or septum. These lesions include cystic carcinomas and require surgical removal.

Reprinted from Israel and Bosniak An update of the Bosniak [28]. With permission from Elsevier
Abbreviation: *F* follow-up
[a]Not measurable enhancement

(Figs. 17.7 and 17.8). Although lesions in category III are "indeterminate," they are worrisome enough to warrant a recommendation for surgical excision (Fig. 17.9). Category IV lesions are clearly malignant on the basis of their imaging characteristics and require surgical removal (Fig. 17.10). Category IIF was added to the original Bosniak classification system because some category II cysts were more complicated than expected yet were not complicated enough to warrant placement in category III. Lesions classified as IIF require follow-up imaging studies to confirm benign status.

Historically, percutaneous biopsy has not been used to evaluate complex cystic renal masses. It is generally believed that a benign diagnosis can only be established after examination of the entire lesion, and a biopsy specimen that does not contain malignant cells does not rule out the possibility of malignancy. Therefore, category III cystic lesions should

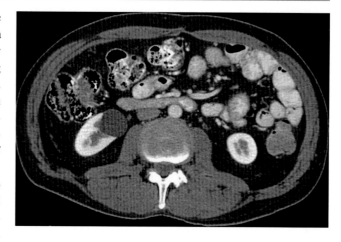

Fig. 17.7 A CT image of the abdomen in a 60-year-old man with a history of gastrointestinal stromal tumor reveals a simple renal cyst in the right kidney

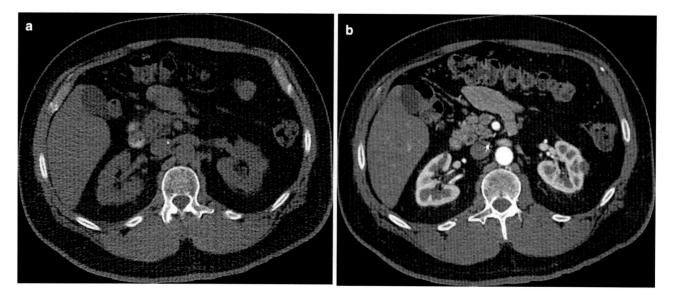

Fig. 17.8 An axial CT image of the abdomen in a 56-year-old man with pancreatic neuroendocrine carcinoma reveals a small hemorrhagic renal cyst in the lateral aspect of the left kidney (**a**). There was no enhancement after administration of intravenous contrast material (**b**)

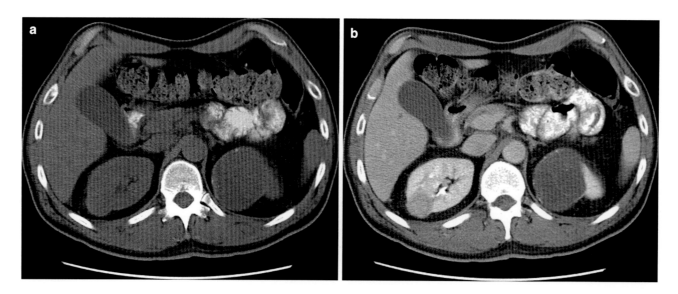

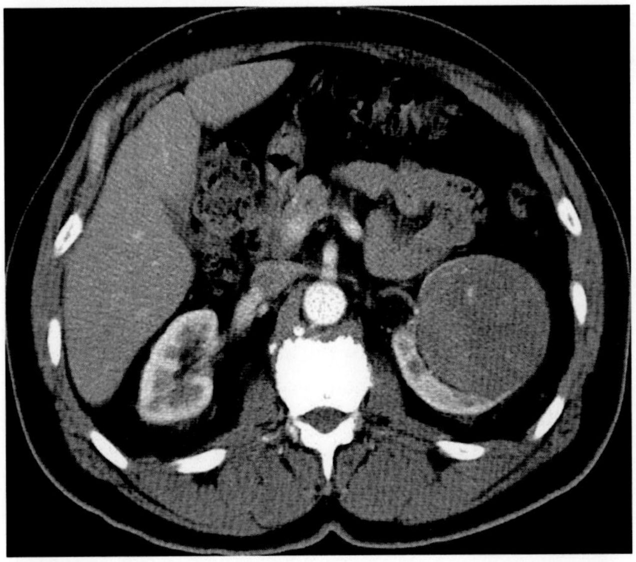

help identify benign causes of indeterminate cystic renal masses, thus obviating surgery in a subset of patients. The major problem with these studies is that it is very difficult to prove negative results [7]. Sampling error remains a potential limitation of biopsy in cases where the cancer may be focal and interspersed with benign cystic spaces. Therefore, biopsy of complex cystic renal masses is probably helpful only in selected cases in which the risk of surgical resection is too high or the patient is considered a candidate for thermal ablative therapies (Fig. 17.11).

Patients with a Solid Renal Mass

Traditionally, most solid enhancing renal masses have been presumed to be primary renal cancer. When a patient presents with a locally invasive renal mass or metastatic disease that is thought to be inoperable, percutaneous needle biopsy is performed to confirm the diagnosis prior to initiation of systemic therapy. Historically, if disease was localized to the kidney and was deemed resectable, preoperative percutaneous needle biopsy was not performed because of concerns about complications and the accuracy of biopsy results [31]. With the widespread use of cross-sectional abdominal imaging (e.g., CT, ultrasonography, and magnetic resonance imaging [MRI]), most renal tumors are now detected incidentally

Fig. 17.10 A 72-year-old man with prostate cancer was found to have a complex solid and cystic mass in his left kidney, Bosniak class IV. A biopsy revealed renal cell carcinoma

be surgically excised. On the other hand, several reports have been published that support using percutaneous biopsy to evaluate an indeterminate cystic renal mass [27, 29, 30]. The authors of these reports argued that percutaneous biopsy can

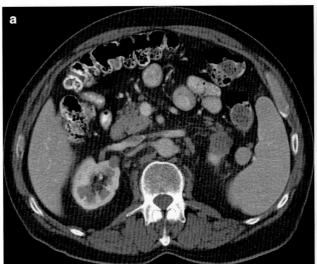

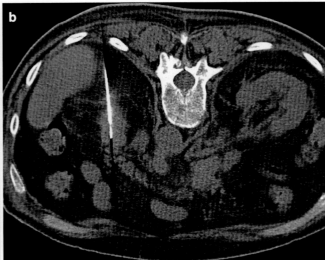

Fig. 17.11 An axial CT image of the abdomen (**a**) in a 70-year-old man with a history of lymphoma reveals a small cyst in the right kidney and a complex cystic mass in the upper pole of the left kidney. A CT-guided biopsy (**b**) of the left upper pole renal mass revealed renal cell carcinoma

Fig. 17.9 Axial CT images before (**a**) and after (**b**) intravenous contrast administration reveal a solid enhancing mass in the right kidney and a Bosniak III cyst involving the upper pole of the left kidney. The left upper pole cystic mass was resected. A pathologic evaluation revealed renal cell carcinoma (60 % clear cells, 40 % eosinophilic cells, Fuhrman nuclear grade 3). A fine-needle aspiration biopsy of the right renal tumor was performed at the time of ablation. A pathologic evaluation revealed renal cell carcinoma. The subtype and nuclear grade could not be determined from the fine-needle aspiration biopsy sample

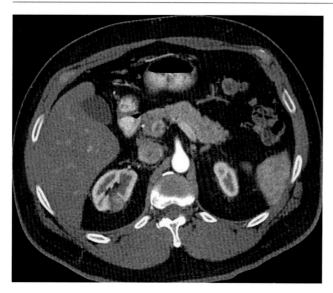

Fig. 17.12 A 56-year-old man with pancreatic neuroendocrine carcinoma was referred for evaluation of a solid enhancing mass involving the right kidney. An axial CT image reveals a 2-cm right renal mass; a biopsy revealed oncocytoma

when they are still small and are confined to the kidney [2]. It is now recognized that small renal masses represent a heterogeneous group of pathologic entities, ranging from benign to malignant. When resected without a preoperative diagnosis, 23 % of tumors smaller than 4 cm were found to be benign (Fig. 17.12) [3]. For smaller tumors, the incidence of benign pathology is even higher. When tumors smaller than 1 cm were resected, 46 % were found to be benign. Aside from traditional nephrectomy, several new treatment options for small renal tumors are now available. Active surveillance, image-guided ablation, and partial nephrectomy are some of the less invasive treatment options that have gained varying degrees of acceptance in the urologic community. As a result, there has been renewed interest in percutaneous image-guided needle biopsy of small renal masses to help guide treatment of these patients (Fig. 17.13). Pretreatment percutaneous biopsy has been shown to decrease the number of unnecessary surgeries for benign disease in 16–44 % of cases [32, 33].

Patients with Suspected RCC Managed with Ablation Therapy

In the recent years, ablation therapies have evolved as an alternative treatment option for patients with small RCCs who may not be suitable candidates for surgery [34–37]. Unlike surgical excision in which the harvested tumor undergoes pathologic evaluation, the ablated tumor

remains in situ after the procedure, precluding pathologic assessment. Because a substantial number of small renal masses are benign, some researchers have suggested that a pre-ablation biopsy should be performed to establish a diagnosis [38]. After the ablation, surveillance imaging studies are conducted to confirm complete ablation of the tumor and lack of recurrence [39]. The lack of enhancement after administration of contrast on CT or MRI is confirmation of technical and clinical success (Fig. 17.14). Over time, the ablation zone will undergo involution, resulting in "shrinkage" of the ablated tumor (Fig. 17.15). Any abnormal enhancement or enlargement of the ablation zone may indicate residual or recurrent tumor and should be further investigated via percutaneous biopsy (Fig. 17.16) [40]. Some researchers have advocated a routine biopsy of the ablated tumor to confirm the absence of any viable cancer cells in the ablation zone [37, 41]. Neither one of these strategies is free of pitfalls. Particularly in cases of radiofrequency ablation wherein the cellular architecture is preserved for some time after ablation, hematoxylin and eosin staining can be misleading with false-positive results [42]. Viability staining (e.g., nicotinamide adenine dinucleotide hydrogenase) may be necessary to confirm complete ablation of the tumor. At the time of this writing, a biopsy of the ablation zone is indicated if any signs of enhancement or enlargement or any unusual or unexpected findings are present on surveillance imaging studies [40].

Contraindications to Renal Mass Biopsy

Percutaneous biopsy of renal masses is a safe procedure with very low risk to the patient. The only contraindication to renal mass biopsy is coagulopathy that cannot be corrected. For decades, the potential for tract seeding was considered a contraindication to percutaneous biopsy of renal masses; however, recent data suggest that the risk of tract seeding after renal mass biopsy is exceedingly low.

Renal Mass Biopsy Techniques

Coagulation Status

To minimize the risk of hemorrhagic complications from renal biopsy, patients are screened for hemorrhagic diathesis. Screening is warranted even in patients with no history of bleeding. In the United States, most radiologists (84 %) routinely obtain a screening history of potential hemostatic defects and have patients undergo relevant laboratory

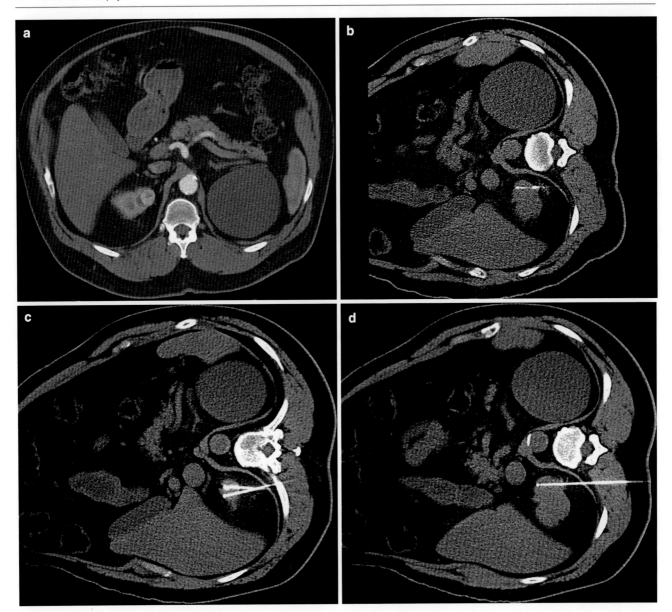

Fig. 17.13 A 62-year-old man with a history of esophageal cancer was found to have a solid enhancing mass in the upper pole of his right kidney (**a**). A CT-guided biopsy (**b**) was performed in the lateral decubitus position. A histological evaluation revealed renal cell carcinoma. He subsequently underwent percutaneous radiofrequency ablation. Axial CT images during the ablation (**c**, **d**) reveal three radiofrequency electrodes in the tumor

tests—81 % request prothrombin time, 78 % request partial thromboplastin time, and 59 % request platelet count [43]. At a minimum, a platelet count and international normalized ratio (INR) should be obtained. Patients are advised to stop taking aspirin and other antiplatelet agents 5–7 days prior to the procedure. Patients taking warfarin are asked to stop taking it 5 days prior to the procedure to allow the INR to return to an acceptable range. While anticoagulation agents are suspended, patients may be given heparin or low-molecular-weight heparin to bridge the gap until warfarin can be restarted. Continuous intravenous heparin infusion should be stopped at least 2 h prior to the procedure. Low-molecular-weight heparin (e.g., Lovenox) is suspended only on the day of the biopsy. Although a normal platelet count and normal INR are desirable, we have more liberal guidelines in our practice and perform renal mass biopsy in patients with platelet counts as low as 50,000 and INRs of 1.5.

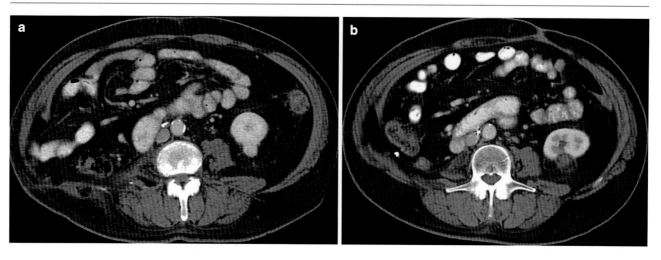

Fig. 17.14 A 77-year-old man with a history of renal cell carcinoma and right nephrectomy was referred for treatment of a new enhancing renal mass involving the lower pole of his left kidney (**a**). An axial CT image of the left kidney 1 year after ablation reveals no enhancement in the tumor (**b**)

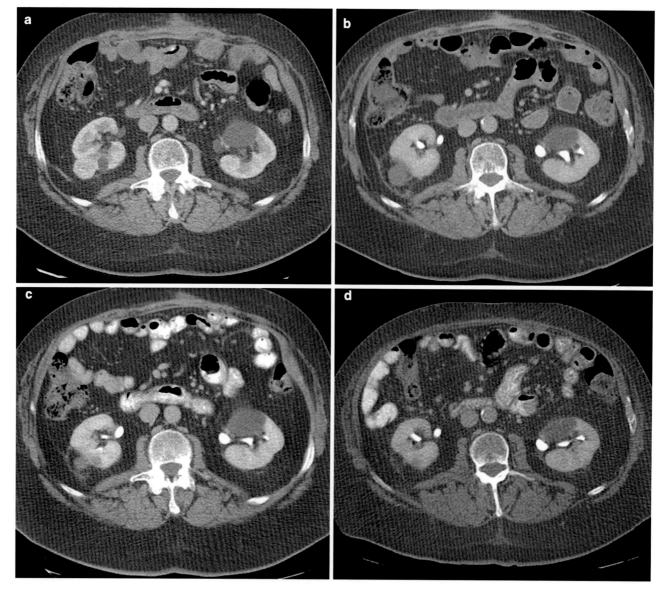

Fig. 17.15 A 68-year-old man underwent cryoablation of a solid enhancing tumor in the posterolateral aspect of the right kidney (**a**). Follow-up CT images at 1 month (**b**), 6 months (**c**), and 29 months (**d**) reveal progressive involution of the ablated tumor and the ablation zone. At 29 months, the tumor has nearly completely disappeared. Tumors treated with radiofrequency ablation demonstrate lesser degrees of involution

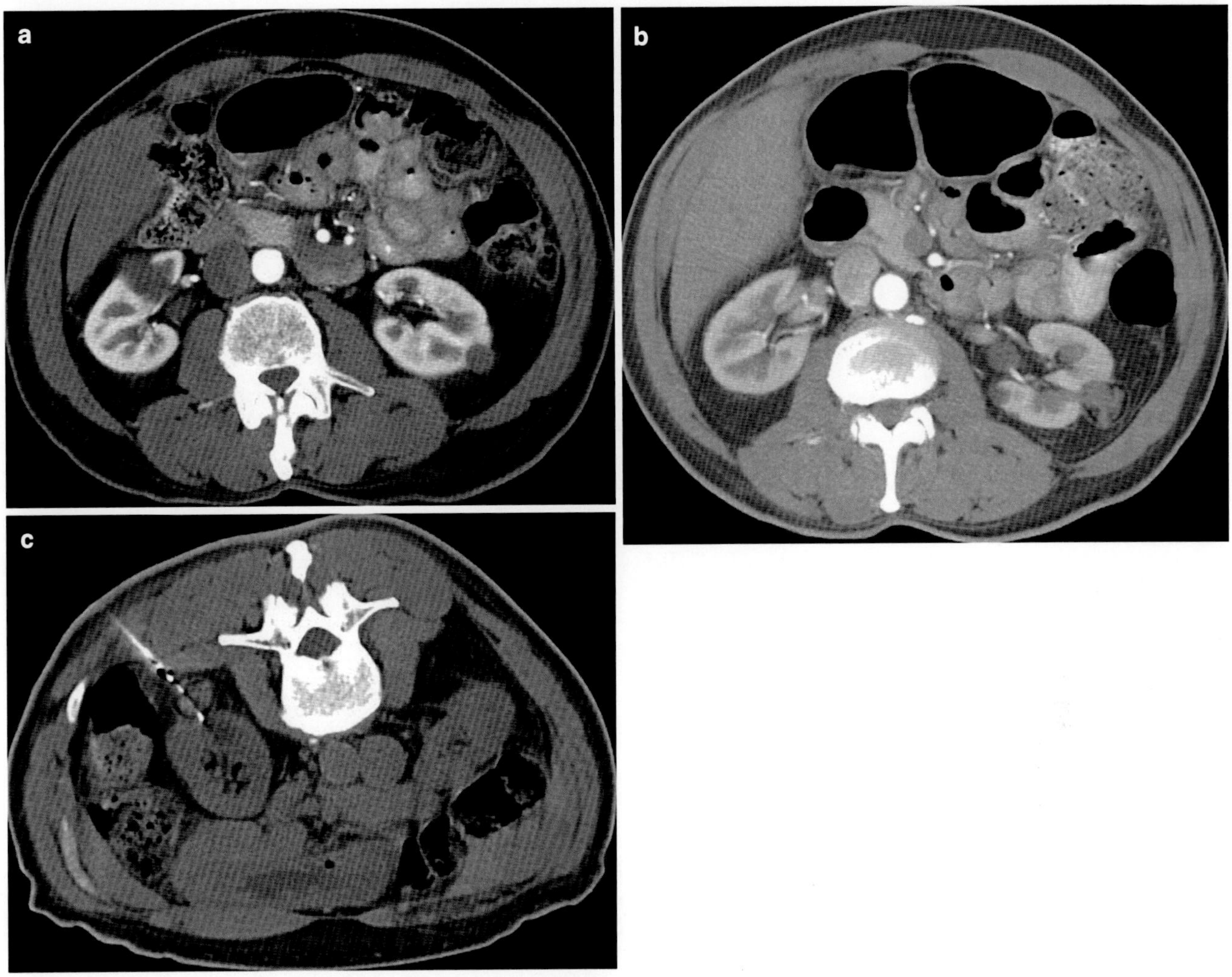

Fig. 17.16 A 66-year-old man with a small left renal cell carcinoma was referred for percutaneous ablation. An axial CT image of the abdomen (**a**) reveals a solid, low-density, left renal tumor. Follow-up CT images at 1 and 6 months (not shown) demonstrated continued involution of the ablation zone. A repeat CT study at 1 year (**b**) reveals enlarging soft tissue density adjacent to the tumor in the ablation zone. The findings were suspicious for a recurrent tumor. A CT-guided biopsy (**c**) of the enlarging portion of the ablation zone revealed recurrent renal cell carcinoma

Imaging

Biopsy of a renal mass can be accomplished using ultrasonography [14, 44–46], CT [14, 29, 38, 44, 47], or MR [38, 48] imaging for guidance. Multiplanar imaging capability and real-time demonstration of the needle tip are major advantages of ultrasound guidance (Fig. 17.17). Because the perinephric fat and the needle are both echogenic, visualization of the needle as it is advanced to the kidney may be difficult under ultrasound guidance, and the utility of ultrasound is limited in obese patients. Also, tumors in the upper pole or medial aspect of the kidney are more difficult to image with ultrasound due to adjacent bowel and intervening lung. Although a nonsedated patient can cooperate with breathing exercises to provide a better window for imaging of the kidney and renal tumors, performing a renal biopsy with breath-hold in deep inspiration is challenging for both the patient and the operator. If patients are sedated during the procedure, it is less likely that they will be able to cooperate with breathing and long breath-hold instructions.

Alternatively, renal biopsies can be performed under CT guidance. Exophytic renal masses change the contour of the kidney and are easily detected with non-contrast CT (Fig. 17.18). Intraparenchymal tumors without an exophytic component may be more difficult to localize on non-contrast CT images if they are isodense with the kidney. In these cases, administration of iodinated contrast medium immediately prior to the biopsy helps delineate the margins of the tumor (Fig. 17.19). Hypervascular tumors such as RCC show intense arterial enhancement, but nearly all tumors become more hypodense than the normal kidney in the excretory phase of the examination. As the normal kidney continues to accumulate and excrete iodinated contrast medium, the difference in density remains perceptible for the duration of the

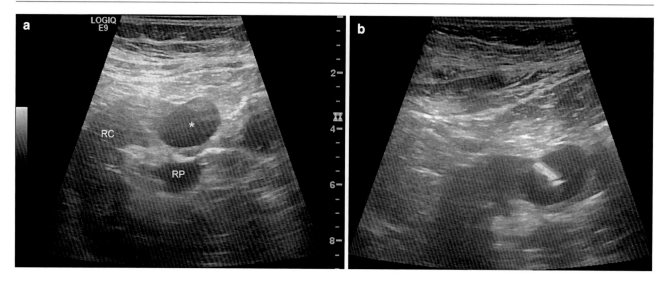

Fig. 17.17 A 53-year-old woman with a history of spindle cell sarcoma of her right iliac bone was found to have a solid mass in the right kidney. A gray-scale sonographic image of the right kidney (**a**) reveals the mass (*) anterior to the renal pelvis (*RP*). The mass is hypoechoic compared with the renal cortex (*RC*). The lesion was targeted under real-time sonographic guidance using the freehand technique. The needle tip is highly echogenic compared to the mass (**b**)

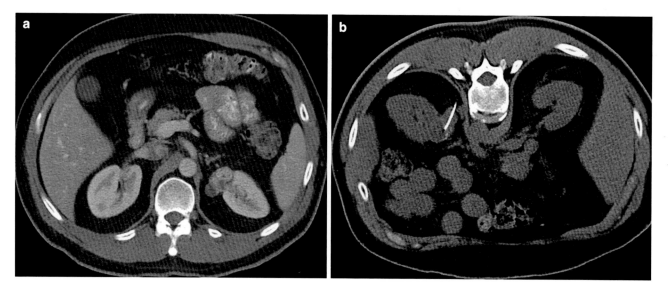

Fig. 17.18 A 42-year-old man with a renal mass was referred for biopsy. A diagnostic CT image (**a**) reveals a hypervascular, exophytic mass that alters the smooth contour of the left kidney. A biopsy was performed under CT guidance (**b**). There was no need for administration of contrast medium because of the exophytic nature of the mass. An out-of-plane technique was used to minimize the risk of pneumothorax. A pathologic evaluation revealed renal cell carcinoma

biopsy, allowing targeting of the tumor. Anatomic structures such as intervening bowel and pleural space that may be hard to visualize on ultrasonography are readily visible on CT. A major drawback of CT guidance for renal mass biopsy is the intermittent nature of imaging in a single axial plane. It may be difficult to image the needle and the tumor in the same plane, particularly in cases of small tumors. Real-time CT fluoroscopy can alleviate some of these challenges but can also increase radiation dose to the patient and the operator.

Ultrasonography and CT guidance can be combined to optimize targeting of renal tumors in difficult cases.

Renal tumors are particularly well suited for biopsy under MRI guidance if an interventional MRI suite is available. Renal tumors often demonstrate high signal intensity on T2-weighted images, allowing easy detection. Any number of imaging planes—such as axial, oblique axial, sagittal, or sagittal oblique—can be used to target the tumor using intermittent or real-time imaging (Fig. 17.20). MRI-compatible

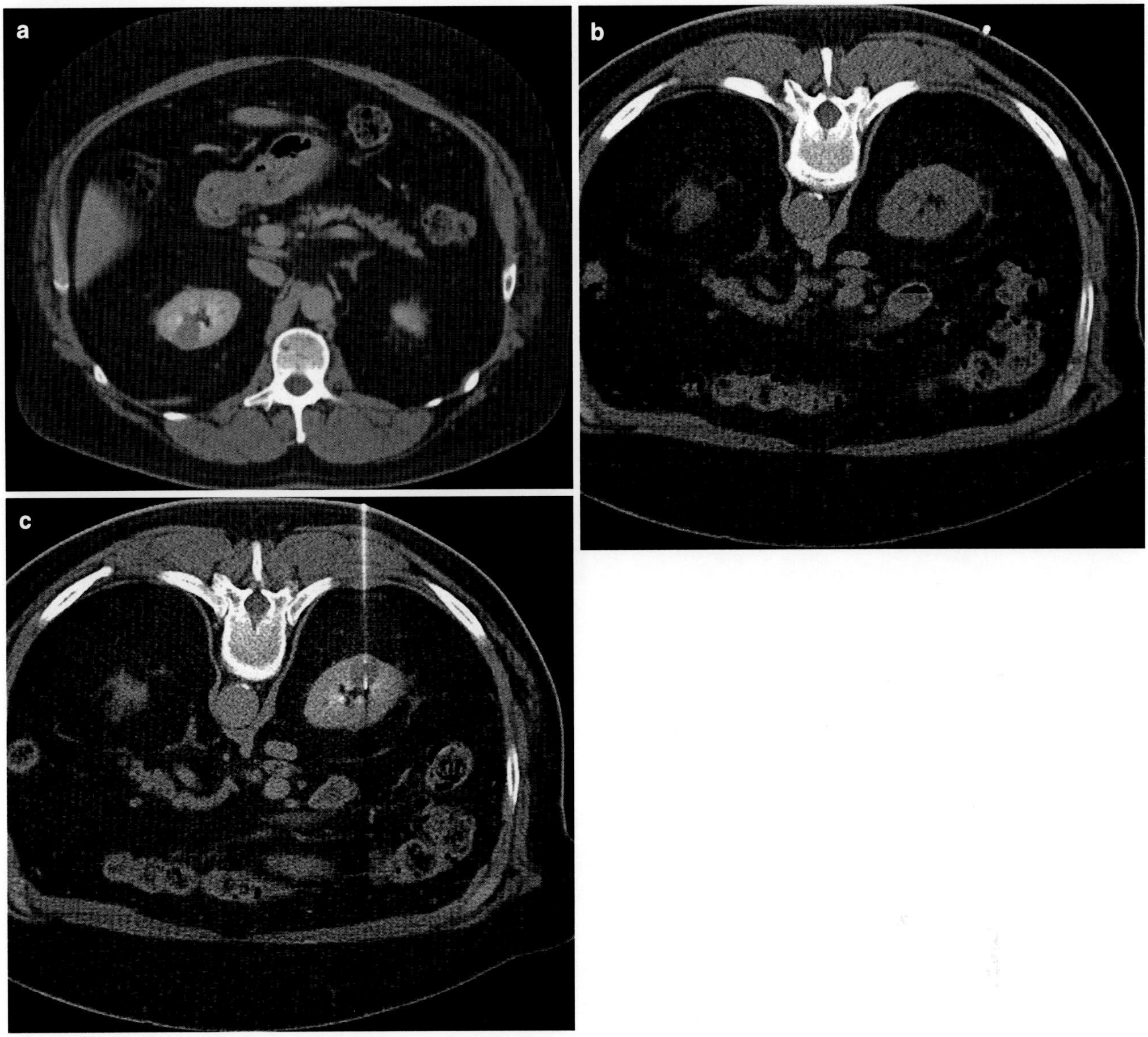

Fig. 17.19 A 68-year-old man with coronary artery disease was referred for biopsy of a right renal mass that was detected incidentally. A diagnostic CT image (**a**) in the late phase of contrast enhancement reveals a relatively low-density solid mass (1.6 cm diameter) that is confined to the renal parenchyma and does not change the contour of the kidney. An axial non-contrast CT image of the right kidney in the prone position (**b**) does not reveal the tumor. After administration of contrast medium, the lesion became conspicuous and was targeted for biopsy (**c**). A pathologic evaluation revealed oncocytoma

needles, constructed of nonferromagnetic alloys, are available for use within the magnetic field. There are no published reports directly comparing the diagnostic success rates of the different imaging modalities used in image-guided renal mass biopsy. Anecdotal reports indicate that diagnostic yield, sensitivity, or negative predictive value for image-guided renal mass biopsy is independent of the imaging modality [14, 49]. Most important, the imaging features of an individual mass along with the experience and personal preference of the operator help determine the most useful method of tumor localization and targeting.

Devices

Renal masses can be sampled both by fine-needle aspiration (FNA) and by tissue-cutting tip needles. FNA samples are obtained using 21-gauge or smaller needles, which are believed to minimize blood contamination of the sample and to yield a larger number of cells. Larger core biopsy samples are obtained using automated "biopsy guns" that are equipped with tissue-cutting tip needles. Both FNA and core biopsies can be performed through a coaxial guide or cannula [50]. Once the guiding cannula is advanced to the surface of the tumor, multiple samples can be obtained without reinserting the sampling needle through a new tract (Fig. 17.21). This technique decreases patient discomfort and shortens the procedure time. The coaxial technique helps avoid repeated contact of a needle that may be contaminated with tumor cells with the overlying abdominal or retroperitoneal tissues, thus reducing the potential risk of

tract seeding. In addition, procoagulants or an absorbable gelatin sponge (Gelfoam) can be injected into the tract to promote hemostasis at the end of the procedure [49]. For most renal biopsies, an 18- to 16-gauge guide needle is used. With this approach, 22-gauge needles can be used in FNA biopsy, and 20- to 18-gauge cutting needles can be used in core biopsy.

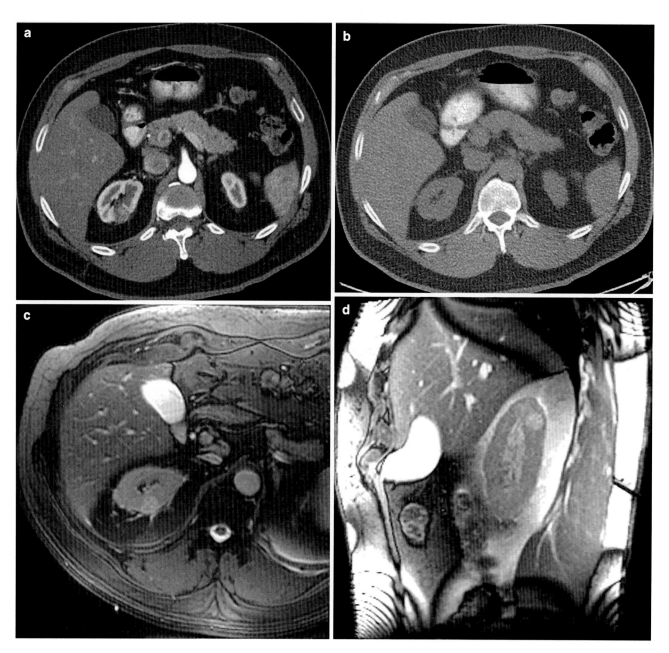

Fig. 17.20 A 56-year-old man was found to have a 1.6-cm mass in his right kidney. The mass was discovered incidentally when a CT scan was performed for a non-urological complaint. Because of his other comorbidities, he was referred for biopsy to determine the need for surgery or other interventions. An axial CT image of the abdomen after administration of contrast material (**a**) reveals a hypervascular mass in the posterior upper pole of the right kidney. The mass could not be

visualized on non-contrast CT images (**b**). An axial trueFISP MRI of the abdomen (**c**) in the prone position reveals a hyperdense tumor in the right kidney. This image also reveals the lung base interposed between the tumor and the chest wall. Sagittal MR images reveal a biopsy trajectory that avoids the lung base (**d–f**). A biopsy revealed oncocytoma. The patient did not require treatment

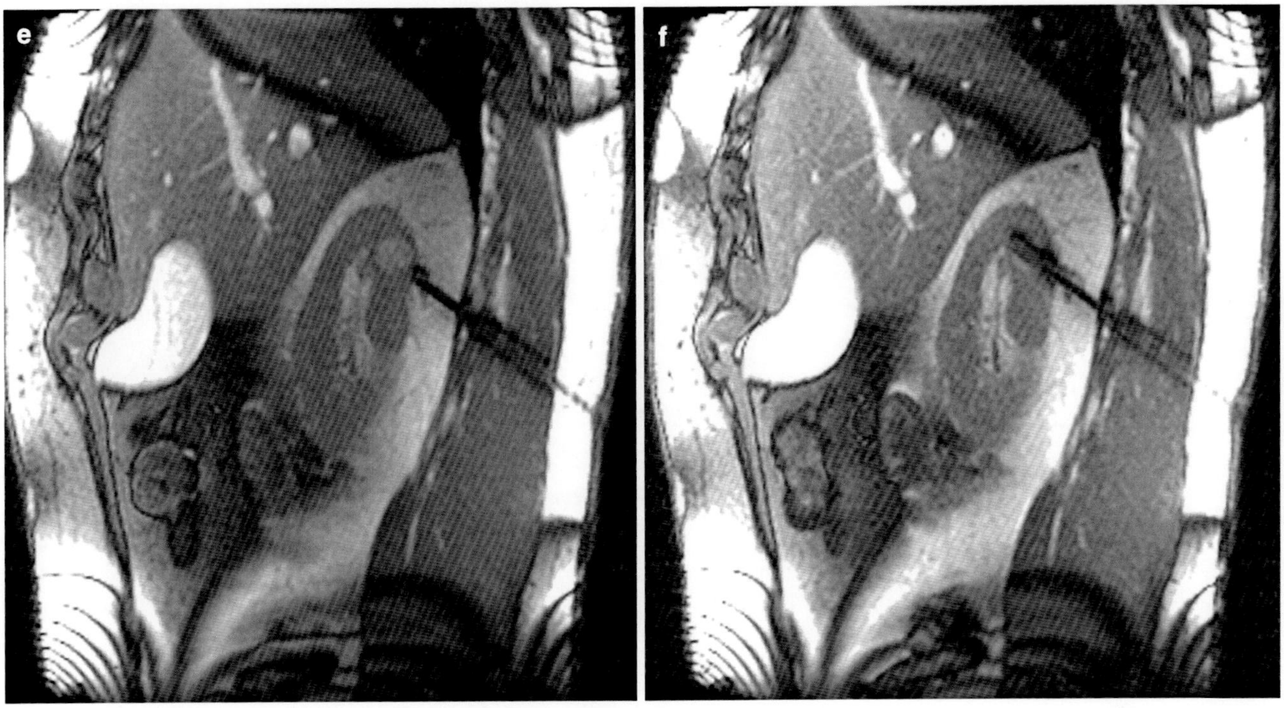

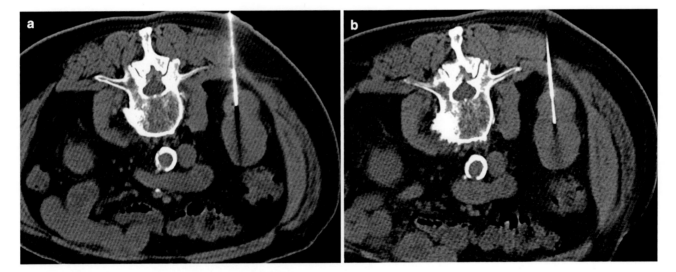

Fig. 17.20 (continued)

Fig. 17.21 An axial CT image of the abdomen (**a**) reveals a guide needle placed in an exophytic mass along the posterior aspect of the right kidney. (**b**) A smaller gauge biopsy (FNA or core) can be advanced in coaxial fashion to obtain a biopsy sample. As long as the guide needle remains in place, the biopsy needle can be reinserted to obtain additional samples

Approach and Relevant Anatomy

Most renal mass biopsies are performed with the patient in a prone (Fig. 17.22), semiprone, or decubitus position. During ultrasound-guided biopsies, the patient can be rotated to an arbitrary oblique position to allow a better window to visualize the tumor or a safer tract for advancing the needle. For CT-guided procedures, an ipsilateral decubitus position helps decrease the volume of the dependent thoracic cavity, thus reducing the lung excursion in the caudal direction (Fig. 17.23). This position provides a safer approach to upper pole tumors and has a lower risk of pneumothorax (Fig. 17.24). Otherwise, the CT gantry may be tilted to allow an oblique axial plane of imaging to avoid traversing the lung base (Fig. 17.25). Occasionally, a large renal mass in a very thin patient can be approached laterally (Fig. 17.26) or

Fig. 17.22 A schematic demonstration of the relevant anatomy with the patient in the prone position. In the prone position, the lung bases are often interposed between the chest wall and the upper pole of the kidneys (**a**). The mid pole (**b**) and lower pole (**c**) of the kidneys are usually surrounded by retroperitoneal fat

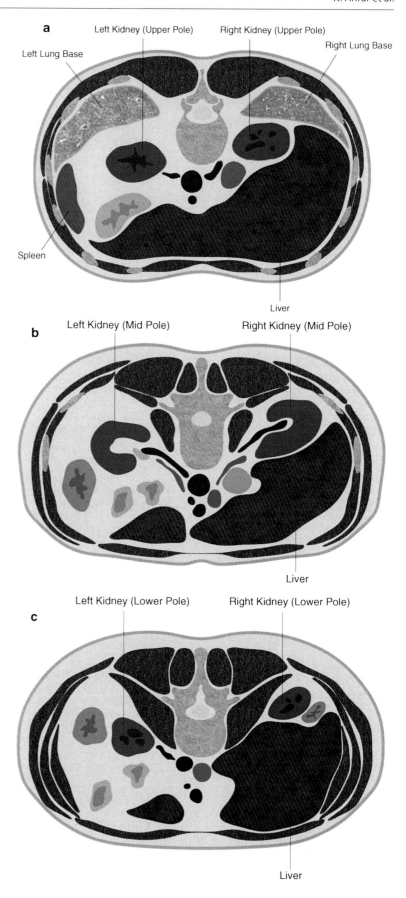

Fig. 17.23 When the patient is placed in an ipsilateral decubitus position, the ipsilateral lung is compressed and the lung base is no longer interposed between the upper pole of the kidney and the chest wall. This will decrease the risk of pneumothorax during CT-guided biopsy of tumors in the upper pole of the kidney

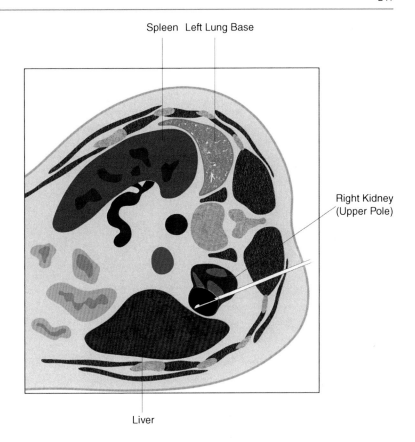

Spleen   Left Lung Base

Right Kidney (Upper Pole)

Liver

anteriorly (Fig. 17.27) with the patient in the supine position. Small tumors in the anterior aspect of the kidney may warrant a lateral approach with the patient in the supine or prone position (Fig. 17.28). If an intercostal approach is needed, care must be taken to avoid injury to the neurovascular bundle that is often located along the inferior margin of the ribs. Transhepatic and transsplenic biopsy of renal masses may be considered if no other needle paths are available, but these approaches are rarely used (Fig. 17.29). Ideally, different areas of the tumor should be targeted to obtain a representative sample. Necrotic areas, usually encountered in the center of large tumors, should be avoided [51]. For tumors smaller than 4 cm, one central and one peripheral core biopsy is recommended, whereas for tumors larger than 4 cm with a potentially necrotic center, two peripheral core biopsies are recommended [51]. Core biopsy samples should be visually inspected to estimate their size and quality. Fragmented or small samples (<1 cm) warrant additional sampling of the tumor [32].

Potential Complications

Some of the largest recent series of renal mass biopsy have reported very few or no major complications [14, 32, 44, 45, 52–54]. In a total of 362 biopsies, there were 17 minor com-

plications (4.7 %) and 1 major complication (0.3 %). Potential complications for renal mass biopsy include perinephric hemorrhage, hematuria, arteriovenous fistula, infection, pneumothorax, and needle tract seeding.

Most renal tumors, particularly RCCs, are hypervascular and such are prone to bleeding after percutaneous biopsy. Small perinephric or subcapsular hematomas accompany these procedures in 44–91 % of cases but are often self-limited, do not cause any symptoms, and do not require additional intervention (Fig. 17.30) [47, 55]. Renal hemorrhage that necessitates hospital admission or blood transfusion occurs in 1–2 % of cases [33, 56]. Subcapsular hematomas are often asymptomatic (Fig. 17.31), but they can be large and may cause significant pain and severe hypertension [57]. Hematuria as a result of renal mass biopsy is also uncommon, but it may lead to ureteral obstruction and pain [58]. An arteriovenous fistula should be considered in cases of persistent bleeding [56, 59]. If careful attention is given to aseptic technique, the risk of infection is minimal. With the patient in the prone position, the posterior sulcus extends over the upper pole of the kidney in most patients. During CT-guided renal mass biopsy, transgression of the pleural space and/or lung may cause a pneumothorax [60, 61]. Placing the patient in an ipsilateral decubitus position or using a triangulation technique with subcostal needle insertion helps reduce the risk of pneumothorax [62].

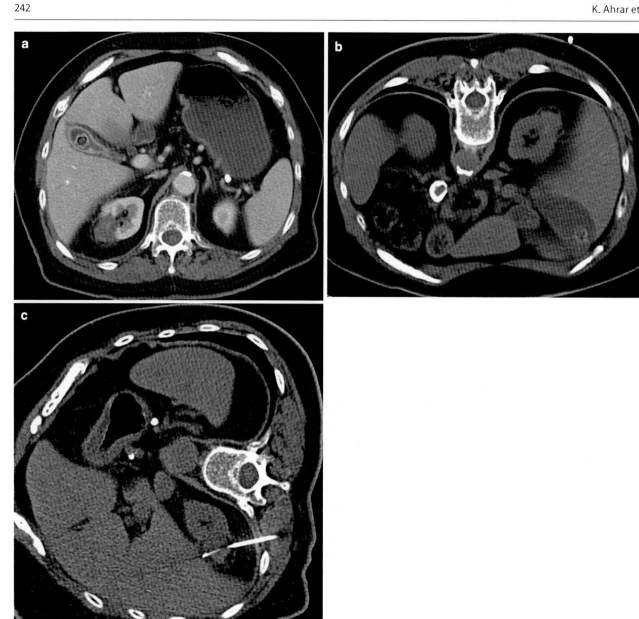

Fig. 17.24 A 77-year-old woman with a history of renal cell carcinoma underwent percutaneous radiofrequency ablation. Follow-up images were suspicious for recurrence. The patient was referred for biopsy. An axial CT image of the abdomen (**a**) reveals the zone of ablation in the lateral aspect of the upper pole of the right kidney. The patient was placed in the prone position for biopsy. An axial CT image of the abdomen (**b**) reveals interposition of the lung parenchyma between the kidney and the intended needle insertion site. The patient was then placed in the right lateral decubitus position. In this position (**c**), the right lung is compressed, the volume of the right hemithorax is decreased, and the lung is no longer in the path of the needle. Core biopsies of the ablation zone revealed necrotic tissue and no viable tumor

Fig. 17.25 A schematic illustration of the approach to upper pole tumors, avoiding the lung base. The CT gantry can be tilted to outline the path of the needle. Alternatively, an out-of-plane approach can be achieved by triangulation. In this case, axial CT images will reveal only a segment of the needle. Using MRI, the entire biopsy can be planned and carried out in the sagittal plane

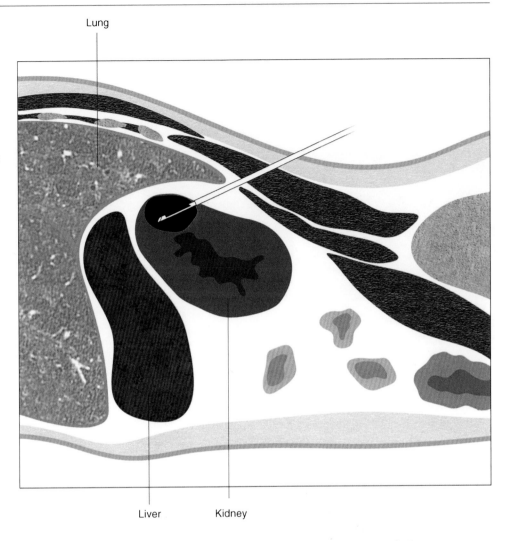

Fig. 17.26 A 67-year-old man was referred for biopsy of a large right renal mass. An axial CT image of the abdomen reveals a large exophytic mass arising from the right kidney (**a**). A CT-guided biopsy was performed in the supine position, using a lateral approach (**b**). Only fine-needle aspiration biopsy samples were obtained. A pathologic evaluation revealed high-grade carcinoma but could not distinguish between renal cell carcinoma and urothelial carcinoma. Core biopsy samples may have been beneficial for establishing a firm diagnosis

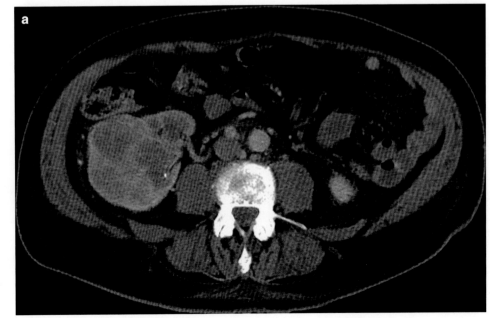

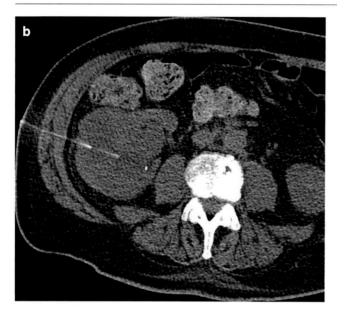

Fig. 17.26 (continued)

For many years, percutaneous renal mass biopsy was considered inappropriate because of fear of needle tract seeding. Although occasional cases of tract seeding have been reported after percutaneous biopsy of renal tumors, the actual incidence is low. The overall estimated risk of needle tract seeding in urologic malignancies is less than 0.01 % [63], which is comparable to risk of this complica-

tion in other abdominal biopsies. In recent series of renal tumor biopsy, no case of needle tract seeding was reported [32, 33, 47, 52, 59, 64–69]. The lack of tract seeding in recent series may be related to the widespread use of the guiding cannula and coaxial technique during image-guided biopsy of renal tumors. It has been reported that urothelial carcinomas are at higher risk of seeding than are RCCs [63, 70], and some researchers have recommended that an infiltrative renal mass should not be biopsied unless lymphoma is a primary consideration [53]. However, we have found very little scientific evidence for this recommendation [70].

Management of Complications

Large or persistent perinephric hemorrhage may cause a drop in hemoglobin levels and may cause symptoms related to blood loss. These symptoms often include one or more of the following: pain, hypotension, tachycardia, diaphoresis, weakness, and drowsiness. Transfusion of packed red blood cells may be warranted if the patient is symptomatic. If the bleeding persists, an angiogram and possible selective embolization may be warranted (Fig. 17.32) [71]. Gross hematuria, if self-limited and asymptomatic, does not require intervention. However, ureteral obstruction may require placement of a stent, preferably retrograde via cystoscopy rather than antegrade via percutaneous nephrostomy.

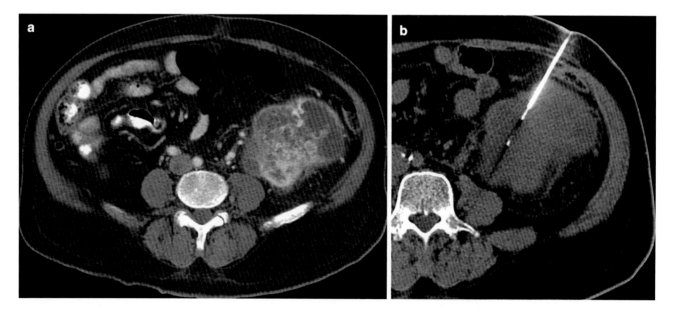

Fig. 17.27 A 72-year-old man with a large left renal mass was referred for biopsy. An axial CT image of the lower abdomen (**a**) reveals a large hypervascular mass arising from the left kidney, with areas of necrosis. A CT-guided biopsy (**b**) was performed from an anterior approach, with the patient in the supine position. A fine-needle aspiration biopsy was performed, and an immediate assessment of the slides revealed viable tumor cells. Core biopsy samples were obtained from the same region. The final cytopathology report was "rare atypical cell clusters, suspicious for renal cell carcinoma." A histological evaluation report of the core biopsy sample revealed renal cell carcinoma, clear cell type, and Furman's nuclear grade 3

Fig. 17.28 A schematic illustration of a lateral approach for an anteriorly located renal tumor (right kidney) compared with a posterior approach for a posteriorly located renal tumor (left kidney)

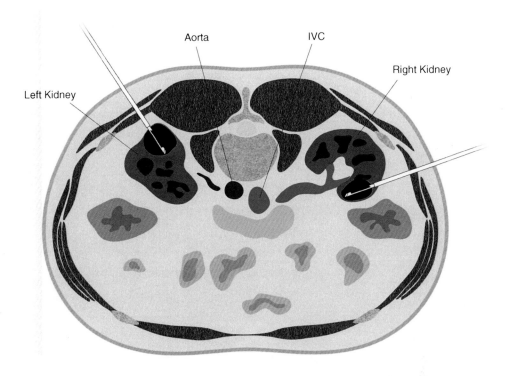

Left Kidney

Aorta

IVC

Right Kidney

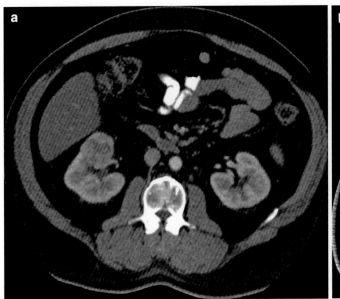

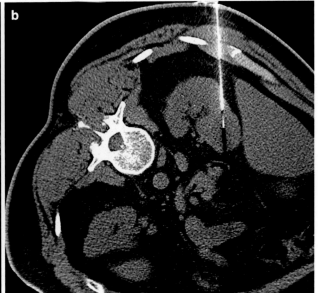

Fig. 17.29 A 57-year-old man was referred for biopsy of a right renal tumor. An axial CT image of the abdomen in the supine position reveals a solid enhancing mass in the anterior aspect of the right kidney (**a**). A

CT-guided biopsy was performed in the lateral decubitus position, with a lateral approach (**b**). This position helped displace the liver anteriorly and provided a safe path for the biopsy needle

Persistent hematuria should be evaluated by angiography to rule out a pseudoaneurysm or arteriovenous fistula. If the course of the needle is close to the base of the lung, observation and chest radiography are warranted after the biopsy. A small pneumothorax may be observed, but an enlarging pneumothorax may require chest tube placement.

Outcomes and Results of Renal Mass Biopsy

In studies published prior to 2001, renal mass biopsy yielded an accurate diagnosis in 88.9 % of 2,474 biopsies for suspected RCC [6] (Table 17.2). More recently, renal mass biopsy has received increasing attention and has played a

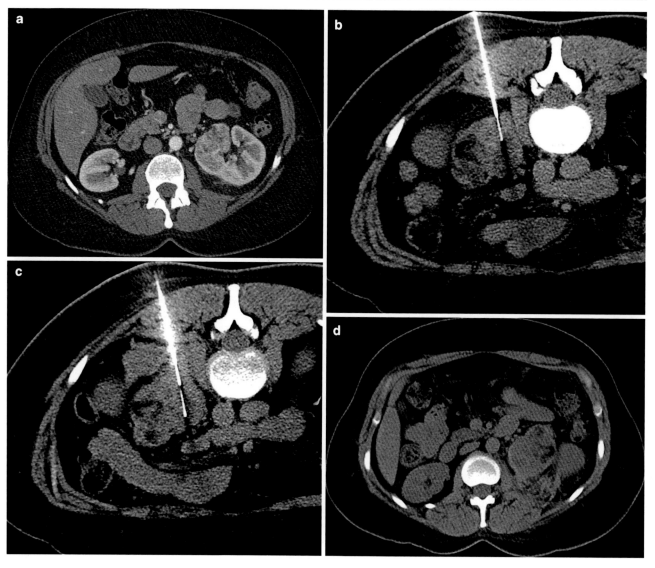

Fig. 17.30 A 47-year-old woman with a history of synovial sarcoma was referred for biopsy of a left renal mass. A diagnostic axial CT image of the abdomen (**a**) reveals a hypervascular mass in the medial aspect of the left kidney. A CT-guided biopsy (**b**) was performed in the prone position. Shortly after the first biopsy sample was obtained, a CT image (**c**) revealed development of a moderate-sized retroperitoneal hematoma. An axial CT image of the abdomen (**d**) 4 h later revealed no change in the size of the retroperitoneal hematoma. The patient was hemodynamically stable and was discharged home with no other interventions

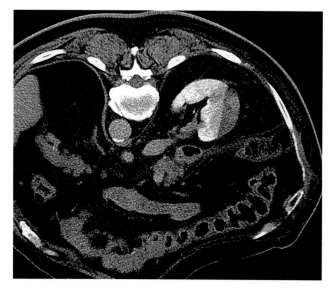

Fig. 17.31 A subcapsular hematoma after a renal mass biopsy is often self-limited and has no major consequences. If the hematoma enlarges sufficiently, it can cause pain or hypertension

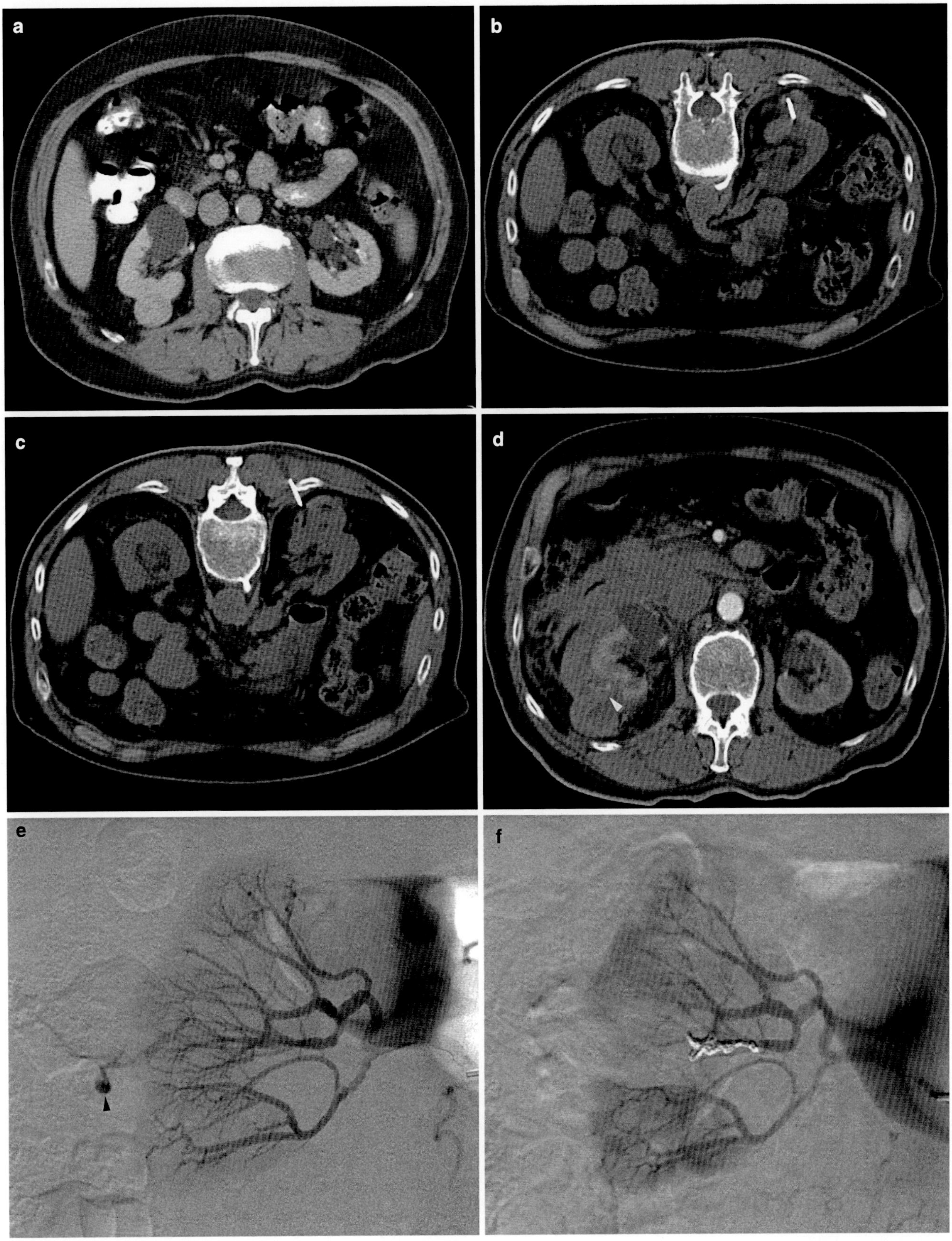

Fig. 17.32 A 79-year-old man with a right renal mass was referred for biopsy to determine the need for surgery or other interventions. A diagnostic CT image of the abdomen reveals a solid enhancing mass in the posterior aspect of the right kidney (**a**). A CT-guided biopsy was performed in the prone position (**b**). During the procedure, the patient developed a hematoma surrounding the tumor (**c**). A contrast-enhanced CT scan was performed because of increasing flank pain during the recovery period (**d**). The image revealed a larger retroperitoneal hematoma, with evidence of active contrast extravasation (*arrowhead* in **d**). A selective right renal artery angiogram (**e**) reveals active bleeding (*arrowhead*). After embolization of the bleeding artery, an angiogram (**f**) revealed no further extravasation

Table 17.2 Studies published before 2001 of renal mass biopsy of solid renal tumors

References	No. of solid tumors	No. of pathologically confirmed (%)	No. of Ca (%)	Needle Size	Needle Type	Biopsies No.	Guidance	No. of biopsy failure (%)[a]	No. of indeterminate pathology (%)[a]	No. of false-neg (%)	No. of false-pos (%)	% Ca accuracy
Kristensen	34	29 (85)	34(100)	1.2 mm	Chiba	NA	US	1 (2.9)	4 (12)	1 (3.0)	0	85
Karp	23	23 (100)	23 (100)	22 G		NA	US	5 (22)	1 (5.6)	1 (5.6)	0	89
Nosher	12	NA	7 (58)	20–22 G		NA	US	0	1 (8.3)		1 (8.3)	83
Helm	31	15 (48)	21 (68)	18 G	Chiba	2	US	4 (13)	0	2 (7.4)	1 (3.7)	89
Nurmi	150	150 (100)	150 (100)	21 G		2	Ex vivo	3 (2.0)	0		0	100
Elder	25	NA	25 (100)	22 G		1	F/US		3 (12)		0	88
Juul	301	NA	218 (72)	23 G		4–5	US	16 (5.3)	0	25 (8.8)	0	91
Murphy	56	37 (66)	41 (73)	17–22 G		2	F	6 (11)	7 (14)	1 (2.0)	1 (2.0)	82
Orell	83	58 (70)	69 (83)	22 G		1–4	F/US/CT	7 (8.4)	0		1 (1.3)	99
Nadel	30	NA	14 (47)	21–14 G	Chiba	1–4	F/US/CT	0	0	1 (3.3)	0	97
Pilotti	132	32 (24)	65 (49)	22 G	Chiba	1–3	F/CT	8 (6.1)	0		1 (0.8)	99
Leiman	120	42 (35)	91 (76)	22 G	Chiba	1–5	US/CT	26 (22)	0		2 (2.1)	98
Haubek	169	NA	137 (81)	18–23 G			NA	8 (4.7)	0	17 (11)	4 (2.5)	87
Torp[b]	134	63 (47)	82 (61)	22,20 G	Chiba, Chiba + Surecut	6	US	3 (2.2), 28 (21)	0	7 (5.3), 8 (7.5)	7 (5.3), 0	89, 93
Cristallini	79	27 (34)	34 (43)	21–22 G	Chiba	NA	US/CT	7 (8.9)	0	4 (5.6)	1 (1.4)	93
Abe	36	21 (58)	31 (86)	14–18 G		NA	US	2 (5.6)	1 (2.8)		0	97
Mondal	92	92 (100)	79 (86)	21 G		NA	US	0	4 (4.3)		2 (2.2)	94
Niceforo	23	6 (26)	17 (74)	22 G		1–3	CT	0	0	3 (13)	0	87
Kelley	43	10 (23)	40 (93)	NA		NA	US/CT	1 (2.3)	6 (14)		1 (2.4)	83
Campbell	25	25 (100)	25 (100)	22 G	Chiba	2	CT	0	9 (36)	6 (24)	0	40
Nguyen	129	NA	57 (44)	NA		1–2	NA	11 (8.5)	0		0	100
Truong	108	94 (87)	62 (57)	23–25 G		1–4	US/CT	17 (16)	11 (12)	1 (1.1)	0	87
Dechet[c]	106	106 (100)	91 (86)	18 G		NA	Ex vivo	0	12–18 (range 11–17)	3–5 (range 2.8–4.7)	4 (3.8)	76–80
Wood	79	41 (52)	54 (68)	17–22 G		2	F/US/CT	5 (6.3)	0		0	100
Richter	205	126 (62)	86 (42)	18–22 G	Chiba	2	F/US/CT	21 (10)	55 (30)	4 (2.2)	2 (1.1)	67
Brierly	42	35 (83)	40 (95)	NA		NA	US/CT	7 (17)	8 (23)	7 (17)	1 (2.9)	54
Lechevallier	73	27 (37)	56 (77)	18 G	Chiba	2–4	CT	15 (21)	2 (3.4)		0	97
Overall	2,474	1,059/1,674 (63.3 %, range 23–100 %)	1,649/2,340 (70.5 %, range 42–100 %)	Median 21 G (range 14–25)		Median 2 (range 1–6)	US 19 CT 13 F 7, ex vivo 2[d]	198/2,218 (8.9 %, range 0–22 %)	112/2,020 (5.5 %, range 0–36 %)	88/2020 (4.4 %, range 0–24 %)	25/2,020 (1.2 %, range 0–8.3 %)	1,795/2,020 (88.9 %, range 40–100 %)

Reprinted from Lane et al. [6]. Copyright 2008, with permission from Elsevier

Abbreviations: *G* gauge, *NA* not available, *US* ultrasonography, *F* fluoroscopy, *CT* computed tomography

[a]Biopsy failure was defined as the inability to obtain tissue sufficient for diagnosis; indeterminate biopsies included cases in which the pathologist could not make a definitive diagnosis using available tissue. In the few studies in which it could not be determined whether biopsies failed or were indeterminate, biopsies were considered indeterminate, which negatively impacted accuracy. Percentage of failed biopsies was based on the total number of biopsies. Percentage of indeterminate, false-negative, and false-positive biopsies was based on the number of successful biopsies. Accuracy for cancer diagnosis or benign pathology was defined as the percent of biopsies with material sufficient for analysis (excluding biopsy failures) in which the diagnosis was accurate, i.e., not indeterminate, false-negative, or false-positive

[b]Biopsies of the same 134 tumors were obtained using fine-needle aspiration with 22- and 20-gauge Chiba or Surecut needle; this series was counted only once to calculate the overall percentage of pathologically confirmed tumors and cancer

[c]The same 106 biopsies were reviewed separately by two independent pathologists, providing two sets of outcomes

[d]Two ex vivo studies were excluded from the overall percentage of biopsy failure, indeterminate pathology, false-negative and false-positive biopsies, and diagnostic accuracy for cancer to determine percutaneous rate

substantial role in the management of patients with renal tumors. Various studies have been published reporting the success rates and accuracy of these biopsies, albeit in an inconsistent manner. There are variations in technique. Several studies reported only core needle biopsy, whereas others reported the results of FNA biopsies, and still others reported success rates for both FNA and core needle biopsies. Most studies used CT and/or ultrasound to guide needle placement, but definitions of nondiagnostic, inadequate, indeterminate, and failed biopsy varied between studies. Nevertheless, the reported rate of technical failure due to insufficient material has dropped from 9 % before 2001 to approximately 4 % in the more recent series [6] (Table 17.3). The rate of indeterminate or inaccurate pathologic findings was reported to be 10 % in earlier studies, but this rate has decreased to 4 % in the more recent series [6]. Given these findings, when initial biopsy results are inconclusive, a repeat biopsy is warranted. A definitive diagnosis can be obtained in 83–100 % of repeat renal mass biopsies [33, 47, 49, 64, 65, 69, 72, 73].

For core needle biopsies, sensitivity ranges from 70–100 % (even in cases of experienced radiologists), and false-negative results do occur. False-positive results are rare, and specificity has been reported as 100 %. The accuracy is frequently greater than 90 % [27, 32, 33, 42, 44, 47, 52, 53, 59, 64, 65, 68]. Several series have reported comparable results in FNA biopsy with high sensitivity, specificity, and accuracy [74–76]. Reportedly, the accuracy of FNA biopsy is highly dependent on the skills of the cytologist. Some investigators have argued that core needle biopsies are complementary to FNA biopsies. A combination of these techniques may result in better accuracy than either technique alone [33, 45, 49].

In a study of 100 renal tumors smaller than 4 cm, multivariate analysis determined larger tumor size and a solid pattern as independent predictors of diagnostic results for image-guided biopsy [49]. Smaller tumors are technically more difficult to target and sample [14]. In tumors larger than 4 cm, the risk of sampling error has been associated with greater incidence of central necrosis [14, 47]. Negative results of a biopsy in a patient with a radiologically suspicious mass should be viewed with caution. Several studies have reported high diagnostic rates for repeat core biopsy when the initial attempt was nondiagnostic [33, 47, 69].

Aside from significant improvements in imaging and biopsy techniques, recent advances in pathology have helped improve the diagnostic yield of renal mass biopsies [7] (Table 17.4). In addition to accurately characterizing a tumor as benign or malignant, biopsy would ideally help determine the tumor subtype and nuclear grade of RCC. This information may help select a more appropriate therapy and may help determine prognosis for a given patient. The most common subtypes of RCC include clear cell, papillary, and

chromophobe. It is believed that the clear cell subtype has a worse prognosis when controlling for TNM stage and Fuhrman grade, whereas no difference in outcome was noted between papillary and chromophobe RCC [77]. However, a more recent multicenter study demonstrated histological subtype was not an independent predictor of survival [78]. Nevertheless, histological classification of RCC is important since different subtypes may respond differently to various therapies [11, 79, 80]. Recent series have reported the concordance of histological subtype determined at biopsy with pathologic results at nephrectomy. In these studies, subtypes of RCC were accurately determined in 94 % of cases [32, 44, 51, 54, 76, 81]. The Fuhrman grading system stratifies tumors based on nuclear morphology into grades 1–4. The role of nuclear grade in prognosis has been well established; low-grade tumors have better survival rates than do high-grade tumors. Fuhrman nuclear grade was accurately characterized in 74–94 % of core biopsies [32, 51, 68]. On the other hand, using FNA biopsy samples, the nuclear grade was correctly predicted in 28 % of cases [68]. Interobserver variability and tumor heterogeneity may negatively affect the accuracy of nuclear grading in biopsy samples [63, 76]. Tumor heterogeneity and grade variability have been documented in up to 25 % of RCCs [63]. However, in cases of discordant nuclear grade, the grade recorded at biopsy was within one grade of that assigned to the nephrectomy specimen [32, 51]. Better agreement between preoperative and postoperative grading can be achieved if tumors are simply defined as low (1–2) or high (3–4) grade [82].

As noted in the preceding discussion, the studies of renal mass biopsy have focused on RCC, for the most part. The literature lacks any large biopsy series in which most cases represent benign renal tumors. Most benign lesions such as simple cysts or angiomyolipomas are diagnosed by imaging, and a biopsy is usually not warranted [7]. On the other hand, in some large series of renal mass biopsies, the pathologists have been able to characterize some benign tumors with confidence. In a series of 88 patients, 14 (15.9 %) biopsies yielded benign diagnoses—10 oncocytomas, 3 angiomyolipomas, and 1 cystadenoma [32].

Despite these results, the role of percutaneous biopsy in the diagnosis of renal oncocytomas remains controversial. Differentiation of oncocytoma from the eosinophilic variant of chromophobe RCC is particularly difficult [42]. Addition of immunohistochemical stains (e.g., Hale's colloidal iron stain, cytokeratin 7, cytokeratin 20, and RCC) to cytologic morphology may help distinguish renal oncocytoma from RCC [42, 83]. When pathologists are faced with equivocal morphology or immunohistochemical studies that do not completely support a diagnosis of oncocytoma, they render a diagnosis of "oncocytic neoplasm," which implies that malignant RCC cannot be excluded [42]. Other ancillary studies such as electron microscopy, microRNA expression, and comparative genomic hybrid-

Table 17.3 Studies published in 2001 and after of renal mass biopsy of solid renal tumors

References	No. of tumors	No. of pathologically confirmed (%)	No. of Ca (%)	Biopsies Needle type (gauge)	No.	Guidance	No. complications Any	Major	No. of biopsy failure (%)	No. of indeterminate pathology (%)	No. of false-neg (%)	No. of false-pos (%)	No. of accuracy/total no. (%)[b] Ca	Histology	Grade
Clinical RMB															
Hara	33	15 (45)	21 (64)	18	NA	US/CT	9	0	0	0	0	0	33/33 (100)	NA	NA
Johnson	44	NA	NA	18–22	1–5	US	4	0	8 (18)	0	NA	NA	36/36 (100)	NA	NA
Caoili	26	7 (27)	19 (73)	18	2–5	US	1	1	0	2 (7.7)	0	0	24/26 (92)	NA	NA
Rybicki	99	58 (59)	94 (95)	18–22 Chiba	3–5	US/CT/MRI	0	0	3 (3.0)	6 (6.3)	1 (1.0)	0	89/96 (93)	NA	NA
Neuzillet	88	62 (70)	71 (81)	18	2 or greater	CT	0	0	3 (3.4)	5 (5.6)	0	0	80/85 (94)	58/63 (92)	44/63 (70)
Eshed	23	14 (61)	15 (65)	18	NA	CT	0	0	1 (4.3)	0	1 (4.5)	0	21/22 (95)	NA	NA
Volpe[c]	49	16 (33)	NA	18	NA	US/CT	3	0	4 (8.2)	0	0	0	45/45 (100)	14/14 (100)	NA
Overall	362	172/318 (54)	220/269 (82)				17 (4.7 %)	1 (0.3 %)	19 (5.2)	13 (3.8)	2 (0.6)	0	326/341 (96)	72/77 (94)	NA
Ex vivo RMB															
Dechet[b]	100	100 (100)	85 (85)	18	NA		NA	NA	0	20–21 (20.5 %)	1–2 (1–2 %)	0–4 (0–4 %)	75–77/100 (76)	NA	NA
Wunderlich	50	50 (100)	46 (92)	18	5		NA	NA	1 (2)	3 (6 %)	0 (0 %)	0 (0 %)	46/49 (94)	46/50 (92)	38/46 (83)
Barocas[d]	77	77 (100)	60 (78)	14	3		NA	NA	7 (9.1)	0 (0 %)	0 (0 %)	0 (0 %)	70/70 (100)	50/60 (90)–57/60 (95)	NA
Overall	227	(100)	(84)				NA	NA	8 (3.5)	23.5 (11)	1.5 (0.7)	2 (0.9)	192/219 (88)	96/110 (87)	NA

Reprinted from Lane et al. [6]. Copyright 2008, with permission from Elsevier

Abbreviations: *RMB* renal mass biopsy, *NA* not available, *US* ultrasonography, *CT* computed tomography, *MRI* magnetic resonance imaging

[a]Biopsy failure was defined as the inability to obtain tissue sufficient for diagnosis; indeterminate biopsies include cases in which the pathologist could not make a definitive diagnosis using available tissue and percentage of failed biopsies was based on the total number of biopsies. Percentage of indeterminate, false-negative, and false-positive biopsies was based on the number of successful biopsies, and accuracy was defined as the percentage of biopsies with sufficient material for analysis (excluding biopsy failures) in which the diagnosis was accurate, i.e., not indeterminate, false-negative, or false-positive. Accuracy of renal mass biopsy for histological subtype and nuclear grade was determined as the final pathologic diagnosis at nephrectomy

[b]The same 100 biopsies were reviewed separately by 2 independent pathologists providing 2 sets of outcomes, and since it could not be determined whether biopsies were failed or indeterminate, these biopsies were considered indeterminate, which negatively impacted accuracy

[c]Histological accuracy was reported for standard histopathology and for histopathology plus reverse transcriptase-polymerase chain reaction for CA-IX, alpha-methylacyl coenzyme A racemase, parvalbumin, and kidney-specific chloride channel

[d]A second study by this group investigating histopathology plus fluorescence in situ hybridization increased the accuracy for identifying histological subtype from 87 to 94 % in 33 cases (92 %) with adequate tissue

Table 17.4 Histochemical, immunocytochemical, and cytogenetic profiles of renal masses

Tumor	Histochemical	Immunocytochemistry					Cytogenetics
	Stain[a]	HMB45	SMA	RCC	CD10	p63	
Angiomyolipoma	—	+	+	—	NK	NK	Normal or trisomy 7
Oncocytoma	—	NK	NK	—	—	NK	−1, -X or Y, 11q13 rearrangement
RCC, clear cell	—	—	—	+	+	—	del 3p
RCC, papillary	—	—	NK	+	+	NK	Trisomies 3, 7, 12, 16, 17, 20
RCC, chromophobe	+	—	NK	—	+	NK	Monosomies 1, 2, 3,6,10, 13, 17, 21
Transitional cell carcinoma	—	—	—	-	±	+	Complex karyotype

Printed with permission from Silverman et al. [7]

Abbreviations: *HMB45* human melanoma black 45; *SMA* smooth muscle actin, *RCC* renal cell carcinoma, + positive, – negative, ± variable results, *NK* not known

Note: False-negative and false-positive results are observed occasionally with immunocytochemistry. Therefore, a profile of several antibodies is recommended when investigating any particular case

[a]Hale colloidal iron stain

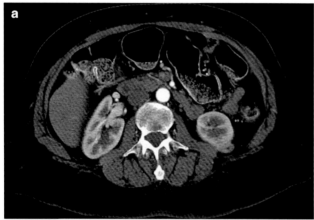

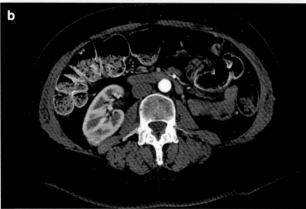

Fig. 17.33 A 61-year-old woman underwent a CT scan for non-urological complaints. She was found to have bilateral renal tumors. A biopsy of the left posterior renal tumor (**a**) revealed angiomyolipoma. A biopsy of the right posterior tumor (**b**) revealed renal cell carcinoma

ization have been reported in the literature to help confidently make a diagnosis of oncocytoma, but they are not commonly used in clinical practice [84–86].

Renal angiomyolipoma is composed of variable proportions of blood vessels, smooth muscle, and adipose tissue

[87]. Presence of macroscopic fat as demonstrated on CT or MRI studies is characteristic of angiomyolipoma (AML). A rare subtype, epithelioid AML, typically does not show macroscopic fat and cannot be distinguished from other renal masses. Epithelioid AML is potentially malignant with aggressive biology leading to recurrence, metastasis, and death. In addition, 5 % of classic triphasic AMLs do not contain macroscopic fat, creating a diagnostic dilemma [88, 89]. These so-called lipid-poor angiomyolipomas cannot be distinguished from RCC on the basis of their imaging characteristics (Fig. 17.33). Percutaneous biopsy can help establish the diagnosis when CT or MRI studies do not show any evidence of macroscopic fat in these tumors. Pathologic diagnosis is based on identification of mature fat cells in association with smooth muscle cell bundles and vascular components. An immunohistochemical profile shows expression of HMB-45, a melanosome-associated protein, but no staining with cytokeratin [87].

In the setting of extrarenal primary cancer, percutaneous biopsy is 90 % sensitive for detection of metastatic disease to the kidney [14, 63].

In summary, percutaneous renal mass biopsy is a safe procedure with low complication rates. Advanced imaging techniques have enabled greater precision in localizing and targeting renal tumors for biopsy. Percutaneous renal mass biopsy has a high diagnostic accuracy, making a significant impact in the management of patients with renal tumors.

References

1. Skinner DG, Colvin RB, Vermillion CD, Pfister RC, Leadbetter WF. Diagnosis and management of renal cell carcinoma. A clinical and pathologic study of 309 cases. Cancer. 1971;28:1165–77.
2. Chow WH, Devesa SS, Warren JL, Fraumeni Jr JF. Rising incidence of renal cell cancer in the United States. JAMA. 1999; 281:1628–31.

3. Frank I, Blute ML, Cheville JC, Lohse CM, Weaver AL, Zincke H. Solid renal tumors: an analysis of pathological features related to tumor size. J Urol. 2003;170:2217–20.

4. Link RE, Bhayani SB, Allaf ME, et al. Exploring the learning curve, pathological outcomes and perioperative morbidity of laparoscopic partial nephrectomy performed for renal mass. J Urol. 2005;173:1690–4.

5. Gill IS, Matin SF, Desai MM, et al. Comparative analysis of laparoscopic versus open partial nephrectomy for renal tumors in 200 patients. J Urol. 2003;170:64–8.

6. Lane BR, Samplaski MK, Herts BR, Zhou M, Novick AC, Campbell SC. Renal mass biopsy–a renaissance? J Urol. 2008; 179:20–7.

7. Silverman SG, Gan YU, Mortele KJ, Tuncali K, Cibas ES. Renal masses in the adult patient: the role of percutaneous biopsy. Radiology. 2006;240:6–22.

8. Volpe A, Jewett MA. Current role, techniques and outcomes of percutaneous biopsy of renal tumors. Expert Rev Anticancer Ther. 2009;9:773–83.

9. Truong LD, Caraway N, Ngo T, Laucirica R, Katz R, Ramzy I. Renal lymphoma. The diagnostic and therapeutic roles of fine-needle aspiration. Am J Clin Pathol. 2001;115:18–31.

10. Gattuso P, Ramzy I, Truong LD, et al. Utilization of fine-needle aspiration in the diagnosis of metastatic tumors to the kidney. Diagn Cytopathol. 1999;21:35–8.

11. Atkins MB. Treatment selection for patients with metastatic renal cell carcinoma: identification of features favoring upfront IL-2-based immunotherapy. Med Oncol. 2009;26 Suppl 1:18–22.

12. Samplaski MK, Zhou M, Lane BR, Herts B, Campbell SC. Renal mass sampling: an enlightened perspective. Int J Urol. 2011;18:5–19.

13. Bracken RB, Chica G, Johnson DE, Luna M. Secondary renal neoplasms: an autopsy study. South Med J. 1979;72:806–7.

14. Rybicki FJ, Shu KM, Cibas ES, Fielding JR, van Sonnenberg E, Silverman SG. Percutaneous biopsy of renal masses: sensitivity and negative predictive value stratified by clinical setting and size of masses. AJR Am J Roentgenol. 2003;180:1281–7.

15. Richmond J, Sherman RS, Diamond HD, Craver LF. Renal lesions associated with malignant lymphomas. Am J Med. 1962;32: 184–207.

16. Hartman DS, David Jr CJ, Goldman SM, Friedman AC, Fritzsche P. Renal lymphoma: radiologic-pathologic correlation of 21 cases. Radiology. 1982;144:759–66.

17. Reznek RH, Mootoosamy I, Webb JA, Richards MA. CT in renal and perirenal lymphoma: a further look. Clin Radiol. 1990;42:233–8.

18. El-Sharkawy MS, Siddiqui N, Aleem A, Diab AA. Renal involvement in lymphoma: prevalence and various patterns of involvement on abdominal CT. Int Urol Nephrol. 2007;39:929–33.

19. Lohse CM, Cheville JC. A review of prognostic pathologic features and algorithms for patients treated surgically for renal cell carcinoma. Clin Lab Med. 2005;25:433–64.

20. Cohen HT, McGovern FJ. Renal-cell carcinoma. N Engl J Med. 2005;353:2477–90.

21. Cho D, Signoretti S, Dabora S, et al. Potential histologic and molecular predictors of response to temsirolimus in patients with advanced renal cell carcinoma. Clin Genitourin Cancer. 2007;5:379–85.

22. Renshaw AA, Granter SR, Cibas ES. Fine-needle aspiration of the adult kidney. Cancer. 1997;81:71–88.

23. Rosenfield AT, Glickman MG, Taylor KJ, Crade M, Hodson J. Acute focal bacterial nephritis (acute lobar nephronia). Radiology. 1979;132:553–61.

24. Nguyen GK. Percutaneous fine-needle aspiration biopsy cytology of the kidney and adrenal. Pathol Annu. 1987;22(Pt 1): 163–91.

25. Lee JK, McClennan BL, Melson GL, Stanley RJ. Acute focal bacterial nephritis: emphasis on gray scale sonography and computed tomography. AJR Am J Roentgenol. 1980;135:87–92.

26. McKinstry CS. Acute lobar nephronia. Br J Radiol. 1985;58:1217–19.

27. Harisinghani MG, Maher MM, Gervais DA, et al. Incidence of malignancy in complex cystic renal masses (Bosniak category III): should imaging-guided biopsy precede surgery? AJR Am J Roentgenol. 2003;180:755–8.

28. Israel GM, Bosniak MA. An update of the Bosniak renal cyst classification system. Urology. 2005;66:484–8.

29. Richter F, Kasabian NG, Irwin Jr RJ, Watson RA, Lang EK. Accuracy of diagnosis by guided biopsy of renal mass lesions classified indeterminate by imaging studies. Urology. 2000;55: 348–52.

30. Lang EK, Macchia RJ, Gayle B, et al. CT-guided biopsy of indeterminate renal cystic masses (Bosniak 3 and 2F): accuracy and impact on clinical management. Eur Radiol. 2002;12:2518–24.

31. Campbell SC, Novick AC, Herts B, et al. Prospective evaluation of fine needle aspiration of small, solid renal masses: accuracy and morbidity. Urology. 1997;50:25–9.

32. Neuzillet Y, Lechevallier E, Andre M, Daniel L, Coulange C. Accuracy and clinical role of fine needle percutaneous biopsy with computerized tomography guidance of small (less than 4.0 cm) renal masses. J Urol. 2004;171:1802–5.

33. Wood BJ, Khan MA, McGovern F, Harisinghani M, Hahn PF, Mueller PR. Imaging guided biopsy of renal masses: indications, accuracy and impact on clinical management. J Urol. 1999;161:1470–4.

34. Gervais DA, McGovern FJ, Arellano RS, McDougal WS, Mueller PR. Radiofrequency ablation of renal cell carcinoma: Part 1, Indications, results, and role in patient management over a 6-year period and ablation of 100 tumors. AJR Am J Roentgenol. 2005;185:64–71.

35. Zagoria RJ, Traver MA, Werle DM, Perini M, Hayasaka S, Clark PE. Oncologic efficacy of CT-guided percutaneous radiofrequency ablation of renal cell carcinomas. AJR Am J Roentgenol. 2007;189:429–36.

36. Atwell TD, Farrell MA, Leibovich BC, et al. Percutaneous renal cryoablation: experience treating 115 tumors. J Urol. 2008;179:2136–40. discussion 2140–2131.

37. Gill IS, Remer EM, Hasan WA, et al. Renal cryoablation: outcome at 3 years. J Urol. 2005;173:1903–7.

38. Tuncali K, vanSonnenberg E, Shankar S, Mortele KJ, Cibas ES, Silverman SG. Evaluation of patients referred for percutaneous ablation of renal tumors: importance of a preprocedural diagnosis. AJR Am J Roentgenol. 2004;183:575–82.

39. Gervais DA, Arellano RS, McGovern FJ, McDougal WS, Mueller PR. Radiofrequency ablation of renal cell carcinoma: Part 2, Lessons learned with ablation of 100 tumors. AJR Am J Roentgenol. 2005;185:72–80.

40. Javadi S, Matin SF, Tamboli P, Ahrar K. Unexpected atypical findings on CT after radiofrequency ablation for small renal-cell carcinoma and the role of percutaneous biopsy. J Vasc Interv Radiol. 2007;18:1186–91.

41. Weight CJ, Kaouk JH, Hegarty NJ, et al. Correlation of radiographic imaging and histopathology following cryoablation and radio frequency ablation for renal tumors. J Urol. 2008;179:1277–81. discussion 1281–1273.

42. Shah RB, Bakshi N, Hafez KS, Wood Jr DP, Kunju LP. Image-guided biopsy in the evaluation of renal mass lesions in contemporary urological practice: indications, adequacy, clinical impact, and limitations of the pathological diagnosis. Hum Pathol. 2005;36:1309–15.

43. Silverman SG, Coughlin BF, Seltzer SE, Swensson RG, Mueller PR. Current use of screening laboratory tests before abdominal

interventions: a survey of 603 radiologists. Radiology. 1991;181:669–73.

44. Hara I, Miyake H, Hara S, Arakawa S, Hanioka K, Kamidono S. Role of percutaneous image-guided biopsy in the evaluation of renal masses. Urol Int. 2001;67:199–202.

45. Johnson PT, Nazarian LN, Feld RI, et al. Sonographically guided renal mass biopsy: indications and efficacy. J Ultrasound Med. 2001;20:749–53. quiz 755.

46. Tang S, Li JH, Lui SL, Chan TM, Cheng IK, Lai KN. Free-hand, ultrasound-guided percutaneous renal biopsy: experience from a single operator. Eur J Radiol. 2002;41:65–9.

47. Lechevallier E, Andre M, Barriol D, et al. Fine-needle percutaneous biopsy of renal masses with helical CT guidance. Radiology. 2000;216:506–10.

48. Silverman SG, Collick BD, Figueira MR, et al. Interactive MR-guided biopsy in an open-configuration MR imaging system. Radiology. 1995;197:175–81.

49. Volpe A, Mattar K, Finelli A, et al. Contemporary results of percutaneous biopsy of 100 small renal masses: a single center experience. J Urol. 2008;180:2333–7.

50. Appelbaum AH, Kamba TT, Cohen AS, Qaisi WG, Amirkhan RH. Effectiveness and safety of image-directed biopsies: coaxial technique versus conventional fine-needle aspiration. South Med J. 2002;95:212–17.

51. Wunderlich H, Hindermann W, Al Mustafa AM, Reichelt O, Junker K, Schubert J. The accuracy of 250 fine needle biopsies of renal tumors. J Urol. 2005;174:44–6.

52. Caoili EM, Bude RO, Higgins EJ, Hoff DL, Nghiem HV. Evaluation of sonographically guided percutaneous core biopsy of renal masses. AJR Am J Roentgenol. 2002;179:373–8.

53. Eshed I, Elias S, Sidi AA. Diagnostic value of CT-guided biopsy of indeterminate renal masses. Clin Radiol. 2004;59:262–7.

54. Volpe A, Kachura JR, Geddie WR, et al. Techniques, safety and accuracy of sampling of renal tumors by fine needle aspiration and core biopsy. J Urol. 2007;178:379–86.

55. Ralls PW, Barakos JA, Kaptein EM, et al. Renal biopsy-related hemorrhage: frequency and comparison of CT and sonography. J Comput Assist Tomogr. 1987;11:1031–4.

56. Nadel L, Baumgartner BR, Bernardino ME. Percutaneous renal biopsies: accuracy, safety, and indications. Urol Radiol. 1986;8:67–71.

57. Chung J, Caumartin Y, Warren J, Luke PP. Acute Page kidney following renal allograft biopsy: a complication requiring early recognition and treatment. Am J Transplant. 2008;8:1323–8.

58. Vassiliades VG, Bernardino ME. Percutaneous renal and adrenal biopsies. Cardiovasc Intervent Radiol. 1991;14:50–4.

59. Maturen KE, Nghiem HV, Caoili EM, Higgins EG, Wolf Jr JS, Wood Jr DP. Renal mass core biopsy: accuracy and impact on clinical management. AJR Am J Roentgenol. 2007;188:563–70.

60. Silver TM, Thornbury JR. Pneumothorax: a complication of percutaneous aspiration of upper pole renal masses. AJR Am J Roentgenol. 1977;128:451–2.

61. Hopper KD, Yakes WF. The posterior intercostal approach for percutaneous renal procedures: risk of puncturing the lung, spleen, and liver as determined by CT. AJR Am J Roentgenol. 1990;154:115–17.

62. vanSonnenberg E, Wittenberg J, Ferrucci Jr JT, Mueller PR, Simeone JF. Triangulation method for percutaneous needle guidance: the angled approach to upper abdominal masses. AJR Am J Roentgenol. 1981;137:757–61.

63. Herts BR, Baker ME. The current role of percutaneous biopsy in the evaluation of renal masses. Semin Urol Oncol. 1995;13:254–61.

64. Lebret T, Poulain JE, Molinie V, et al. Percutaneous core biopsy for renal masses: indications, accuracy and results. J Urol. 2007;178:1184–8. discussion 1188.

65. Vasudevan A, Davies RJ, Shannon BA, Cohen RJ. Incidental renal tumours: the frequency of benign lesions and the role of preoperative core biopsy. BJU Int. 2006;97:946–9.

66. Brierly RD, Thomas PJ, Harrison NW, Fletcher MS, Nawrocki JD, Ashton-Key M. Evaluation of fine-needle aspiration cytology for renal masses. BJU Int. 2000;85:14–8.

67. Beland MD, Mayo-Smith WW, Dupuy DE, Cronan JJ, DeLellis RA. Diagnostic yield of 58 consecutive imaging-guided biopsies of solid renal masses: should we biopsy all that are indeterminate? AJR Am J Roentgenol. 2007;188:792–7.

68. Schmidbauer J, Remzi M, Memarsadeghi M, et al. Diagnostic accuracy of computed tomography-guided percutaneous biopsy of renal masses. Eur Urol. 2008;53:1003–11.

69. Somani BK, Nabi G, Thorpe P, N'Dow J, Swami S, McClinton S. Image-guided biopsy-diagnosed renal cell carcinoma: critical appraisal of technique and long-term follow-up. Eur Urol. 2007;51:1289–95. discussion 1296–1287.

70. Slywotzky C, Maya M. Needle tract seeding of transitional cell carcinoma following fine-needle aspiration of a renal mass. Abdom Imaging. 1994;19:174–6.

71. Jain V, Ganpule A, Vyas J, et al. Management of non-neoplastic renal hemorrhage by transarterial embolization. Urology. 2009; 74:522–6.

72. Shannon BA, Cohen RJ, de Bruto H, Davies RJ. The value of preoperative needle core biopsy for diagnosing benign lesions among small, incidentally detected renal masses. J Urol. 2008;180:1257–61. discussion 1261.

73. Wang R, Wolf Jr JS, Wood Jr DP, Higgins EJ, Hafez KS. Accuracy of percutaneous core biopsy in management of small renal masses. Urology. 2009;73:586–90. discussion 590–581.

74. Truong LD, Todd TD, Dhurandhar B, Ramzy I. Fine-needle aspiration of renal masses in adults: analysis of results and diagnostic problems in 108 cases. Diagn Cytopathol. 1999;20:339–49.

75. Garcia-Solano J, Acosta-Ortega J, Perez-Guillermo M, Benedicto-Orovitg JM, Jimenez-Penick FJ. Solid renal masses in adults: image-guided fine-needle aspiration cytology and imaging techniques–"two heads better than one?". Diagn Cytopathol. 2008;36:8–12.

76. Cajulis RS, Katz RL, Dekmezian R, el-Naggar A, Ro JY. Fine needle aspiration biopsy of renal cell carcinoma. Cytologic parameters and their concordance with histology and flow cytometric data. Acta Cytol. 1993;37:367–72.

77. Cheville JC, Lohse CM, Zincke H, Weaver AL, Blute ML. Comparisons of outcome and prognostic features among histologic subtypes of renal cell carcinoma. Am J Surg Pathol. 2003;27:612–24.

78. Patard JJ, Leray E, Rioux-Leclercq N, et al. Prognostic value of histologic subtypes in renal cell carcinoma: a multicenter experience. J Clin Oncol. 2005;23:2763–71.

79. Upton MP, Parker RA, Youmans A, McDermott DF, Atkins MB. Histologic predictors of renal cell carcinoma response to interleukin-2-based therapy. J Immunother. 2005;28:488–95.

80. Atkins M, Regan M, McDermott D, et al. Carbonic anhydrase IX expression predicts outcome of interleukin 2 therapy for renal cancer. Clin Cancer Res. 2005;11:3714–21.

81. Barocas DA, Rohan SM, Kao J, et al. Diagnosis of renal tumors on needle biopsy specimens by histological and molecular analysis. J Urol. 2006;176:1957–62.

82. Al-Aynati M, Chen V, Salama S, Shuhaibar H, Treleaven D, Vincic L. Interobserver and intraobserver variability using the Fuhrman grading system for renal cell carcinoma. Arch Pathol Lab Med. 2003;127:593–6.

83. Liu J, Fanning CV. Can renal oncocytomas be distinguished from renal cell carcinoma on fine-needle aspiration specimens? A study of conventional smears in conjunction with ancillary studies. Cancer. 2001;93:390–7.

84. Fridman E, Dotan Z, Barshack I, et al. Accurate molecular classification of renal tumors using microRNA expression. J Mol Diagn. 2010;12:687–96.

85. Vieira J, Henrique R, Ribeiro FR, et al. Feasibility of differential diagnosis of kidney tumors by comparative genomic hybridization of fine needle aspiration biopsies. Genes Chromosomes Cancer. 2010;49:935–47.

86. Johnson NB, Johnson MM, Selig MK, Nielsen GP. Use of electron microscopy in core biopsy diagnosis of oncocytic renal tumors. Ultrastruct Pathol. 2010;34:189–94.

87. L'Hostis H, Deminiere C, Ferriere JM, Coindre JM. Renal angiomyolipoma: a clinicopathologic, immunohistochemical, and follow-up study of 46 cases. Am J Surg Pathol. 1999;23:1011–20.

88. Kim JK, Park SY, Shon JH, Cho KS. Angiomyolipoma with minimal fat: differentiation from renal cell carcinoma at biphasic helical CT. Radiology. 2004;230:677–84.

89. Jinzaki M, Tanimoto A, Narimatsu Y, et al. Angiomyolipoma: imaging findings in lesions with minimal fat. Radiology. 1997;205:497–502.

Percutaneous and Transjugular Kidney Biopsy

Judy U. Ahrar, Sanaz Javadi, and Kamran Ahrar

18

Background

Percutaneous sampling of renal cortical tissue, usually referred to as percutaneous renal biopsy (PRB), is performed to establish a diagnosis in acute kidney disease, to help decide if therapy is warranted, to help determine appropriate therapy, and to determine the degree of active (potentially reversible) or chronic (irreversible) kidney disease. When chronic changes predominate, a positive response to therapy is less likely. When patients are appropriately selected, the results of percutaneous renal biopsy affect the management of patients in up to 60 % of cases [1–4]. This chapter will cover the indications, contraindications, and techniques for percutaneous and transjugular renal biopsy as well as potential complications, management of complications, and outcomes and results.

Indications

Unexplained Acute Renal Failure

In most cases, acute renal failure is related to prerenal disease, acute tubular necrosis, or urinary tract obstruction. Clinical presentation, signs, symptoms, imaging studies, and laboratory tests are often adequate to identify the underlying pathology of acute renal failure; however, for assessment of acute renal failure of an unknown origin, most nephrologists perform a percutaneous renal biopsy [5]. In a worldwide survey of nephrologists, 20 % of respondents said they would perform a biopsy in the early stages of acute renal failure, 26 % said they would perform a biopsy after 1 week of nonrecovery, and 40 % said they would perform a biopsy after 4 weeks of nonrecovery [5].

Acute Nephritic Syndrome

Nephritic syndrome is characterized by hematuria, red blood cell casts in the urine, mild proteinuria, hypertension, and varying degrees of renal insufficiency. Acute nephritic syndrome may be caused by a variety of systemic diseases. A renal biopsy is often required to establish a specific diagnosis and to determine appropriate therapy.

Acute Nephrotic Syndrome

Nephrotic syndrome is characterized by severe proteinuria ($\geq$3.5 g/day), hypoalbuminemia, hyperlipidemia, and edema. When acute nephrotic syndrome is associated with amyloidosis, long-term diabetes mellitus, or hypertension, biopsy is not necessary. Renal biopsy is warranted in patients with active lupus nephritis. In the absence of a plausible cause for the development of nephrotic syndrome, renal biopsy can help determine the disease's etiology and can help determine appropriate therapy. In one study, renal biopsy for acute

J.U. Ahrar, MD
Department of Interventional Radiology,
The University of Texas MD Anderson Cancer Center,
1515 Holcombe Blvd., Unit 1471, Houston, TX 77030, USA
e-mail: judy.ahrar@mdanderson.org

S. Javadi, MD
Department of Radiology, Baylor College of Medicine,
One Baylor Plaza, Unit 360, Houston, TX 77030, USA
e-mail: sjavadi@bcm.edu

K. Ahrar, MD, FSIR (✉)
Department of Interventional Radiology,
Department of Thoracic and Cardiovascular Surgery,
The University of Texas MD Anderson Cancer Center,
1515 Holcombe Boulevard, Unit 1471, Houston, TX 77030, USA
e-mail: kahrar@mdanderson.org

K. Ahrar, S. Gupta (eds.), *Percutaneous Image-Guided Biopsy*,
DOI 10.1007/978-1-4614-8217-8_18, © Springer Science+Business Media New York 2014

nephrotic syndrome in adults altered management of the disease in 86 % of patients who were diagnosed with nephrotic syndrome [1].

Isolated Glomerular Hematuria

Renal biopsy is not necessary in patients who have isolated microscopic hematuria but are asymptomatic [5]. Renal biopsy in asymptomatic patients rarely changes the clinical management of the disease [1]. However, if a patient develops proteinuria or renal insufficiency during the follow-up period, a biopsy may be warranted.

Isolated Low-Grade Proteinuria

Isolated low-grade proteinuria (0.5–1.0 g/day) in the absence of glomerular hematuria or renal insufficiency does not warrant a renal biopsy; however, an increase in proteinuria or serum creatinine in the absence of a systemic disease such as diabetes warrants a renal biopsy.

Systemic Lupus Erythematosus

Nearly 50 % of patients with systemic lupus erythematosus develop renal disease within a year of diagnosis. Renal manifestations of various classes of systemic lupus erythematosus include asymptomatic hematuria, asymptomatic proteinuria, nephrotic syndrome, nephritic syndrome, acute renal failure, and chronic renal failure [6]. When a patient with systemic lupus erythematosus has any renal involvement, a renal biopsy is indicated to establish an initial pathologic diagnosis early in the course of the disease. The biopsy will determine the severity, activity, and chronicity of disease and will identify specific glomerular lesions as well as other concomitant lesions. Serial biopsies provide prognostic information that can guide therapy decisions and predict outcome in patients who may have a transformation to either a more aggressive or a less active form of the disease.

Chronic Renal Disease

The role of renal biopsy in patients with chronic kidney disease is more controversial. When significant parenchymal scarring is the predominant feature in the biopsy samples, pathologists may not be able to render a specific diagnosis, and the biopsy may not contribute greatly to the management of the disease. Moreover, the risk of bleeding from biopsy is higher in patients with chronic kidney disease [7]. On the other hand, a few studies have shown that even in patients with end-stage renal failure, a clinically unsuspected histology may be diagnosed in 10–48 % of patients with chronic kidney disease who underwent renal biopsy [8–10]. In other studies, renal biopsy led to a change in therapy in 23–40 % of patients with chronic kidney disease [1, 3, 11]. In general, renal biopsy is associated with a greater incidence of bleeding complications and fewer opportunities for therapy in patients who have prolonged (>6 months) elevated levels of serum creatinine [7].

Transplant Kidneys

Most nephrologists biopsy a transplanted kidney only in cases of graft failure, acute renal failure, slow but progressive deterioration of renal function, or nephritic proteinuria [5]. At some institutions, however, protocol dictates that biopsies be performed during periods of stable allograft renal function to detect subclinical acute rejection, a cause of graft failure, as treatment of subclinical acute rejection prolongs graft survival [12, 13]. Also, chronic allograft nephropathy, another cause of graft failure, can be detected on biopsy long before initial symptoms of renal dysfunction [14], and serial biopsies can quantify the progression of chronic transplant nephropathy in seemingly stable renal allografts [15]. Although some physicians believe that biopsy of renal allografts poses a significant risk to the patient and that the risk is greater than the benefit, a multicenter study of renal allograft biopsies demonstrated that the incidence of complications after biopsy of a stable renal transplant was low [12].

Contraindications

In the past, absolute contraindications for percutaneous renal biopsy included uncontrolled severe hypertension, uncontrollable bleeding diathesis, an uncooperative patient, and a solitary native kidney [16]. Previously, risk of significant hemorrhage leading to nephrectomy was believed to be too high to allow percutaneous biopsy of a solitary native kidney, and an open biopsy was recommended. More recent studies have demonstrated that percutaneous renal biopsy is safe and is well tolerated in patients with a solitary kidney [17, 18]. In fact, complication rates are higher with open renal biopsy than with percutaneous renal biopsy [7]. Other relative contraindications include small hyperechoic kidneys (<9 cm) suggestive of chronic irreversible disease, multiple bilateral renal cysts or tumors, hydronephrosis, active renal or perirenal infection, and anatomic abnormalities of the kidney that may increase the risk of complications. Old age and pregnancy are not contraindications for percutaneous renal biopsy as renal biopsy can be safely performed in very elderly patients and in pregnant patients when necessary [19–27].

Technique

Imaging

Currently, most percutaneous renal biopsies are performed using real-time ultrasonography guidance [17, 28]. The operator visualizes the kidney on ultrasound, measures the length of the kidney, notes any anatomic abnormalities (including cysts, tumors, or hydronephrosis), and identifies an appropriate target for tissue sampling (usually the lower pole of the kidney) (Fig. 18.1). The real-time guidance provided by ultrasonography places the needle accurately in the target renal parenchyma and avoids injury to the kidney or nearby organs (Fig. 18.2) [29, 30]. With markedly obese patients or small echogenic kidneys, ultrasonography may be of limited utility. Under these circumstances, computed tomography can be used for needle guidance (Fig. 18.3) [28].

Devices

When percutaneous renal biopsy was first introduced, 14-gauge manual needles (e.g., Tru-Cut) were used to obtain large samples of renal cortical tissue. Subsequently, spring-loaded biopsy

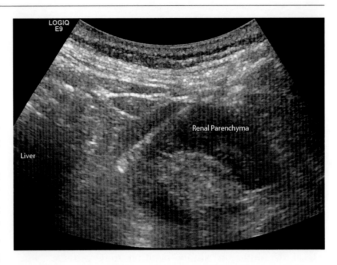

Fig. 18.2 A 47-year-old woman with multiple myeloma and renal dysfunction. Ultrasound-guided biopsy of the right renal cortex

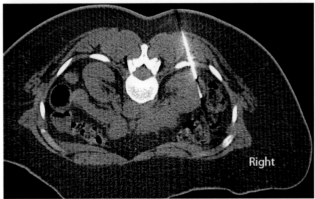

Fig. 18.3 A 73-year-old woman with morbid obesity and renal dysfunction of unknown etiology. CT guidance was chosen for biopsy of the right renal cortex due to the patient's body habitus. Axial CT image of the abdomen in prone position shows the biopsy needle inserted into the lateral aspect of the right kidney

needles were introduced to clinical practice and have increasingly gained popularity. Large-gauge (14 gauge) manual needles provide a large number of glomeruli per core biopsy sample [31, 32]. Automated needles provide more glomeruli per core biopsy than provided by manual biopsy needles of the same gauge [33, 34]. For needles of similar gauge, there is no difference in the number of complications between manual and spring-loaded needles [33], but when 14-gauge manual needles were compared to smaller automated needles, there were fewer complications with the smaller automated needles [31, 35, 36]. In addition to the needle size and mechanism of action, the number of cores taken during the biopsy helps determine the success of the procedure. Some investigators recommend obtaining at least two core biopsy samples from the kidney [17, 28, 37].

For patients at high risk of bleeding complications, a transjugular biopsy was recommended using a modified Colapinto transjugular hepatic biopsy system [38]. More

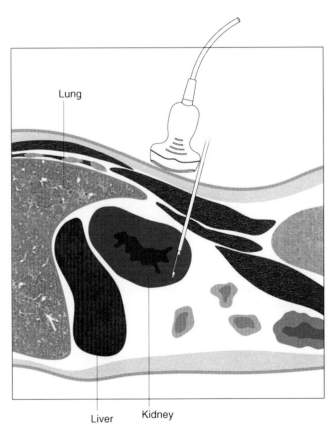

Fig. 18.1 Illustration of an ultrasound-guided renal biopsy in the sagittal plane shows sampling of the renal cortex from the inferior pole. The right kidney is most commonly selected due to its more caudal location, compared to the left

recently, 19-gauge, 70-cm, side-cutting, spring-loaded biopsy needles have become available for transjugular renal biopsy [39].

Approaches, Relevant Anatomy, and Technical Considerations

Percutaneous renal biopsies are usually performed with the patient in a prone position, providing access to both kidneys (Fig. 18.3). In patients with systemic disease affecting the kidneys, either kidney can be biopsied to determine a diagnosis. However, care must be taken to avoid an atrophic kidney with an underlying chronic abnormality. Occasionally, a lateral decubitus or sitting position may provide better access, a safer approach, or more comfort for an obese or pregnant patient (Fig. 18.4). The lower pole of the kidney is usually selected for nontarget renal biopsy to decrease the risk of hemorrhagic complications (Fig. 18.1). Imaging immediately prior to the biopsy can help identify renal cysts and tumors; ideally, renal cysts or tumors should not be traversed to reach the renal cortex. Biopsy may be performed with or without the use of a coaxial guide needle.

A transvenous renal biopsy has been advocated for patients who have thrombocytopenia, coagulopathy, or a solitary kidney; who are morbidly obese, in whom percutaneous biopsy has failed; or who may require simultaneous renal and hepatic or cardiac biopsy (Fig. 18.5) [39–41]. The risk of perinephric bleeding is reduced because the renal capsule is not punctured in transjugular renal biopsy. For transjugular renal biopsy, the patient is placed in a supine position on the angiography table. Ultrasonography is used to access the jugular vein. The right internal jugular vein is preferred, but either the right or left internal or external jugular vein may serve as the initial access site. Initial reports of the transjugular technique described aspiration of renal tissue through a modified Colapinto needle [38]. More recently, a spring-loaded biopsy gun with a 19-gauge side-cutting needle has produced good results [39, 41]. The renal access and biopsy set (RABS-100; Cook, Bloomington, IN) has several components: a 7-French introducer sheath with stiffening cannula, a 5-French 90-cm multipurpose catheter, and a 19-gauge 70-cm Quick-Core biopsy needle. After gaining access to the jugular vein, a 9-French introducer sheath is placed. The renal vein is selected using the multipurpose catheter. The right renal vein is preferred owing to the more favorable angle and shorter course from the inferior vena cava. A subcortical vein in the lower pole of the kidney is then selected. With the catheter pushed into the periphery of the selected vein, contrast medium is injected to opacify a wedge of renal parenchyma. Over a guidewire, the catheter is removed, and the 7-French introducer sheath with stiffening cannula is advanced to the same location. Next, the Quick-Core spring-loaded needle

is inserted into the cannula. The cannula is rotated laterally and posteriorly. The needle is advanced into the renal cortex and a tissue sample is obtained. Several tissue samples can be obtained while maintaining access with the cannula. In one study, up to five tissue samples were obtained [39]. In another study, See et al. reported a modification of this technique using a long flexible 7-French sheath instead of the stiff cannula [41]. The sheath was advanced over a guidewire into the peripheral subcortical vein. In absence of the stiff metallic cannula, the needle tip must be protected by a catheter prior to insertion into the sheath. A 70-cm-long 19-gauge Quick-Core biopsy needle was loaded into a 60- or 65-cm 5-French straight catheter with the catheter covering the tip of the needle. The assembly was then loaded into the 7-French sheath and was advanced to the biopsy target area. The catheter was pulled back exposing the needle tip to obtain a tissue sample.

Potential Complications

Varying degrees of bleeding may be encountered after percutaneous renal biopsy [17, 18, 28, 37, 42–44] (Table 18.1). Percutaneous renal biopsy often results in perinephric hemorrhage. Generally, perinephric bleeding is slight and self-limiting and does not require therapy (Fig. 18.6). However, a retroperitoneal hematoma can enlarge rapidly and cause signs and symptoms of blood loss (Fig. 18.7). Both percutaneous and transjugular renal biopsy may also cause bleeding into the collecting system, resulting in microscopic or gross hematuria, but this form of hemorrhage is often self-limiting. Gross hematuria may result in blood clots that can cause ureteral obstruction. Persistent hematuria may be a sign of arteriovenous fistula formation. In up to 18 % of patients who underwent renal biopsy, arteriovenous fistulas were identified using color Duplex sonography [17, 45]. Although most of these arteriovenous fistulas resolve spontaneously with time [35], occasionally persistent hematuria, hypertension, or high-output heart failure may be encountered. In a transplanted kidney, arteriovenous fistula may cause renal insufficiency [45]. Finally, a subcapsular hematoma, if large enough, may exert pressure on the renal parenchyma, leading to pain and pressure. In a Page kidney, a large subcapsular hematoma exerts sufficient pressure to induce ischemia, activating the renin-angiotensin system, which can lead to chronic hypertension [46–48]. Most clinically significant bleeding complications are identified within 24 h [49]. Major risk factors for bleeding include thrombocytopenia, coagulopathy, hypertension, renal insufficiency, and anemia [28, 43, 49–51]. The risk of mortality from percutaneous renal biopsy is less than 0.1 % [28, 44, 52].

Some researchers have recommended that patients should be observed in a supine position for 4–6 h and then remain

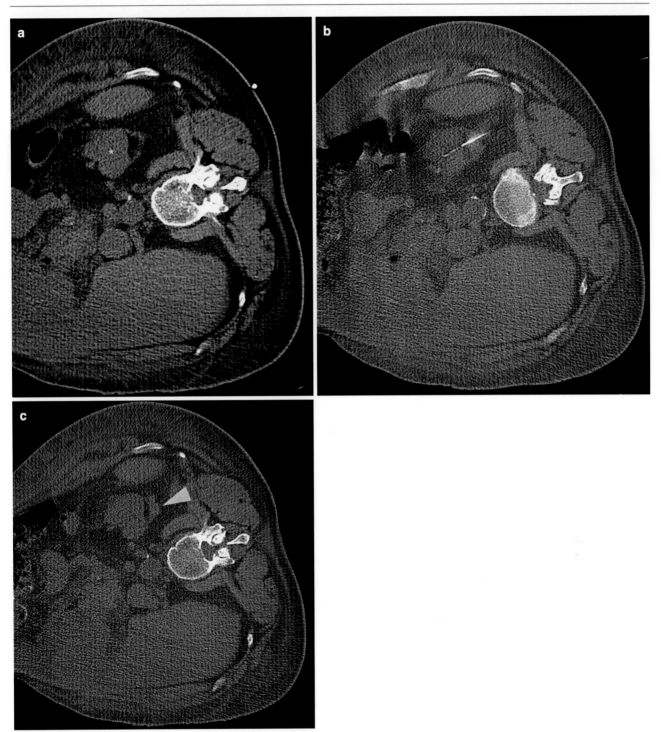

Fig. 18.4 A 62-year-old man with colon carcinoma and renal dysfunction. CT-guided renal biopsy was performed in the right decubitus position due to the patient's body habitus. Axial CT image of the abdomen in right lateral decubitus position (**a**) shows the left renal parenchyma (*) surrounded by perinephric fat. CT image during the biopsy (**b**) shows small perinephric hemorrhage. The hematoma (*arrowhead*) remained stable several minutes after removing the biopsy needle (**c**)

on bed rest overnight. Close to 90 % of complications are identified within 12 h after biopsy [49], and over 90 % of complications are detected within 24 h after biopsy. Determining the optimum observation time after renal biopsy

requires consideration of both healthcare cost and patient safety [53]. Several studies have claimed that observation for 12 h after renal biopsy is safe and cost-effective [51, 54, 55]. In a study of 44 patients, postrenal biopsy hematuria was

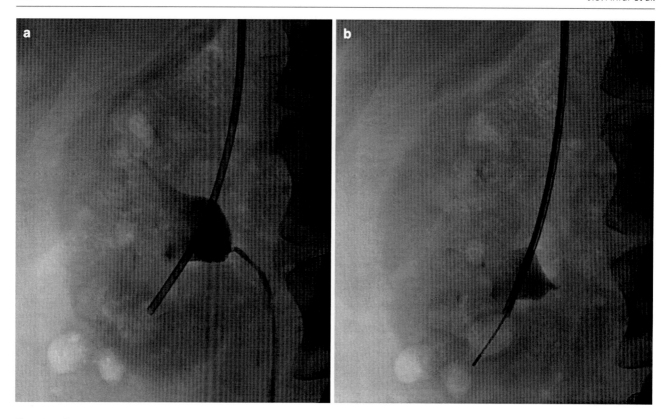

Fig. 18.5 Transjugular kidney biopsy. Fluoroscopic image of the right kidney (**a**) shows the introducer sheath in the lower pole of the kidney. The core biopsy needle with a blunt tip (**b**) is inserted into the renal cortex to obtain a biopsy sample (Images courtesy of Sanjay Misra, M.D.)

Table 18.1 Incidence of bleeding after percutaneous renal biopsy

Type of bleeding	Incidence
Transient microscopic hematuria	Nearly 100 %
Transient gross hematuria	3–18 %
Decrease in hemoglobin 1 g/dL or more	Nearly 50 %
Severe bleeding causing hypotension	1–2 %
Severe bleeding requiring transfusion	Up to 6 %
Surgery required to control bleeding	0.1–0.4 %
Severe bleeding leading to nephrectomy	Nearly 0.3 %
Risk of mortality	0.02–0.1 %

detected in 52 % of patients within ≤2 h, 85 % within ≤4 h, and 97.7 % within ≤6 h after biopsy [55].

Management of Complications

In the past, surgery was recommended to control severe or persistent bleeding caused by percutaneous renal biopsy and may have resulted in nephrectomy in a small number of patients [56]. At the time of this writing, angiography and selective embolization is the treatment of choice in patients with life-threatening or persistent bleeding and/or symptomatic arteriovenous fistula. In most cases, selective embolization guided by angiography can easily manage the bleeding and preserve the remainder of the kidney (Fig. 18.8) [57].

Outcomes and Results

In cases of kidney disease, renal biopsy samples are routinely evaluated by light microscopy, immunofluorescent microscopy, and electron microscopy following optimal preservation, thin-tissue sectioning (2–3 μm thick), and use of special stains (e.g., periodic acid-Schiff, Jones' silver, or trichome) [6, 58]. The goal is to comprehensively evaluate all components of the renal parenchyma including glomeruli, tubules, vessels, and interstitium. An adequate tissue sample is a prerequisite for successful pathologic evaluation. However, the definition of tissue adequacy varies among studies. It is almost impossible to arrive at an absolute number of glomeruli necessary to make a definitive diagnosis in every case. Some investigators believe that up to 20 glomeruli are needed for complete qualitative and quantitative evaluation of interstitial tubular and glomerular parameters [59]. Others believe that an adequate sample contains at least five glomeruli [60]. For most cases, tissue samples are considered adequate if they contain five or more glomeruli for light microscopy, two or more glomeruli for immunofluorescent microscopy, and at least one glomerulus for electron microscopy. Immunofluorescent studies require fresh tissue from a frozen sample, but the immunoperoxidase technique may be used instead to utilize tissue that was fixed in formalin [61]. When automated biopsy needles that are 18-gauge or larger

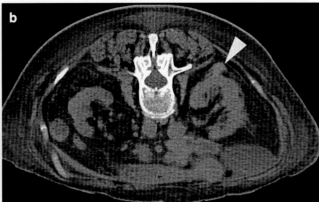

Fig. 18.6 An 82-year-old woman with toxic goiter and acute renal failure was referred for percutaneous renal biopsy. Axial CT image of the patient in prone position (**a**) shows small left kidney; biopsy samples were obtained from the right kidney. Immediately after the biopsy, CT image of the abdomen (**b**) shows a small right perinephric hematoma (*arrowhead*). There were no clinical consequences

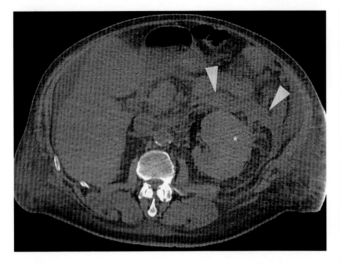

Fig. 18.7 The patient in Fig. 18.4 returned to the emergency center 3 days after the renal biopsy complaining of left flank pain. A non-contrast CT of the abdomen reveals a large retroperitoneal (*arrowheads*) and subcapsular (***) hematoma. He was admitted for conservative management with transfusion of packed red blood cells

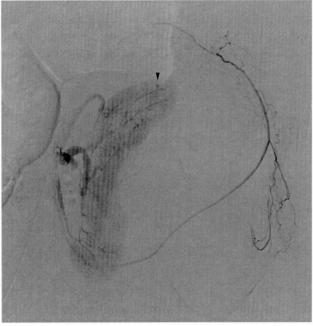

Fig. 18.8 The patient from Fig. 18.4 failed to stabilize after 3 days of conservative management and transfusion. An angiogram was performed. Diagnostic left renal angiogram in the parenchymal phase shows a small pseudoaneurysm (*arrowhead*) in the superior pole of the kidney, in the region of the biopsy. The arterial branch was successfully embolized with no further clinical evidence of bleeding. Note the stretching of the capsular artery and deformation of the renal parenchyma from the large subcapsular hematoma

are used to obtain at least two tissue samples from the kidney, adequate tissue can be obtained in the majority of cases [29–36, 62, 63] (Table 18.2). Automated 18-gauge biopsy needles that are currently used pose less risk of postbiopsy hemorrhage than by the manual 14-gauge biopsy needles used in the past [35, 60]. Riehl et al. also found that complication rates were lower in biopsies of transplanted kidneys than in biopsies of native kidneys [35].

Transjugular renal biopsy has been shown to be effective in obtaining adequate tissue samples in high-risk patients [38, 39, 41, 64–68] (Table 18.3). In one study, 1 to 5 (mean 1.8) core biopsies were obtained using an automated biopsy gun with a 19-gauge needle [39]. Overall, the amount of renal tissue was sufficient to make a firm diagnosis in 92 % of the patients. On average, tissue samples examined by light microscopy contained 5 glomeruli, samples examined by immunofluorescent microscopy contained 2 glomeruli, and samples examined by electron microscopy contained 2.2 glomeruli.

In summary, image-guided biopsy of renal cortex is an important tool in the workup and follow-up of patients with medical renal disease and those with transplant kidneys. Up to

Table 18.2 Percutaneous renal biopsy outcomes

Reference	Number of biopsies	Needle size	Number of glomeruli	Percentage diagnostic biopsy
Wiseman et al. [29]	24	14 G, 18 G	12 per specimen	96 %
Doyle et al. [31]	69	14 G Tru-Cut, 18 G	21.7 per core	96 %
	86		16.7	99 %
Kim et al. [32]	67	14 G Tru-Cut, 18 G	15.3 ± 8.4 per core	100 %
	99		9.95 ± 6.9	
Burstein et al. [33]	232	14 G Tru-Cut, 18 G	28 ± 15 per bx	93.5 % total
	91		21 ± 13	
Feneberg et al. [34]	252	Silverman 14 G, Tru-Cut 14 G, automated 14 G	22.3 ± 14.4 per core	95.8 %[a]
	568		26.6 ± 13.1	95.7 %
	262		32.1 ± 12.4	96 %
Riehl et al. [35]	231	14 G Tru-Cut, 18 G	9.5 ± 4.9 per core	93.5 %
	227		8.7 ± 5.6	96.5 %
Nyman et al. [36]	235	Tru-Cut, Gun bx	>15 g: Tru-Cut 46 %(107), Gun bx 45 %(96)	90 %
	213		6–15 g: Tru-Cut 33 %(78), Gun bx 39 %(84)	95 %
			1–5 g: Tru-Cut 11 %(26), Gun bx 13 %(27)	
			0 g: Tru-Cut 10 %(24), Gun bx 3 %(6)	
Maya et al. [54]	100	16 G, 18 G	12.7 ± 9.7 per patient	100 %
Nicholson et al. [62]	33	14 G	14.5 ± 8.9	88 %
	33	16 G	11.2 ± 8.3	94 %
	34	18 G	8.5 ± 5.8	88 %
Pasquariello et al. [63]	249	14 G	22 per specimen	92 %

Abbreviations: *G* gauge, *bx* biopsy, *g* glomeruli
[a]Results reported in native kidneys

Table 18.3 Transjugular renal biopsy outcomes

Reference	Patients/ biopsies	Needle size	Number of glomeruli	Percentage diagnostic biopsies
Cluzel et al. [38]	400/383	18 G	9.8 ± 7.6 per core	95 %
Misra et al. [39]	39/38	19 G	5 ± 3.8 per core	92 %
See et al. [41]	59/56	Quick-Core (19 G)	10.3 per bx	94.6 %
Abbott et al. [64]	9/10	Quick-Core (14 G)	9 ± 8 per core	90 %
Jouet et al. [65]	70/70	15 G	10 ± 1 per bx	78.6 %
Mal et al. [66]	195/200	15 G	10 ± 6 per core	90 %[a]
Sam et al. [67]	29/29	18 G	19.4 ± 12.2 per bx	96.5 %
Thompson et al. [68]	23/23	18 or 19 G	9.9 per bx	91.3 %

Abbreviations: *G* gauge, *bx* biopsy, *g* glomeruli
[a]Renal tissue samples were obtained in 176 of 200 patients (88 %); renal tissue samples were histologically diagnostic in 159 of 176 patients (90 %)

6 % of patients undergoing percutaneous biopsy may develop severe hemorrhage. Transjugular renal biopsy of native kidneys may be used in patients with high risk of bleeding.

References

1. Richards NT, Darby S, Howie AJ, Adu D, Michael J. Knowledge of renal histology alters patient management in over 40% of cases. Nephrol Dial Transplant. 1994;9:1255–9.
2. Pfister M, Jakob S, Frey FJ, Niederer U, Schmidt M, Marti HP. Judgment analysis in clinical nephrology. Am J Kidney Dis. 1999;34:569–75.
3. Cohen AH, Nast CC, Adler SG, Kopple JD. Clinical utility of kidney biopsies in the diagnosis and management of renal disease. Am J Nephrol. 1989;9:309–15.
4. McGregor DO, Lynn KL, Bailey RR, Robson RA, Gardner J. Clinical audit of the use of renal biopsy in the management of isolated microscopic hematuria. Clin Nephrol. 1998;49:345–8.
5. Fuiano G, Mazza G, Comi N, et al. Current indications for renal biopsy: a questionnaire-based survey. Am J Kidney Dis. 2000;35:448–57.
6. Seshan SV, Jennette JC. Renal disease in systemic lupus erythematosus with emphasis on classification of lupus glomerulonephritis: advances and implications. Arch Pathol Lab Med. 2009;133:233–48.
7. Joseph AJ, Compton SP, Holmes LH, et al. Utility of percutaneous renal biopsy in chronic kidney disease. Nephrology (Carlton). 2010;15:544–8.

8. Curtis JJ, Rakowski TA, Argy Jr WP, Schreiner GE. Evaluation of percutaneous kidney biopsy in advanced renal failure. Nephron. 1976;17:259–69.

9. Kropp KA, Shapiro RS, Jhunjhunwala JS. Role of renal biopsy in end stage renal failure. Urology. 1978;12:631–4.

10. Sobh M, Moustafa F, Ghoniem M. Value of renal biopsy in chronic renal failure. Int Urol Nephrol. 1988;20:77–83.

11. Turner MW, Hutchinson TA, Barre PE, Prichard S, Jothy S. A prospective study on the impact of the renal biopsy in clinical management. Clin Nephrol. 1986;26:217–21.

12. Furness PN, Philpott CM, Chorbadjian MT, et al. Protocol biopsy of the stable renal transplant: a multicenter study of methods and complication rates. Transplantation. 2003;76:969–73.

13. Rush D, Nickerson P, Gough J, et al. Beneficial effects of treatment of early subclinical rejection: a randomized study. J Am Soc Nephrol. 1998;9:2129–34.

14. Seron D, Moreso F, Ramon JM, et al. Protocol renal allograft biopsies and the design of clinical trials aimed to prevent or treat chronic allograft nephropathy. Transplantation. 2000;69:1849–55.

15. Moreso F, Lopez M, Vallejos A, et al. Serial protocol biopsies to quantify the progression of chronic transplant nephropathy in stable renal allografts. Am J Transplant. 2001;1:82–8.

16. Health and Public Policy Committee, American College of Physicians. Clinical competence in percutaneous renal biopsy. Ann Intern Med. 1988;108:301–3.

17. Madaio MP. Renal biopsy. Kidney Int. 1990;38:529–43.

18. Mendelssohn DC, Cole EH. Outcomes of percutaneous kidney biopsy, including those of solitary native kidneys. Am J Kidney Dis. 1995;26:580–5.

19. Haas M, Spargo BH, Wit FJ, Meehan SM. Etiologies and outcome of acute renal insufficiency in older adults: a renal biopsy study of 259 cases. Am J Kidney Dis. 2000;35:433–47.

20. Kohli HS, Jairam A, Bhat A, et al. Safety of kidney biopsy in elderly: a prospective study. Int Urol Nephrol. 2006;38:815–20.

21. Uezono S, Hara S, Sato Y, et al. Renal biopsy in elderly patients: a clinicopathological analysis. Ren Fail. 2006;28:549–55.

22. Moutzouris DA, Herlitz L, Appel GB, et al. Renal biopsy in the very elderly. Clin J Am Soc Nephrol. 2009;4:1073–82.

23. Packham D, Fairley KF. Renal biopsy: indications and complications in pregnancy. Br J Obstet Gynaecol. 1987;94:935–9.

24. Chen HH, Lin HC, Yeh JC, Chen CP. Renal biopsy in pregnancies complicated by undetermined renal disease. Acta Obstet Gynecol Scand. 2001;80:888–93.

25. Kuller JA, D'Andrea NM, McMahon MJ. Renal biopsy and pregnancy. Am J Obstet Gynecol. 2001;184:1093–6.

26. Lindheimer MD, Davison JM. Renal biopsy during pregnancy: 'to b… or not to b…?'. Br J Obstet Gynaecol. 1987;94:932–4.

27. Day C, Hewins P, Hildebrand S, et al. The role of renal biopsy in women with kidney disease identified in pregnancy. Nephrol Dial Transplant. 2008;23:201–6.

28. Korbet SM. Percutaneous renal biopsy. Semin Nephrol. 2002;22:254–67.

29. Wiseman DA, Hawkins R, Numerow LM, Taub KJ. Percutaneous renal biopsy utilizing real time, ultrasonic guidance and a semiautomated biopsy device. Kidney Int. 1990;38:347–9.

30. Maya ID, Maddela P, Barker J, Allon M. Percutaneous renal biopsy: comparison of blind and real-time ultrasound-guided technique. Semin Dial. 2007;20:355–8.

31. Doyle AJ, Gregory MC, Terreros DA. Percutaneous native renal biopsy: comparison of a 1.2-mm spring-driven system with a traditional 2-mm hand-driven system. Am J Kidney Dis. 1994;23:498–503.

32. Kim D, Kim H, Shin G, et al. A randomized, prospective, comparative study of manual and automated renal biopsies. Am J Kidney Dis. 1998;32:426–31.

33. Burstein DM, Korbet SM, Schwartz MM. The use of the automatic core biopsy system in percutaneous renal biopsies: a comparative study. Am J Kidney Dis. 1993;22:545–52.

34. Feneberg R, Schaefer F, Zieger B, Waldherr R, Mehls O, Scharer K. Percutaneous renal biopsy in children: a 27-year experience. Nephron. 1998;79:438–46.

35. Riehl J, Maigatter S, Kierdorf H, Schmitt H, Maurin N, Sieberth HG. Percutaneous renal biopsy: comparison of manual and automated puncture techniques with native and transplanted kidneys. Nephrol Dial Transplant. 1994;9:1568–74.

36. Nyman RS, Cappelen-Smith J, al Suhaibani H, Alfurayh O, Shakweer W, Akhtar M. Yield and complications in percutaneous renal biopsy. A comparison between ultrasound-guided gun-biopsy and manual techniques in native and transplant kidneys. Acta Radiol. 1997;38:431–6.

37. Appel GB. Renal biopsy: how effective, what technique, and how safe. J Nephrol. 1993;6:4.

38. Cluzel P, Martinez F, Bellin MF, et al. Transjugular versus percutaneous renal biopsy for the diagnosis of parenchymal disease: comparison of sampling effectiveness and complications. Radiology. 2000;215:689–93.

39. Misra S, Gyamlani G, Swaminathan S, et al. Safety and diagnostic yield of transjugular renal biopsy. J Vasc Interv Radiol. 2008;19:546–51.

40. Stiles KP, Yuan CM, Chung EM, Lyon RD, Lane JD, Abbott KC. Renal biopsy in high-risk patients with medical diseases of the kidney. Am J Kidney Dis. 2000;36:419–33.

41. See TC, Thompson BC, Howie AJ, et al. Transjugular renal biopsy: our experience and technical considerations. Cardiovasc Intervent Radiol. 2008;31:906–18.

42. Stratta P, Canavese C, Marengo M, et al. Risk management of renal biopsy: 1387 cases over 30 years in a single centre. Eur J Clin Invest. 2007;37:954–63.

43. Shidham GB, Siddiqi N, Beres JA, et al. Clinical risk factors associated with bleeding after native kidney biopsy. Nephrology (Carlton). 2005;10:305–10.

44. Parrish AE. Complications of percutaneous renal biopsy: a review of 37 years' experience. Clin Nephrol. 1992;38:135–41.

45. Harrison KL, Nghiem HV, Coldwell DM, Davis CL. Renal dysfunction due to an arteriovenous fistula in a transplant recipient. J Am Soc Nephrol. 1994;5:1300–6.

46. Patel MD, Phillips CJ, Young SW, et al. US-guided renal transplant biopsy: efficacy of a cortical tangential approach. Radiology. 2010;256:290–6.

47. McCune TR, Stone WJ, Breyer JA. Page kidney: case report and review of the literature. Am J Kidney Dis. 1991;18:593–9.

48. Bakri RS, Prime M, Haydar A, Glass J, Goldsmith DJ. Three 'Pages' in a chapter of accidents. Nephrol Dial Transplant. 2003;18:1917–19.

49. Whittier WL, Korbet SM. Timing of complications in percutaneous renal biopsy. J Am Soc Nephrol. 2004;15:142–7.

50. Nass K, O'Neill WC. Bedside renal biopsy: ultrasound guidance by the nephrologist. Am J Kidney Dis. 1999;34:955–9.

51. Eiro M, Katoh T, Watanabe T. Risk factors for bleeding complications in percutaneous renal biopsy. Clin Exp Nephrol. 2005;9:40–5.

52. Schow DA, Vinson RK, Morrisseau PM. Percutaneous renal biopsy of the solitary kidney: a contraindication? J Urol. 1992;147:1235–7.

53. Yuan CM, Jindal RM, Abbott KC. Biopsy: observation time after kidney biopsy: when to discharge? Nat Rev Nephrol. 2009;5:552–4.

54. Maya ID, Allon M. Percutaneous renal biopsy: outpatient observation without hospitalization is safe. Semin Dial. 2009;22(4):458–61.

55. Al-Hweish AK, Abdul-Rehaman IS. Outpatient percutaneous renal biopsy in adult patients. Saudi J Kidney Dis Transpl. 2007;18:541–6.

56. Toledo K, Perez MJ, Espinosa M, et al. Complications associated with percutaneous renal biopsy in Spain, 50 years later. Nefrologia. 2010;30:539–43.

57. Jain V, Ganpule A, Vyas J, et al. Management of non-neoplastic renal hemorrhage by transarterial embolization. Urology. 2009;74:522–6.

58. Haas M. A reevaluation of routine electron microscopy in the examination of native renal biopsies. J Am Soc Nephrol. 1997; |8:70–6.

59. Oberholzer M, Torhorst J, Perret E, Mihatsch MJ. Minimum sample size of kidney biopsies for semiquantitative and quantitative evaluation. Nephron. 1983;34:192–5.

60. Bolton WK. Nonhemorrhagic decrements in hematocrit values after percutaneous renal biopsy. JAMA. 1977;238:1266–8.

61. Molne J, Breimer ME, Svalander CT. Immunoperoxidase versus immunofluorescence in the assessment of human renal biopsies. Am J Kidney Dis. 2005;45:674–83.

62. Nicholson ML, Wheatley TJ, Doughman TM, et al. A prospective randomized trial of three different sizes of core-cutting needle for renal transplant biopsy. Kidney Int. 2000;58:390–5.

63. Pasquariello A, Innocenti M, Batini V, et al. Theoretical calculation of optimal depth in the percutaneous native kidney biopsy to drastically reduce bleeding complications and sample inadequacy for histopathological diagnosis. Nephrol Dial Transplant. 2007;22:3516–20.

64. Abbott KC, Yuan CM, Batty DS, Lane JD, Stiles KP. Transjugular biopsy in patients with combined renal and liver disease: making every organ count. Am J Kidney Dis. 2001;37:1304–7.

65. Jouet P, Meyrier A, Mal F, et al. Transjugular renal biopsy in the treatment of patients with cirrhosis and renal abnormalities. Hepatology. 1996;24:1143–7.

66. Mal F, Meyrier A, Callard P, Kleinknecht D, Altmann JJ, Beaugrand M. The diagnostic yield of transjugular renal biopsy. Experience in 200 cases. Kidney Int. 1992;41:445–9.

67. Sam R, Leehey DJ, Picken MM, et al. Transjugular renal biopsy in patients with liver disease. Am J Kidney Dis. 2001;37:1144–51.

68. Thompson BC, Kingdon E, Johnston M, et al. Transjugular kidney biopsy. Am J Kidney Dis. 2004;43:651–62.

Nodes and Soft Tissue Masses Involving the Retroperitoneum, Mesentery, Omentum, and Peritoneal Ligaments

19

Colette M. Shaw, Bruno C. Odisio, Rony Avritscher, and David C. Madoff

Background

Disease within the intraperitoneal and retroperitoneal spaces is usually the result of a systemic process or local organ pathology. Primary pathological processes are uncommon and often elude detection in the early stages of disease. Clinical symptoms and signs, when present, are frequently nonspecific. The detection, characterization, and staging of disease in the soft tissues of the abdominal cavity are almost entirely dependent on cross-sectional imaging.

The intraperitoneal and retroperitoneal spaces, the mesenteries, and peritoneal ligaments are usually not apparent on imaging studies unless distended or outlined by fluid or air. Rapid acquisition times and thin slice collimation available with multidetector computed tomography (MDCT) enable assessment of blood vessels, lymph nodes, and fascial planes within these anatomical spaces. The radiologist's ability to identify subtle peritoneal disease and distinguish tumor deposits and lymph nodes from adjacent vessels and

bowel has been enhanced by the development of picture archiving systems, digitalized image interpretation, and post-processing tools, e.g., multiplanar reformatting.

This chapter addresses the percutaneous biopsy of soft tissue masses within the retroperitoneum and the mesenteries of the peritoneal cavity. The discussion begins with a brief overview of the relevant anatomy, the mechanisms by which disease may spread between and within these spaces, and a reminder of the diverse differential diagnoses for a mass lesion in these anatomic regions.

Anatomy

The peritoneal cavity is a potential space between the parietal and visceral peritoneum and comprises the greater and lesser sacs (Fig. 19.1). Within the peritoneal cavity are a number of double-layered folds of peritoneum. These include the small bowel mesentery, the transverse and sigmoid mesocolons, the greater and lesser omentum, and several peritoneal ligaments. The mesentery encloses an organ and connects it to the abdominal wall. An omentum is a multilayered fold of peritoneum that extends from the stomach to adjacent organs. The lesser omentum joins the lesser curve of the stomach and proximal duodenum to the liver. The greater omentum is a 4-layered fold of peritoneum that hangs from the greater curve of the stomach [1].

The retroperitoneum lies between the parietal peritoneum anteriorly and the transversalis fascia posteriorly. It is divided into three compartments by well-defined fascial planes. The perirenal space is enclosed by Gerota's fascia. It extends across the midline, abuts the bare area of the liver on the right, and the subphrenic space on the left. It communicates with the mediastinum via the diaphragmatic hiatus. The posterior pararenal space is open toward the pelvis inferiorly but bound superiorly by fusion of the quadratus lumborum fascia and the posterior perirenal fascia. The anterior pararenal space communicates across the midline, superiorly it extends to the dome of the diaphragm and mediastinum, inferiorly it

C.M. Shaw, MD
Division of Interventional Radiology,
Thomas Jefferson University Hospital,
132 South 10th Street Suite 766 Main Building,
Philadelphia, PA 19107, USA
e-mail: colette.shaw@jefferson.edu

B.C. Odisio, MD • R. Avritscher, MD
Department of Interventional Radiology,
Division of Diagnostic Imaging,
The University of Texas MD Anderson Cancer Center,
Houston, TX 77030, USA
e-mail: bruno.odisio@gmail.com;
rony.avritscher@mdanderson.org

D.C. Madoff, MD (✉)
Division of Interventional Radiology,
Department of Radiology,
New York-Presbyterian Hospital/
Weill Cornell Medical Center, 525 E 68th Street,
New York, NY 10065, USA
e-mail: dcm9006@med.correll.edu

K. Ahrar, S. Gupta (eds.), *Percutaneous Image-Guided Biopsy*,
DOI 10.1007/978-1-4614-8217-8_19, © Springer Science+Business Media New York 2014

Fig. 19.1 Ligaments and
peritoneal spaces in upper
abdomen. *A* – lesser omentum,
B – greater peritoneal cavity,
C – gastrosplenic ligament,
D – lesser sac, *E* – splenorenal
ligament, *K* – kidney, *L* – liver,
S – spleen, *St* – stomach

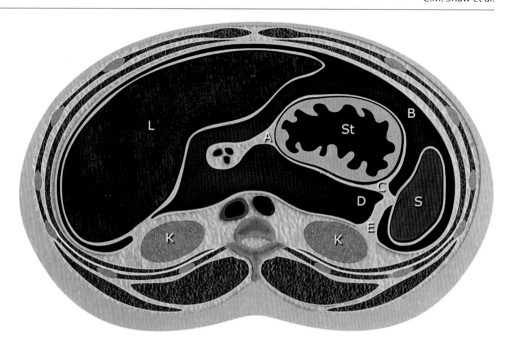

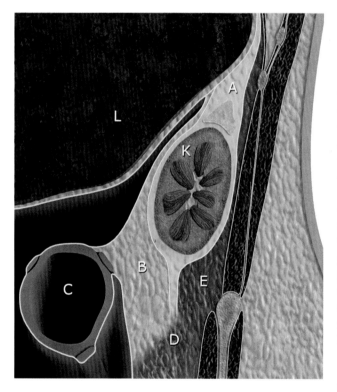

Fig. 19.2 Retroperitoneal compartments. *A* – perirenal space contains
the kidney, the adrenal gland, the proximal ureter, and fat; *B* – anterior
pararenal space contains the pancreas, duodenum, ascending and
descending colon, and fat; *C* – transverse colon; *D* – infrarenal retroperitoneal space; *E* – posterior pararenal space contains fat, lymph
nodes, nerves, and blood vessels; *K* – kidney; *L* – liver

communicates with the pelvis, and below the inferior renal
cone it communicates with the posterior pararenal space
(Fig. 19.2) [2].

Pathways for Spread of Disease in the Abdominal Cavity

An understanding of the possible mechanisms by which disease can spread within the abdominal cavity can greatly
enhance the radiologist's ability to identify the epicenter of a
disease process and predict the likely path of disease progression. Pathways for disease transmission within the
abdominal cavity include hematogenous, transperitoneal,
and subperitoneal spread [3]. Transperitoneal dissemination
is confined to the peritoneal cavity and includes ascites,
abscesses, pneumoperitoneum, and peritoneal tumor deposits. Subperitoneal spread of disease refers to disease spread
within the ligaments, mesentery, mesocolon, or under the
peritoneal surface of the organs [4]. This interconnecting
potential space represents a significant conduit for bidirec-
tional spread of disease within and between the peritoneal
and retroperitoneal compartments. Subperitoneal spread
may also follow the lymphatic drainage of organs along the
blood vessels in the mesentery, mesocolon, and ligaments.

Pathology

Retroperitoneal and mesenteric lymphadenopathy can be an
unexpected imaging finding and represent the first sign of
disease. Given the increased frequency with which lymph
nodes are identified on cross-sectional imaging and the wide
differential diagnosis for lymphadenopathy in these regions,
a careful evaluation of lymph node imaging characteristics
(size, distribution, CT attenuation coefficient, signal changes
on MRI, post-contrast enhancement) should be performed.

Correlation with the patient's clinical history should be made in an effort to rule out a neoplastic condition. Bulky retroperitoneal lymphadenopathy in association with mesenteric lymphadenopathy is suggestive of lymphoma. Abdominal lymphadenopathy, disproportionately involving the mesentery, is suggestive of tuberculosis [5].

The most common soft tissue masses to affect the retroperitoneum and peritoneal structures are metastases and lymphoma [6]. Metastases to the retroperitoneum most commonly originate in the pelvis (rectum, cervix, prostate) [7]. Peritoneal carcinomatosis and metastases to omentum and mesentery frequently arise from tumors of the ovary, colon, stomach, pancreas, uterus, and bladder [8–11]. Tuberculosis can closely mimic peritoneal carcinomatosis radiologically. Forty to eighty percentage of gastrointestinal carcinoid tumors metastasize directly or via lymphatic spread to the mesentery [12, 13]. The infiltrative pattern of mesenteric disease seen with carcinoid, desmoid tumors, retractile mesenteritis, and peritoneal mesothelioma can sometimes be difficult to differentiate on CT.

Primary neoplasms of the retroperitoneum are uncommon and are derived from mesenchyme, neurogenic tissue, or embryonic rests. Primary malignant tumors are about four times more common than benign neoplasms [14]. Liposarcoma and leiomyosarcoma account for over 90 % of malignant tumors. Approximately two-thirds of omental tumors are benign and include leiomyomas, lipomas, and neurofibromas. Malignant tumors include leiomyosarcoma, liposarcoma, fibrosarcoma, mesothelioma, and hemangiopericytoma [6, 15]. Primary peritoneal tumors are a rare group of tumors that arise from the mesothelial and submesothelial layers of the peritoneum [16]. They include malignant mesothelioma, multicystic mesothelioma, primary peritoneal serous carcinoma, leiomyomatosis peritonealis disseminata, and desmoplastic small round cell tumor. Many of these tumors have imaging findings similar to peritoneal carcinomatosis.

Indications

For many patients, the information provided by the clinical history and imaging studies is insufficient to exclude a malignancy. The imaging features of many primary neoplasms of the retroperitoneum and peritoneum are nonspecific. While the presence of calcifications, fat, necrosis, or cystic components are key to providing a differential diagnosis, there is often considerable overlap between neoplastic and nonneoplastic lesions and between benign and malignant tumors. Moreover, cytological analysis of ascitic fluid rarely results in site-specific tumor diagnoses in cases of peritoneal carcinomatosis [17]. Percutaneous needle biopsy of the retroperitoneum, mesentery, or omentum may be

required to establish the benign or malignant nature of a lesion, to obtain material for microbiologic analysis in patients with known or suspected infections, and to stage patients with known or suspected malignancy when local spread or distant metastasis is suspected. A repeat biopsy may be required if there is a strong clinical suspicion of malignancy and the previous biopsy result was negative or inconclusive, or the result is discordant with the clinical and imaging findings.

At our institution, one of the most common indications for percutaneous biopsy of a retroperitoneal or mesenteric soft tissue mass is for the diagnosis, staging, and restaging of lymphoma. While the clinical practice guidelines issued by the European Society of Medical Oncology recommend *excision* biopsy for the diagnosis of newly diagnosed and relapsed lymphoma (except in emergency circumstances) [18], numerous studies support the use of core biopsy in providing a definitive histological diagnosis. Core biopsy diagnostic rates of 83–88 % for lymphoma have been quoted for nodes inside and outside of the retroperitoneum [19–22]. Controversy also surrounds the diagnosis of retroperitoneal soft tissue sarcomas. In the past, definitive diagnosis and treatment of these tumors was achieved with surgical resection. High local recurrence rates of 50–60 % at 5 years and 90 % at 10 years have led to efforts to downstage the disease with preoperative and intraoperative radiotherapy [23–26]. In this patient, population pretreatment percutaneous biopsy is appropriate. While surgical excision is the treatment of choice for many cystic masses in the retroperitoneum and mesentery, percutaneous needle aspiration can be useful to confirm the nature of a nonneoplastic cystic mass, e.g., urinoma, lymphocele, hematoma, or pseudocyst.

The radiologist's pre-procedure evaluation should include a review of the patient's clinical history and physical examination and correlation with available imaging studies. With a differential diagnosis in hand, the radiologist must determine if a diagnosis is possible with the evidence available, whether the diagnosis can be confirmed by less invasive means or that biopsy is indeed indicated. Not all lesions identified by imaging need to be biopsied, (e.g., FDG-avid mesenteric lymph nodes on PET-CT may be sufficient to confirm the presence of metastatic disease; an enhancing soft tissue mass involving bowel, with linear areas of soft tissue attenuation radiating outward in the mesenteric fat, is a CT finding strongly suggestive of carcinoid tumor). In order to avoid unnecessary and possibly hazardous interventions, the radiologist must be familiar with common "pseudotumors" and normal variants. Left-sided paraortic lymphadenopthy can mimic duplication of or left inferior vena cava (IVC). Retrocrural lymphadenopathy may mimic an enlarged azygos vein in the retrocrural space. Retroperitoneal lymphadenopthy can mimic circumaortic left renal vein. Retroperitoneal fibrosis is an inflammatory disorder that may be misinterpreted as a

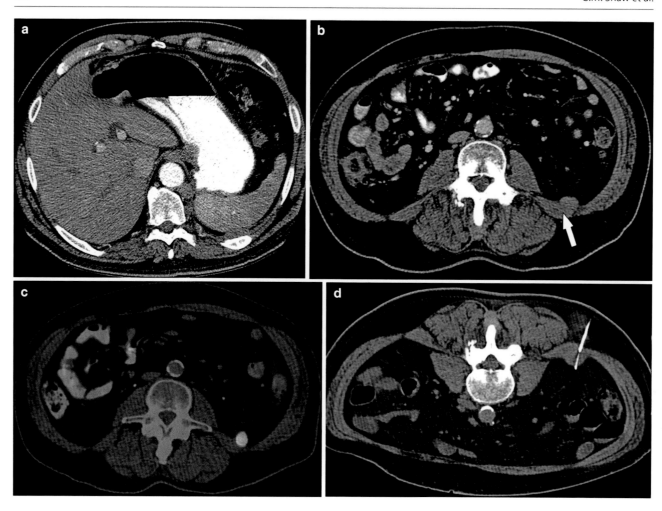

Fig. 19.3 A 66-year-old male with lymphadenopathy worrisome for lymphoproliferative disorder. (**a**) Contrast-enhanced CT abdomen axial image shows retrocrural lymph node. (**b**, **c**) Review of the PET CT revealed a more superficial and metabolically active lesion (*arrow*) contiguous with the quadrates lumborum fascia in the posterior pararenal space. (**d**) CT-guided biopsy was performed of this alternative site using a posterior approach. Pathology revealed a large B-cell lymphoma

malignant process, as it envelops the aorta and IVC, often displacing and encasing the ureters. Other nonneoplastic entities that can have a mass-like appearance on CT include cystic masses (hematoma, urinoma, lymphocele, pseudocyst, duplication cyst), omental torsion, omental infarction, and inflammatory pseudotumor.

Patient Selection and Pre-procedure Planning

Before embarking upon biopsy of a deep retroperitoneal or mesenteric lesion, consideration should be given to biopsy of more accessible sites, e.g., the axillary or inguinal regions in the case of lymphadenopathy (Fig. 19.3). To minimize the risks associated with biopsy of deep lesions, the safest and shortest needle trajectory should be identified. A careful risk-benefit assessment should be performed prior to trans-intestinal biopsy of deep mesenteric lesions or trans-caval biopsy of retroperito-

neal lesions. Biopsy may be contraindicated if the lesion is highly vascular. Markedly hypervascular tumors include paragangliomas and hemangiopericytomas. Moderately hypervascular tumors include some of the soft tissue sarcomas including leiomyosarcoma which can also be partly intravascular. Hypervascular retroperitoneal lymphadenopathy is a feature of Kaposi's sarcoma and Castleman disease.

Many retroperitoneal and deep mesenteric biopsies are performed with the patient. Close proximity to viscera, e.g., kidneys or bowel, may require breath holding during the procedure. The patient's ability to cooperate and lie supine or prone should be assessed. Patient comfort and cooperation may be optimized with the use of moderate sedation administered by dedicated nursing staff. At our institution, respiratory compromise, decompensated cardiac failure, morbid obesity and diagnosed sleep apnea, pregnancy, pediatric patient, and inability to lie in the required position for the procedure are among some of the reasons that referral to anesthesia may be required.

A history of anticoagulation therapy and antiplatelet agents should be obtained. The Society of Interventional Radiology provides guidelines for the cessation of these drugs in patients undergoing percutaneous biopsy [27]. At our institution, aspirin and clopidogrel are held 5 days and coumadin 3–5 days prior to percutaneous biopsy. Coagulation status is tested in those on coumadin therapy and those with known or suspected liver disease. If the risks associated with complete cessation of anticoagulation are high, the patient is converted to unfractionated heparin (biological half-life 1–2 h). Patients on low molecular weight heparin have one dose held prior to the procedure. In patients with malignancy, biopsy of mesenteric and retroperitoneal lesions may involve additional risks owing to treatment-related coagulation disorders or the cancer itself, e.g., chemotherapy-induced thrombocytopenia. Although numerous studies have demonstrated a relatively low predictive value of abnormal laboratory screening parameters in predicting bleeding, laboratory criteria for biopsy at our institution include a platelet count greater than 50×10^9 and an international normalized ratio of less than 1.6 within 1 month before the procedure.

Contraindications [27]

There are no absolute contraindications for percutaneous needle biopsy. Relative contraindications may include:

1. Significant coagulopathy that cannot be adequately corrected
2. Severely compromised cardiopulmonary function or hemodynamic instability
3. Lack of a safe pathway to the lesion

4. Inability of the patient to cooperate with, or to be positioned for, the procedure
5. Pregnancy in cases when imaging guidance involves ionizing radiation

Imaging Modality

The choice of imaging modality is based on equipment availability, radiologist preference, the size and location of the target lesion, patient body habitus, potential access routes, the ability to visualize the lesion, and cost. Factors to be considered in a patient with a high body mass index include the maximum weight load of the CT/MRI table, the ability to visualize the lesion on ultrasonography, and the ability of the interventional radiologist to compress the subcutaneous tissue with the ultrasound probe while performing the biopsy. Although many interventional radiologists prefer to perform CT-guided biopsies of retroperitoneal and mesenteric lesions in obese patients, ultrasound-guided biopsy has been demonstrated to be very effective in this subset of patients [28].

CT

CT is traditionally used as the modality for image-guided biopsy of retroperitoneal and deep mesenteric lesions [29, 30]. CT provides high spatial and contrast resolution and excellent delineation of intervening structures, such as vessels and bowel, thus enabling accurate needle localization (Fig. 19.4). The operator can easily correlate the findings on CT and functional imaging (e.g., positron emission tomography (PET)) to target the appropriate part of the mass for

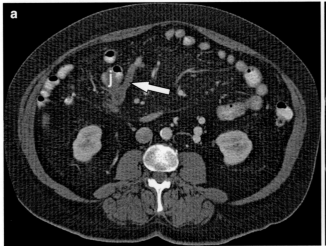
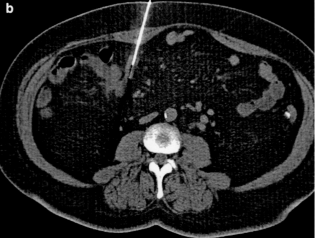

Fig. 19.4 A 65-year-old female status post right hemicolectomy for colonic carcinoma. (**a**) Contrast-enhanced CT abdomen axial image demonstrated a mass (*arrow*) involving the proximal small bowel mesentery and adjacent loop of jejunum (*j*). (**b**) CT-guided tissue sampling demonstrated metastatic colorectal carcinoma

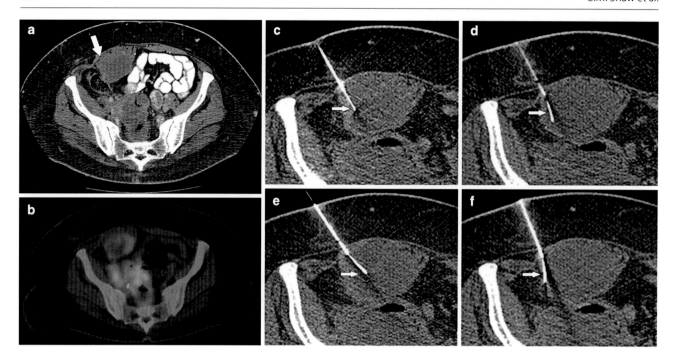

Fig. 19.5 A 62-year-old male with a history of sigmoid carcinoma treated with sigmoid colectomy and adjuvant chemotherapy. (**a**) Contrast-enhanced CT abdomen axial image demonstrated a partly necrotic mass involving the right rectus abdominis muscle (*arrow*). (**b**) PET CT shows greater metabolic activity the periphery of the mass.

(**c**) CT-guided biopsy using coaxial technique was performed. (**d–f**) By curving the tip of the core biopsy needle (*arrows*), it was possible to acquire sufficient tissue for a diagnosis of metastatic mucin-producing adenocarcinoma

biopsy and to avoid areas of necrosis (Fig. 19.5). Performing CT-guided biopsies is associated with a shorter learning curve than performing ultrasound-guided biopsies, increasing the reliability of CT-guided biopsy among the general population of radiologists. Standard CT acquisition parameters for mesenteric/retroperitoneal biopsies are 3–5-mm-thick contiguous transverse sections.

CT fluoroscopy combines the advantages of the high-resolution imaging of CT with the real-time imaging of fluoroscopy. CT fluoroscopy can be especially useful for needle placement in omental or mesenteric lesions that move when the patient breathes or that may be intermittently surrounded by bowel loops [31, 32]. When using this modality, the operator should be aware of the available techniques to reduce radiation exposure for both the operator and the patient, including dedicated needle holders to keep the operator's hand away from the gantry, using a low tube potential and low tube current, and using CT fluoroscopy intermittently during needle advancement instead of continuously [33–37].

Ultrasonography

In many countries in Europe and Asia, ultrasonography is the preferred guidance technique for biopsy in many regions of the body, including the mesentery (Fig. 19.6) [28, 38–41]. Advantages of ultrasonography include real-time imaging capabilities, the ability of color Doppler to delineate major

vascular structures in and around the target lesion, the capacity to identify alternative access routes to the target lesion by angling the probe away from the axial plane, lack of exposure to ionizing radiation, decreased procedure time, and lower cost. Application of transducer pressure can displace and compress overlying fat or bowel loops, thus reducing the needle-path distance. In experienced hands, ultrasound-guided biopsy has been demonstrated to be as effective as CT-guided biopsy in establishing site-specific diagnosis in patients with peritoneal carcinomatosis [42].

The major drawback of ultrasound-guided biopsy is the fact that it is an operator-dependent method and thus may have low reproducibility. For those less experienced in ultrasound-guided interventions, a needle guide can facilitate visualization of the needle, reduce the time spent searching for the needle tip, and enable biopsy to be performed during a single breath-hold. This technique also ensures that the sampling is limited to the lesion.

Other drawbacks include the poor visualization of small or deep lesions and lesions overlying bowel or bone [43, 44]. While deep mesenteric and retroperitoneal lesions are often accessed via CT guidance, some authors have reported that ultrasonography is an accurate and safe guidance technique in the biopsy of small or deep lesions or lesions obscured by overlying bowel or bone [28, 45]. A number of new innovative ultrasound tools are now available that are likely to increase radiologist confidence in interventional studies. Fusion of ultrasound images with previously acquired imag-

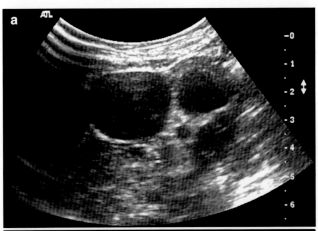

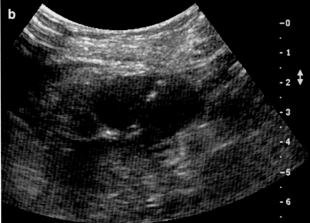

Fig. 19.6 A 31-year-old female presented with abdominal distension. (**a**) Ultrasound abdomen showed multiple hypoechoic mesenteric masses worrisome for lymphoma. (**b**) Ultrasound-guided biopsy was performed of a more superficial lesion located beneath the anterior abdominal wall. Pathology confirmed a diagnosis of B-cell lymphoma

ing modalities like CT and MR combines the advantages of real-time ultrasound imaging with the high spatial and contrast resolution of CT, MR, or PET. The development of a "GPS-like technology" enables the radiologist to track and mark a patient's anatomy during the ultrasound exam and in particular to track "hot spots" found on previous CT, MRI, or PET CT studies. These tools may be particularly beneficial for guiding biopsy of deep-seated lymph nodes and small soft tissue masses. Ultrasound-guided biopsy of deep lesions is usually performed with a convex probe. High-frequency linear probes are reserved for thin patients or superficial peritoneal lesions.

MRI

The superb soft tissue contrast resolution achieved with MRI makes it a useful diagnostic tool for localizing and staging retroperitoneal and mesenteric soft tissue masses. MRI guidance of percutaneous biopsies is becoming more popular with the advent of new open-configuration MRI systems, continuing

development in the field of MRI-compatible instruments, and ultrafast MRI sequences that allow real-time imaging [46, 47]. Other advantages of MRI include its multiplanar capabilities, the lack of ionizing radiation, and its ability to visualize vessels without a contrast agent. Multiplanar imaging allows the radiologist to identify the safest trajectory for biopsy and maintain continuous visualization of the needle trajectory in that plane throughout the procedure. This is particularly relevant for posterior paraspinal and anterior approaches to deep retroperitoneal and mesenteric lesions that lie in close proximity to vessels and bowel loops. The higher cost associated with MR-guided interventions is largely attributed to the cost of MR-compatible instruments. With increased use, it is likely that the cost differential will diminish. These characteristics, in addition to a low complication rate and a high rate of adequate specimens, make MRI-guided biopsy a reasonable alternative to CT-guided biopsy [48].

Techniques

Retroperitoneal and mesenteric lesions can be accessed from an anterior or posterior approach. When the posterior approach is performed, the needle usually passes alongside or through the quadratus lumborum and psoas muscles (Fig. 19.7). Although this is a safe trajectory, the operator should be aware that passing the needle through these muscles decreases the possibility of correct needle trajectory. Some proponents of a posterior paraspinal approach argue that in the event of a bleeding complication, the result would be a contained retroperitoneal hematoma rather than free intraperitoneal hemorrhage [49].

Due to limited visualization from a posterior paraspinal approach, ultrasound-guided biopsy of deep-seated nodes and soft tissue masses is usually performed from an anterior approach. The major limitation of the anterior approach is that bowel may be traversed. Traversing bowel is not a contraindication to percutaneous biopsy if small caliber needles are used [45, 49–51]. Application of abdominal compression during ultrasound-guided biopsies of mesenteric lesions can help displace the intervening bowel loops. Compression also improves depiction of deep lesions, shortens the needle path, and helps fix mobile masses.

A number of techniques have been described to enable safe CT-guided biopsy of lesions in difficult locations. These include the triangulation method, angling the gantry, and/or tilting the patient [52, 53]. Angulation of the gantry may be required to minimize the risk of transgressing the pleura in a posterior approach or to avoid bowel loops and mesenteric vessels that lie in an anterior trajectory. For some lesions, angulation in both the sagittal and axial planes may be required. In order to simplify the needle approach and optimize the precision of needle placement, obliquity in the axial plane may be achieved by tilting the patient.

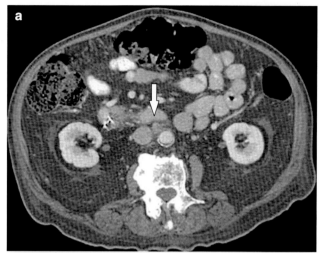

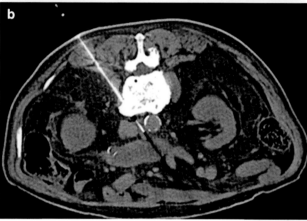

Fig. 19.7 A 78-year-old male undergoing chemotherapy for pancreatic carcinoma. (**a**) Contrast-enhanced CT axial image demonstrates aorto-caval lymph node (*open arrow*) suspicious for malignancy. (**b**) CT-guided biopsy using a posterior approach was performed avoiding the aorta (*a*) and the IVC (*ivc*). Pathology confirmed metastatic adenocarcinoma

Biopsies may be acquired using a coaxial or a tandem technique. At our institution, the coaxial technique is preferred for mesenteric and retroperitoneal lesions [54]. A thin-walled guide needle (typically 18 G) is placed close to the target lesion, and the biopsy needle (20 G) is then placed through the guide needle to obtain tissue samples. This method allows multiple samples to be obtained without additional passes through the overlying tissue, decreasing the risk of complications and minimizing patient discomfort. The coaxial method also shortens the duration of the procedure and, consequently, reduces radiation exposure in CT-guided biopsies. One potential limitation of the coaxial technique is that after the first pass, subsequent passes tend to be directed to the same location in the lesion and thus yield little additional tissue. To avoid this limitation, custom-made curved core and FNA biopsy needles may be used, potentially increasing the tissue yield and avoiding injury to vital structures close to the target lesion (Fig. 19.5) [55, 56].

The tandem method is an alternative approach in which a small-gauge needle (e.g., 25 gauge) is used to work out the appropriate angle of access to the target lesion, followed by a larger-gauge device (e.g., 20 G) placed immediately adjacent and parallel to the first (Fig. 19.8).

Devices

An extensive variety of needles differing in caliber, length, tip configuration, and mechanism of sample acquisition are available for percutaneous biopsies. For retroperitoneal and mesenteric biopsies, an 18- or 19-gauge thin-walled guide needle is placed close to the target lesion. A smaller caliber (20 Gauge) cutting needle passed through the guide needle is usually adequate for core biopsies. A 22-gauge fine needle may be used to obtain cytologic specimens. Use of larger (14- to 16-gauge) cutting needles to perform biopsies in peritoneal tissue has been reported without complications, even when multiple passes are made [57]. Using a Hawkins needle with a blunt trocar tip in the retroperitoneal and peritoneal space reduces the risk of injury to bowel, major vessels, and nerves in the needle path and also helps displace nontarget organs from the needle's path (Fig. 19.9) [58–60]. Saline solution may be injected to displace intervening bowel loops and to create a safe path for the needle [32, 61].

The accuracy of FNA biopsy of peritoneal lesions has been a point of controversy, but some studies have suggested that FNA biopsy has an equal or greater sensitivity than core biopsy for peritoneal lesions [62]. If on-site cytologic review is available during the procedure, both FNA and core biopsies may be performed during the same procedure. At our institution, FNA biopsy is performed first to assess the presence of adequate tissue in the target lesion, and then a core biopsy is performed to study the architectural features of the lesion and to collect tissue for immunohistochemical analysis.

If lymphoma is suspected, a large amount of tissue may be required for cytogenetic, immunohistochemical, and flow cytometry analysis. To obtain an adequate number of cells for these studies, circumferentially sharpened needles, such as Franseen, Greene, and Turner needles (Cook Medical Inc, Bloomington, IN), can provide a larger specimen yield for cytologic analysis.

Complications

Complications related to image-guided biopsy of retroperitoneal and mesenteric lesions are rare, and in most cases, conservative treatment is sufficient. Several studies have demonstrated the safety of image-guided percutaneous mesenteric and retroperitoneal biopsies [63, 64]. The two most common complications are pain at the puncture site and

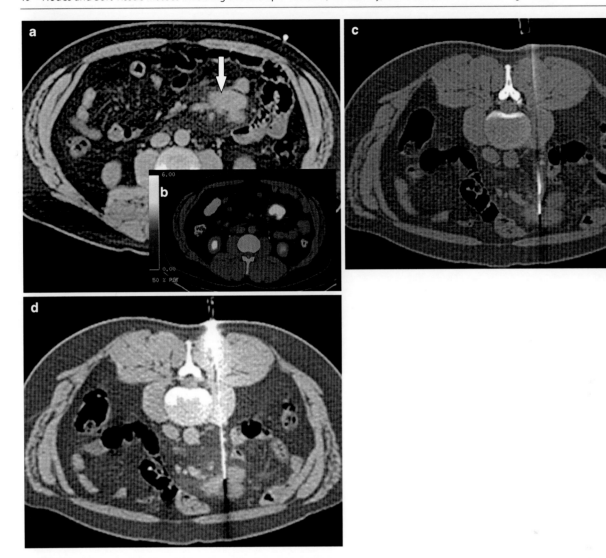

Fig. 19.8 A 51-year-old male with a history of lymphoma. (**a**) Non-contrast CT abdomen (axial image) demonstrated mesenteric lymphadenopathy. (**b**) PET CT showed increased metabolic activity associated with this lesion. Biopsy from an anterior approach was not possible without traversing small bowel. (**c**, **d**) The patient was turned prone, and a safe trajectory was identified via a posterior paraspinal approach. The depth of the needle trajectory required the use of a tandem technique for core biopsy

hemorrhage of the target lesion or along the needle trajectory (Fig. 19.10). The possibility of bowel injury or peritonitis due to inadvertent transgression of bowel loops is greatest when ultrasound-guided biopsy is performed, owing to ultrasonography's limitations in distinguishing compressed bowel from omental or fat tissue [28, 45, 65]. However, only one study in the literature reported a case of colonic perforation during ultrasound-guided FNA biopsy of a colonic wall lesion [66], while other large series have demonstrated the safety and effectiveness of this approach, even if unintentional transgression of the bowel occurred [28]. Based on current data, the risk of peritonitis associated with bowel transgression when small caliber needles are used (18–20 gauge) appears to be very small; however, transgressing the colon or small bowel should be avoided whenever possible.

Avoiding vessels during biopsies is advisable; however, a trans-caval approach using a 22-gauge needle has been demonstrated to be a safe technique [67, 68]. Neoplastic dissemination resulting from biopsy has been described in the literature, but is anecdotal in view of the number of biopsies performed, with an estimated risk of 0.005 % [69].

Management of Complications

Localized pain after retroperitoneal and mesenteric biopsy is generally self-limiting and can be managed with oral analgesics. Pain usually subsides in the 24 h after the procedure. Hemorrhagic events are generally also self-limiting and can be managed conservatively by closely monitoring hematocrit

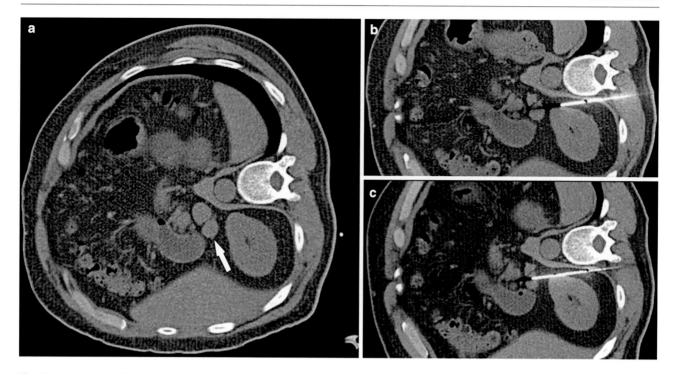

Fig. 19.9 A 61-year-old male status post left nephrectomy for the treatment of renal cell carcinoma. (**a**) Limited non-contrast CT axial image identified right adrenal nodule (*arrow*) suspicious for metastatic disease. A direct approach to the mass would require traversing the renal parenchyma. Biopsy was performed using the blunt tip of an 18-gauge Hawkins needle. (**b** and **c**) After traversing the right diaphragmatic crura, the needle displaces the right kidney laterally enabling access to the mass

levels. CT or ultrasonography studies may be acquired if necessary. If clinically significant hemorrhage occurs during the biopsy procedure, one possible approach is to embolize the bleeding site with Gelfoam particles through the needle biopsy orifice [70, 71]. If bleeding relates to injury to a nearby vessel or organ, intra-arterial embolization may be indicated. Surgical treatment is required in a minority of cases.

Outcomes and Results

While there is no randomized data comparing different imaging modalities or biopsy techniques, a large number of retrospective studies support the use of image-guided biopsy for the diagnosis and staging of retroperitoneal and mesenteric disease. Hewitt et al. showed image-guided biopsy to be safe and accurate for providing site-specific diagnoses in women with peritoneal carcinomatosis [42]. The initial ultrasound-guided biopsy was diagnostic for 54 of 60 women (90 %), and the initial CT-guided biopsy was diagnostic in 81 of 89 women (91 %). In 56 % (18/32) of women with a previous malignancy, a new primary malignancy was identified. A review of 49 patients who underwent CT-guided core biopsy of non-organ-bound retroperitoneal lesions using a coaxial technique showed this approach to be 95.2 % sensitive, 100 % specific, and 95.9 % accurate [19]. The correct lymphoma subtype was revealed in 20 of 23 cases (87.0 %). In a study by

Ho et al. sonography-guided percutaneous biopsy of mesenteric lesions was 95 % (18/19) sensitive and 100 % (4/4) specific in distinguishing benign from malignant disease [45].

The accuracy and reliability of image-guided biopsies of mesenteric and retroperitoneal masses depends on the type, site and size of the lesions, as well as the approach and type of biopsy performed (FNA biopsy or core biopsy). The diagnosis of mesenteric or retroperitoneal lesions, particularly lymphadenopathy, requires that adequate tissue specimens be obtained for histologic evaluation, immunophenotyping, and cytogenetic and molecular profile studies. Thus, precise localization of the biopsy site and collection of an adequate number and quality of tissue samples is essential.

Summary

The increased frequency with which disease is identified in the retroperitoneum and mesenteries has led to a greater demand for percutaneous tissue sampling of lesions within these regions. The percutaneous biopsy of retroperitoneal and peritoneal masses can be challenging. Lesions may be small, deep seated, and within close proximity of bowel loops and blood vessels. Technical and clinical success can only be achieved after a thorough assessment of the clinical and imaging information available, and an appropriate pre-procedure plan is put in place.

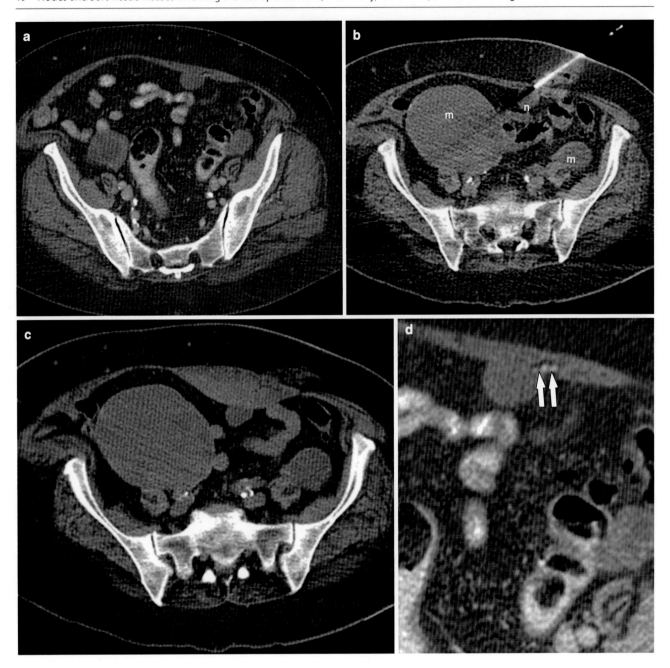

Fig. 19.10 A 42-year-old female with bilateral adnexal masses. (**a** and **b**) CT pelvis axial image showed bilateral adnexal masses (*m*) and peritoneal nodule (*n*) beneath the anterior abdominal wall. CT-guided biopsy of the peritoneal nodule (*n*) was performed. (**c**) The procedure was complicated by a hematoma in the left rectus abdominis muscle. This was managed conservatively. (**d**) Contrast-enhanced CT pelvis axial image shows the close relationship between the epigastric vessels (*arrows*) and the peritoneal nodule

References

1. Healy JC, Reznek RH. Peritoneal anatomy. Imaging. 2000;12:1–9.
2. Burkill GJC, Healy JC. Anatomy of the retroperitoneum. Imaging. 2000;12:10–20.
3. Meyers MA, Oliphant M, Berne AS, Feldberg MA. The peritoneal ligaments and mesenteries: pathways of intraabdominal spread of disease. Radiology. 1987;163(3):593–604.
4. Gore RM, Newmark GM, Thakrar KH, Mehta UK, Berlin JW, Mehta UK, et al. Pathways of abdominal tumour spread: the role of the subperitoneal space. Cancer Imaging. 2009;9:112–20.
5. Hulnick DH, Megibow AJ, Naidich DP, Hilton S, Cho KC, Balthazar EJ. Abdominal tuberculosis: CT evaluation. Radiology. 1985;157:199–204.
6. Adams JT. Abdominal wall, omentum, mesentery, and retroperitoneum. In: Schwartz SI, editor. Principles of surgery. 4th ed. New York: McGraw-Hill; 1984. p. 1421–56.
7. Park JM, Charnsangavej C, Yoshimitsu K, Herron DH, Robinson TJ, Wallace S. Pathways of nodal metastases from pelvic tumors: CT demonstration. Radiographics. 1994; 14:1309–21.
8. Whitley NO, Bohlman ME, Baker LP. CT patterns of mesenteric disease. J Comput Assist Tomogr. 1982;6:490–6.

9. Silverman PM, Baker ME, Cooper C, Kelvin FM. Computed tomography of mesenteric disease. Radiographics. 1987;7:309–20.

10. Walkey MM, Friedman AC, Sohotra P, Radecki PD. CT manifestations of peritoneal carcinomatosis. AJR Am J Roentgenol. 1988;150:1035–41.

11. Yeh HC. Ultrasonography of peritoneal tumors. Radiology. 1979;133:419–24.

12. Pantongrag-Brown L, Buetow PC, Carr NJ, Lichtenstein JE, Buck JL. Calcification and fibrosis in mesenteric carcinoid tumor: CT findings and pathologic correlation. AJR Am J Roentgenol. 1995;164:387–91.

13. Burke AP, Thomas RM, Elsayed AM, Sobin LH. Carcinoids of the jejunum and ileum: an immunohistochemical and clinicopathologic study of 167 cases. Cancer. 1997;79:1086–93.

14. Johnson AH, Searls HH, Grimes OF. Primary retroperitoneal tumors. Am J Surg. 1954;88(1):155–61.

15. Stout AP, Hendry J, Purdie FJ. Primary solid tumors of the greater omentum. Cancer. 1963;16:231–43.

16. Robbins SL, Cotran RS. Peritoneum. In: Pathologic basis of disease. Philadelphia: Saunders; 1979. p. 1003–5.

17. Karoo R, Lloyd T, Garcea G, Redway H, Robertson G. How valuable is ascitic cytology in the detection and management of malignancy? Postgrad Med J. 2003;79(931):292–4.

18. Tilly H, Dreyling M. ESMO Guidelines Working Group. Diffuse large B-cell non-Hodgkin's lymphoma: ESMO Clinical Practice Guidelines for diagnosis, treatment and follow-up. Ann Oncol. 2010;21(S5):172–4.

19. Stattaus J, Kalkmann J, Kuehl H, Metz KA, Nowrousian MR, Forsting M, et al. Diagnostic yield of computed tomography-guided coaxial core biopsy of undetermined masses in the free retroperitoneal space: single-center experience. Cardiovasc Intervent Radiol. 2008;31(5):919–25.

20. de Kerviler E, Guermazi A, Zagdanski AM, Meignin V, Gossot D, Oksenhendler E, et al. Image-guided core-needle biopsy in patients with suspected or recurrent lymphomas. Cancer. 2000;89(3):647–52.

21. Pappa VI, Hussain HK, Reznek RH, Whelan J, Norton AJ, Wilson AM, et al. Role of image-guided core-needle biopsy in the management of patients with lymphoma. J Clin Oncol. 1996;14(9):2427–30.

22. Agid R, Sklair-Levy M, Bloom AI, Lieberman S, Polliack A, Ben-Yehuda D, et al. CT-guided biopsy with cutting-edge needle for the diagnosis of malignant lymphoma: experience of 267 biopsies. Clin Radiol. 2003;58(2):143–7.

23. Storm FK, Mahvi DM. Diagnosis and management of retroperitoneal soft-tissue sarcoma. Ann Surg. 1991;214(1):2–10.

24. Windham TC, Pisters PW. Retroperitoneal sarcomas. Cancer Control. 2005;12(1):36–43.

25. Pawlik TM, Pisters PW, Mikula L, Feig BW, Hunt KK, Cormier JN. Long-term results of two prospective trials of preoperative external beam radiotherapy for localized intermediate- or high-grade retroperitoneal soft tissue sarcoma. Ann Surg Oncol. 2006;13(4):508–17.

26. Tzeng CW, Fiveash JB, Popple RA, Arnoletti JP, Russo SM, Urist MM, et al. Preoperative radiation therapy with selective dose escalation to the margin at risk for retroperitoneal sarcoma. Cancer. 2006;107(2):371–9.

27. Gupta S, Wallace MJ, Cardella JF, Kundu S, Miller DL, Rose SC. Quality improvement guidelines for percutaneous needle biopsy. J Vasc Interv Radiol. 2010;21:969–75.

28. Memel DS, Dodd 3rd GD, Esola CC. Efficacy of sonography as a guidance technique for biopsy of abdominal, pelvic, and retroperitoneal lymph nodes. AJR Am J Roentgenol. 1996;167(4):957–62.

29. Gazelle GS, Haaga JR. Guided percutaneous biopsy of intraabdominal lesions. AJR Am J Roentgenol. 1989;153(5):929–35.

30. Welch TJ, Sheedy 2nd PF, Johnson CD, Johnson CM, Stephens DH. CT-guided biopsy: prospective analysis of 1,000 procedures. Radiology. 1989;171(2):493–6.

31. Sauthier PG, Bélanger R, Provencher DM, Gauthier P, Drouin P. Clinical value of image-guided fine needle aspiration of retroperitoneal masses and lymph nodes in gynecologic oncology. Gynecol Oncol. 2006;103(1):75–80.

32. Gupta S. Role of image-guided percutaneous needle biopsy in cancer staging. Semin Roentgenol. 2006;41(2):78–90.

33. Kato R, Katada K, Anno H, Suzuki S, Ida Y, Koga S. Radiation dosimetry at CT fluoroscopy: physician's hand dose and development of needle holders. Radiology. 1996;201(2):576–8.

34. Nawfel RD, Judy PF, Silverman SG, Hooton S, Tuncali K, Adams DF. Patient and personnel exposure during CT fluoroscopy-guided interventional procedures. Radiology. 2000;216(1):180–4.

35. Paulson EK, Sheafor DH, Enterline DS, McAdams HP, Yoshizumi TT. CT fluoroscopy-guided interventional procedures: techniques and radiation dose to radiologists. Radiology. 2001;220(1):161–7.

36. Daly B, Templeton PA. Real-time CT fluoroscopy: evolution of an interventional tool. Radiology. 1999;211(2):309–15.

37. Froelich JJ, Wagner HJ. CT-fluoroscopy: tool or gimmick? Cardiovasc Intervent Radiol. 2001;24(5):297–305.

38. Buscarini L, Cavanna L. Ultrasound and ultrasonically guided biopsy in oncohematology. Haematologica. 1991;76(1):53–64.

39. Nagano T, Nakai Y, Taniguchi F, Suzuki N, Wakutani K, Ohnishi T, et al. Diagnosis of paraaortic and pelvic lymph node metastasis of gynecologic malignant tumors by ultrasound-guided percutaneous fine-needle aspiration biopsy. Cancer. 1991;68(12):2571–4.

40. Sistrom CL, Abbitt PL, Feldman PS. Ultrasound guidance for biopsy of omental abnormalities. J Clin Ultrasound. 1992;20(1):27–36.

41. Spencer JA, Swift SE, Wilkinson N, Boon AP, Lane G, Perren TJ. Peritoneal carcinomatosis: image-guided peritoneal core biopsy for tumor type and patient care. Radiology. 2001;221(1):173–7.

42. Hewitt MJ, Anderson K, Hall GD, Weston M, Hutson R, Wilkinson N, et al. Women with peritoneal carcinomatosis of unknown origin: Efficacy of image-guided biopsy to determine site-specific diagnosis. BJOG. 2007;114(1):46–50.

43. Nyman RS, Cappelen-Smith J, von Sinner W, Kagevi I. Yield and complications in ultrasound-guided biopsy of abdominal lesions. Acta Radiol. 1995;36(5):485–90.

44. Nolsoe C, Nielsen L, Torp-Pederson S, Holm HH. Major complications and deaths due to interventional ultrasonography: a review of 8000 cases. J Clin Ultrasound. 1990;18(3):179–84.

45. Ho LM, Thomas J, Fine SA, Paulson EK. Usefulness of sonographic guidance during percutaneous biopsy of mesenteric masses. AJR Am J Roentgenol. 2003;180(6):1563–6.

46. Günther RW, Bücker A, Adam G. Interventional magnetic resonance: realistic prospect or wishful thinking? Cardiovasc Intervent Radiol. 1999;22(3):187–95.

47. Hinks RS, Bronskill MJ, Kucharczyk W, Bernstein M, Collick BD, Henkelman RM. MR systems for image-guided therapy. J Magn Reson Imaging. 1998;8(1):19–25.

48. Zangos S, Eichler K, Wetter A, Lehnert T, Hammerstingl R, Diebold T. MR-guided biopsies of lesions in the retroperitoneal space: technique and results. Eur Radiol. 2006;16(2):307–12.

49. Fisher AJ, Paulson EK, Sheafor DH, Simmons CM, Nelson RC. Small lymph nodes of the abdomen, pelvis, and retroperitoneum: usefulness of sonographically guided biopsy. Radiology. 1997;205(1):185–90.

50. Gottlieb RH, Tan R, Widjaja J, Fultz PJ, Robinette WB, Rubens DJ. Extravisceral masses in the peritoneal cavity: sonographically guided biopsies in 52 patients. AJR Am J Roentgenol. 1998;171(3):697–701.

51. Farmer KD, Harries SR, Fox BM, Maskell GF, Farrow R. Core biopsy of the bowel wall: efficacy and safety in the clinical setting. AJR Am J Roentgenol. 2000;175(6):1627–30.

52. Van Sonnenberg E, Wittenberg J, Ferrucci Jr JT, Mueller PR, Simeone JF. Triangulation method for percutaneous needle guidance: the angled approach to upper abdominal masses. AJR Am J Roentgenol. 1981;137(4):757–61.

53. Hussain S, Santos-Ocampo RS, Silverman SG, Seltzer SE. Dual-angled CT-guided biopsy. Abdom Imaging. 1994;19(3): 217–20.

54. Jeffrey Jr RB. Coaxial technique for CT-guided biopsy of deep retroperitoneal lymph nodes. Gastrointest Radiol. 1988;13(3):271–2.

55. Gupta S, Ahrar K, Morello Jr FA, Wallace MJ, Madoff DC, Hicks ME. Using a coaxial technique with a curved inner needle for CT-guided fine-needle aspiration biopsy. AJR Am J Roentgenol. 2002;179(1):109–12.

56. Singh AK, Leeman J, Shankar S, Ferrucci JT. Core biopsy with curved needle technique. AJR Am J Roentgenol. 2008;191(6): 1745–50.

57. Griffin N, Grant LA, Freeman SJ, Jimenez-Linan M, Berman LH, Earl H, et al. Image-guided biopsy in patients with suspected ovarian carcinoma: a safe and effective technique? Eur Radiol. 2009;19(1):230–5.

58. Gupta S, Nguyen HL, Morello Jr FA, Ahrar K, Wallace MJ, Madoff DC, et al. Various approaches for CT-guided percutaneous biopsy of deep pelvic lesions: anatomic and technical considerations. Radiographics. 2004;24(1):175–89.

59. de Bazelaire C, Farges C, Mathieu O, Zagdanski AM, Bourrier P, Frija J. Blunt-Tip coaxial introducer: a revisited tool for difficult CT-guided biopsy in the chest and abdomen. AJR Am J Roentgenol. 2009;193(2):144–8.

60. Akins EW, Hawkins Jr IF, Mladinich C, Tupler R, Siragusa RJ, Pry R. The blunt needle: a new percutaneous access device. AJR Am J Roentgenol. 1989;152(1):181–2.

61. Langen HJ, Jochims M, Günther RW. Artificial displacement of kidneys, spleen, and colon by injection of physiologic saline and CO2 as an aid to percutaneous procedures: experimental results. J Vasc Interv Radiol. 1995;6(3):411–16.

62. Souza FF, Mortelé KJ, Cibas ES, Erturk SM, Silverman SG. Predictive value of percutaneous imaging-guided biopsy of peritoneal and omental masses: results in 111 patients. AJR Am J Roentgenol. 2009;192(1):131–6.

63. Layfield LJ, Gopez EV. Percutaneous image-guided fine-needle aspiration of peritoneal lesions. Diagn Cytopathol. 2003;28(1): 6–12.

64. Jaeger HJ, MacFie J, Mitchell CJ, Couse N, Wai D. Diagnosis of abdominal masses with percutaneous biopsy guided by ultrasound. BMJ. 1990;301(6762):1188–91.

65. Gupta S, Rajak CL, Sood BP, Gulati M, Rajwanshi A, Suri S. Sonographically guided fine needle aspiration biopsy of abdominal lymph nodes: experience in 102 patients. J Ultrasound Med. 1999;18(2):135–9.

66. Javid G, Gulzar GM, Khan B, Shah A, Khan MA. Percutaneous sonography-guided fine needle aspiration biopsy of colonoscopic biopsy-negative colonic lesions. Indian J Gastroenterol. 1999;18(4): 146–8.

67. Gupta S, Ahrar K, Morello Jr FA, Wallace MJ, Hicks ME. Masses in or around the pancreatic head: CT-guided coaxial fine-needle aspiration biopsy with a posterior transcaval approach. Radiology. 2002;222(1):63–9.

68. Sofocleous CT, Schubert J, Brown KT, Brody LA, Covey AM, Getrajdman GI. CT-guided transvenous or transcaval needle biopsy of pancreatic and peripancreatic lesions. J Vasc Interv Radiol. 2004;15(10):1099–104.

69. Carmignani CP, Sugarbaker TA, Bromley CM, Sugarbaker PH. Intraperitoneal cancer dissemination: mechanisms of the patterns of spread. Cancer Metastasis Rev. 2003;22(4):465–72.

70. Fandrich CA, Davies RP, Hall PM. Small gauge Gelfoam plug liver biopsy in high risk patients: safety and diagnostic value. Australas Radiol. 1996;40(3):230–4.

71. Sakr MA, Desouki SE, Hegab SE. Direct percutaneous embolization of renal pseudoaneurysm. J Endourol. 2009;23(6):875–8.

Biopsy of Pelvic Lesions

Efe Ozkan and Sanjay Gupta

Background

Image-guided biopsy has become established as a safe, effective procedure. However, deep pelvic masses pose problems for interventional radiologists because the overlying bowel, bladder, vessels, and bones, as well as the uterus and adnexa in female patients, can preclude safe access to these lesions [1]. The success and safety of image-guided pelvic biopsy depends on good access route planning, which requires a thorough understanding of the cross-sectional anatomy of the pelvis. Different approaches have been described for needle biopsy of pelvic lesions under computed tomography (CT) and ultrasound (US) guidance [1–10]. The best technique to use for each patient, including the most appropriate imaging type, needle type, and approach, depends on the characteristics and exact location of the patient's lesion. This article describes the various approaches and techniques of image-guided pelvic biopsy and discusses the advantages and limitations of each approach and technique. A review of the pelvic anatomy relevant to performing these biopsies is also included.

E. Ozkan, MD
Department of Radiology, The Ohio State University,
395 West 12th Avenue, Columbus, OH 43210, USA
e-mail: efeoz@msn.com

S. Gupta, MD, DNB (✉)
Department of Interventional Radiology,
Department of Diagnostic Radiology,
The University of Texas MD Anderson
Cancer Center, 1515 Holcombe Blvd.,
Unit 1471, Houston, TX 77030, USA
e-mail: sgupta@mdanderson.org

Indications

Despite recent advances in imaging technology, a definite histologic diagnosis of a pelvic mass is rarely possible with noninvasive imaging alone. Thus, image-guided biopsy is required for patients presenting with undiagnosed pelvic masses or enlarged pelvic lymph nodes.

The differential diagnosis of a pelvic mass includes inflammatory processes as well as a variety of primary and metastatic neoplastic conditions. The pelvic lymph nodes are commonly involved with hematologic malignancies or metastases from various local and distant cancers. Image-guided pelvic lymph node biopsy can help differentiate reactive nodal hyperplasia from neoplastic involvement as well as determine the type of malignancy. Primary and metastatic tumors of the peritoneum and omentum may also present as pelvic masses, and the pelvis is a common site for soft tissue recurrence of colorectal cancer and gynecologic tumors after surgical resection. Imaging features alone are not sufficient to differentiate recurrent carcinoma from postoperative fibrosis; hence, tissue diagnosis is generally required prior to institution of further chemotherapy, radiation therapy, or repeat surgery.

Diagnosis of a primary malignant tumor of the ovary is generally made with open or laparoscopic surgery because of the potential risk of peritoneal seeding associated with image-guided biopsy. However, patients who have advanced disease or poor performance status may not be able to undergo radical cytoreductive surgery, and in these cases image-guided biopsy is used to establish a histologic diagnosis prior to initiation of chemotherapy. Image-guided biopsy is also used in patients with a history of cancers (e.g., breast cancer, gastrointestinal tumors, melanoma) that are known to metastasize to the ovaries and present as ovarian masses mimicking primary ovarian cancers.

K. Ahrar, S. Gupta (eds.), *Percutaneous Image-Guided Biopsy*,
DOI 10.1007/978-1-4614-8217-8_20, © Springer Science+Business Media New York 2014

Technique

Imaging Guidance

Percutaneous pelvic biopsies are currently performed primarily under CT guidance because it allows precise localization and documentation of the biopsy needle and the targeted lesion. CT offers excellent delineation of intervening vital structures, permitting safe biopsy path planning. With CT, the operator can target the appropriate part of the mass and avoid areas of necrosis.

US guidance can be used for percutaneous biopsy of large pelvic masses that are in contact with the abdominal wall and for percutaneous biopsy of superficial inguinal and anterior abdominal wall lesions. US-guided transvaginal or transrectal approaches are used for deep pelvic masses that are not accessible via percutaneous biopsy. The advantages of US guidance are that it provides real-time, continuous monitoring of the needle during advancement and sampling; allows the operator to use oblique needle paths; and can be used at the bedside of critically ill patients [11]. The major drawbacks of US guidance are its poor visualization of deep or small lesions and its inability to penetrate through air or bone, which can lead to obscuration of lesions by overlying bowel or bone.

CT fluoroscopy (CTF) combines the high resolution of CT with the real-time imaging capability of fluoroscopy. CTF can be used to guide percutaneous biopsies of masses with difficult or narrow access routes; it can be especially useful for biopsies of lesions that are intermittently surrounded by bowel loops. However, CTF is not uniformly accepted by all interventional radiologists because of concerns about the increased radiation exposure associated with it.

The use of magnetic resonance imaging (MRI) guidance for percutaneous biopsies has become more popular with the advent of new, open-configuration MRI systems, continuing development of MRI-compatible instruments, and availability of ultrafast MRI sequences, including magnetic resonance fluoroscopy that allows real-time imaging. The advantages of MRI as a guidance modality for percutaneous biopsy procedures include its high-contrast resolution, multiplanar imaging capacity, ability to visualize vessels without the need for contrast agent administration, lack of ionizing radiation, and 2- and 3-dimensional imaging capabilities. MRI can use various nonorthogonal oblique planes, which allows the interventional radiologist to see the entire needle length and the relationship of the needle to the target lesion and the surrounding vital structures in a single image.

Recently introduced magnetic field-based electronic guidance systems use a low magnetic field with position sensors on the patient and the needle shaft to provide virtual, real-time guidance for needle placement during CT-guided biopsy procedures. A computer-generated trajectory map allows accurate calculation of the depth, position, and angle of inclination of the needle before it is actually placed. As the needle is advanced toward the target lesion, the relative location, orientation, and virtual trajectory of the needle are displayed and continually updated as an overlay on the corresponding CT images. This system has the potential to decrease procedural time by facilitating rapid, single-pass needle placement, especially for difficult-to-reach lesions and out-of-plane procedures.

Biopsy Needles

A variety of needles differing in caliber and mechanism of sample acquisition are available for pelvic biopsies. Aspiration needles, ranging in size from 20 to 23 gauge, provide specimens for cytologic evaluation. Cutting needles, ranging from 14 to 20 gauge, provide core specimens for histologic evaluation. Small-caliber (18- to 20-gauge), automated cutting needles consistently provide high-quality histopathologic specimens adequate for histologic diagnosis in most cases. The use of large-caliber (14- or 16-gauge) needles is generally reserved for musculoskeletal and soft tissue neoplasms.

Needle selection in any given case depends on a number of factors, including the size and location of the target lesion, intervening structures in the planned biopsy path, experience and preference of the interventional radiologist, availability of on-site cytopathologists for immediate assessment, and suspected likely diagnosis. The preferences of the pathologists and oncologists at one's institution also play a major role in the decision to use fine-needle aspiration biopsy or core biopsy. The roles of cytologic and histologic analysis remain complementary, and several studies suggest that analyzing both a histologic specimen and a cytologic specimen for each patient can increase the overall accuracy of the diagnosis. Some radiologists routinely obtain both cytologic and histologic specimens, whereas others obtain histologic specimens only if the cytologic specimens are inadequate or a more detailed characterization of the malignant lesion is required.

Percutaneous pelvic biopsies can be performed with the single-needle or the coaxial technique. The coaxial technique, involving initial placement of a guide needle close to the target lesion followed by advancement of the biopsy needle through this needle to obtain tissue samples, is the most commonly used technique for pelvic biopsies. This method allows multiple samples of tissue to be obtained without the need for additional passes through overlying tissues, thus decreasing the risk of complications and patient discomfort. Unlike the single-needle technique, the coaxial technique requires the precise placement of only the guide needle, thus substantially decreasing the duration of the procedure and the number of images required, especially for deep lesions with difficult access routes. Also, the coaxial technique allows both core biopsies and fine-needle aspiration biopsies to be performed through the same guide needle.

Relevant Anatomy

Planning a safe access route for image-guided biopsy of deep pelvic lesions requires a thorough knowledge of the complex anatomy of this region. Familiarity with the appearance and location of various structures on cross-sectional CT images is especially important (Fig. 20.1a–e).

The bony walls of the pelvis consist of the innominate bones anteriorly and laterally and the sacrum and coccyx posteriorly. The abdominal muscles, including the rectus abdominis, external oblique, internal oblique, and transverse abdominal muscles, form the anterior and anterolateral walls of the pelvis. The iliacus and psoas muscles join to form the iliopsoas muscle, which courses anterolaterally through the pelvis, medial to the iliac wing. The greater sciatic foramen is bounded by the iliac bone superiorly, the sacrospinous ligament inferiorly, the sacrum posteriorly, and the ischium anteriorly. The sacrospinous

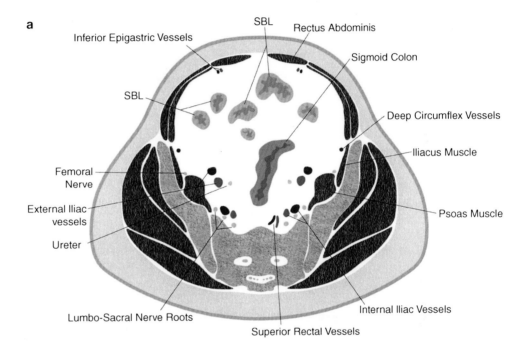

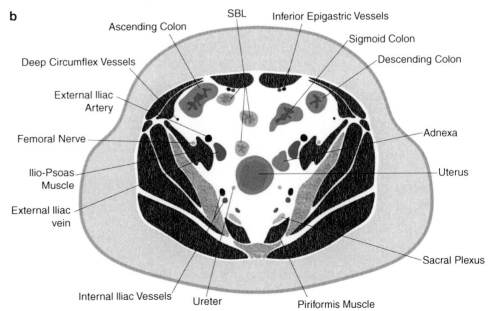

Fig. 20.1 Schematic drawing showing axial cross-sectional anatomy at various levels in the pelvic region: (**a**, **b**) upper pelvis; (**c**) upper, (**d**) mid-, and (**e**) lower greater sciatic foramen levels

Fig. 20.1 (continued)

c

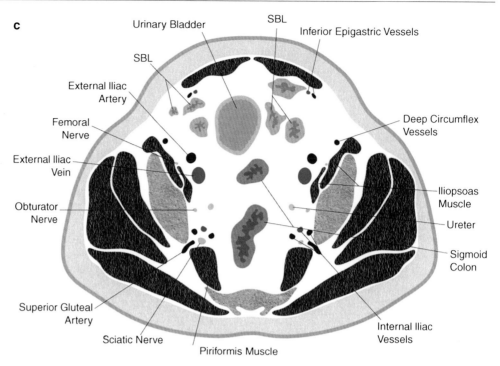

d

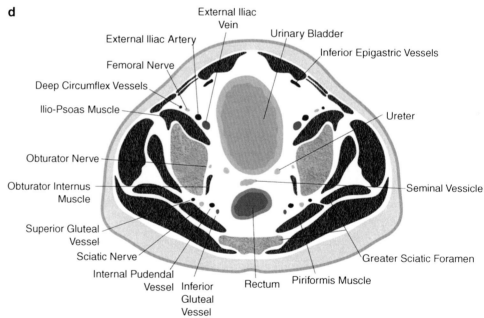

Fig. 20.1 (continued)   **e**

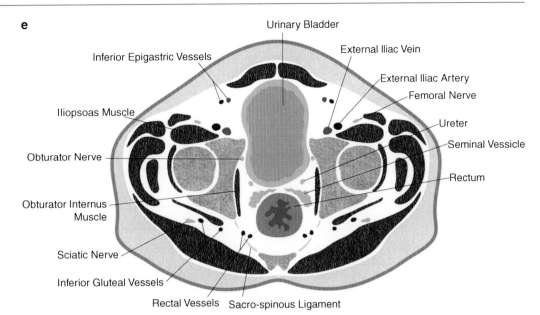

ligament divides the greater sciatic foramen into the superior and inferior portions. The important vasculature and nerve bundles exit the greater sciatic bundle cephalad to the level of the sacrospinous ligament. The piriformis muscle originates from the lateral sacrum, exits the pelvis through the greater sciatic foramen, and inserts into the greater trochanter of the femur. The internal obturator muscle forms the lateral wall of the pelvis and the ischiorectal fossa. The gluteal muscles lie posterior to the innominate bones.

Major intrapelvic visceral structures include the urinary bladder, rectum, and sigmoid colon in all patients, the uterus and ovaries in female patients, and the prostate and seminal vesicles in male patients. In addition, the superior portion of the pelvis is occupied by variable amounts of small-bowel loops and the ascending, descending, and sigmoid colon. The uterus is seen as a soft tissue density structure between the bladder and rectum. Although the position of the ovaries is highly variable, they are usually located posterolateral to the uterus, between the external iliac vessels and the ureter. In the upper part of the pelvis, the ureters are anterior to the common iliac vessels and anteromedial to the psoas muscle. The ureters then course inferiorly and posteriorly and at mid-pelvis level are located posterior to the external iliac vessels, anterior to the internal iliac vessels, and medial to the obturator nerve and artery. At the level of the sciatic foramen, the ureters turn medially toward the lateral angle of the bladder.

The common iliac arteries course downwards and laterally on the anterolateral surface of the fourth and fifth lumbar vertebrae along the medial aspect of the psoas muscles before dividing into the internal and external iliac arteries. The external iliac arteries run along the anteromedial border of the psoas muscles and continue as the common femoral arteries below the level of the inguinal ligament. The internal iliac arteries lie

posteriorly, in close relation to the lumbosacral plexus, before dividing into multiple branches at the level of the greater sciatic foramen. The external iliac veins are situated posteromedial to the arteries. The right common iliac vein is posterolateral to the corresponding artery, and the left common iliac vein ascends obliquely from the medial side of the left common iliac artery to pass posterior to the right common iliac artery.

At the level of the pelvis, the testicular/ovarian vessels are located laterally on the psoas muscles and lateral to the ureters. The inferior epigastric artery runs superiorly within the lateral umbilical fold and then along the posterior surface of the rectus abdominis muscle. The deep circumflex iliac artery, along with the accompanying vein, ascends along the anterior abdominal wall laterally near the iliac crest, and it is located just medial to the anterior portion of the iliacus muscle. The superior gluteal arteries arise from the posterior division of the internal iliac vessels and exit the greater sciatic foramen anterior and cephalad to the piriformis muscle. The internal pudendal and inferior gluteal vessels exit the greater sciatic foramen between the piriformis and the coccygeal muscle through the inferior part of the greater sciatic foramen.

The major pelvic nerve trunks can be visualized on CT sections. The greater sciatic nerve is formed from the sacral plexus. The nerve courses inferiorly on the ventral aspect of the piriformis muscle, exits the greater sciatic foramen below the piriformis muscle, and courses immediately posterior to the acetabulum. The femoral nerve can be seen posterior to the psoas muscle at about the L5 level. The nerve travels anteriorly and laterally in a fat plane between the iliacus and psoas muscles; in this location it is difficult to differentiate it from the iliac fascia. The femoral nerve then joins the external iliac vessels and is located lateral to the common femoral artery below the inguinal ligament. The obturator nerve emerges from the medial edge of the psoas muscle above the pelvic brim and courses inferiorly, in front of the internal iliac and obturator vessels and behind the external iliac vessels. The sacral canal contains 5 pairs of sacral nerve roots that exit through the sacral foramina. All the major nerve roots exit anteriorly; the dorsal foramina carry only minor cutaneous nerves.

Approaches to Pelvic Biopsy

Various approaches can be used for percutaneous needle biopsy of deep pelvic lesions using CT guidance. These include the anterior or anterolateral transabdominal approach, transgluteal approach, anterolateral extraperitoneal approach, and transosseous approach (Fig. 20.2a–e). For deep pelvic

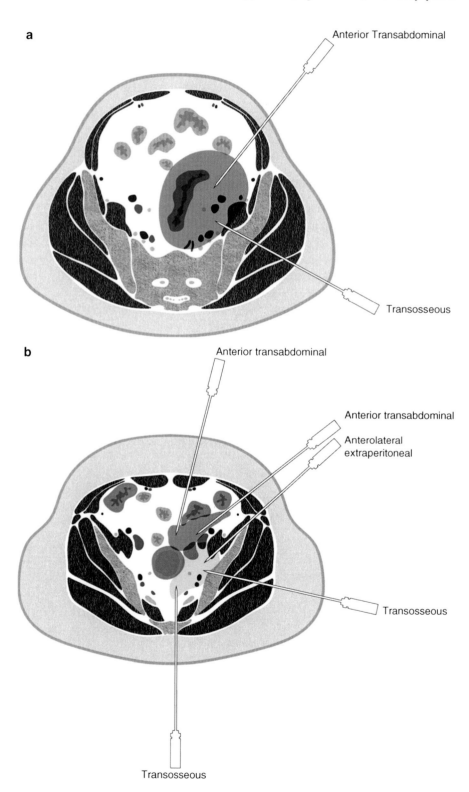

Fig. 20.2 Schematic drawing showing possible needle trajectories for pelvic biopsies at various levels in the pelvic region: (**a**, **b**) upper pelvis; (**c**) upper, (**d**) mid-, and (**e**) lower greater sciatic notch levels

Fig. 20.2 (continued)

c

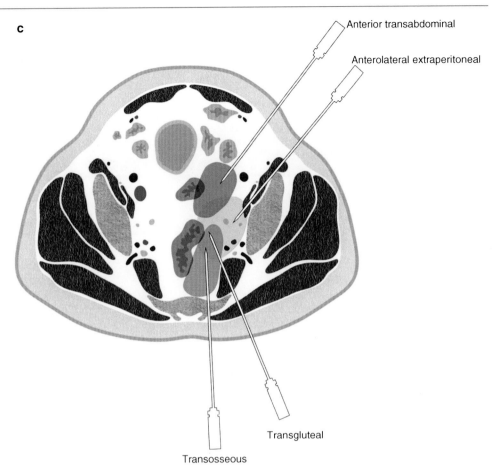

Anterior transabdominal

Anterolateral extraperitoneal

Transgluteal

Transosseous

d

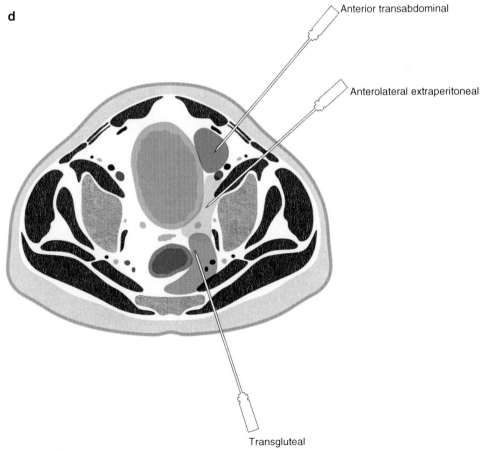

Anterior transabdominal

Anterolateral extraperitoneal

Transgluteal

Fig. 20.2 (continued)

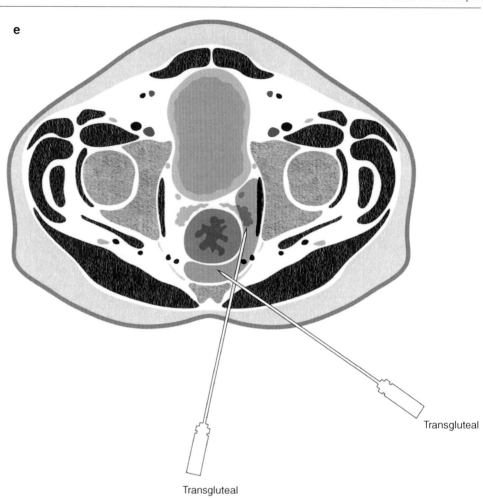

Transgluteal

Transgluteal

masses that are not accessible via percutaneous biopsy, the US-guided transvaginal or transrectal approach can be used.

Anterior or Anterolateral Transabdominal Approach

For this approach, the needle is inserted through the lower anterior or lateral abdominal wall muscles and the peritoneum. The inferior epigastric vessels located immediately behind the rectus abdominis muscle and the deep circumflex iliac vessels that are located more laterally are easy to identify on CT scans and should be avoided (Fig. 20.3). The transabdominal approach is suitable for lesions anterior or lateral to the bladder and is commonly used for biopsy of lymph nodes along the common iliac vessels, lesions that are located anterior or lateral to the psoas muscles, lower mesenteric masses, and, occasionally, anterior external iliac nodes.

Deep pelvic lesions are often difficult to reach by the transabdominal approach because of the intervening bowel and bladder, as well as the uterus and adnexa in female patients. A custom-tailored, curved 22-gauge needle advanced

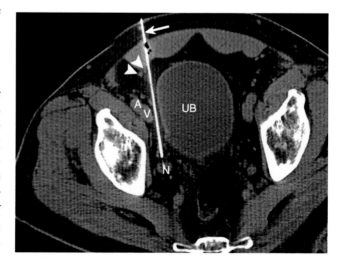

Fig. 20.3 Anterior abdominal approach. A computed tomographic scan shows the biopsy needle (*arrow*) advanced between the urinary bladder (*UB*) and the external iliac vessels (*A* and *V*) to biopsy a small internal iliac node (*N*). Note the presence of inferior epigastric vessels (*arrowheads*) immediately lateral to the needle trajectory

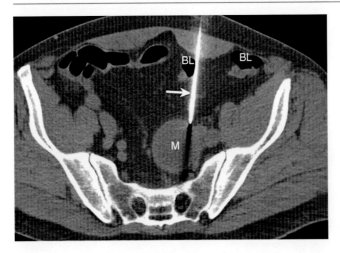

Fig. 20.4 Anterior abdominal approach. A computed tomographic scan shows an 18-gauge needle (*arrow*) advanced between the bowel loops (*BL*) to sample a presacral lesion (*M*)

coaxially through a straight guide needle can be used to circumvent intervening structures [1, 11]. The tip of the needle is grasped with a hemostat and bent to impart a curve. Occasionally, emptying the urinary bladder may allow access to deep lesions. CTF can also be used to assist percutaneous biopsy of masses with difficult or narrow access routes, especially lesions that are intermittently surrounded by bowel loops [12]. Angling of the CT gantry is another technique that can be used to help the radiologist avoid intervening structures in CT-guided biopsies of the abdomen [13].

Bowl loops occupy a major portion of the upper pelvis. Although transgression of bowel loops with a thin 22-gauge needle is generally considered safe, an attempt should be made to avoid transgression of the bowel loops. Bowel loops may change position and shape during the course of the biopsy, and bowel peristalsis may deflect the needle from its projected path. Hence, CT scans should be obtained between incremental needle advancements in order to determine the exact location of the needle with respect to the bowel loops (Fig. 20.4). Placing the patient in a lateral decubitus position may help displace the bowel loops from the projected needle path [1]. Alternatively, administration of saline through the guide needle can be used to displace intervening bowel loop and allow safe access to an otherwise unreachable lesion (Fig. 20.5).

With the transabdominal approach, the potential risk of inadvertent transgression of bowel loops limits the size of biopsy needle that can be used, precluding the option of obtaining a core specimen in most patients. This approach can also be painful for the patient because of the peritoneal transgression. The presence of abdominal wounds, dressings, or colostomy bags may preclude access in patients who have just had surgery.

Transgluteal Approach

For the transgluteal approach, the patient is usually placed in a prone, prone oblique, or lateral decubitus position. This approach is also called the trans-sciatic approach because the needle traverses the greater sciatic foramen. Care should be taken to avoid the neurovascular structures (branches of internal iliac arteries and sciatic nerve) coursing in the sciatic foramen. The needle should be inserted through the sacrospinous ligament in the caudal part of the notch below the level of the piriformis muscle to avoid injury to the gluteal vessels and the sacral plexus, which lie anterior to the muscle. It is generally recommended that the needle be placed close to the edge of the sacrum to avoid injury to the sciatic nerve and gluteal vessels that exit the pelvis in the anterior portion of the notch, close to the ischium [3, 6, 7].

The transgluteal approach is generally used for posterior pelvic lesions in the lower part of the pelvis at the level of the greater sciatic foramen that are difficult to access by an anterior approach because of the intervening bowel, bladder, uterus, and iliac vessels (Fig. 20.6). Lesions located in the presacral and perirectal regions, lesions located posterior or posterolateral to the urinary bladder (Fig. 20.7), and adnexal masses can be accessed with this technique.

Cranial needle angulation allows the transgluteal approach to be used for accessing upper pelvic lesions located cranial to the level of the greater sciatic foramen. Using a triangulation method, the physician estimates the needle angle from contiguous axial CT scans obtained from the level of the planned skin entry site to the level of the target lesion. The needle is inserted below the level of the lesion and advanced cranially and medially through the greater sciatic foramen, and axial CT scans are obtained to check the needle tip position and angulation (Fig. 20.8).

Alternatively, a magnetic field-based electronic guidance system can be used to facilitate this out-of-plane access to pelvic lesions. The system uses a low magnetic field, with position sensors on the patient and the needle shaft to provide virtual real-time guidance for needle placement. This works by overlaying real-time instrument tracking information on an existing CT or positron emission tomographic-CT image. As the needle is advanced toward the target lesion, the relative location, orientation, and virtual trajectory of the needle are displayed and continually updated.

The transgluteal approach avoids peritoneal transgression and potential injury of the bladder, bowel loops, and external iliac vessels. Although the sciatic nerve, gluteal vessels, and branches of the sacral plexus can be injured in the transgluteal approach, the risk is extremely low. Also, a needle advanced through the gluteal muscles is more stable and less prone to needle deflection than it is in the transabdominal approach. However, a distended rectum can block the needle path, and obese patients or patients with abdominal wounds,

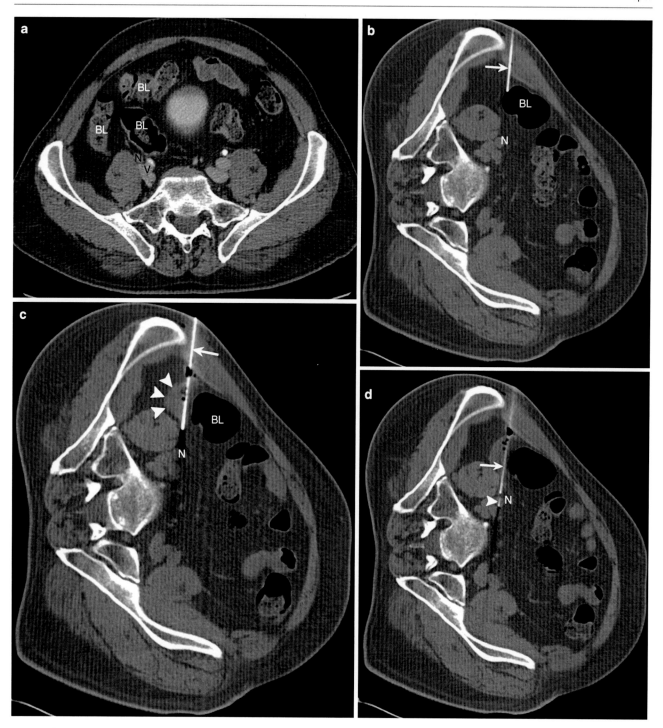

Fig. 20.5 Lateral abdominal approach. (**a**) A computed tomographic scan of the patient in the supine position shows bowel loops (*BL*) anterior to a common iliac node (*N*), which is located anterolaterally to the common iliac vessels (*V*). (**b**) Placing the patient in the left lateral decubitus position created a small window lateral to the bowel loop (*BL*) allowing initial needle (*arrow*) insertion. However, further advancement of the needle is not possible because of the presence of bowel. (**c**) Injection of saline (*arrowheads*) through the 18-gauge Hawkins needle (*arrow*) resulted in displacement of the bowel (*BL*), allowing safe advancement of the needle up to the target node (*N*). (**d**) A 22-gauge needle (*arrowhead*) was advanced through the Hawkins needle (*arrow*) to sample the node (*N*)

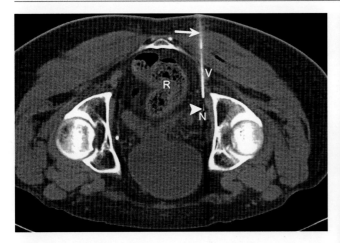

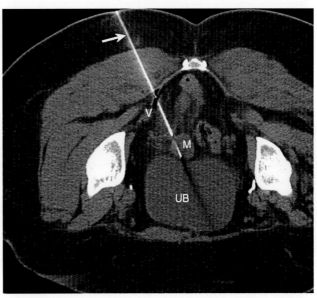

Fig. 20.6 Transgluteal approach. A computed tomographic scan shows the coaxial technique, with a 22-gauge inner needle (*arrowhead*) advanced through an 18-gauge guide needle (*arrow*) to biopsy an obturator lymph node (*N*). The needle is passing through the sacrospinous ligament and between the rectum (*R*) and vessels (*V*)

Fig. 20.7 Transgluteal approach. A computed tomographic scan shows the needle (*arrow*) passing through the sacrospinous ligament, posterior to the inferior gluteal vessels (*V*), for biopsy of a soft tissue mass (*M*) located posterior to the urinary bladder (*UB*)

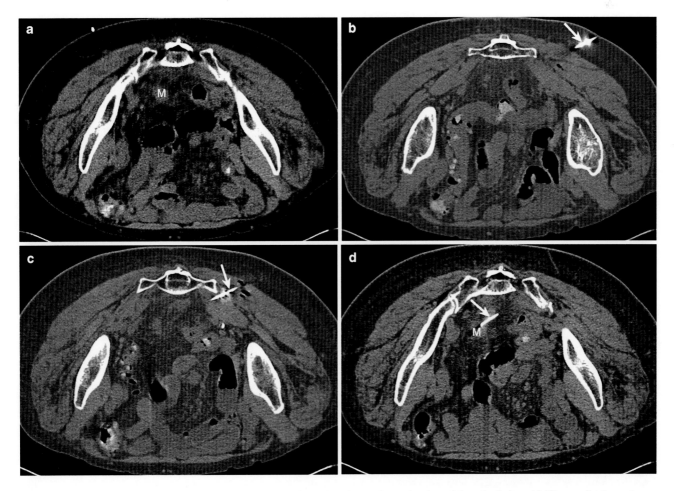

Fig. 20.8 Transgluteal out-of-plane approach. (**a**) A computed tomographic (*CT*) scan with the patient in the prone position shows a soft tissue mass (*M*) in the posterior pelvis. Direct transgluteal access is not possible because the lesion is located cranially to the level of the greater sciatic foramen. (**b**) A CT scan shows the biopsy needle (*arrow*) inserted at a level caudal to the lesion. (**c**) The needle (*arrow*) was advanced through the greater sciatic foramen in a cranial direction using the triangulation method. (**d**) A CT scan at a more cranial level shows the needle tip (*arrow*) within the mass (*M*)

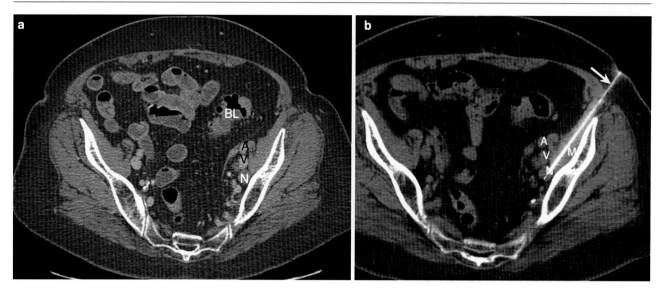

Fig. 20.9 Anterolateral approach. (**a**) A computed tomographic (*CT*) scan shows that an anterior approach to the deep external iliac lymph node (*N*) was obstructed by bowel loops (*BL*) and the external iliac artery (*A*) and vein (*V*). A transgluteal approach was obstructed by the sacrum. (**b**) A CT scan shows safe biopsy of the node (*N*) with a needle (*arrow*) advanced through the iliopsoas muscle (*M*), medial to the external iliac artery (*A*) and vein (*V*)

multiple surgical dressings, drainage tubes, or colostomy bags may not be able to lie in the prone position.

Anterolateral Extraperitoneal Approach

The anterolateral extraperitoneal approach involves needle transgression through the iliopsoas muscle [8, 14]. The biopsy needle is inserted medial to the iliac crest and advanced through the iliopsoas muscle toward the target lesion, using CT to check the needle's trajectory and ensure that the needle remains lateral to the iliac vessels (Fig. 20.9). The deep circumflex iliac vessels are located just medial to the anterior portion of the iliacus muscle and should be avoided.

The anterolateral extraperitoneal approach provides safe access to the obturator or deep external iliac, anterior external iliac, and internal iliac lymph nodes. The anterior transabdominal approach to these nodes is obstructed by the intervening bladder, bowel, uterus, and iliac vessels. These nodes are also usually not accessible by the posterior transgluteal approach because of the presence of osseous structures or internal iliac vessel branches in the needle path. Also, a transgluteal approach to internal iliac or obturator nodes often requires needle placement close to the ischial tuberosity, which increases the risk of injury to the sciatic nerve and gluteal vessels.

The anterolateral extraperitoneal approach can also be used to access adnexal masses, soft tissue masses or loculated fluid collections along the lateral pelvic side wall, and common iliac nodes located posterior to the vessels. It can also be used for biopsy of posteriorly located lesions in patients who have difficulty lying in a prone position because of recent surgery, colostomy bags, or abdominal wounds [14].

For most patients the preliminary noncontrast-enhanced CT scans are sufficient for biopsy planning. However, contrast administration is occasionally necessary to differentiate vessels from lymph nodes [14]. Care should be taken to avoid puncturing the ureter, which is located posterior to the external iliac vessels and anterior to the internal iliac vessels before coursing medially to enter the base of the urinary bladder. When the location of the external iliac vessels and the slope of the iliac wing preclude a straight route to the target lesion, a curved 22-gauge needle advanced coaxially through the straight 18-gauge guide needle can be used to obtain a biopsy specimen (Fig. 20.10).

The anterolateral approach through the iliopsoas muscle is less painful and better tolerated by patients than the anterior transabdominal approach because it avoids transgression of the peritoneum. Because the anterolateral approach does not pose a risk of bowel or bladder injury, the use of large-caliber needles for core biopsies is possible. The iliac bone prevents lateral deviation of the needle, allowing accurate needle placement. Advancement of the biopsy needle through the iliopsoas muscle stabilizes the needle, permitting long needle paths without the risk of needle deflection because of anterior abdominal wall movement or bowel peristalsis, which is a potential problem with the anterior transabdominal approach.

On the other hand, approach via the iliopsoas muscle poses a risk of injury to the femoral nerve, which runs in the fat plane separating the iliacus and psoas muscles. Injury is unlikely, however, because the femoral nerve is located at the medial end of the fissure between the muscles, whereas the needle usually passes through the lateral portion of the fis-

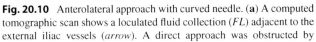

Fig. 20.10 Anterolateral approach with curved needle. (**a**) A computed tomographic scan shows a loculated fluid collection (*FL*) adjacent to the external iliac vessels (*arrow*). A direct approach was obstructed by bowel loops (*B*). (**b**) A curved 22-gauge needle (*arrow*) was advanced through a straight 18-gauge guide needle (*curved arrow*) and passed anterior to the iliac vessels (*arrowhead*) into the fluid collection (*FL*)

sure. Also, the guide needle is much more likely to displace the nerve than to puncture it.

Transosseous Approach

For the transosseous approach, the needle can be advanced through the sacrum or through the iliac bone [1]. The trans-sacral approach can be used for biopsy of presacral and posterior pelvic lesions that are not accessible via the transgluteal approach either because they are located above the level of the greater sciatic foramen or because of the presence of intervening vascular structures. The trans-sacral approach can also be used for biopsy of small presacral masses when the transgluteal approach would entail a prohibitively long needle path through the buttock fat and gluteal muscles, especially in obese patients. Care should be taken to avoid the sacral foramina and sacral canal to avoid injury to sacral nerve roots and the sacral plexus. It is especially important to avoid the ventral neural foramina, which contain the major nerve roots. The needle can be advanced through the medial portion of the sacrum between the central canal and the foramina, or it can go through the extreme lateral part of the sacrum. Occasionally, bone involvement by tumor extension may create a path for the needle.

A transosseous approach through the iliac bone can be used to access lesions in relation to the iliopsoas muscle not approachable by other routes. The use of this approach for biopsy of common iliac or external iliac nodes or adnexal cystic lesions has been reported [1]. For the transiliac approach, if possible, the needle should be advanced through the narrow part of the iliac wing (Fig. 20.11). The needle subsequently passes through the iliopsoas muscle on its way to the lesion. It is important to identify and avoid the ureters and gonadal vessels, which course anterior and medial to the psoas muscle, close to the common iliac vessels.

Any of the commercially available 16- or 18-gauge needles allow easy transosseous access through the iliac wing or the caudal part of the sacrum. However, if required, large-bore (11- or 13-gauge) bone-biopsy needles or a bone drill can be used for transosseous access [2]. Bone transgression can occasionally be painful; however, this can be avoided by generous infiltration of anesthetic agent into the periosteum before attempting bone penetration.

Transvaginal or Transrectal Approach

An US-guided transvaginal or transrectal approach is used for biopsy of deep pelvic masses that are not accessible via percutaneous approach.

The transvaginal approach is an optimal route to deep pelvic masses owing to the proximity of the vaginal fornices to these lesions. However, it is infrequently used because the primary diagnosis of ovarian and adnexal masses is usually made with open or laparoscopic surgery. Controversies regarding risk of peritoneal seeding, spread of malignant cells, and false-negative results in cystic malignancies limit the use of transvaginal biopsy. Currently, it is performed in patients who are not surgical candidates because of poor performance status or inoperable disease and who have a primary malignancy outside the pelvis with suspected ovarian metastasis [15]. Transvaginal biopsy is also used to confirm recurrent ovarian or adnexal malignancies before initiation of chemotherapy. Recurrent malignancies at the cervix or vaginal cuff, where the anatomy could be distorted if the patient has had radiotherapy, are also readily imaged and biopsied using the transvaginal approach [16].

For the transvaginal approach, the patient is placed in the lithotomy position for insertion of the US transducer. An initial US is performed to evaluate the mass and to determine the shortest and safest route to avoid the intervening bowel,

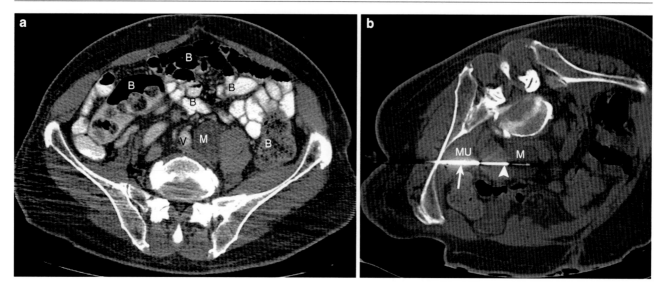

Fig. 20.11 Transosseous approach. (**a**) A computed tomographic scan with the patient in the supine position shows that multiple bowel loops (*B*) obstruct a straight path to a mass (*M*) located lateral to the left common iliac vessel (*V*). (**b**) With the patient in the prone position, the biopsy needle was advanced through iliac bone and the iliacus and psoas muscles (*MU*) to sample the mass (*M*)

bladder, and vessels. Once the biopsy route is planned, the perineum and the vagina are prepared with povidone-iodine. Antibiotic prophylaxis is not routinely required. The transvaginal transducer is covered with a sterile cover and a special guide needle is attached to the transducer. The guide needle-transducer assembly is then covered with a second sterile cover and applied against the vaginal fornix with steady pressure. The procedure is performed under moderate sedation because it is usually not possible to adequately anesthetize the needle tract. The biopsy needle is directed to the lesion through the guide needle using the coaxial technique. Subsequently, the vaginal forniceal wall is traversed with a short, rapid thrust of the needle to minimize tenting of the vaginal wall [17]. Aspiration needles ranging from 20 to 22 gauge are used for cytologic evaluation and cutting needles ranging from 16 to 20 gauge for histologic evaluation. When the lesion is predominantly cystic, complete aspiration is important to decrease the risk of infection and recurrence. Lesions with features suggestive of a dermoid cyst should not be aspirated because they require surgical removal.

The transrectal approach is well established for prostate biopsy in routine clinical urology practice today, although it is rarely used for biopsy of other pelvic masses. The transrectal approach is especially useful for pelvic masses close to the iliac vessels, the most common site for nodal metastasis from pelvic malignancies [18]. Transrectal US has also been shown to be highly accurate in differentiating between normal vaginal vault thickness and tumor recurrence. The transrectal approach may be favored over the transvaginal approach in patients with postsurgical/ postmenopausal vaginal shortening and post-radiation vaginal fibrosis or atrophy [19].

Transrectal biopsy is performed with the patient in the left lateral decubitus position for the insertion of the transrectal transducer. Infection is the most feared complication; therefore, routine antibiotic prophylaxis is recommended. Local anesthetic is infiltrated using a 22-gauge needle along the projected needle tract to decrease patient discomfort and pain. Biopsy is usually performed with an 18-gauge cutting needle through the guide needle-transducer assembly using the coaxial technique.

Outcome and Results

Image-guided biopsy is widely employed in daily clinical practice. It is a safe, cost-effective, and accurate procedure for cytohistologic diagnosis of most pelvic lesions (ovarian and adnexal lesions are usually diagnosed with open or laparoscopic surgery instead).

CT guidance is routinely used for percutaneous biopsy of pelvic lesions and has a reported diagnostic accuracy ranging from 88 to 97 % in large series [10, 20, 21]. Technical success rates are 96–100 % and no complications are reported in these series. At some institutions, US guidance is preferred over CT guidance for percutaneous biopsy of pelvic lesions whenever feasible. Studies using US guidance demonstrate diagnostic accuracy rates as high as 95–98 % and technical success rates of 94–95 % when adequate specimens are obtained [15, 22]. Although US guidance has slightly higher rates of accuracy and sensitivity than CT guidance, the difference is not statistically significant [22, 23].

US guidance also offers alternative routes, such as the transvaginal or transrectal approach, to deep pelvic lesions that may not be accessible via CT-guided percutaneous approach. In a series of 101 patients, sensitivity was 76 and 91 % for transvaginal fine-needle aspiration biopsy and core biopsy, respectively, and accuracy was 83 and 91 % (no false-positive results were obtained) [24].

There are few studies evaluating transrectal biopsy for pelvic lesions. In a study of 17 patients with recurrent cervical carcinoma, transrectal biopsy provided histologic diagnosis of recurrence in 16 patients [19]. In another study of 11 patients with primary and secondary pelvic malignancies, transrectal biopsy was adequate for histologic diagnosis in all patients [18]. Pathologic diagnoses included 6 nodal metastases from transitional cell carcinoma, 1 nodal metastasis from prostate cancer, 1 paravesical recurrence of cervical cancer, 1 metastasis from cecal cancer, and 2 cases of paravesical metastasis of gastric cancer [18]. No major complications have been reported in several studies of both transvaginal and transrectal biopsies [25].

Summary

Several approaches and various imaging techniques can be used for image-guided pelvic biopsy. Familiarity with the cross-sectional pelvic anatomy facilitates planning of a safe access route for biopsy of deep-seated lesions and helps avoid injury to major neurovascular structures and other viscera. Knowing the advantages and disadvantages of each approach allows the clinician to choose the most appropriate one. Additionally, techniques such as saline injection, change in patient position, or the use of a curved needle may allow safe access to seemingly "unapproachable" lesions.

References

1. Gupta S, Nguyen HL, Morello Jr FA, et al. Various approaches for CT-guided percutaneous biopsy of deep pelvic lesions: anatomic and technical considerations. Radiographics. 2004;24(1):175–89.
2. Bodne DJ, Carrasco CH, Richli WR. Transosseous air contrast CT-guided needle biopsy of a cystic neoplasm. Cardiovasc Intervent Radiol. 1993;16(2):122–3.
3. Butch RJ, Mueller PR, Ferrucci Jr JT, et al. Drainage of pelvic abscesses through the greater sciatic foramen. Radiology. 1986;158(2):487–91.
4. Carlson P, Crummy AB, Wojtowycz M, McDermott JC. A safe route for deep pelvic biopsy with distention of the iliacus muscle. J Vasc Interv Radiol. 1991;2(2):277–8.
5. Guo Z, Kurtycz DF, De Las Casas LE, Hoerl HD. Radiologically guided percutaneous fine-needle aspiration biopsy of pelvic and retroperitoneal masses: a retrospective study of 68 cases. Diagn Cytopathol. 2001;25(1):43–9.
6. Harisinghani MG, Gervais DA, Hahn PF, et al. CT-guided transgluteal drainage of deep pelvic abscesses: indications, technique, procedure-related complications, and clinical outcome. Radiographics. 2002;22(6):1353–67.
7. Pardes JG, Schneider M, Koizumi J, Engel IA, Auh YH, Rubenstein W. Percutaneous needle biopsy of deep pelvic masses: a posterior approach. Cardiovasc Intervent Radiol. 1986;9(2):65–8.
8. Phillips VM, Bernardino M. The parallel iliac approach: a safe and accurate technique for deep pelvic node biopsy. J Comput Tomogr. 1984;8(3):237–8.
9. Rapport 2nd RL, Ferguson GS. Dorsal approach to presacral biopsy: technical case report. Neurosurgery. 1997;40(5):1087–8.
10. Triller J, Maddern G, Kraft P, Heidar A, Vock P. CT-guided biopsy of pelvic masses. Cardiovasc Intervent Radiol. 1991;14(1):63–8.
11. Gupta S, Ahrar K, Morello Jr FA, Wallace MJ, Madoff DC, Hicks ME. Using a coaxial technique with a curved inner needle for CT-guided fine-needle aspiration biopsy. Am J Roentgenol. 2002;179(1):109–12.
12. Schweiger GD, Yip VY, Brown BP. CT fluoroscopic guidance for percutaneous needle placement into abdominopelvic lesions with difficult access routes. Abdom Imaging. 2000;25(6):633–7.
13. Yueh N, Halvorsen Jr RA, Letourneau JG, Crass JR. Gantry tilt technique for CT-guided biopsy and drainage. J Comput Assist Tomogr. 1989;13(1):182–4.
14. Gupta S, Madoff DC, Ahrar K, et al. CT-guided needle biopsy of deep pelvic lesions by extraperitoneal approach through iliopsoas muscle. Cardiovasc Intervent Radiol. 2003;26(6):534–8.
15. Fischerova D, Cibula D, Dundr P, et al. Ultrasound-guided tru-cut biopsy in the management of advanced abdomino-pelvic tumors. Int J Gynecol Cancer. 2008;18(4):833–7.
16. Scanlan KA, Propeck PA, Lee Jr FT. Invasive procedures in the female pelvis: value of transabdominal, endovaginal, and endorectal US guidance. Radiographics. 2001;21(2):491–506.
17. O'Neill MJ, Rafferty EA, Lee SI, et al. Transvaginal interventional procedures: aspiration, biopsy, and catheter drainage. Radiographics. 2001;21(3):657–72.
18. Rinnab L, Kufer R, Hautmann RE, Gottfried HW. Use of transrectal ultrasound-guided biopsy in the diagnosis of pelvic malignancies. J Clin Ultrasound. 2006;34(9):440–5.
19. Roy D, Kulkarni A, Kulkarni S, Thakur MH, Maheshwari A, Tongaonkar HB. Transrectal ultrasound-guided biopsy of recurrent cervical carcinoma. Br J Radiol. 2008;81(971):902–6.
20. Oyen RH, Van Poppel HP, Ameye FE, Van de Voorde WA, Baert AL, Baert LV. Lymph node staging of localized prostatic carcinoma with CT and CT-guided fine-needle aspiration biopsy: prospective study of 285 patients. Radiology. 1994;190(2):315–22.
21. Welch TJ, Sheedy 2nd PF, Johnson CD, Johnson CM, Stephens DH. CT-guided biopsy: prospective analysis of 1,000 procedures. Radiology. 1989;171(2):493–6.
22. Yarram SG, Nghiem HV, Higgins E, Fox G, Nan B, Francis IR. Evaluation of imaging-guided core biopsy of pelvic masses. Am J Roentgenol. 2007;188(5):1208–11.
23. Griffin N, Grant LA, Freeman SJ, et al. Image-guided biopsy in patients with suspected ovarian carcinoma: a safe and effective technique? Eur Radiol. 2009;19(1):230–5.
24. Zanetta G, Brenna A, Pittelli M, Lissoni A, Trio D, Riotta S. Transvaginal ultrasound-guided fine needle sampling of deep cancer recurrences in the pelvis: usefulness and limitations. Gynecol Oncol. 1994;54(1):59–63.
25. Zanetta G, Lissoni A, Franchi D, Pittelli MR, Cormio G, Trio D. Safety of transvaginal fine needle puncture of gynecologic masses: a report after 500 consecutive procedures. J Ultrasound Med. 1996;15(5):401–4.

MRI-Guided Prostate Biopsy

R. Jason Stafford, Stephen E. McRae, and Kamran Ahrar

Background

Prostate cancer was the most prevalent non-cutaneous cancer diagnosis in men in the United States in 2011 and was the second most deadly cancer, increasing several percentage points in recent years to account for roughly 29 % (240,890) of cases and 11 % (33,720) of cancer-related deaths [1]. On the basis of data collected between 1996 and 2004, 91 % of newly diagnosed cases are staged as localized or regional, for which the 5-year relative survival rate approaches 100 % [2, 3].

Patient management in the era of early detection is an area of discussion and research, with a focus on potential overdiagnosis and overtreatment of disease versus quality of life. Modern prostate cancer screening is accomplished by measuring prostate-specific antigen (PSA) levels, a nonspecific test, and digital rectal examinations (DREs) [4–8]. Taking into account the lack of solid evidence that early detection substantially influences outcomes, the current recommendation is to discuss and consider the benefits of annual screening in men >50 years with a life expectancy of at least 10 years and screening in men ≤50 years with risk factors for prostate cancer [6].

Abnormal PSA or DRE findings are standard indicators for prostate biopsy, or in the case of posttreatment changes, the prostate bed. Transrectal ultrasound (TRUS) has become the standard image-guidance modality for prostate interventions after having been introduced in 1968 [9]. With TRUS, procedures can often be performed by urologists in an office setting, using a relatively inexpensive, portable ultrasound device that is placed in the rectum to provide real-time imaging of the prostate to facilitate systemic sampling across the gland. The optimal biopsy strategy for prostate cancer remains an area of research, but the current standard is to use an 18-gauge biopsy gun to sample at least six, but more often 10–14, cores distributed across the base, mid-gland, and apex of the prostate [10]. Often, additional lateral sampling is performed to ensure proper sampling of the peripheral zone, in which approximately 70 % of prostate cancer is diagnosed. Positive biopsy rates using TRUS guidance are 30–40 % [11, 12], with approximately 35 % of cancers being missed on the first biopsy [13].

Prostate biopsy samples are sent for histopathologic analysis, from which the Gleason score is calculated [14]. The Gleason system uses a five-level scale to score observed cellular differentiation, with 1 having the most differentiation and 5 the least. The score is the addition of the most prevalent and second-most prevalent scores from the tissue samples (e.g., $3+4=7$). High scores are associated with a poor prognosis. The Gleason score, in conjunction with the number and percentage of tumor-involved cores, is a standard primary prognostic indicator for patient management decisions [15].

Unfortunately, TRUS-guided prostate biopsy is associated with a significant number of false-negative findings, often leading to repeated biopsies in men with persistently abnormal PSA results. A high incidence of cancer is detected on subsequent TRUS biopsies, indicating that TRUS-guided biopsy has a poor negative predictive value. In addition, the

R.J. Stafford, PhD (✉)
Department of Imaging Physics,
The University of Texas MD Anderson
Cancer Center, Houston, TX, USA
e-mail: jstafford@mdanderson.org

S.E. McRae, MD
Department of Interventional Radiology,
The University of Texas MD Anderson
Cancer Center, Houston, TX, USA

Department of Diagnostic Radiology,
Division of Diagnostic Imaging,
The University of Texas MD Anderson
Cancer Center, Houston, TX, USA

K. Ahrar, MD, FSIR
Department of Interventional Radiology,
Department of Thoracic and Cardiovascular Surgery,
The University of Texas MD Anderson Cancer Center,
1515 Holcombe Boulevard, Unit 1471,
Houston, TX 77030, USA
e-mail: kahrar@mdanderson.org

K. Ahrar, S. Gupta (eds.), *Percutaneous Image-Guided Biopsy*,
DOI 10.1007/978-1-4614-8217-8_21, © Springer Science+Business Media New York 2014

current approach to random biopsy can result in underestimation of the Gleason grade [16]. This deficiency has resulted in a substantial amount of research on more advanced imaging modalities and techniques to identify potential regions of focal disease.

Magnetic Resonance Imaging of the Prostate

Although TRUS remains the current standard for guidance of prostate interventions, targeted guidance of prostate biopsies on the basis of sonographic imaging findings has been shown to be less effective at cancer detection than systemic approaches [17, 18]. However, incorporating sonographic imaging information into systemic biopsy approaches may lead to higher sensitivity [19].

This potential to dramatically increasing diagnostic power by incorporating additional imaging information has been a strong motivation for incorporating magnetic resonance imaging (MRI) results into biopsy planning. MRI has multiple soft-tissue contrast mechanisms that can be exploited to evaluate the prostate and surrounding anatomy, establishing it as one of the best imaging modalities for detecting and staging prostate cancer. The potential for MRI to identify the most suspicious areas and increase the chance of obtaining comprehensive results has led many research groups to investigate the use of MR guidance for biopsy targeting and other prostate interventions, such as brachytherapy, photodynamic therapy, and thermal ablative therapy [20, 21]. In this chapter, we briefly outline the diagnostic imaging procedures for prostate MRI. More nuanced reviews are recommended for a more detailed discussion of prostate MRI [22].

Diagnostic MRI of the prostate is usually performed with the patient supine and oriented feet first into a 1.5 T or 3.0 T scanner. A carefully placed endorectal receiver coil is used, in conjunction with anterior and posterior pelvic phased-array receiver coils, to increase the signal-to-noise ratio (SNR). Endorectal coils are usually relatively inexpensive, single-use coils that connect to the system through a special surface coil connector interface that must be purchased from the MRI vendor that provides automatic coil tuning.

The position of the endorectal coil must be confirmed via localization images and adjusted to ensure proper alignment and coverage prior to proceeding with the examination. The signal from the endorectal coil also falls off precipitously with distance from the coil, introducing substantial shading into the image that should be removed during post-processing. Poor bowel preparation and air between the endorectal coil balloon and rectum can also be sources of poor image quality and motion artifacts. The balloon used to keep the endorectal coil in place can compress the prostate, distorting the appearance of local anatomical structures. Because of these technical hindrances, the endorectal coil is often omitted for detection and localization purposes, such as for radiotherapy or brachytherapy planning or for image-guided interventions.

The prostate gland is approximately 4 cm in diameter and is generally abutted between the urogenital diaphragm at the apex of the gland and the bladder at the base. The anatomy of the prostate gland is usually described in terms of zones [23]. The centermost zone is the transition zone, which surrounds the urethra, consists of approximately 5 % glandular tissue, and houses 25 % of prostate tumors. Although the zonal interface is not discernible on imaging, it is surrounded by the central zone, which is 20 % glandular tissue, with a 5 % tumor incidence. The central zone contains the ejaculatory ducts, which connect the urethra to the seminal vesicles at the base of the prostate, posterior to the bladder. Because the transition and central zones cannot be distinguished on imaging, the entire region is often referred to as the central gland. The outermost zone is the peripheral zone, which is primarily glandular tissue (70–80 %) and houses approximately 70 % of prostate cancers. A non-glandular fibromuscular stroma lies anterior to the peripheral zone, and the gland is encapsulated by fibrous tissue. Tumor extending beyond this region is referred to as extraprostatic extension. The neurovascular bundles are located posterolateral to the capsule that encompasses the peripheral zone. The bundles penetrate the capsule at the apex and base and are a common area of extraprostatic extension.

High-resolution, T2-weighted (fast spin echo with TR: 3,000–4,000 ms; TE: 120–140 ms) anatomical imaging is a primary diagnostic and localization tool in prostate MRI; it provides the most accurate representation of zonal prostate anatomy and surrounding critical structures, with contrast that is unmatched by any other current imaging modality [22, 24]. The central gland tends to be hypointense but can be of mixed intensity in the presence of benign prostatic hyperplasia. In contrast, the peripheral zone tends to be hyperintense to isointense, making a usually hypointense prostate carcinoma more conspicuous in the peripheral zone than in the central gland. However, other pathologic conditions can also present as hypointense on T2-weighted images, including benign prostatic hyperplasia, chronic prostatitis, radiation or hormonal treatment effects, calcifications, smooth muscle or fibromuscular hyperplasia, and biopsy hemorrhage [25]. To minimize interpretation errors due to biopsy, waiting at least 6–8 weeks is recommended [26]. In addition, because of the anatomical contrast, T2-weighted images are useful for evaluating extracapsular extension and seminal vesicle invasion (Fig. 21.1).

An extremely valuable functional imaging complement to T2-weighted imaging is diffusion-weighted imaging (DWI). DWI usually uses a lower-resolution echo-planar imaging acquisition sequence, which can be prone to distortion and susceptibility artifacts from nearby air-tissue or metal interfaces. Large gradients are applied that strongly attenuate freely diffusing water molecules in tissue. Prostate carcinoma is often

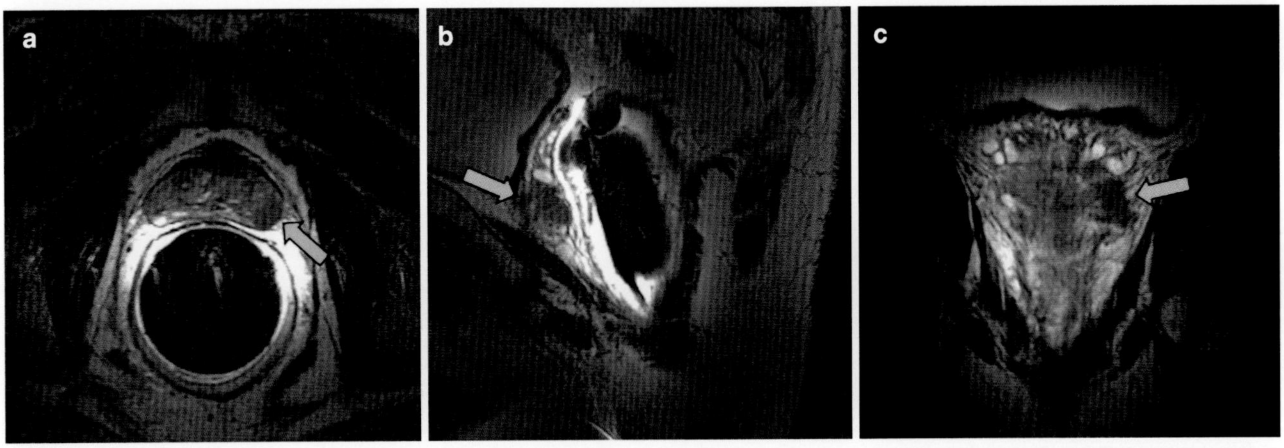

Fig. 21.1 Axial (**a**), sagittal (**b**), and coronal (**c**) T2-weighted images of the prostate in a 66-year-old with increasing PSA levels. The images were acquired at 1.5 T, with an endorectal coil for staging, and diagnosed as stage T2a prostate adenocarcinoma, with a PSA of 2 and Gleason score of 7 (3 + 4). The suspicious lesion (*arrows*) presents as a hypointense region in the left posterolateral aspect of the mid-gland and base, extending almost to the apex

characterized by high cellularity, which restricts water diffusion and results in hyperintensity on DWI. Fluid regions, such as cysts, have extremely high signals to start with; thus, the residual signal may also appear hyperintense on DWI. To remove this "T2 shine-through" effect, maps of the apparent diffusion coefficient (ADC) are generally constructed using two or more weighting values ("b-values"), generally of 0–1,000 s/mm². Most modern scanners automatically generate these maps as a separate series to the DWI if the option is purchased and turned on in the protocol. These ADC maps are reflective of the diffusion coefficient itself; therefore, contrast is inverted with respect to DWI (i.e., restricted diffusion lesions appear hypointense on ADC maps). Although these derived ADC maps may appear noisier than DWI, they can be essential to the proper interpretation of DWI findings (Fig. 21.2).

T1-weighted images do not have a similar level of anatomical or zonal contrast, and the gland tends to be isointense. Hemorrhage often appears hyperintense against this background, making T1-weighted images useful for interpreting regions of hypointensity on T2-weighted images. Because of this and because of the usefulness of T1-weighted images in evaluating regional lymphadenopathies, periprostatic structure invasion, and bone lesions, T1-weighted imaging is usually performed in only one plane, with a larger field of view for diagnostic imaging (Fig. 21.3).

Static pre- and post-contrast T1-weighted imaging is not useful for tumor evaluation because of nonspecific contrast uptake in the gland [27, 28]. Dynamic contrast-enhanced (DCE) MRI of the prostate provides a means to observe contrast uptake kinetics via the change in the T1-weighed signal over time (Fig. 21.3) [29]. The time course of the signal is usually analyzed using a workstation with dedicated software that also generates metrics on the basis of the contrast kinetics in the tissue. Tissue with rapid uptake and contrast agent

washout are suspicious for malignancy [30]. Although techniques vary widely and the practice is evolving, acquisitions usually incorporate a rapid (<8 s per volume), 3D gradient-recalled echo technique after an injection of gadolinium-based contrast agent (~3 ml/s). In a manner analogous to incorporating color and power Doppler in conventional TRUS-guided biopsy, DCE-MRI may play a role in biopsy cases, aiding in further increasing the sensitivity of the technique and reducing the number of samples required to obtain a diagnostic result [31]. However, post-biopsy changes are still difficult to interpret, with some investigators suggesting the use of MR spectroscopy to aid in localizing suspicious regions [32].

MR spectroscopy of the prostate is a 2D or 3D acquisition technique that suppresses water and lipid signals to observe alternative metabolites that have signal-producing protons (Fig. 21.4). Each metabolite resonates at a slightly different frequency on the basis of its chemical environment; thus, results are often shown in terms of a spectrum. The acquisition is of low spatial resolution, and 15–20 min is usually required to acquire a low-resolution 3D volume through the prostate. Maps of certain metabolites may be generated by vendor software by quantifying the signal in windows that approximately isolate these metabolites. Citrate (~2.6 ppm) is a by-product of normal gland metabolism that should dominate in the normal gland but is often highly attenuated in tumors. Choline (~3.2 ppm) is a by-product of cell membrane construction and maintenance that tends to increase with the proliferative cell activity associated with prostate carcinoma, whereas creatine (~3.0 ppm) does not. The variable amount of spermine in the prostate is associated with polyamine (~3.15 ppm) metabolite signals between choline and creatine that tend to make quantification of choline alone difficult on clinical scanners. Therefore, a common metric for characterizing

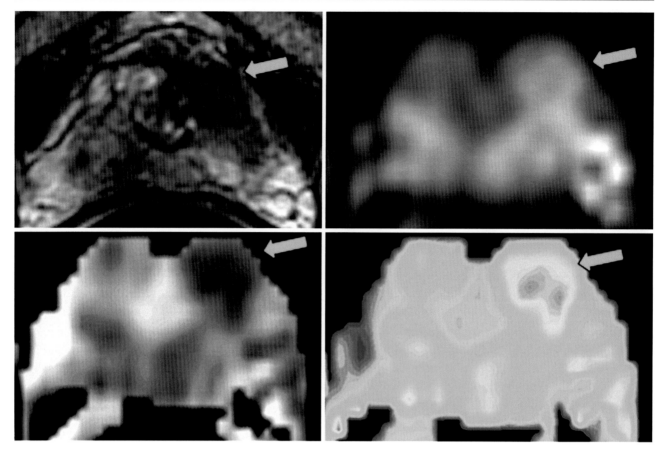

Fig. 21.2 Diffusion-weighted imaging ($b=0,700$ s/mm²) of the prostate in a 74-year-old, acquired at 1.5 T with an endorectal coil. The lesion, which had a Gleason score of 7 (3 + 4), was in the transition zone 12 weeks after TRUS-guided biopsy. The T2-weighted images demonstrate the lesion (*arrow*) as an abnormally hypointense region. The lower-resolution diffusion-weighted image (700 s/mm²) reveals a coinciding region of hyperintensity (*arrow*). The calculated apparent diffusion coefficient (*ADC*) map depicts a region of reduced diffusion (0.80×10^{-3} mm²/s) on the left (*arrow*) versus the contralateral side of the gland (1.6×10^{-3} mm²/s). The ADC can be presented as an "exponential ADC" map to mimic the positive contrast characteristics of the DWI image, but without the T2 "shine-through" effects

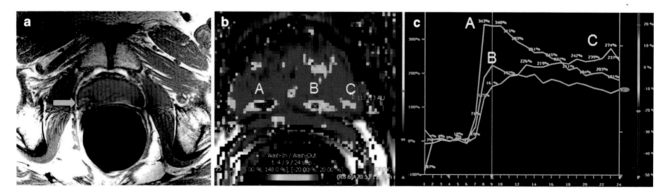

Fig. 21.3 T1-weighted, fast spin-echo imaging is useful for depicting hemorrhage, which appears hyperintense against the isointense prostate gland (**a**). In a different patient, dynamic contrast-enhanced imaging using a fast gradient-recalled echo technique reveals contrast kinetics in the prostate that can be used in conjunction with T2-weighted or DWI to aid in localizing potential lesions (**b**). The false color map in (**b**) shows rapid washout as *red*. The points at several suspicious locations in the peripheral zone (*A*, *B*, and *C*) can be *plotted* to visually assess the kinetics (**c**)

prostate spectroscopy is the ratio of the choline-to-creatine signal to the citrate signal. The larger this ratio becomes, the more suspicious the voxel is for cancer. However, despite

the recent success of numerous single center trials, a rigidly controlled, prospective multicenter study of 110 patients (mean PSA level = 5.9 ng/ml and median Gleason score = 7)

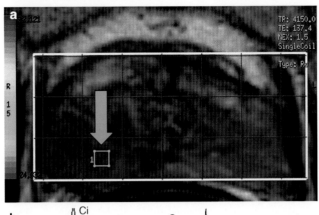

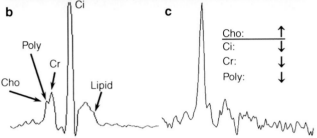

Fig. 21.4 1.5 T MR spectroscopy using an endorectal coil is a low-resolution technique that provides relative metabolite concentrations in the region of interest. 3D MR spectroscopy is usually prescribed from an axial anatomical image. The spectrum from each voxel in the grid (**a**) can be analyzed independently or displayed as a montage of spectrums; alternatively, specific metabolite maps can be derived and shown. A typical prostate MR spectroscopy voxel has components of choline (*Cho*), polyamines (*Poly*), creatine (*Cr*), and citrate (*Ci*) and may have lipid contamination (**b**). Voxels containing tumor (*arrow* in (**a**)) exhibit altered metabolism, often characterized by increased levels of choline and decreased levels of other metabolites (**c**)

conducted by the American College of Radiology Imaging Network determined there was no quantifiable benefit of combined endorectal MRI and MR spectroscopic imaging at 1.5 T versus endorectal MR imaging alone for sextant localization of peripheral zone prostate cancer [24]. Although the authors reasoned that this could be partly due to selection bias, it is important to realize that endorectal coil MR spectroscopy was still an emerging technology when these studies were conducted. Both the sensitivity and resolution of spectroscopy increase at 3 T. This, coupled with advancements in the number, fidelity, and dynamic range of modern multichannel systems, as well as more widespread use of higher order shimming and advanced spectroscopy analysis packages, are promising.

MRI Guidance for Prostate Biopsy

Because of its ability to visualize suspicious lesions for targeting, substantial interest has developed in the use of MRI guidance for prostate biopsy, particularly in patients with

negative TRUS biopsies and persistent clinical indicators for prostate cancer [22, 33]. Several research groups have evaluated the value of MRI versus TRUS-guided biopsy and have found that MRI can enhance or is superior to the predictive capabilities of TRUS-guided biopsy [34–36]. A review of the recent medical literature revealed an accuracy rate of 69–82 % for T2-weighted imaging and 86–89 % for DWI using endorectal coil MRI at 1.5 T [37]. There is a trend toward incorporating a multimodal approach that includes T2-weighted imaging with DWI and sometimes DCE or MRS to localize prostate carcinoma [38].

Indications and Patient Selection

Because of early detection with modern screening, most patients do not present with clinical symptoms of advanced prostate cancer, such as urethral obstruction, but instead tend to be asymptomatic. General indications for a prostate biopsy include an abnormal PSA test on the basis of patient age and abnormal findings on a DRE. Repeat biopsy may be indicated when the sample is not satisfactory for pathological analysis, contains too little tissue, or is of insufficient quality. Repeat biopsy may also be indicated for patients with a previous normal biopsy and persistently abnormal or increasing PSA levels and patients with a suspicious previous biopsy result, such as high-grade prostatic intraepithelial neoplasia or atypical small acinar proliferation. High-grade prostatic intraepithelial neoplasia is associated with undetected cancer in 50–80 % of cases [39, 40], whereas atypical small acinar proliferation is associated in 40–50 %.

The role of MRI-guided prostate biopsy is currently being investigated, in patients with one or more negative TRUS-guided biopsy results [34]. Repeatedly negative TRUS biopsies in patients with persistently abnormal or increasing PSA levels can be difficult for patients and urologists. Subsequent conventional TRUS biopsies result in low detection rates, which have been reported to be 14–22 %, 10–15 %, 5–10 %, and 4 % for first, second, third, and fourth repeated biopsies, respectively [41, 42]. The results of subsequent studies in men with abnormal PSA levels (4–10 ng per 100 ml) indicate that TRUS has an approximately 40–45 % detection rate for a standard 10–12-core transrectal approach [43, 44]. Although third and fourth repeated biopsies often result in a lower grade and stage, first and second repeated biopsies detect localized cancers of equivalent stage and grade as in the initial biopsy [45]. Saturation biopsies have been suggested to increase sensitivity and are associated with more accurate Gleason scores [46]; however, they do not significantly increase detection rates on first biopsy [47, 48]. Most recent studies of MRI-guided prostate biopsy have included patients with high PSA levels (>4.0 ng/mL) and one or more negative TRUS biopsy results.

Contraindications to MRI-Guided Prostate Biopsy

Prostate biopsy may be contraindicated in patients taking oral anticoagulants or anti-inflammatories and in those with thrombocytopenia. For transrectal approaches, periproctal abscesses and rectal tumors are contraindications, as is acute, painful perianal disorder and hemorrhagic diathesis. Prostate biopsy is also contraindicated in patients with suspected acute bacterial prostatitis within 6 weeks of intervention because of the potential complication of seeding the bacterial infection in adjacent organs, which may result in gram-negative sepsis.

Any contraindications for MRI preclude MRI-guided biopsy. Patients should be carefully screened for contraindicated implants and devices. A surgically absent rectum, severe hemorrhoids, or previous colorectal surgery may preclude the use of an endorectal coil or transrectal route. Contraindications for intravenous gadolinium administration and anesthesia and the effect of other urinary or medical conditions should also be considered.

Potential Complications

The complications associated with prostate biopsy include the risk of infection (sepsis or urinary tract or prostate infection), hemorrhage at the biopsy site, and urinary retention [49]. TRUS-guided transrectal or transperineal biopsies of the prostate are generally well-tolerated procedures, with minor pain and morbidity. Minor complications are reported in 3–5 % of patients [10]. Routine post-biopsy complications that manifest acutely include rectal bleeding and mild to severe hematuria, whereas delayed hemorrhagic complications include hematospermia and mild hematuria. Repeat biopsies performed at least 6 weeks later do not appear to be associated with any significantly different complications. Of the minor hemorrhagic complications, only hematospermia tends to demonstrate a significant positive correlation with the number of cores taken (6 versus 10) [50]. A prospective study of morbidity and quality of life after 6- versus 12-core approaches found no substantial increase in morbidity [51, 52].

MRI-Guided Approaches

Early approaches to adapting MRI for prostate interventions were generally performed using low magnetic field systems (i.e., 0.2–0.5 T), allowing for significant patient access and resulting in fewer biopsy equipment artifacts [53, 54]. However, to achieve the image quality needed for optimal prostate visualization and targeting, higher fields were required. Many early studies of MRI-guided biopsy were performed using these systems,

which often substituted T1-weighted imaging for guidance over T2-weighted imaging. Generally, there has been a transition toward performing prostate interventions at standard clinical field strengths (i.e., 1.5–3.0 T) to obtain better image quality. However, it is important to note that the availability of a prior diagnostic MRI performed with an endorectal coil is invaluable when the goal is to target a specific suspicious area, as it can save additional imaging time, allowing faster sequences to be used for targeting.

Most current approaches to MRI-guided prostate biopsy use phased-array radiofrequency coils to obtain appropriate reception for pelvic imaging without the need for an additional endorectal coil, although commercial biopsy systems that incorporate endorectal coils are being developed [55]. Given the location at which most radiofrequency coils attach to the MRI scanner, the most appropriate position of the patient will often be feet first. The patient may lie supine or prone, primarily on the basis of the approach. Practitioners considering transrectal or transperineal approaches should note that in this position the ability to work from the back of a short-bore MRI scanner can be critical to patient access.

Transrectal Approach

In the transrectal approach to MRI-guided prostate biopsy, an applicator is placed directly into the rectum under MRI guidance, and a needle is passed directly through the rectal mucosa for biopsy sampling. A recent review of TRUS-guided biopsy studies reported that most urologists prescribe a cleansing enema for bowel preparation to reduce the bacterial load in the rectal mucosa [49], despite little evidence of effectiveness [10]. However, this procedure also reduces discomfort and image quality issues associated with the presence of fecal matter if an endorectal coil is used.

Antibiotics, such as fluoroquinolone, may be prescribed as early as 30–60 min prior to the biopsy and up to 12 h after the biopsy aid in infection control [10, 56]. Most transrectal biopsy infections are caused by *Escherichia coli* or *Enterococcus* species.

Cessation of anti-inflammatory or anticoagulant therapies (e.g., aspirin or warfarin) 7–10 days prior to the procedure is a common practice. However, it should be noted that research indicates that such practices have a negligible effect on hemorrhagic complications [57–59].

One benefit of the transrectal approach is the reduced need for general anesthesia. Varying local anesthesia techniques have been reported in the medical literature, but many studies have found that periprostatic lidocaine is superior to intrarectal lidocaine [10, 56], and that peristalsis can be suppressed with the intravenous administration of butylscopolaminebromide and an intramuscular administration of butylscopolaminebromide and glucagon [60].

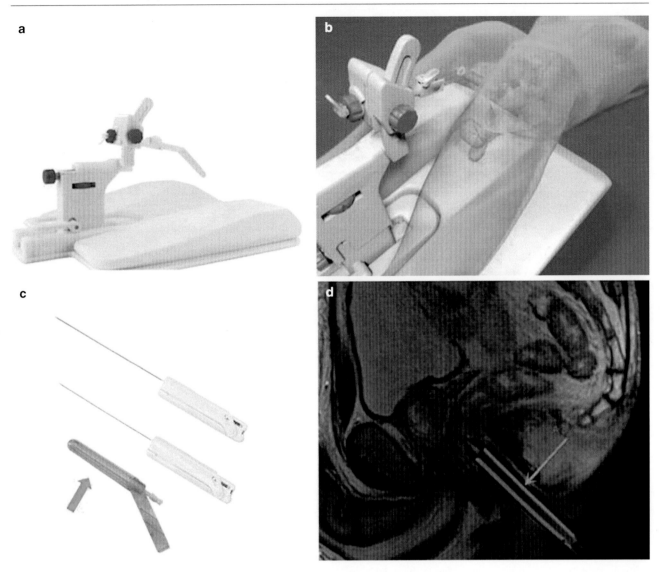

Fig. 21.5 An example of a commercialized system designed for transrectal MRI-guided prostate biopsy is illustrated. An articulating arm, clamped to a baseplate (**a**), is used to hold an MRI-visible needle sleeve (*arrows*), which is positioned in the patient's rectum (**b**). The disposable needle sleeve (**c**) is used as both a fiducial and a guide for the biopsy needles. An example of two forward throw, automatic 18-gauge biopsy guns (15 and 17.5 cm) is shown in (**c**). A sagittal MRI illustrates the needle sleeve in a patient for planning (**d**) (Courtesy of Invivo Corporation)

Patients are positioned supine in the MRI, in a partial lithotomy position. Because of the difficulty of manually maintaining the position of the needle guide during the entire navigation process, robotic assistance in the form of an articulating arm is often necessary. An example of a commercially available device designed for safe MRI use is shown in Fig. 21.5. With this approach, the patient can be positioned supine or prone on the table after undergoing a DRE to verify an unobstructed approach to the prostate (Fig. 21.5).

In the transrectal approach, the patient sits atop a reusable padded polyoxymethylene baseplate to which an articulating arm is clamped (Fig. 21.5b); their weight helps secure the position of the system on the table. A disposable, MR-visible needle sleeve filled with a gadolinium-based contrast agent is inserted gently into the rectum and attached to the articulating arm. This sleeve acts as a fiducial to illustrate the path of the biopsy needle (Fig. 21.5c, d). Sagittal planning images of the prostate, including the sleeve, are acquired, and gross adjustments are made to ensure that the needle sleeve is appropriately located near the prostate. New sagittal images are obtained, followed by axial images that better demonstrate the anatomy. For these purposes, a fast sequence with T2-like weighting is used, such as a balanced, steady-state, free-precession (bSSFP) sequence, which provides T2-like weighting, at a high resolution, in seconds. However, if the contrast of the sequence is not adequate for initial targeting, a high-resolution, T2-weighted, fast spin-echo approach, with an acquisition time of several minutes, should be used.

These sequences can be used to iteratively fine-tune the position of the needle sleeve and plan the needle insertion. Because this can be a time-consuming process, software can guide the adjustments on the basis of the sagittal visualization of the needle sleeve and target region on the axial images. Once the orientation of the needle sleeve is dialed into the articulating arm, a verification image should be acquired. This procedure is followed by inserting the biopsy needle to the anticipated depth. If a guide needle is used, the location of the guide needle with respect to the throw of the biopsy gun can be evaluated. Biopsy guns suitable for use in the MRI environment (Fig. 21.5c) can then be inserted and cores acquired. No support exists for the biopsy gun; thus, a verification image of the needle location will be unavailable if the radiologist does not have sufficient access. If there is access to the patient, real-time imaging may be useful to manually fine-tune the sampling position and verify the location prior to acquiring the tissue sample. If multiple sites of interest exist, the next site of interest is planned, and the procedure is executed again.

Beyersdorff et al. [35] were one of the first research groups to report on this approach and investigated a real-time guided transrectal approach in a cylindrical bore 1.5 T scanner using a pre-market version of this device and no guidance software. Patients ($n=12$) had negative TRUS biopsy results and increasing PSA levels. They were positioned prone, and the MRI-visible needle guide (Invivo Corp., Schwering, Germany) was placed rectally and connected to an MRI-compatible articulating arm mounted to a baseplate. A telescoping rod was used to facilitate needle manipulation from outside the bore under real-time MRI guidance. High-resolution, fast spin-echo, T2-weighted images were acquired for initial planning, and a T2-weighted, single-shot, fast spin-echo acquisition was used to guide the needle during the procedure. In five patients, MRI-guided biopsy was performed immediately after a diagnostic endorectal coil MRI. Seven patients returned after <2 weeks for a separate MRI-guided biopsy session that did not include additional imaging. In all cases, MRI guidance for biopsy used torso array coils but no endorectal coil. An eight-core biopsy strategy was used, with sampling being directed at the most suspicious area of each sextant on the basis of the targeting MRI. Procedure durations of <60 min were reported. Approximately 50 % of biopsies directed at the most suspicious locations on T2-weighted MRI were diagnosed as prostate cancer, versus 33 and 3.5 % of biopsies in moderately and not suspicious areas, respectively. Overall, prostate cancer was diagnosed in 42 % of patients.

Engelhard et al. [61] used a similar transrectal MRI-guided biopsy methodology in a clinical closed-bore 1.5 T scanner using the same device. In this study, patients ($n=37$) were positioned supine in a closed-bore clinical 1.5 T MRI. Endorectal coil-based diagnostic T2-weighted images were acquired prior to biopsy. Localization of the needle sleeve was performed using fast bSSFP sequences to guide and document the needle position prior to sampling. The 4–9 MRI-directed locations per patient took up to 150 min and resulted in a prostate cancer diagnosis in 37 % of patients. Another similar study in 27 patients by Anastasiadis et al. reported prostate cancer detection in 55 % of patients [62]. Hambrock et al. evaluated a large cohort of patients ($n=71$) with increasing PSA levels and two or more negative TRUS biopsy results; using a clinical 3 T scanner and a multiparametric imaging approach, they found a 59 % detection rate with a median of four cores [63].

Investigators at the National Institutes of Health and Johns Hopkins independently designed and demonstrated the feasibility of a transrectal biopsy system that facilitates real-time needle guidance in a standard cylindrical bore 1.5 T scanner via a robotically assisted transrectal approach [55]. A dedicated endorectal coil was developed that could accommodate transrectal biopsy, enabling simultaneous diagnostic-quality MRI via a transrectal approach. Instead of passive-contrast fiducials, active tracking coils were embedded. The primary goal of the study was fiducial placement in previously diagnosed patients for radiotherapy, but three patients underwent a biopsy procedure to demonstrate the system. Patients were positioned prone; the procedure was performed using local anesthesia and lasted a mean of 76 min. The needle (14 gauge) placement accuracy was reported to be 1.8 mm. This system has been further developed into a complete system by Sentinelle Medical, and further results are anticipated.

Transperineal Approach

In the transperineal approach, the needle does not pass directly through the rectum; therefore, fecal contamination is not as critical an issue as with transrectal biopsy (Fig. 21.6). If an endorectal coil is not used, an enema is not necessary, as it is in transrectal approaches. This approach is also useful for patients in whom a rectal approach is contraindicated.

A recent study of TRUS-guided transperineal approaches recommended antibiotic prophylaxis in patients at high risk for infection, those of poor general health, and those with cardiac valve problems, prosthetics, an indwelling catheter, or high post-voiding residual urine [49]. As with the transrectal approach, fluoroquinolones are the antibiotic of choice. Lidocaine has been locally administered in transperineal approaches [64] that rely on one or two penetrations; however, general anesthesia is preferred. This is particularly true in the MRI environment because of the potential duration of the procedure and the potential for multiple cores or targets to be sampled, particularly if stereotactic grid targeting and planning is used.

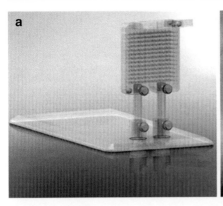
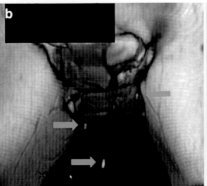
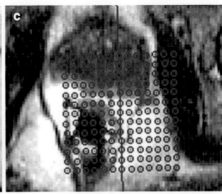

Fig. 21.6 Perineal grids (**a**) for the MRI environment are commercially available to facilitate transperineal approaches to prostate biopsy. The grid above has integrated MRI-visible markers (*arrows*) that can be visualized by fast T2-weighted MRI acquisition; (**b**) the marker coordinates are fed into proprietary vendor software, operating on a stand-alone workstation, to provide a planning grid (**c**) (Courtesy of Visualase, Inc.)

Transperineal TRUS-guided biopsy has been found to detect prostate cancer at a rate of 45 % in men with elevated PSA levels using a 12-core technique [65], 36 % using a 14-core technique [66], and 43 % using a saturation technique (9–33 cores) [67]. Similar detection rates have been found for secondary biopsies, with reports of 43 % [68] and 42.2 % [69]. In a recent study, Taira and colleagues found a 75 % detection rate for primary biopsy versus 55.5 %, 41.7 %, and 34.4 % in men with negative first, second, and third biopsies, respectively, when using a template technique that identified 24 locations, with 1–3 cores taken per location on the basis of prostate size [70]. Most of the cancers were multifocal, with 61.1 % of the men diagnosed having ≥5 positive cores and 25.3 % having ≥12 positive cores.

The transperineal approach is amenable to a single point of entry, followed by a "fan" sampling approach under real-time guidance. However, using a template-based grid approach in cylindrical bore magnets allows the incorporation of stereotaxy, in conjunction with intermittent imaging, in place of real-time imaging, such as in cases in which patient access is limited or specific site targeting is desired. Several research groups have had success with this approach. A potential source of error during needle placement is prostate motion or rotation, which has been shown to be substantial [71].

Some of the earliest research into transperineal MRI-guided procedures was conducted by the research group at Brigham and Women's Hospital in Boston in a 0.5 T scanner (Signa SP, GE Healthcare Technologies, Waukesha, WI). Patients had at least one previous negative biopsy and persistently abnormal PSA levels. A transperineal approach was used, with the patient supine in the dorsal lithotomy position. The use of real-time needle guidance and fast spin-echo imaging for T2-weighted images established the feasibility of the technique in two case studies [53, 54, 72]. This group has performed 40 procedures with this system, with a reported detection rate of 30 % [21].

A research team working at Johns Hopkins University, in collaboration with a team from the National Institutes of Health, reported on a transperineal technique performed using a standard cylindrical bore 1.5 T scanner (60-cm bore aperture). Custom-built targeting software and a perineal template grid affixed to an MRI-compatible arm were used to guide the biopsy needles transperineally into the prostate, with the patient in the decubitus position. An endorectal coil was used to provide high SNR images of the prostate anatomy and the 32 needle placements performed over eight procedures in four patients. The mean needle placement accuracy was 2.1 mm, with 95 % of needle placement errors <4.0 mm; the maximum needle placement error was 4.4 mm [73].

Figure 21.6 shows an MRI from an example transperineal MRI-guided prostate biopsy using a commercially available grid and planning software (Visualase, Inc., Houston, TX). The procedure was performed under general anesthesia. A Foley catheter was placed and the patient was positioned in a 1.5 T MRI clinical scanner (MAGNETOM Espree, Siemens Medical Systems, Erlangen, Germany). The spine and body arrays were used for signal reception, with no additional endorectal coil. High-resolution, axial, T1- and T2-weighted images were obtained, followed by DWI with calculated ADC maps. These images revealed no regions immediately suspicious for prostate cancer.

Fast (<1 s per image) axial bSSFP images were acquired to register the template coordinates to the MRI coordinate system. With the template coordinates overlaid on the vendor's stand-alone workstation, several suitable areas of the prostate were chosen for biopsy. Axial bSSFP images were used to verify the appropriate position of the needle (Fig. 21.7). Unlike in typical percutaneous biopsies in the MRI environment, in which the needle is perpendicular to the static magnetic field, the needle was fairly parallel to the field in the transperineal approach and had a much smaller artifact, which can be difficult to see without orthogonal views. To make the artifact larger, the bandwidth was decreased from the usual value, in excess of 500–250 Hz/pixel.

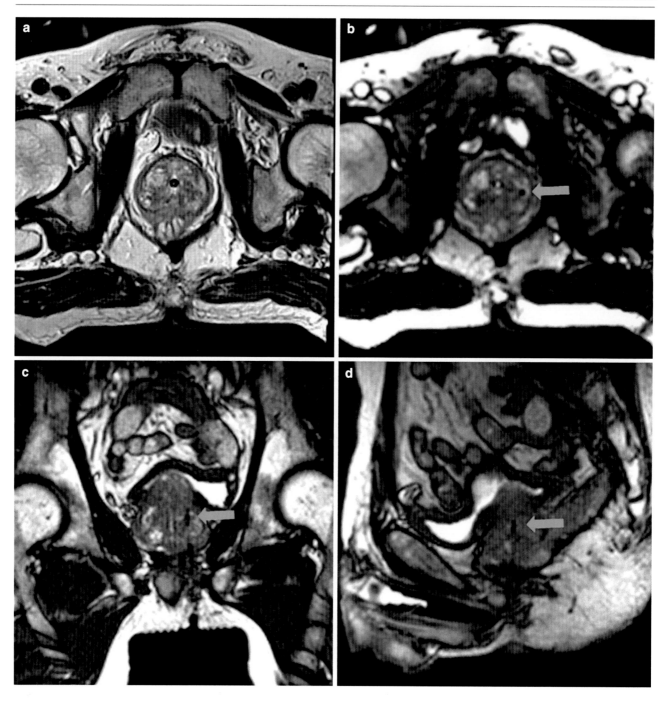

Fig. 21.7 An MRI-guided transperineal prostate template biopsy in a 77-year-old man who had undergone resection of the rectum. The patient had elevated PSA levels and was referred for MRI-guided biopsy. High-resolution T2-weighted fast spin-echo imaging (TR/TE = 4,000 ms/92 ms; acquisition time = 3:08 min) using surface phased-array receiver coils only was used to visualize the anatomy (**a**). Fast bSSFP imaging (TR/TE/FA = 3.8 ms/1.6 ms/72; acquisition time = 0.75 s per image) was used to register the grid to the MRI coordinate system and visualize the needle (*arrows*) with respect to prostate anatomy on axial, coronal, or sagittal images (**b**–**d**). Note that the interface between the perineal grid and perineum is clearly visible on coronal images (**c**). Seven locations were sampled, with one core containing a 1.5-mm prostate cancer focus with a Gleason score of 6 (3 + 3)

Core biopsies were obtained from the left central gland, left anterior peripheral zone (base), left mid-gland peripheral zone, and left posterior peripheral zone (apex). On the right side, biopsies were obtained from the right central gland, right anterior peripheral zone (base), and right mid-gland peripheral zone (mid-gland and base). T1-weighted images were obtained, and no significant peri-prostatic or intraprostatic hemorrhage was observed. The patient was extubated and transferred to the recovery unit. He experienced post-procedure urinary retention that

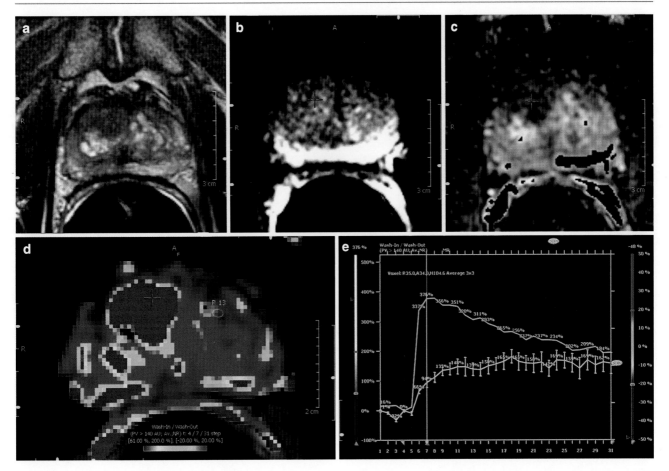

Fig. 21.8 A diagnostic endorectal coil prostate MRI examination, performed at 1.5 T, revealed a suspicious region in a 71-year-old man who had undergone multiple TRUS biopsies and had elevated PSA levels. A large hypointense region (cross hairs) was observed on T2-weighted fast spin-echo imaging (**a**) that was well correlated with suspicious regions observed on DWI (**b**) and ADC (**c**) and DCE-derived washin and washout maps (**d**). The suspicious region was found to have rapid washin and washout of contrast versus the contralateral gland (**e**). The patient was subsequently referred for MRI-guided prostate biopsy (see Fig. 21.9)

required extended catheterization, but no other immediate complications were associated with the procedure.

Transgluteal Approach

A transgluteal approach to prostate biopsy much more closely mimics the standard approach to percutaneous biopsy in the MRI environment (Figs. 21.8 and 21.9). Transgluteal approaches under computed tomographic guidance have been demonstrated to be safe and effective in patients in whom a standard TRUS-guided approach is not feasible or desired [74]. The standard considerations for patient preparation apply, including cessation of anticoagulant or anti-inflammatory therapies; local anesthesia using lidocaine is appropriate, although general anesthesia may be considered for patients who cannot tolerate the procedure.

A transgluteal approach was used by Zangos et al. in a 0.2 T open magnet, with patients in the decubitus position [64]. MRI-directed biopsy was performed at a low magnetic field after an endorectal coil diagnostic prostate examination had been performed at a higher field. All 25 patients had increasing PSA levels, but only 17 had had previous negative TRUS biopsy results. Low-resolution T1-weighted gradient echo images with an acquisition time of 18 s were used to localize the low-field magnet because the needle was not easily visualized with T2-weighted sequences. Cancer was detected in 40 % of patients using this technique, with a mean of 3.8 cores per patient and a reported intervention duration of 11 min. This research group has since developed and investigated the use of a pneumatically driven robot for transgluteal approaches in higher-field, closed-bore systems; however, detection rates have yet to be reported for patient procedures [75, 76].

Images from a transgluteal MRI-guided prostate biopsy, performed in a wide-bore, compact-length 1.5 T MRI scanner, are shown in Figs. 21.8 and 21.9. In brief, a 71-year-old with a history of elevated PSA levels and a prostate nodule, identified on 1.5 T endorectal coil MRI (Fig. 21.8), underwent a percutaneous transgluteal MRI-guided prostate

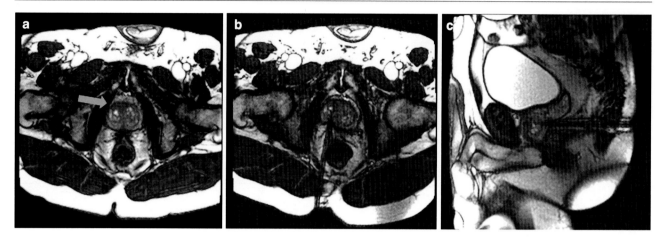

Fig. 21.9 An MRI-guided transgluteal prostate biopsy was performed in a 71-year-old man who had undergone multiple TRUS biopsies and had elevated PSA levels; he was referred for MRI-guided biopsy after a suspicious lesion was identified on endorectal coil MRI (Fig. 21.8). The index lesion was identifiable (*arrow*) on the planning bSSFP images (**a**). Intermittent MRI guidance of a 16-gauge needle facilitated sampling by an 18-gauge core at a depth of approximately 13 cm, as visualized on axial (**b**) and sagittal (**c**) bSSFP imaging. The core was positive for prostate cancer, with a Gleason score of 7 (3+4)

biopsy. The patient was anesthetized and positioned prone. The suspicious region, identified on the previous diagnostic examination, was easily identified on fast bSSFP planning images, using spine and body arrays for signal reception (Fig. 21.9); thus, no further planning images were acquired. The skin was marked, and the area of interest was prepped and draped. The body array, which was not sterilized, was placed atop the sterile keyhole drape and covered with another sterile keyhole drape. Lidocaine (1 %) was given as local anesthesia. A 16-gauge needle was advanced into the anterior superior aspect of the prostate using intermittent axial bSSFP updates (Fig. 21.9) until the target region was reached. An 18-gauge needle was used to obtain samples for surgical pathologic evaluation. No complications were reported. The pathologic diagnosis was prostate cancer on three foci, with a Gleason score of 7 (3+4).

Future Developments

During MRI-guided biopsies in high-field systems (≥1.5 T), the bore aperture (≤60 cm) and length (≥150 m) of a standard cylindrical MRI scanner limits physicians' ability to manipulate needles and applicators under real-time guidance. One solution to this dilemma is large-bore, compact-length MRI, which facilitates patient access. Commercially available scanners are available with bore apertures of 70 cm and lengths of 125 cm.

In conventional cylindrical bore scanners, patients are moved in and out of the scanner intermittently so that image feedback can be obtained during the intervention, which is performed outside the gantry. Innovations in MRI-compatible materials and robotics may lead to a solution to this problem.

MRI-compatible robots that can operate in the scanner under real-time MRI guidance are being developed, from basic manipulation devices to fully automated robotic assistance systems [75–78].

Fully incorporating multiparametric MRI data into the process provides additional localization benefits. Franiel et al. studied the effect of incorporating DWI, DCE, and MRS into MRI-guided transrectal biopsy in patients (*n* = 54) with two negative TRUS biopsy results and increasing PSA levels. A detection rate of 70 % was reported for T2-weighted imaging only. When coupled with DWI, DCE, or MRS, the rate increased to 85 %, 83 %, and 81 %, respectively. With three independent methods, 94 % of all lesions were detected, while simultaneously, the number of suspicious areas that required sampling decreased by 13 % [79].

Summary

Significant advancements have been made in the quality of prostate MR imaging, resulting in more effective diagnostic and staging capabilities that in turn has fueled an increased interest in using MRI to direct prostate interventions. In the current paradigm, T2-weighted imaging remains the workhorse for MRI lesion localization, with DWI and DCE MRI providing synergistic functional information. In addition, although MRS does not lead to increased prostate cancer detection, it may play a role in localization. The focus of research remains on advancements in acquisition techniques, post-processing, and hardware using high-field (≥1.5 T) systems. In addition, ancillary equipment that can facilitate these procedures in closed-bore systems is reaching the marketplace, although longer guide needles and biopsy guns are needed that can be used in the MRI environment.

Because of the logistic issues involved in adopting this technology, no larger scale multi-site studies have been performed. Therefore, the specific role of and approaches to MRI-guided biopsy are rapidly evolving. A transrectal approach has been used in most patients in prospective clinical trials. The most studied patients are those with increasing PSA levels and one or more negative TRUS biopsy results.

The initial results of these studies suggest that MRI guidance is beneficial in prostate biopsy. However, the length and cost of this procedure, as well as limited access to patient and the need for specialized equipment, will play as large a role in the technique's future as its effectiveness. The preliminary evidence suggests that MRI-guided biopsy will lead to increased prostate cancer detection, supporting the theory that this technique, regardless of the approach, is a viable prostate biopsy method in patients who have clinical and MRI findings that are suspicious for prostate cancer but negative TRUS biopsy results.

References

1. Siegel R, Ward E, Brawley O, Jemal A. Cancer statistics. The impact of eliminating socioeconomic and racial disparities on premature cancer deaths. CA Cancer J Clin. 2011;61(4):212–36.
2. Jemal A, Siegel R, Ward E, Hao Y, Xu J, Thun MJ. Cancer statistics, 2009. CA Cancer J Clin. 2009;59(4):225–49.
3. Tewari A, Divine G, Chang P, et al. Long-term survival in men with high grade prostate cancer: a comparison between conservative treatment, radiation therapy and radical prostatectomy–a propensity scoring approach. J Urol. 2007;177(3):911–15.
4. Brawley OW, Ankerst DP, Thompson IM. Screening for prostate cancer. CA Cancer J Clin. 2009;59(4):264–73.
5. Boyle P, Brawley OW. Prostate cancer: current evidence weighs against population screening. CA Cancer J Clin. 2009;59(4):220–4.
6. Smith RA, Cokkinides V, Brawley OW. Cancer screening in the United States, 2009: a review of current American Cancer Society guidelines and issues in cancer screening. CA Cancer J Clin. 2009;59(1):27–41.
7. Andriole GL, Crawford ED, Grubb 3rd RL, et al. Mortality results from a randomized prostate-cancer screening trial. N Engl J Med. 2009;360(13):1310–19.
8. Schroder FH, Hugosson J, Roobol MJ, et al. Screening and prostate-cancer mortality in a randomized European study. N Engl J Med. 2009;360(13):1320–8.
9. Watanabe H. History and applications of transrectal sonography of the prostate. Urol Clin North Am. 1989;16(4):617–22.
10. Sadeghi-Nejad H, Simmons M, Dakwar G, Dogra V. Controversies in transrectal ultrasonography and prostate biopsy. Ultrasound Q. 2006;22(3):169–75.
11. Eskicorapci SY, Baydar DE, Akbal C, et al. An extended 10-core transrectal ultrasonography guided prostate biopsy protocol improves the detection of prostate cancer. Eur Urol. 2004;45(4):444–8; discussion 448–9.
12. Karam JA, Shulman MJ, Benaim EA. Impact of training level of urology residents on the detection of prostate cancer on TRUS biopsy. Prostate Cancer Prostatic Dis. 2004;7(1):38–40.
13. Djavan B, Ravery V, Zlotta A, et al. Prospective evaluation of prostate cancer detected on biopsies 1, 2, 3 and 4: when should we stop? J Urol. 2001;166(5):1679–83.
14. Gleason DF. Histologic grading of prostate cancer: a perspective. Hum Pathol. 1992;23(3):273–9.
15. Iczkowski KA, Lucia MS. Current perspectives on Gleason grading of prostate cancer. Curr Urol Rep. 2011;12(3):216–22.
16. Noguchi M, Stamey TA, McNeal JE, Yemoto CM. Relationship between systematic biopsies and histological features of 222 radical prostatectomy specimens: lack of prediction of tumor significance for men with nonpalpable prostate cancer. J Urol. 2001;166(1):104–9; discussion 109–10.
17. Hodge KK, McNeal JE, Terris MK, Stamey TA. Random systematic versus directed ultrasound guided transrectal core biopsies of the prostate. J Urol. 1989;142(1):71–4; discussion 74–5.
18. Onur R, Littrup PJ, Pontes JE, Bianco Jr FJ. Contemporary impact of transrectal ultrasound lesions for prostate cancer detection. J Urol. 2004;172(2):512–14.
19. Heijmink SW, van Moerkerk H, Kiemeney LA, Witjes JA, Frauscher F, Barentsz JO. A comparison of the diagnostic performance of systematic versus ultrasound-guided biopsies of prostate cancer. Eur Radiol. 2006;16(4):927–38.
20. Atalar E, Menard C. MR-guided interventions for prostate cancer. Magn Reson Imaging Clin N Am. 2005;13(3):491–504.
21. Tempany C, Straus S, Hata N, Haker S. MR-guided prostate interventions. J Magn Reson Imaging. 2008;27(2):356–67.
22. Hoeks CM, Barentsz JO, Hambrock T, et al. Prostate cancer: multiparametric MR imaging for detection, localization, and staging. Radiology. 2011;261(1):46–66.
23. Kundra V, Silverman PM, Matin SF, Choi H. Imaging in oncology from the University of Texas M. D. Anderson Cancer Center: diagnosis, staging, and surveillance of prostate cancer. Am J Roentgenol. 2007;189(4):830–44.
24. Weinreb JC, Blume JD, Coakley FV, et al. Prostate cancer: sextant localization at MR imaging and MR spectroscopic imaging before prostatectomy–results of ACRIN prospective multi-institutional clinicopathologic study. Radiology. 2009;251(1):122–33.
25. Ahmed HU, Kirkham A, Arya M, et al. Is it time to consider a role for MRI before prostate biopsy? Nat Rev Clin Oncol. 2009;6(4):197–206.
26. Qayyum A, Coakley FV, Lu Y, et al. Organ-confined prostate cancer: effect of prior transrectal biopsy on endorectal MRI and MR spectroscopic imaging. Am J Roentgenol. 2004;183(4):1079–83.
27. Huisman HJ, Engelbrecht MR, Barentsz JO. Accurate estimation of pharmacokinetic contrast-enhanced dynamic MRI parameters of the prostate. J Magn Reson Imaging. 2001;13(4):607–14.
28. Alonzi R, Padhani AR, Allen C. Dynamic contrast enhanced MRI in prostate cancer. Eur J Radiol. 2007;63(3):335–50.
29. Bonekamp D, Macura KJ. Dynamic contrast-enhanced magnetic resonance imaging in the evaluation of the prostate. Top Magn Reson Imaging. 2008;19(6):273–84.
30. Franiel T, Ludemann L, Rudolph B, et al. Evaluation of normal prostate tissue, chronic prostatitis, and prostate cancer by quantitative perfusion analysis using a dynamic contrast-enhanced inversion-prepared dual-contrast gradient echo sequence. Invest Radiol. 2008;43(7):481–7.
31. Ito H, Kamoi K, Yokoyama K, Yamada K, Nishimura T. Visualization of prostate cancer using dynamic contrast-enhanced MRI: comparison with transrectal power Doppler ultrasound. Br J Radiol. 2003;76(909):617–24.
32. Kaji Y, Kurhanewicz J, Hricak H, et al. Localizing prostate cancer in the presence of postbiopsy changes on MR images: role of proton MR spectroscopic imaging. Radiology. 1998;206(3):785–90.
33. Pondman KM, Futterer JJ, ten Haken B, et al. MR-guided biopsy of the prostate: an overview of techniques and a systematic review. Eur Urol. 2008;54(3):517–27.
34. Hambrock T, Somford DM, Hoeks C, et al. Magnetic resonance imaging guided prostate biopsy in men with repeat negative biopsies and increased prostate specific antigen. J Urol. 2010;183(2):520–7.
35. Beyersdorff D, Winkel A, Hamm B, Lenk S, Loening SA, Taupitz M. MR imaging-guided prostate biopsy with a closed MR unit at 1.5 T: initial results. Radiology. 2005;234(2):576–81.

36. Roethke M, Anastasiadis AG, Lichy M, et al. MRI-guided prostate biopsy detects clinically significant cancer: analysis of a cohort of 100 patients after previous negative TRUS biopsy. World J Urol. 2011;30(2):213–18.

37. Heijmink SW, Futterer JJ, Strum SS, et al. State-of-the-art uroradiologic imaging in the diagnosis of prostate cancer. Acta Oncol. 2011;50 Suppl 1:25–38.

38. Tanimoto A, Nakashima J, Kohno H, Shinmoto H, Kuribayashi S. Prostate cancer screening: the clinical value of diffusion-weighted imaging and dynamic MR imaging in combination with T2-weighted imaging. J Magn Reson Imaging. 2007;25(1):146–52.

39. Schoenfield L, Jones JS, Zippe CD, et al. The incidence of high-grade prostatic intraepithelial neoplasia and atypical glands suspicious for carcinoma on first-time saturation needle biopsy, and the subsequent risk of cancer. BJU Int. 2007;99(4):770–4.

40. Wills ML, Hamper UM, Partin AW, Epstein JI. Incidence of high-grade prostatic intraepithelial neoplasia in sextant needle biopsy specimens. Urology. 1997;49(3):367–73.

41. Djavan B, Milani S, Remzi M. Prostate biopsy: who, how and when. An update. Can J Urol. 2005;12:44.

42. Lujan M, Paez A, Santonja C, Pascual T, Fernandez I, Berenguer A. Prostate cancer detection and tumor characteristics in men with multiple biopsy sessions. Prostate Cancer Prostatic Dis. 2004;7(3):238–42.

43. Eichler K, Hempel S, Wilby J, Myers L, Bachmann LM, Kleijnen J. Diagnostic value of systematic biopsy methods in the investigation of prostate cancer: a systematic review. J Urol. 2006;175(5):1605–12.

44. Jones JS. Saturation biopsy for detecting and characterizing prostate cancer. BJU Int. 2007;99(6):1340–4.

45. Djavan B, Fong YK, Ravery V, et al. Are repeat biopsies required in men with PSA levels < or =4 ng/ml? A Multiinstitutional Prospective European Study. Eur Urol. 2005;47(1):38–44; discussion 44.

46. Mian BM, Lehr DJ, Moore CK, et al. Role of prostate biopsy schemes in accurate prediction of Gleason scores. Urology. 2006;67(2):379–83.

47. Jones JS, Patel A, Schoenfield L, Rabets JC, Zippe CD, Magi-Galluzzi C. Saturation technique does not improve cancer detection as an initial prostate biopsy strategy. J Urol. 2006;175(2):485–8.

48. Pepe P, Aragona F. Saturation prostate needle biopsy and prostate cancer detection at initial and repeat evaluation. Urology. 2007;70(6):1131–5.

49. Galfano A, Novara G, Iafrate M, et al. Prostate biopsy: the transperineal approach. EAU-EBU Update Series. 2007;5(6):241–9.

50. Berger AP, Gozzi C, Steiner H, et al. Complication rate of transrectal ultrasound guided prostate biopsy: a comparison among 3 protocols with 6, 10 and 15 cores. J Urol. 2004;171(4):1478–80; discussion 1480–1471.

51. Naughton CK, Miller DC, Yan Y. Impact of transrectal ultrasound guided prostate biopsy on quality of life: a prospective randomized trial comparing 6 versus 12 cores. J Urol. 2001;165(1):100–3.

52. Naughton CK, Ornstein DK, Smith DS, Catalona WJ. Pain and morbidity of transrectal ultrasound guided prostate biopsy: a prospective randomized trial of 6 versus 12 cores. J Urol. 2000;163(1):168–71.

53. D'Amico AV, Tempany CM, Cormack R, et al. Transperineal magnetic resonance image guided prostate biopsy. J Urol. 2000;164(2):385–7.

54. Hata N, Jinzaki M, Kacher D, et al. MR imaging-guided prostate biopsy with surgical navigation software: device validation and feasibility. Radiology. 2001;220(1):263–8.

55. Susil RC, Menard C, Krieger A, et al. Transrectal prostate biopsy and fiducial marker placement in a standard 1.5T magnetic resonance imaging scanner. J Urol. 2006;175(1):113–20.

56. Djavan B, Margreiter M. Biopsy standards for detection of prostate cancer. World J Urol. 2007;25(1):11–7.

57. Maan Z, Cutting CW, Patel U, et al. Morbidity of transrectal ultrasonography-guided prostate biopsies in patients after the continued use of low-dose aspirin. BJU Int. 2003;91(9):798–800.

58. Giannarini G, Mogorovich A, Valent F, et al. Continuing or discontinuing low-dose aspirin before transrectal prostate biopsy: results of a prospective randomized trial. Urology. 2007;70(3):501–5.

59. Halliwell OT, Yadegafar G, Lane C, Dewbury KC. Transrectal ultrasound-guided biopsy of the prostate: aspirin increases the incidence of minor bleeding complications. Clin Radiol. 2008;63(5):557–61.

60. Yakar D, Hambrock T, Hoeks C, Barentsz JO, Futterer JJ. Magnetic resonance-guided biopsy of the prostate: feasibility, technique, and clinical applications. Top Magn Reson Imaging. 2008;19(6):291–5.

61. Engelhard K, Hollenbach HP, Kiefer B, Winkel A, Goeb K, Engehausen D. Prostate biopsy in the supine position in a standard 1.5-T scanner under real time MR-imaging control using a MR-compatible endorectal biopsy device. Eur Radiol. 2006;16(6):1237–43.

62. Anastasiadis AG, Lichy MP, Nagele U, et al. MRI-guided biopsy of the prostate increases diagnostic performance in men with elevated or increasing PSA levels after previous negative TRUS biopsies. Eur Urol. 2006;50(4):738–48; discussion 748–39.

63. Hambrock T, Hoeks C, Hulsbergen-van de Kaa C, et al. Prospective assessment of prostate cancer aggressiveness using 3-T diffusion-weighted magnetic resonance imaging-guided biopsies versus a systematic 10-core transrectal ultrasound prostate biopsy cohort. Eur Urol. 2012;61(1):177–84.

64. Zangos S, Eichler K, Engelmann K, et al. MR-guided transgluteal biopsies with an open low-field system in patients with clinically suspected prostate cancer: technique and preliminary results. Eur Radiol. 2005;15(1):174–82.

65. Emiliozzi P, Longhi S, Scarpone P, Pansadoro A, DePaula F, Pansadoro V. The value of a single biopsy with 12 transperineal cores for detecting prostate cancer in patients with elevated prostate specific antigen. J Urol. 2001;166(3):845–50.

66. Kawakami S, Kihara K, Fujii Y, Masuda H, Kobayashi T, Kageyama Y. Transrectal ultrasound-guided transperineal 14-core systematic biopsy detects apico-anterior cancer foci of T1c prostate cancer. Int J Urol. 2004;11(8):613–18.

67. Furuno T, Demura T, Kaneta T, et al. Difference of cancer core distribution between first and repeat biopsy: In patients diagnosed by extensive transperineal ultrasound guided template prostate biopsy. Prostate. 2004;58(1):76–81.

68. Igel TC, Knight MK, Young PR, et al. Systematic transperineal ultrasound guided template biopsy of the prostate in patients at high risk. J Urol. 2001;165(5):1575–9.

69. Merrick GS, Gutman S, Andreini H, et al. Prostate cancer distribution in patients diagnosed by transperineal template-guided saturation biopsy. Eur Urol. 2007;52(3):715–23.

70. Taira AV, Merrick GS, Galbreath RW, et al. Performance of transperineal template-guided mapping biopsy in detecting prostate cancer in the initial and repeat biopsy setting. Prostate Cancer Prostatic Dis. 2009;13(1):71–7.

71. Lagerburg V, Moerland MA, Lagendijk JJ, Battermann JJ. Measurement of prostate rotation during insertion of needles for brachytherapy. Radiother Oncol. 2005;77(3):318–23.

72. Cormack RA, D'Amico AV, Hata N, Silverman S, Weinstein M, Tempany CM. Feasibility of transperineal prostate biopsy under interventional magnetic resonance guidance. Urology. 2000;56(4):663–4.

73. Susil RC, Camphausen K, Choyke P, et al. System for prostate brachytherapy and biopsy in a standard 1.5 T MRI scanner. Magn Reson Med. 2004;52(3):683–7.

74. Cantwell CP, Hahn PF, Gervais DA, Mueller PR. Prostate biopsy after ano-rectal resection: value of CT-guided trans-gluteal biopsy. Eur Radiol. 2008;18(4):738–42.

75. Zangos S, Melzer A, Eichler K, et al. MR-compatible Assistance System for Biopsy in a High-Field-Strength System: Initial Results in Patients with Suspicious Prostate Lesions. Radiology. 2011;1:2011.

76. Zangos S, Herzog C, Eichler K, et al. MR-compatible assistance system for punction in a high-field system: device and feasibility of transgluteal biopsies of the prostate gland. Eur Radiol. 2007;17(4):1118–24.

77. Macura KJ, Stoianovici D. Advancements in magnetic resonance-guided robotic interventions in the prostate. Top Magn Reson Imaging. 2008;19(6):297–304.

78. Mozer PC, Partin AW, Stoianovici D. Robotic image-guided needle interventions of the prostate. Rev Urol. 2009;11(1):7–15.

79. Franiel T, Stephan C, Erbersdobler A, et al. Areas suspicious for prostate cancer: MR-guided biopsy in patients with at least one transrectal US-guided biopsy with a negative finding—multiparametric MR imaging for detection and biopsy planning. Radiology. 2011;259(1):162–72.

Biopsy of the Spine

22

Sanjay Gupta

Background

Image-guided percutaneous biopsy of the spine is a safe, accurate, and widely used technique for obtaining tissue samples from spinal or paraspinal lesions. Before the advent of modern imaging modalities, spinal biopsies were performed as open surgical procedures. Since the initial reports in the 1930s demonstrating the feasibility and efficacy of obtaining biopsy specimens from bone lesions using small-caliber needles [1–3], the technique for percutaneous needle biopsy of the spine has evolved considerably. The use of image guidance for needle biopsy of the spine was first reported in 1949 [4]. Initially, percutaneous spinal biopsy was performed with radiographic or fluoroscopic guidance using relatively large-bore needle systems; as a result, these procedures were generally limited to the lower thoracic and lumbar segments of the spine [4]. The use of computed tomography (CT) guidance for spinal biopsy was first reported in the 1980s [5, 6]. Rapid advances in imaging technology, including the clinical introduction of multidetector wide-bore CT along with advances in the design of needle biopsy systems, have enabled image-guided percutaneous biopsy to be used safely today at virtually all levels of the spine. This chapter will review the indications and contraindications for image-guided percutaneous biopsy of the spine; the techniques, devices, and relevant considerations; and outcomes and results documented from the literature.

S. Gupta, MD, DNB
Department of Interventional Radiology,
Department of Diagnostic Radiology,
The University of Texas MD Anderson
Cancer Center, 1515 Holcombe Blvd., Unit 1471,
Houston, TX 77030, USA
e-mail: sgupta@mdanderson.org

Indications and Patient Selection

Common indications for percutaneous spinal biopsy include (1) a focal vertebral lesion in a symptomatic or asymptomatic patient, (2) a destructive vertebral lesion in a patient with or without a known primary tumor, (3) clinically or radiologically suspected osteomyelitis/discitis, (4) isolation of an organism in a patient with a diagnosis of osteomyelitis/discitis, (5) a new vertebral bony compression fracture of unknown etiology, and (6) a previously treated vertebral lesion needing evaluation for tumor viability [7].

Contraindications

The only absolute contraindication for spinal biopsy is an uncorrectable coagulation disorder in the patient. Relative contraindications include hypervascular lesions at risk of bleeding into confined spaces (such as epidural or precervical spaces), infected soft tissues in the needle path, uncooperative patient, pregnancy, and severe allergy to any medication required to perform the procedure.

Although certain locations (e.g., the anterior arch of C1 and the dens) previously were considered inaccessible, with the newer imaging modalities there are few, if any, lesions that cannot be successfully and safely biopsied by trained and experienced interventional radiologists.

Technique

Image Guidance

Percutaneous biopsies of the spine are commonly done with fluoroscopic or CT guidance. The choice of imaging modality is based on the preference of the physician, the size and location of the target lesion, the potential access routes, the ability to visualize the lesion, and the availability and cost of the equipment. Some of the advantages associated with

K. Ahrar, S. Gupta (eds.), *Percutaneous Image-Guided Biopsy*,
DOI 10.1007/978-1-4614-8217-8_22, © Springer Science+Business Media New York 2014

fluoroscopic guidance are real-time visualization of needle position in both the anteroposterior and cephalocaudal direction, inexpensive cost, and short procedure times [7–9]. Fluoroscopy, however, requires the use of ionizing radiation and provides poor visualization of soft tissue, which increases the risk of needle damage to major vessels, nerves, and spinal structures, especially in the cervical region. CT imaging precisely delineates the vertebral lesions, any associated soft-tissue components, and the lesion's relationship to adjacent structures, thus enabling the selection of a safe approach for biopsy [7, 10–12]. CT also helps distinguish necrotic from solid lesions and unequivocally document position of the needle tip. However, CT-guided percutaneous biopsy is limited by the long duration of the procedure and the inability to monitor the needle continuously during insertion and sampling. CT fluoroscopy (CTF) combines the advantages of conventional fluoroscopy with nearly real-time visualization. One of the major concerns about CTF, however, is that it exposes both the patient and the operator to a high level of radiation.

Magnetic resonance imaging (MRI) guidance can also been used for biopsies of spinal lesions. The potential advantages of MRI as a guidance modality for percutaneous biopsy procedures include its high-contrast resolution, multiplanar imaging capacity, ability to visualize vessels without the need to administer a contrast agent, lack of ionizing radiation, and 2- and 3-dimensional imaging capabilities. The superior contrast resolution of MRI may allow visualization of lesions not readily apparent on other imaging modalities.

Sonographic guidance is not routinely used for biopsies of spinal and other skeletal regions because of the inability of the ultrasound beam to penetrate an intact cortex. However, destructive or lytic bony lesions with a break in the overlying cortex and lesions with extraosseous soft-tissue extensions can be visualized with sonography, enabling the biopsy needle to be passed into the lesion under real-time guidance [13–15]. However, patients with sclerotic vertebral or small lytic bone lesions without a cortical break or extraosseous soft-tissue extension are not candidates for a sonographically guided procedure; in these cases, CT or fluoroscopic guidance is necessary.

In a study by Gupta et al., sonographic guidance was found to be particularly useful for cervical spinal biopsies [13, 14]. Real-time sonography allows continuous monitoring of the needle tip and surrounding structures and thus reduces the risk of injury to the many vital structures located in the neck. In addition, cervical lesions involving any part of the vertebra, including the body, transverse process, articular processes, or posterior elements, are accessible to sonographic visualization and hence to sonographically guided fine-needle aspiration biopsy (FNAB). However, in thoracic, lumbar, and sacral regions, the role of sonographically guided FNAB is limited mostly to lesions involving the posterior elements. In rare instances, however, in thin patients, lumbar spinal lesions within the vertebral body and those with paravertebral soft-tissue components can be safely approached from the anterior aspect; with real-time sonographic monitoring, the anteriorly located vessels and other vital structures can be avoided easily [13, 14].

Bone Biopsy Needles

A variety of needle systems for biopsy of bone are commercially available, and any of these is adequate for obtaining biopsy specimens from spinal lesions[7]. Detailed descriptions of all available biopsy systems are beyond the scope of this chapter, but we will describe a few bone-specific biopsy systems to illustrate the general technique for obtaining tissue specimens.

Bone-specific biopsy systems generally use needles with trephine tips, which have a serrated edge for cutting tissue specimens for histologic analysis [6, 16, 17]. Most of the available trephine bone biopsy systems consist of a large-caliber (8- to 16-gauge) outer cannula fitted with an inner stylet or obturator, which is advanced to the proximal edge of the lesion. After removing the stylet, the hollow trephine needle is placed through the cannula and advanced with a clockwise (drilling) motion through the lesion to obtain a core specimen. Most systems come with a metal obturator to push the core sample from inside the trephine needle. Once the outer cannula has been advanced through the cortex, it can also serve as a coaxial guide needle for obtaining FNAB and cutting-needle biopsies using any of the commercially available needles of various calibers. The Craig (10-gauge; Becton Dickinson, Rutherford, NJ) and the Ackerman (12-gauge; Cook Inc., Bloomington, IN) bone biopsy needles have the configuration described above and allow large-core bone biopsies. The Elson bone biopsy set (Cook Inc) is a modification of the Ackerman set that allows initial placement of a thin, 22-gauge, 25-cm needle with removable hub close to the periosteal margin of the vertebra at the selected location. After removing the hub and inner stylet from the 22-gauge needle, a 2-piece biopsy system consisting of an outer 12-gauge cannula with a tapered inner cannula is advanced over the 22-gauge needle to the proximal margin of the lesion. The main advantage of initially introducing the thin needle is that it provides a safe pathway for the larger-caliber needles, and this is especially useful in high-risk areas such as the upper thoracic and cervical spine. This method also facilitates infiltration of local anesthetic into the periosteum at the intended puncture site. The Geremia biopsy system (16-gauge; Cook Inc) is similar to the Elson system and comes with a 40-cm stiffener wire that can be advanced through the 22-gauge, 25-cm introducer needle; this allows sufficient exchange length so that the wire is exposed at all times during coaxial advancement of the biopsy needle [18].

In some biopsy systems, the outer cannula has a sharp beveled edge for cutting through the bone. In these systems, after using the outer cannula for obtaining multiple coaxial biopsies, the outer cannula itself (without the inner stylet) can be advanced into the lesion to obtain a large-core sample. Many of these biopsy systems have T-shaped interlocking handles attached to the inner and outer needles that fit easily into the operator's hand, allowing increased control during insertion of the needle. The needle is advanced using a manual clockwise rotary (drilling) motion with forward pressure or by tapping on the needle handle with a sterile surgical hammer. The Temno bone biopsy needle system (Bauer Medical Inc, Clearwater, FL) consists of an 8- to 13-gauge outer cannula with a T-shaped handle and a diamond-tip inner stylet. The outer cannula has a sharp beveled tip for cutting through the bone. In the Jamshidi needle system (Manan Medical Products, Northbrook, IL), the 8- to 13-gauge outer cannula has a T-shaped handle and a triple-crown trephine cutting edge, and the inner stylet has a trocar tip. Osteo-Site Bone Access Needle Sets (Cook Inc) are available in 11- and 13-gauge calibers. The outer cannula has a beveled cutting edge and T-shaped handle and is fitted with a diamond-tip inner stylet. The Ostycut bone biopsy needle (CR Bard, Covington, GA) has a threaded outer cannula with a sharp beveled cutting tip and a trocar-point stylet; the needle has the dual advantages of having strength to allow it to be advanced through normal bone or overlying intact cortex to provide access and also having the capability of obtaining a core specimen. The Osteo-Rx needle (Cook Inc) is a modification of the Osteo-Site and consists of a 10-gauge outer cannula and a steerable 13-gauge nitinol needle with a 90° curved tip that allows sampling of multiple locations within the vertebra from a single access site. The Bonopty coaxial bone biopsy system (CR Bard) consists of a 14-gauge cannula and a 15-gauge drill. The eccentrically cutting drill tip is ideally suited for penetrating intact cortical bone.

The choice of a biopsy needle system depends on the availability and cost of the system, the location of the target lesion, the suspected pathology, the integrity of the overlying bone cortex, the internal consistency of the target lesion, the availability of on-site pathology support, and, most important, the experience and familiarity of the operator with the given needle system [7].

Once the outer cannula has been placed in or at the edge of the target lesion, the internal consistency of the lesion determines the choice of needles used to obtain the tissue samples. For lesions that are sclerotic, calcified, ossified, or composed of intact trabeculae infiltrated with tumor cells, large-caliber (15-gauge or larger) stiff bone-cutting needles (such as the trephine needles) are necessary for obtaining core specimens. Once the trephine needle has created a space in the hard lesion, 22-gauge needles can be used to obtain fine-needle aspiration samples. On the other hand, for "soft" bone lesions or soft-tissue mass lesions, use of bone-cutting needles is unlikely to yield tissue. Any of the commercially available FNAB needles and spring-driven slotted cutting needles can be used in such cases to obtain biopsy specimens.

Approaches to Spinal Biopsy and Anatomic Considerations

Cervical Spine

Different approaches for cervical spinal biopsy include the anterolateral, posterolateral, posterior, transoral, and paramaxillary approaches (Fig. 22.1a–c) [19, 20].

Anterolateral Approach

The anterolateral approach allows access to lesions of the mid and lower cervical vertebrae (C4–C7) and discs and to lesions in the prevertebral space [10, 21]. This approach allows easier access to the anterior aspect of the vertebral body and also allows access to the intervertebral disc because it is not hidden by the uncovertebral joint, which is located more posterolaterally. This approach can also be used to access lesions involving the transverse process of the vertebrae as long as the vertebral artery is not in the needle path [22].

For the anterolateral approach, the patient is placed in the supine position with the head turned toward the opposite side, with the neck in extension, and with a pillow or bolster under the shoulders. The needle is inserted anterior to the sternocleidomastoid muscle and is advanced posteromedially between the visceral space and the carotid space (Fig. 22.2) [10, 13, 14, 21]. Care should be taken to avoid the hypopharynx and especially the piriform fossa and esophagus. In some cases, it may be helpful to manually retract the great vessels laterally, especially if the procedure is performed with fluoroscopic guidance [19, 20].

As the needle is pushed posteriorly toward the vertebral body, care should be taken to avoid the vertebral artery. From the subclavian artery, the vessel goes upward toward the foramen in the base of the transverse process of the sixth cervical vertebra and then passes upward through the canal in the transverse processes. Between the foramina, the vertebral artery is located lateral to the mid or posterior part of the vertebral body or disc; care should be taken to avoid the lateral aspect of the vertebral body. Because the needle is directed posteriorly and medially in this approach, theoretically, the spinal canal could be penetrated through the neural foramina, which are directed anterolaterally. However, the use of intermittent CT scans to check the position and trajectory of the needle tip can protect against the penetration of the spinal canal and prevent possible damage to vascular and neural structures. Furthermore, the presence of the carotid

Fig. 22.1 (**a–c**) Schematic drawings showing the needle trajectories for the anterolateral, posterolateral, and posterior approaches at the (**a**) C4 and (**b**) C6 vertebral levels. (**c**) Schematic drawing showing needle trajectories for the paramaxillary approach for C1 and C2 lesions

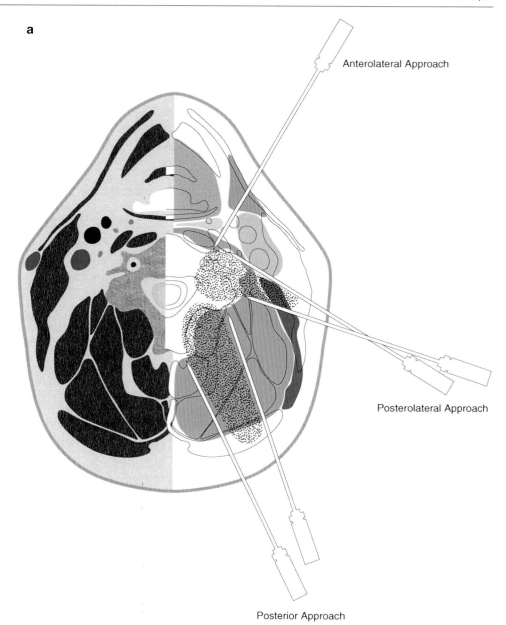

a

Anterolateral Approach

Posterolateral Approach

Posterior Approach

Fig. 22.1 (continued)

b

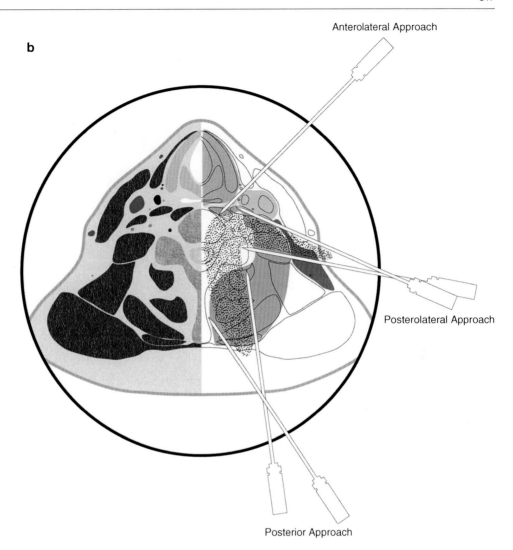

Anterolateral Approach

Posterolateral Approach

Posterior Approach

Fig. 22.1 (continued)

c

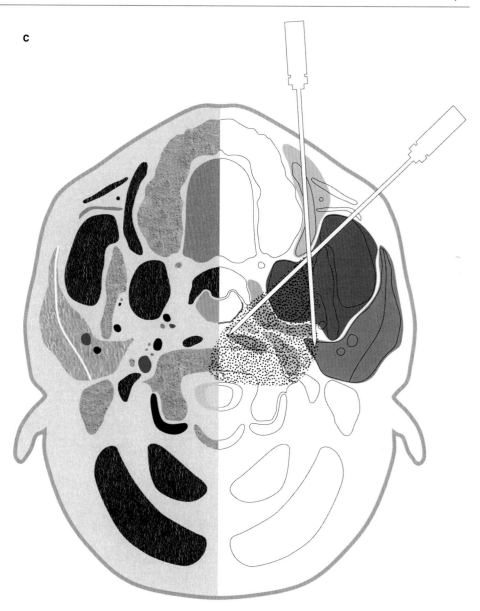

sheath tends to keep the needle pointed medially and away from the neural foramen and the vertebral artery [22].

Other important structures that could be in the needle path when this approach is used include the superior and middle thyroid vessels, the superior and inferior laryngeal nerves, the loop of the hypoglossal nerve, and the cervical ganglia of the sympathetic system. However, the small-caliber needles used for the biopsy are unlikely to cause serious damage to the blood vessels or nerves.

Posterolateral Approach

The posterolateral approach is used for sampling lower cervical (C4–C7) vertebral lesions that involve the transverse process, pedicle, articular pillar, or lamina and for sampling

lesions in the prevertebral and lateral paraspinal portions of the perivertebral space [7, 19]. This approach can also be used for sampling lateral masses involving C1 and C2.

With the patient in the supine, prone, or lateral decubitus position, the needle is inserted through the sternocleidomastoid muscle and the posterior cervical space and advanced posterior to the carotid sheath (Fig. 22.3). Depending on the vertebral level (mid vs. lower cervical), the patient's position, and the size and location of the carotid sheath, the needle may be advanced anteromedially or posteromedially. The soft tissues overlying the clavicles and shoulder may interfere with needle placement in the lower neck, particularly in patients with prominent clavicles and short necks. An out-of-plane angled approach with a caudal needle angulation can

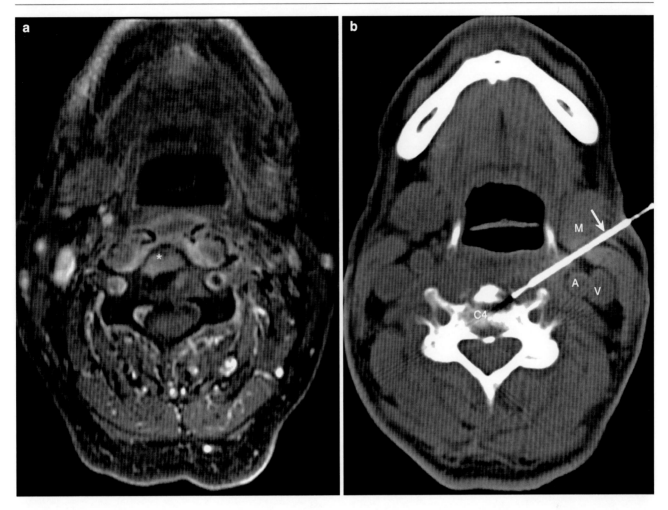

Fig. 22.2 (**a, b**) Cervical spine. Anterolateral approach. (**a**) Contrast-enhanced axial magnetic resonance image shows an abnormal area of enhancement (*asterisk*) in a C4 vertebral body. (**b**) Computed tomography image during the biopsy procedure shows the biopsy needle (*arrow*) inserted through the sternocleidomastoid muscle (*M*) and advanced medial to the carotid artery (*A*) and jugular vein (*V*) into the C4 vertebral body

be used in this situation; the needle is inserted in a plane cranial to the level of the target lesion and advanced caudally and medially (Fig. 22.4).

With this approach, the vertebral artery is the structure most vulnerable to injury during the biopsy, especially at levels between the transverse foramina, where the vessel is located lateral to the vertebral body and disc. Also, a needle inserted behind the carotid sheath and advanced posteromedially toward a lesion involving the seventh cervical vertebra could potentially injure the vertebral artery. Using contrast medium to identify the vertebral artery can reduce the risk of injury. Because the intervertebral foramina run from the spinal canal in an oblique medial-to-lateral and posterior-to-anterior direction, penetrating the spinal canal with this approach is not possible. Furthermore, a small-caliber needle puncture of the brachial or cervical plexus as it runs between the scalene muscles is not dangerous, although it may cause

transient pain. When this approach is used for biopsy of C1 and C2 lesions, care should be taken to identify and avoid the vertebral artery (Fig. 22.5).

Posterior Approach

The posterior approach is used for biopsy of lesions involving the spinous process, lamina, and articular pillars and processes of the cervical vertebrae as well as lesions in the posterior and lateral paraspinal portions of the perivertebral space [22]. This approach also can be used occasionally for sampling lateral masses involving C1 and C2, provided care is taken to identify and avoid the vertebral artery[22].

With the patient in the prone or lateral decubitus position, the needle is advanced through the posterior paraspinal muscles in an anterior direction toward the target lesion (Fig. 22.6). Risk of injury to major vessels or nerves with this approach is extremely low. During biopsy of lesions involving

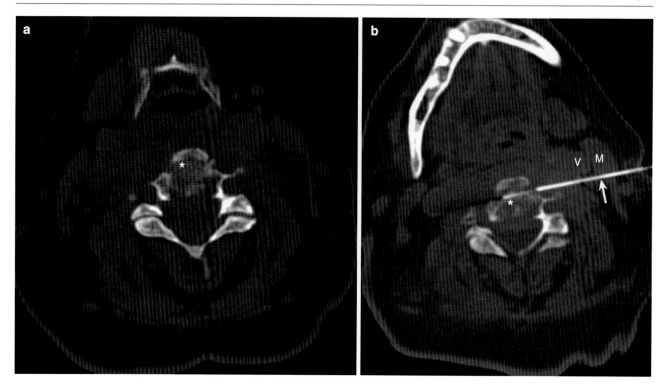

Fig. 22.3 (a, b) Cervical spine. Posterolateral approach. (a) Computed tomography (*CT*) scan shows a lytic process (*asterisk*) involving the C3 vertebral body. (b) CT image during the biopsy procedure shows the biopsy needle (*arrow*) inserted through the sternocleidomastoid muscle (*M*) and advanced posterior to the carotid sheath vessels (*V*) into the C3 lesion (*asterisk*)

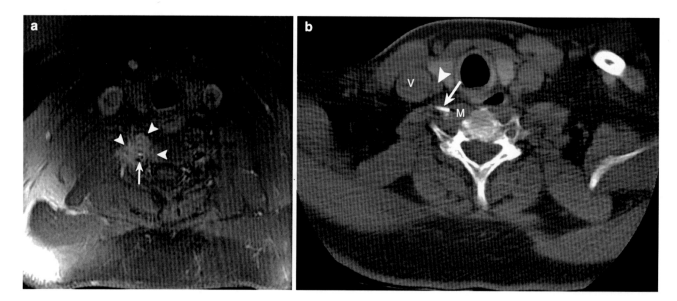

Fig. 22.4 (a, b) Cervical spine. Angled posterolateral approach. (a) Magnetic resonance image shows a hyperintense lesion (*arrowheads*) involving the right transverse process of the C6 vertebra extending into the prevertebral space. The vertebral artery (*arrow*) is immediately posterior to the mass. (b) CT scan shows the needle tip (*arrow*) in the prevertebral portion of the mass (*M*). The needle was inserted at a more cranial level, directed caudally, and advanced posterior to the internal jugular vein (*V*) and the common carotid artery (*arrow*)

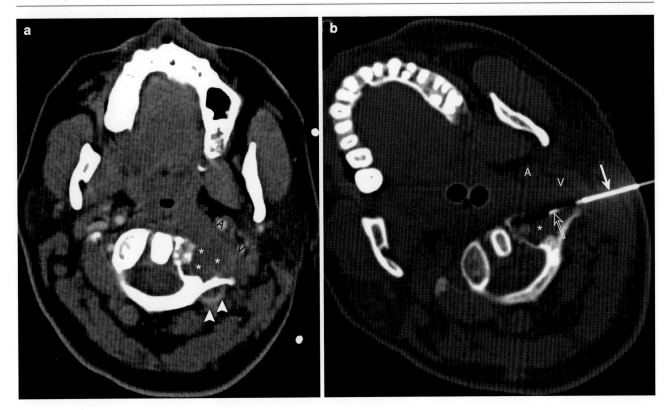

Fig. 22.5 Cervical spine. Posterolateral approach. Use of contrast agent to identify and avoid the vertebral artery. (**a**) Contrast-enhanced computed tomography scan with the patient in a supine position shows a lytic lesion with soft-tissue extension (*asterisks*) involving the lateral mass of the C1 vertebra. The carotid artery (*A*) and jugular vein (*V*) are displaced anteriorly by the mass. Note the posterior location of the vertebral artery (*arrowheads*). (**b**) Computed tomography scan shows the coaxial biopsy system with an outer guide needle (*arrow*) and an inner core biopsy needle (*open arrow*) advanced posterior to the carotid artery (*A*) and jugular vein (*V*) into the mass (*asterisk*)

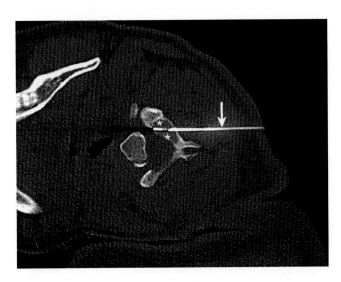

Fig. 22.6 Cervical spine. Posterior approach. Computed tomography scan with the patient in the decubitus position shows the needle (*arrow*) passing through the posterior paravertebral muscles into a lytic process (*asterisks*) involving the left lamina of C3 vertebra

the laminae, care should be taken to ensure that the needle does not penetrate the spinal canal or thecal sac. For sampling lesions involving a lateral mass of C1 using a posterior approach, the needle should be advanced under the lamina, not above it [22]. The vertebral artery, after exiting the C1 foramen, courses posteriorly along the upper surface of the C1 lamina. If necessary, intravenous administration of contrast medium can be used to help identify and avoid the vertebral artery (Fig. 22.7).

Transoral Approach

The transoral approach can be used for percutaneous access to lesions involving the anterior portions of the C1 and C2 vertebrae, including the odontoid [19, 22, 23]. The use of this approach requires general anesthesia. An otolaryngologic retractor is placed in order to provide adequate visibility of the oropharyngeal space. The uvula is pushed away with a retractor or a nasal tube. Some operators recommend placement of an inflatable bronchial blocker into the esophagus to prevent antiseptic fluids or blood from entering the stomach. The oral pharynx and cavity is prepared with antiseptic solution. The posterior pharyngeal wall is sprayed and infiltrated with local anesthetic. The needle is inserted through the posterior pharyngeal mucosa and is advanced posteriorly through the retropharyngeal space and prevertebral muscles

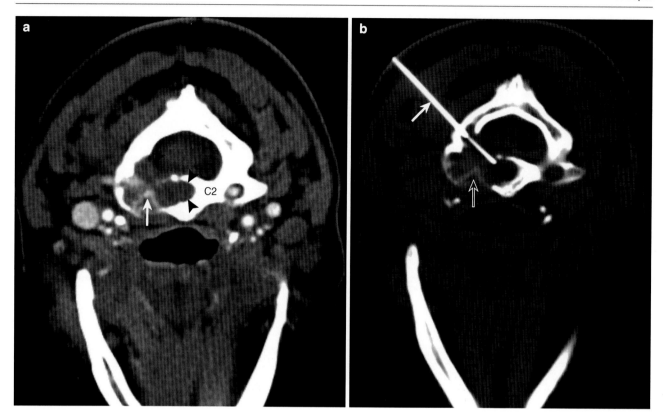

Fig. 22.7 Cervical spine. Posterior approach. Use of contrast administration to identify and avoid the vertebral artery. (**a**) Contrast-enhanced computed tomography scan with the patient in a prone position shows a lytic lesion (*arrowheads*) involving the body and lateral mass of C2 vertebra. Note the vertebral artery (*arrow*) encased and narrowed by the lesion. (**b**) Computed tomography scan shows the biopsy needle (*arrow*) passing through the anterior portion of the lamina into the lesion posterior to the expected location of the vertebral artery (*open arrow*)

toward the target lesion (Fig. 22.8). This is a relatively safe approach because no important structure lies between the posterior pharyngeal wall and the bone. Use of antibiotics in this setting is recommended because of the difficulty in maintaining a sterile field with the transoral approach.

Paramaxillary Approach

Although the presence of facial skeleton precludes the use of the standard anterolateral approach for C1 and C2 lesions, a transfacial paramaxillary approach offers safe anterior access to anterior C1 and C2 lesions [22]. The needle is inserted inferior to the zygomatic process of the maxilla and advanced posteriorly through the buccal space between the maxilla and mandible. The needle is advanced through the lateral and medial pterygoid muscles and the parapharyngeal and retropharyngeal spaces for accessing C1 and C2 lesions (Fig. 22.9).

It is important to avoid the carotid artery; administration of contrast may occasionally be required to visualize this artery. Other structures present in the needle path that could

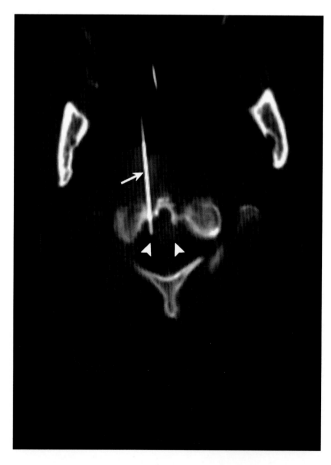

Fig. 22.8 Transoral approach. Computed tomography scan shows the needle (*arrow*) inserted through an open mouth and advanced through the retropharyngeal and prevertebral tissues into a soft-tissue mass (*arrowheads*) involving the tip of the odontoid and the anterior arch of atlas

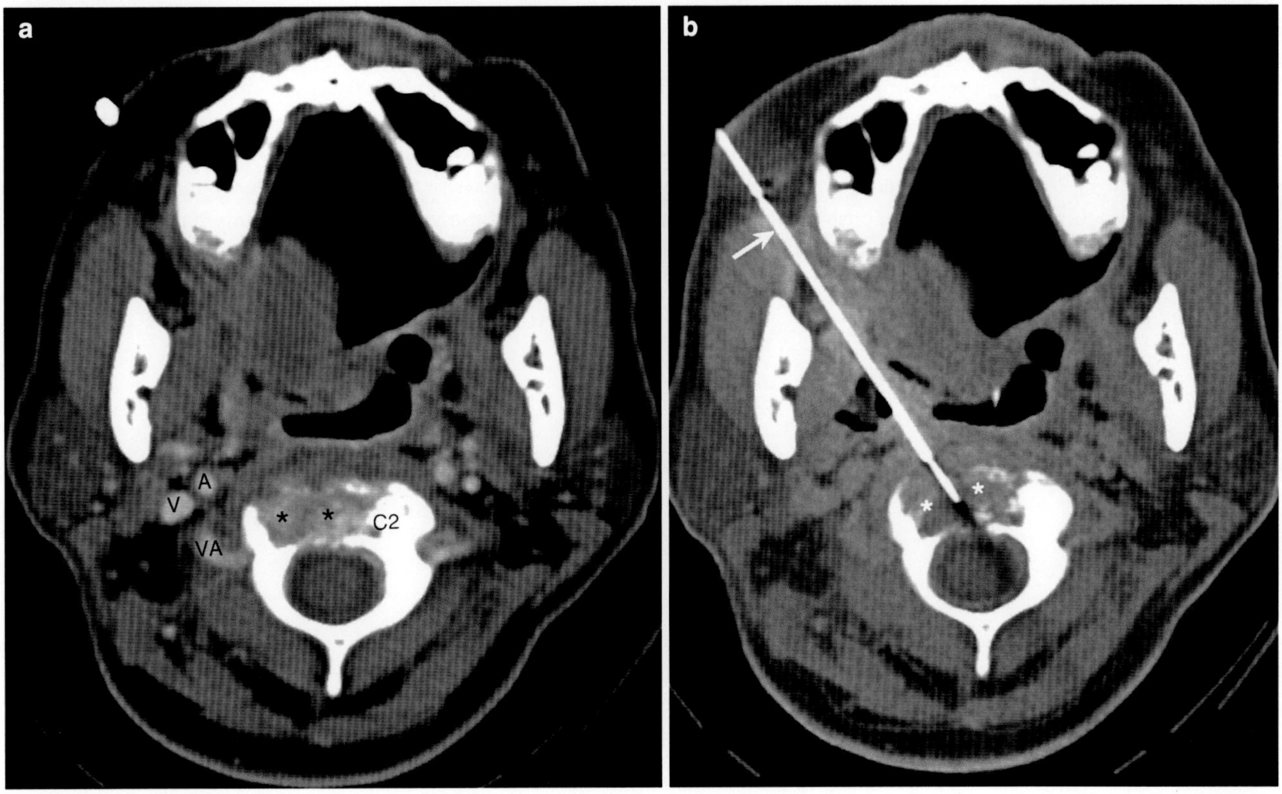

Fig. 22.9 Cervical spine. Paramaxillary approach. (**a**) Contrast-enhanced computed tomography scan with the patient in a supine position shows a lytic lesion (*asterisks*) involving the body of C2 vertebra. Note the position of the carotid artery (*A*), jugular vein (*V*), and the vertebral artery (*VA*). (**b**) Computed tomography scan shows the biopsy needle (*arrow*) advanced through the masticator, parapharyngeal spaces, and prevertebral muscles into a lytic lesion (*asterisks*) involving the C2 vertebral body

potentially be injured with this approach include the facial artery, internal maxillary artery and its branches, the pterygoid venus plexus, branches of the mandibular and maxillary nerves, and the external carotid artery as it courses laterally deep to the lateral pterygoid muscle. Using a Hawkins-Akins needle (Meditech, Westwood, MA) with a blunt-tip stylet as the outer guiding needle decreases the risk of injury to the vessels and nerves in these spaces [22].

Thoracic Spine

Various approaches can be used for thoracic vertebral biopsies (Fig. 22.10). The vertebral level, the location of the lesion in or adjacent to the vertebral body, and the lesion size are the major determinants to use in selecting an approach. Selection of an approach is also affected by the body habitus and the presence and severity of kyphosis and scoliosis.

Transpedicular Approach

The pedicle provides a short and safe path to the vertebral body [24]. A transpedicular approach is generally used for lesions located within or just anterior to the pedicle (Fig. 22.11). This approach is also the preferred approach for lesions that involve the entire vertebral body.

The transpedicular approach avoids risk of injury to major vessels, the thecal sac and the cord, and the nerve roots [25, 26]. Another advantage of the transpedicular approach

is that the needle is perpendicular to the bone cortex at the point of entry. In addition, the cortical bone of the posterior pedicle is typically thin, thus facilitating needle insertion. Since the pedicle is attached to the cranial half of the vertebral body, this approach is generally suitable for lesions involving the upper part of the vertebral body. However, the use of craniocaudal needle angulation with this approach, wherein the needle entering the cranial part of the pedicle is angled caudally, allows access to lesions involving the mid to lower part of the vertebral body (Fig. 22.12).

The transverse diameter of the thoracic pedicle is smaller than that of the lumbar pedicle, leaving less room for error when placing a large-caliber needle through the pedicle [27, 28]. The transverse diameter of the pedicle is smallest (4.6 mm on average) at the T5 level. Thus, a biopsy needle with an outside diameter of 3 mm might injure the medial walls of the pedicle [25]. The small size of the pedicle also restricts the entry angle of the biopsy needle. Although thoracic pedicles generally will accommodate an 11-gauge needle, smaller gauge needles may be preferable, especially at upper and middle thoracic vertebral levels.

Thoracic transpedicular biopsy can be performed with fluoroscopic or CT guidance. Because of the occasional difficulty in visualizing the small thoracic pedicle with X-ray fluoroscopy, CT guidance is the preferred method.

Costovertebral/Transcostovertebral/Costotransverse Joint Approach

For the transcostovertebral approach, the needle is inserted laterally and advanced anteromedially, passing in between the tubercle of the rib and the corresponding transverse process (Fig. 22.10b) [29]. The needle enters the posterolateral aspect of the vertebral body across the costotransverse ligament (Fig. 22.13). CT guidance is necessary to directly visualize accurate needle positioning between the transverse process and the rib.

The needle trajectory is dependent on the orientation and the thickness of the rib and transverse process. With this approach, the bony structures do not leave much room for needle angulation. The head of the rib articulates with the superior costal facet of the corresponding thoracic vertebra, which is located in posterolateral aspect of the upper half of the vertebra immediately caudal to the superior end plate. Thus, this approach allows access to lesions involving the upper part of the vertebral body. This approach allows access to lesions involving posterior or

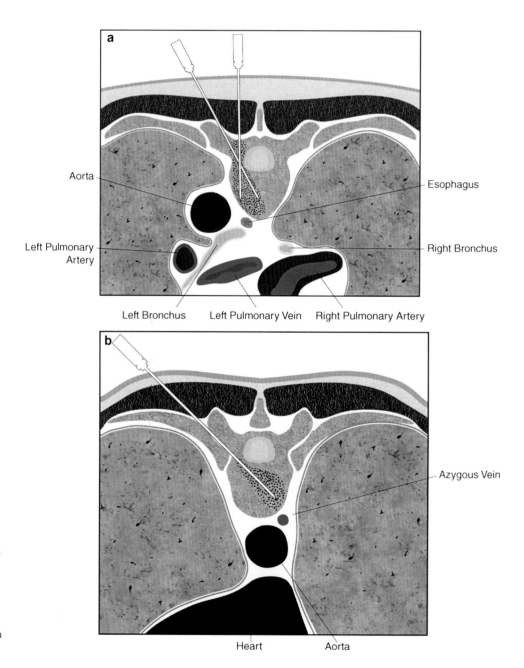

Fig. 22.10 (**a–d**) Schematic drawing showing needle trajectories for the transpedicular (**a**), costotransverse (**b**), costovertebral groove (**c**), and intercostal (**d**) approaches for thoracic vertebral lesions. The shaded areas represent the region that can be accessed with each approach

Fig. 22.10 (continued)

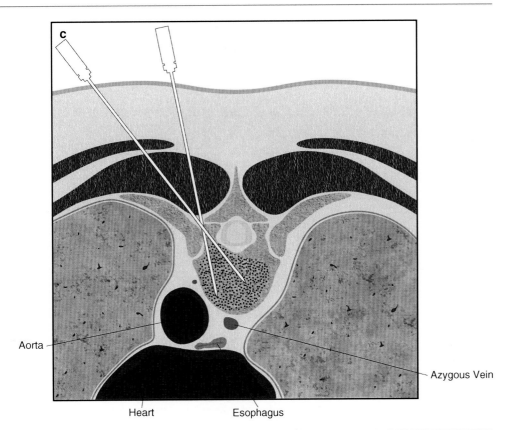

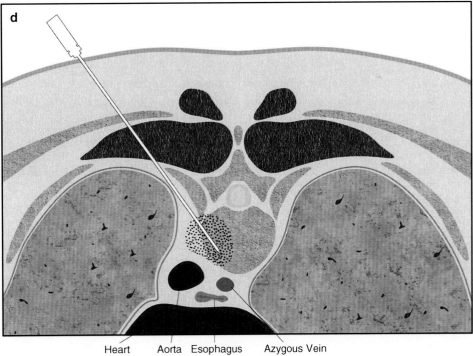

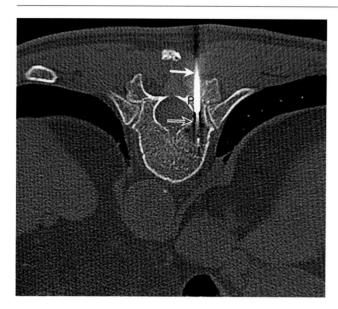

Fig. 22.11 Thoracic spine. Transpedicular approach. Computed tomography scan with the patient in the prone position shows the guide needle (*arrow*) and the coaxially inserted core biopsy needle (*open arrow*) advanced through the right pedicle (*P*) of the T11 vertebra for biopsy of a lytic lesion (*asterisks*) located immediately anterior to the pedicle

posterolateral parts of the vertebral body on the ipsilateral side (Fig. 22.13) and also to lesions involving the anterior part of the ipsilateral pedicle (Fig. 22.10b). However, lesions involving the ipsilateral anterior or anterolateral portion of the vertebral body cannot be reached with this approach. However, this approach allows access to a much larger area of the vertebral body, including the anterior half, on the side contralateral to the needle insertion (Fig. 22.14). This approach can also be used to access the intervertebral disc one level above the level of the corresponding thoracic vertebra.

With this approach, the bony structures (namely, the transverse process and the rib) keep the biopsy needle away from the lung, pleura, and the exiting nerve roots. The presence of rib anterior to the needle path prevents inadvertent pleural transgression and prevents the needle from sliding forward along the lateral cortex of the vertebral body. The transverse process prevents passage of the needle into the spinal canal. Damage to the costotransverse articulation remains a theoretical possibility with this approach.

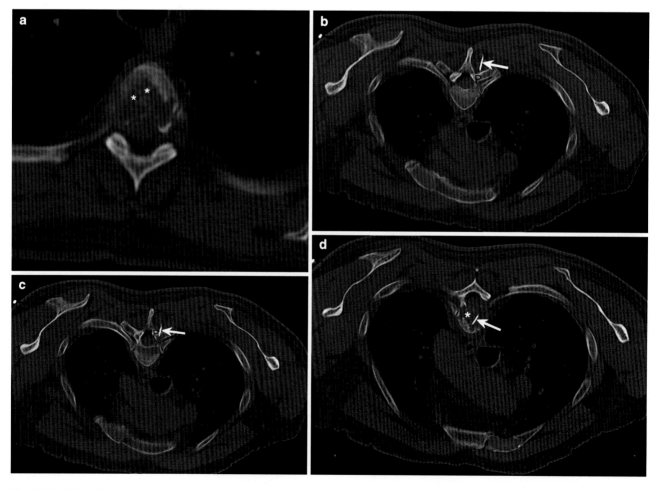

Fig. 22.12 Thoracic spine. Angled transpedicular approach. (**a**) Computed tomography scan with the patient in the supine position shows a lytic process (*asterisks*) involving the T5 vertebral body. Note the lesion is located caudal to the level of the pedicle, precluding a direct transpedicular approach. (**b–d**) The needle (*arrow*) was inserted at a level cranial to the lesion and directed caudally through the pedicle (*P*) into the lesion (*asterisk*)

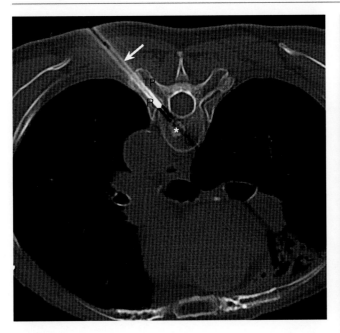

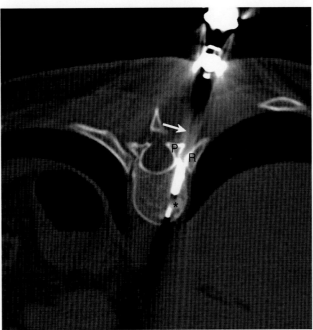

Fig. 22.13 Thoracic spine. Costotransverse approach. Computed tomography scan with the patient in the prone position shows the biopsy needle (*arrow*) advanced in between the left ninth rib (*R*) and the transverse process (*TP*) for biopsy of a sclerotic lesion (*asterisk*) involving the left posterior part of the T9 vertebral body

Fig. 22.15 Thoracic spine. Costovertebral groove approach. Computed tomography scan with the patient in the prone position shows the biopsy needle (*arrow*) advanced in between the head of right eleventh rib (*R*) and the pedicle (*P*) for biopsy of a sclerotic lesion (*asterisk*) involving the ipsilateral anterior part of the T11 vertebral body

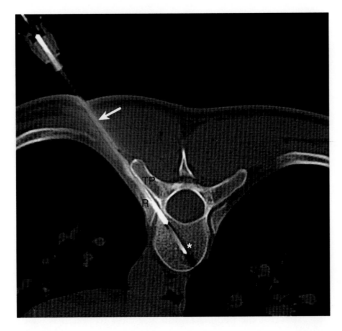

Fig. 22.14 Thoracic spine. Costotransverse approach. Computed tomography scan with the patient in the prone position shows the biopsy needle (*arrow*) advanced in between the left tenth rib (*R*) and the transverse process (*TP*) for biopsy of a lytic lesion (*asterisk*) involving the right anterior part of the T10 vertebral body

Costovertebral Groove Approach

Costovertebral groove approach is a modification of the costotransverse approach. With this approach, the needle is advanced in the groove between the vertebral pedicle (upper portion) and the head of the rib, entering the posterolateral edge of the vertebral body (Fig. 22.10c). This groove/space is located at a level immediately above the level of the transverse process. Because of the absence of transverse process at this level, there is more room for needle angulation than in the costotransverse approach, allowing easy access to larger areas of the vertebral body, including the anterior half of the vertebral body on the ipsilateral side (Fig. 22.15). However, similar to the costotransverse approach, this approach allows access only to lesions involving the upper portion of the vertebral body and the adjoining disc space (Fig. 22.16). When this approach is used with CT guidance, and the needle is advanced in the same axial plane, this allows access only to lesions involving the upper portion of the vertebral body and the adjoining disc space. However, if a craniocaudal angulation is used, this approach can also allow access to lesions in the middle or lower part of the vertebral body. Gantry tilt may be used to align the needle path in one axial plane.

Posterolateral Intercostal Approach

The intercostal approach involves needle placement in the posteromedial intercostal space, anterior to the head of the rib and costovertebral joint (Fig. 22.10d). This approach is generally used for biopsy of paravertebral soft-tissue masses or lateral vertebral body masses (Fig. 22.17) [30]. This approach is also used for lesions located in the lower part of the vertebral body, as these lesions cannot be accessed easily by the

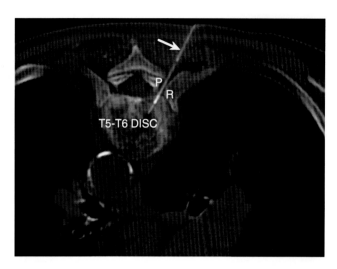

Fig. 22.16 Thoracic intervertebral disc. Costovertebral groove approach. Computed tomography scan with the patient in the prone position shows the biopsy needle (*arrow*) advanced in between the head of the rib (*R*) and the pedicle (*P*) for biopsy of the T5–T6 disc space

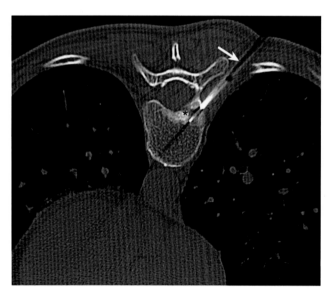

Fig. 22.17 Thoracic spine. Intercostal approach. Computed tomography scan with the patient in the prone position shows the biopsy needle (*arrow*) advanced via the intercostal space for biopsy of a sclerotic lesion (*asterisk*) involving the posterolateral part the T9 vertebral body

standard transpedicular or transcostovertebral approaches. Posterolateral approach can also be used for biopsy of lesions located predominantly in the intervertebral disc. Lesions located in the posterior part of the vertebral body, especially posterocentral lesions, are difficult to access with this approach and there is a risk of inadvertent lung puncture as well. However, injection of saline solution into the paravertebral soft tissues can be used to push the pleura and lung forward, allowing safe needle placement. In addition, the needle may cause injury to the intercostal vessels or paraspinal veins, increasing the risk of paraspinal hematoma.

Transforaminodiscal approach

A transforaminodiscal approach that involves accessing the vertebral body through the intervertebral disc above has also been described [31]. The needle is directed from a superior to inferior direction and from a lateral to medial direction to pass through the intervertebral foramen between the targeted vertebra and the superior vertebra. Since the biopsy needle passes through the inferior half of the foramen, there is almost no risk of injuring the nerve root, because the roots course very close to the inferior edge of the upper pedicle and exit in the upper half portion of the foramen. It is important to ensure that the needle trajectory does not cross the medial pedicular line before entering the intervertebral space; this avoids the possibility of penetrating the dural sac. The entire vertebral body, except for the extreme superomedial aspect, can be sampled with this approach. However, this is a complex pathway requiring more images and prebiopsy calculations, lengthening the average total procedure time.

Posterior Approach

A direct posterior approach is used for lesions involving the posterior elements of the thoracic vertebra.

Lumbar Spine

Approaches to lumbar vertebral lesions include transpedicular, posterolateral, lateral, and posterior methods (Fig. 22.18). Selection of a particular approach depends on the location of the lesion within the vertebra.

Transpedicular Approach

The transpedicular approach provides safe passageway to the vertebral body and is used if a lesion is within the pedicle or central vertebral bodies [24–26, 32]. The pedicle selected for the vertebral biopsy depends on the location of the lesion within the vertebra. Transpedicular approach is also the preferred approach for lesions involving the entire vertebral body. Lesions of the intervertebral discs cannot be reached using this route.

Some of the advantages of a transpedicular biopsy include the following: (a) the needle tract is shorter, (b) the acute angle between the transverse process and the mamillary process helps guide the needle tip toward the pedicle, (c) the biopsy needle is perpendicular to the cortex of the bone at the point of entry, and (d) the cortical bone along the posterior aspect of the pedicle is thin and easy to penetrate with the biopsy needle.

For a CT-guided transpedicular approach, the patient is placed in a prone position. The needle entry site is determined by extrapolating the long axis of the pedicle to the skin surface. It is important to anesthetize the subcutaneous soft tissues up to the level of the periosteum. The course of biopsy needle should be along the long axis of the pedicle. Care should be taken to keep the needle away from the cortical

Fig. 22.18 (**a**, **b**) Schematic drawing showing needle trajectories for the transpedicular (**a**) and posterolateral (**b**) approaches to lumbar vertebral lesions. The *shaded areas* represent the region that can be accessed with each approach

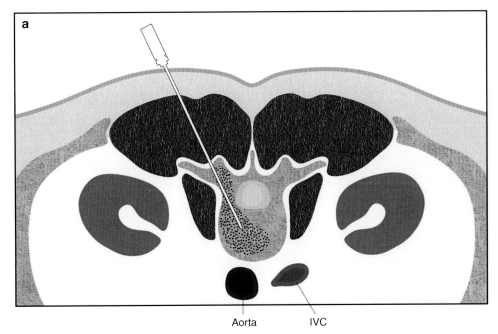

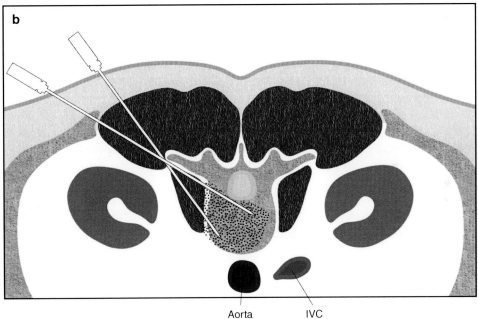

bone of the pedicle, especially along the medial and inferior aspect of the pedicle. This is important to prevent the spread of hematoma, infection, or tumor inside the spinal canal.

Biplane fluoroscopy is useful for the transpedicular approach, because it permits simultaneous visualization of the position of the needle in both the frontal and lateral views. The patient is placed in a prone position on the fluoroscopy table and the C-arm is angled along the inclination of the pedicle selected for the biopsy to obtain an end-on view of the center of the pedicle. The needle track is anesthetized using 1 % lidocaine hydrochloride, and the periosteum surrounding the pedicle and the area at the junction of transverse process and superior facet are anesthetized. The biopsy needle is placed on the skin and angulated to obtain an end-on view in the center of the pedicle (the bull's-eye) on the fluoroscopic image. With the use of a mallet, the guide needle is tapped gently through the pedicle and into the lesion intended for biopsy as determined by fluoroscopy on frontal and lateral views. This is important to ensure that the biopsy needle is in a central position in the pedicle and not near the cortical bone. Puncture of the medial or inferior walls of the pedicle can potentially result in spinal canal damage or nerve root injury.

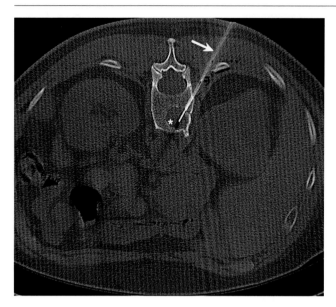

Fig. 22.19 Lumbar spine. Posterolateral approach. Computed tomography scan with the patient in the prone position shows the biopsy needle (*arrow*) advanced via a posterolateral approach for biopsy of a lytic lesion (*asterisk*) involving the anterior part of the L1 vertebral body

Modified Transpedicular Approach for Accessing Disc Lesions

A modified transpedicular approach has been described that allows sampling of the intervertebral disc space as well as both vertebral end plates adjacent to the involved disc [33]. This is an exaggerated oblique transpedicular approach similar to that described for vertebroplasty procedures. The traditional transpedicular approach generally places the needle in a horizontal plane, making access to the disc space and adjacent vertebral bodies impossible. In the modified approach, the needle is placed in the caudal part of the pedicle with a caudal-to-cranial angulation; this allows improved access to the intervertebral disc space.

Posterolateral Paravertebral Approach

With the patient in the prone position, the needle is introduced 5–8 cm lateral to the midline and advanced anteromedially (Fig. 22.19) [4]. The needle passes anterior to the transverse process toward the lateral aspect of the vertebral body [11, 34]. Careful attention should be given to avoid the nerve roots, kidney, renal vessels, and large vessels.

This approach is also useful for accessing disc space lesions. This approach is also useful when a lesion is located in the lower part of the vertebral body, as these lesions are difficult to access with the transpedicular approach. However, lesions located in the pedicle or in the posterior part of the vertebral body are difficult to access with this approach.

Lateral Approach

A lateral approach with the patient in lateral decubitus has also been described, allowing access to the vertebral body, disc, and paraspinal soft tissues [35]. Lateral decubitus positioning results in anterior displacement of abdominal viscera, thereby providing a clear view of the lateral aspect of the lumbar spine. The main advantage of this approach is that the needle is generally a safe distance away from the nerve roots, kidneys, renal pedicle, and large vessels.

Posterior Approach

A direct posterior approach is used for lesions involving the posterior elements of the lumbar vertebra.

Sacrum

Sacral lesions are generally accessed from a posterior approach (Fig. 22.20). A direct anterior approach may occasionally be used for presacral lesions and lesions involving the anterior body of the sacrum. However, presence of bowel loops, bladder, and other viscera makes this a difficult approach.

Complications

The incidence of complications after image-guided percutaneous spine biopsy is less than 1–3 % [7, 36]. The risk of potential complications is greater with cervical spine biopsies than for biopsies of the lumbar and thoracic regions because of the proximity to many vital structures surrounding the cervical spine [20, 21].

Pneumothorax is a potential complication that can be seen with biopsy of the lower cervical or thoracic vertebral lesions [37]. Neural injury, particularly of the spinal cord and nerve roots, is a serious complication that can result in foot drop, transient paresis, transient paraplegia, and paraplegia [5, 38]. However, with careful attention in selecting the needle path and the use of image guidance for needle placement, any serious neural injury is rare. Nerve injury can be caused by direct nerve root injury with the biopsy needle or by anesthesia. Paresis or paralysis resulting from anesthetizing major motor nerves generally dissipates within 3–4 h [39].

Bleeding can occur from needle injury to vertebral arteries, paraspinal veins, azygos veins, or, rarely, the aorta, resulting in paraspinal hematomas [40]. Most of the hematomas are small, clinically insignificant, and do not require any treatment [32, 39]. Paravertebral pseudoaneurysm formation has been reported but is extremely rare; this injury can be treated with arterial embolization or percutaneous injection of thrombin [41, 42]. Injury of paravertebral vessels is more common with a paravertebral approach and can be avoided by using a transpedicular approach whenever possible. Biopsy of hypervascular tumors that involve the posterior vertebral body cortex and extend into the central canal can result in bleeding into the canal, causing cord compression.

Other complications that have been reported rarely after percutaneous vertebral biopsy include fracture,

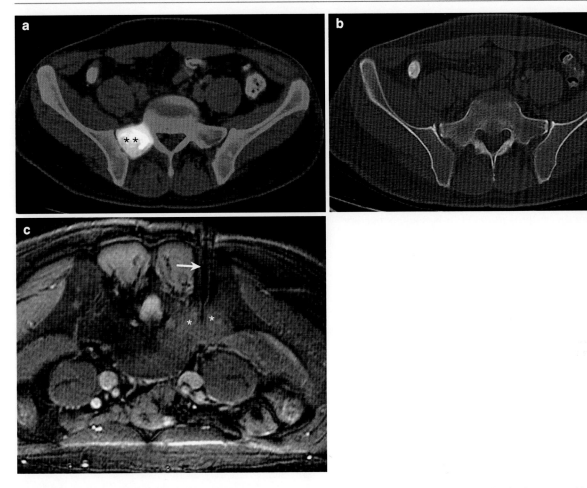

Fig. 22.20 Sacrum. Posterior approach. (**a**) Positron-emission tomography-computed tomography image shows fluorodeoxyglucose (*FDG*)-avid lesion in the right sacrum (*asterisks*). (**b**) Computed tomography scan shows no corresponding abnormality in the sacrum. (**c**) Magnetic resonance imaging during the biopsy procedure shows the needle (*arrow*) used to sample the abnormal signal intensity area in the right sacrum (*asterisk*)

vasovagal reaction, puncture of the thecal sac, disc space infection, osteomyelitis, meningitis, epidural hematoma, tumor seeding along the needle tract, and death [7, 25, 26, 36, 43–52].

Use of CT guidance for needle placement for vertebral biopsies has greatly enhanced the safety of the procedure. CT imaging, with its high-contrast and spatial resolution, shows the relationship of the vertebral lesion to adjacent vital structures, allowing the selection of a safe route.

Outcome and Results

The reported accuracy of imaging-guided percutaneous biopsy of vertebral lesions ranges from 67–100 % [7, 25, 26, 36, 43–52]. The diagnostic accuracy of percutaneous vertebral biopsy varies according to the site biopsied, needle used, radiographic appearance of the biopsied lesions, underlying pathology, and operator's experience.

Sampling errors during percutaneous needle biopsy can lead to false-negative results; therefore, negative results should be viewed with caution. Crushing artifacts and insufficient tissue samples are two major limitations of needle biopsies that can lead to false-negative diagnoses [53]. It is also difficult to obtain sufficient samples in necrotic or cystic lesions [39].

In many patients, the vertebral lesion may be seen only through MRI or positron-emission tomography (PET) imaging, with no radiographically visible changes apparent on CT scans [47]. In these situations, a discrepancy in counting vertebral levels may lead to sampling the wrong vertebra [40]. A false-negative biopsy result in such patients may also result from sampling the wrong part of the involved vertebra because of lack of a visible target.

Another reason for nondiagnostic sampling is biopsy of infectious spondylodiscitis, as tissue specimens generally show nonspecific histologic features. Also, the ability to culture from an infection is generally poor, even more so in patients with fungal discitis [54, 55]. This is especially true if the infection is chronic or if the patient has been treated with broad-spectrum antimicrobials [52]. Improper handling of specimens and failure to perform appropriate microbiologic testing may also result in nondiagnostic sampling [56]. Paravertebral abscesses or fluid obtained from the intervertebral space or vertebral bodies in spondylitis are often sterile. Brugieres et al. [49] described a series of 89 spinal biopsies in which a pathogenic organism was found in 53 % of cases. Michel et al. [55] showed that CT-guided spinal biopsy produced positive bacteriologic examinations in 61 % of patients with spondylitis.

FNAB of vertebral lesions has been shown to have a lower success rate than core biopsy [57]. Core needle biopsy and FNAB are generally considered to be complementary techniques, and combined use of the two techniques can potentially increase the diagnostic yield of vertebral biopsy procedures. In one reported study, the positive predictive value of combined needle aspiration and core biopsy was 82 % and the negative predictive value 100 % [58].

A relationship between the spinal level and the accuracy of biopsy results has been reported in some studies [34, 36, 46]. Nondiagnostic biopsies are more frequently seen with biopsies of cervical and thoracic vertebral lesions than with those at lumbar and sacral levels; this is probably related to the small vertebral body size and technical difficulties associated with achieving percutaneous access to these lesions [34, 36, 46]. The increased accuracy rate with the lower lumbar and sacrum biopsies is likely due to easier access and the absence of vital structures (e.g., spinal cord or major vessels), which allows the use of larger needles and more aggressive sampling of lesions. However, other studies have found no difference in diagnostic accuracy rates based on spinal level [50, 52, 59].

Sclerotic or densely osteoblastic lesions generally have lower diagnostic yields [47]. Brugieres et al. [49] reported higher accuracy rates with osteolytic (94 %) than with osteosclerotic lesions (75 %), whereas Ghelman et al. observed an accuracy rate of 95 % for lytic lesions and 42 % for mixed lesions [34]. Stoker and Kissin also reported lower accuracy rates for sclerotic lesions [50]. The lower diagnostic yield in patients with sclerotic lesions is probably related to the fact that the actual tumor volume that leads to reactive bony sclerosis is very small, and it is impossible to tell which part of the sclerosis represents the tumor. Using large-bore trephine needles, sampling the least-dense portions of the sclerotic lesions, obtaining multiple samples, and sampling different portions of the sclerotic area are some of the methods that can potentially increase the diagnostic yield in such patients.

The histologic type of the target lesion also influences the diagnostic accuracy of image-guided percutaneous biopsy [60]. Diagnostic accuracy rates of metastatic lesions are generally higher than those of primary bone tumors and fractures [59]. Benign bone tumors are associated with a high incidence of false-negative biopsy results [43, 60].

False-negative results are also frequent with biopsies of bone involvement in hematopoietic malignant disorders such as lymphoma. Since these tumors tend to cause diffuse infiltration of bone rather than focal lesions, needle biopsy may not yield sufficient amounts of representative samples. False-negative biopsies in such cases have also been attributed to prolonged decalcification during the histologic preparation of the obtained material, resulting in negative results from immunohistochemical analysis [36].

Summary

Percutaneous needle biopsy of the spine using CT or fluoroscopic guidance is a safe, accurate, and widely used method for establishing the correct pathologic diagnosis in patients presenting with undiagnosed vertebral and paravertebral lesions. Various approaches can be used for spinal biopsies; the choice of approach is generally determined by the vertebral level, the location of the lesion in or adjacent to the vertebral body, and the lesion size.

References

1. Martin HE, Ellis EB. Biopsy by needle puncture and aspiration. Ann Surg. 1930;92:169–81.
2. Coley BLSG, Ellis EB. Diagnosis of bone tumors by aspiration. Am J Surg. 1931;13:215–24.
3. Robertson RCBR. Destructive spine lesions: diagnosis by needle biopsy. J Bone Joint Surg. 1935;17:749.
4. Siffert RS, Arkin AM. Trephine biopsy of bone with special reference to the lumbar vertebral bodies. J Bone Joint Surg Am. 1949;31A:146–9.
5. Adapon BD, Legada Jr BD, Lim EV, Silao Jr JV, Dalmacio-Cruz A. CT-guided closed biopsy of the spine. J Comput Assist Tomogr. 1981;5:73–8.
6. Mick CA, Zinreich J. Percutaneous trephine bone biopsy of the thoracic spine. Spine (Phila Pa 1976). 1985;10:737–40.
7. Geremia G, Joglekar S. Percutaneous needle biopsy of the spine. Neuroimaging Clin N Am. 2000;10:503–33.
8. Pierot L, Boulin A. Percutaneous biopsy of the thoracic and lumbar spine: transpedicular approach under fluoroscopic guidance. AJNR Am J Neuroradiol. 1999;20:23–5.
9. Murphy WA, Destouet JM, Gilula LA. Percutaneous skeletal biopsy 1981: a procedure for radiologists–results, review, and recommendations. Radiology. 1981;139:545–9.
10. Kattapuram SV, Rosenthal DI. Percutaneous biopsy of the cervical spine using CT guidance. AJR Am J Roentgenol. 1987;149:539–41.
11. Babu NV, Titus VT, Chittaranjan S, Abraham G, Prem H, Korula RJ. Computed tomographically guided biopsy of the spine. Spine (Phila Pa 1976). 1994;19:2436–42.
12. Kang M, Gupta S, Khandelwal N, Shankar S, Gulati M, Suri S. CT-guided fine-needle aspiration biopsy of spinal lesions. Acta Radiol. 1999;40:474–8.
13. Gupta RK, Gupta S, Tandon P, Chhabra DK. Ultrasound-guided needle biopsy of lytic lesions of the cervical spine. J Clin Ultrasound. 1993;21:194–7.
14. Gupta S, Takhtani D, Gulati M, et al. Sonographically guided fine-needle aspiration biopsy of lytic lesions of the spine: technique and indications. J Clin Ultrasound. 1999;27:123–9.

15. Civardi G, Livraghi T, Colombo P, Fornari F, Cavanna L, Buscarini L. Lytic bone lesions suspected for metastasis: ultrasonically guided fine-needle aspiration biopsy. J Clin Ultrasound. 1994;22: 307–11.

16. Debnam JW, Staple TW. Trephine bone biopsy by radiologists: results of 73 procedures. Radiology. 1975;116:607–9.

17. Laredo JD, Bard M. Thoracic spine: percutaneous trephine biopsy. Radiology. 1986;160:485–9.

18. Geremia GK, Charletta DA, Granato DB, Raju S. Biopsy of vertebral and paravertebral structures with a new coaxial needle system. AJNR Am J Neuroradiol. 1992;13:169–71.

19. Ottolenghi CE, Schajowicz F, Deschant FA. Aspiration biopsy of the cervical spine. Technique and results in thirty-four cases. J Bone Joint Surg Am. 1964;46:715–33.

20. Tampieri D, Weill A, Melanson D, Ethier R. Percutaneous aspiration biopsy in cervical spine lytic lesions. Indications and Technique. Neuroradiology. 1991;33:43–7.

21. Brugieres P, Gaston A, Voisin MC, Ricolfi F, Chakir N. CT-guided percutaneous biopsy of the cervical spine: a series of 12 cases. Neuroradiology. 1992;34:358–60.

22. Gupta S, Henningsen JA, Wallace MJ, et al. Percutaneous biopsy of head and neck lesions with CT guidance: various approaches and relevant anatomic and technical considerations. Radiographics. 2007;27:371–90.

23. Patil AA. Transoral stereotactic biopsy of the second cervical vertebral body: case report with technical note. Neurosurgery. 1989;25:999–1001; discussion 1001–1002.

24. Renfrew DL, Whitten CG, Wiese JA, el-Khoury GY, Harris KG. CT-guided percutaneous transpedicular biopsy of the spine. Radiology. 1991;180:574–6.

25. Ashizawa R, Ohtsuka K, Kamimura M, Ebara S, Takaoka K. Percutaneous transpedicular biopsy of thoracic and lumbar vertebrae–method and diagnostic validity. Surg Neurol. 1999;52:545–51.

26. Stringham DR, Hadjipavlou A, Dzioba RB, Lander P. Percutaneous transpedicular biopsy of the spine. Spine (Phila Pa 1976). 1994;19:1985–91.

27. Zindrick MR, Wiltse LL, Doornik A, et al. Analysis of the morphometric characteristics of the thoracic and lumbar pedicles. Spine (Phila Pa 1976). 1987;12:160–6.

28. Misenhimer GR, Peek RD, Wiltse LL, Rothman SL, Widell Jr EH. Anatomic analysis of pedicle cortical and cancellous diameter as related to screw size. Spine (Phila Pa 1976). 1989;14:367–72.

29. Brugieres P, Gaston A, Heran F, Voisin MC, Marsault C. Percutaneous biopsies of the thoracic spine under CT guidance: transcostovertebral approach. J Comput Assist Tomogr. 1990;14:446–8.

30. Bender CE, Berquist TH, Wold LE. Imaging-assisted percutaneous biopsy of the thoracic spine. Mayo Clin Proc. 1986;61:942–50.

31. Sucu HK, Bezircioglu H, Cicek C, Ersahin Y. Computerized tomography-guided percutaneous transforaminodiscal biopsy sampling of vertebral body lesions. J Neurosurg. 2003;99:51–5.

32. Jelinek JS, Kransdorf MJ, Gray R, Aboulafia AJ, Malawer MM. Percutaneous transpedicular biopsy of vertebral body lesions. Spine (Phila Pa 1976). 1996;21:2035–40.

33. Layton KF, Thielen KR, Wald JT. A modified vertebroplasty approach for spine biopsies. AJNR Am J Neuroradiol. 2006;27:596–7.

34. Ghelman B, Lospinuso MF, Levine DB, O'Leary PF, Burke SW. Percutaneous computed-tomography-guided biopsy of the thoracic and lumbar spine. Spine (Phila Pa 1976). 1991;16:736–9.

35. Garces J, Hidalgo G. Lateral access for CT-guided percutaneous biopsy of the lumbar spine. AJR Am J Roentgenol. 2000;174:425–6.

36. Rimondi E, Staals EL, Errani C, et al. Percutaneous CT-guided biopsy of the spine: results of 430 biopsies. Eur Spine J. 2008;17:975–81.

37. Metzger CS, Johnson DW, Donaldson 3rd WF. Percutaneous biopsy in the anterior thoracic spine. Spine (Phila Pa 1976). 1993;18:374–8.

38. McLaughlin RE, Miller WR, Miller CW. Quadriparesis after needle aspiration of the cervical spine. Report of a case. J Bone Joint Surg Am. 1976;58:1167–8.

39. Kattapuram SV, Rosenthal DI. Percutaneous biopsy of skeletal lesions. AJR Am J Roentgenol. 1991;157:935–42.

40. Olscamp A, Rollins J, Tao SS, Ebraheim NA. Complications of CT-guided biopsy of the spine and sacrum. Orthopedics. 1997;20: 1149–52.

41. Kulkarni K, Matravers P, Mehta A, Mitchell A. Pseudoaneurysm following vertebral biopsy and treatment with percutaneous thrombin injection. Skeletal Radiol. 2007;36:1195–8.

42. Stevens KJ, Gregson RH, Kerslake RW. False aneurysm of a lumbar artery following vertebral biopsy. Eur Spine J. 1997;6: 205–7.

43. Dupuy DE, Rosenberg AE, Punyaratabandhu T, Tan MH, Mankin HJ. Accuracy of CT-guided needle biopsy of musculoskeletal neoplasms. AJR Am J Roentgenol. 1998;171:759–62.

44. Schweitzer ME, Deely DM. Percutaneous biopsy of osteolytic lesions: use of a biopsy gun. Radiology. 1993;189:615–16.

45. Nourbakhsh A, Grady JJ, Garges KJ. Percutaneous spine biopsy: a meta-analysis. J Bone Joint Surg Am. 2008;90:1722–5.

46. Kornblum MB, Wesolowski DP, Fischgrund JS, Herkowitz HN. Computed tomography-guided biopsy of the spine. A review of 103 patients. Spine (Phila Pa 1976). 1998;23:81–5.

47. Lis E, Bilsky MH, Pisinski L, et al. Percutaneous CT-guided biopsy of osseous lesion of the spine in patients with known or suspected malignancy. AJNR Am J Neuroradiol. 2004;25:1583–8.

48. Donaldson 3rd WF, Johnson DW. Percutaneous biopsy of the thoracic spine. Neurosurg Clin N Am. 1996;7:135–44.

49. Brugieres P, Revel MP, Dumas JL, Heran F, Voisin MC, Gaston A. CT-guided vertebral biopsy. A report of 89 cases. J Neuroradiol. 1991;18:351–9.

50. Stoker DJ, Kissin CM. Percutaneous vertebral biopsy: a review of 135 cases. Clin Radiol. 1985;36:569–77.

51. Akhtar I, Flowers R, Siddiqi A, Heard K, Baliga M. Fine needle aspiration biopsy of vertebral and paravertebral lesions: retrospective study of 124 cases. Acta Cytol. 2006;50:364–71.

52. Heyer CM, Al-Hadari A, Mueller KM, Stachon A, Nicolas V. Effectiveness of CT-guided percutaneous biopsies of the spine: an analysis of 202 examinations. Acad Radiol. 2008;15:901–11.

53. Zornoza J. Needle biopsy of metastases. Radiol Clin North Am. 1982;20:569–90.

54. Laredo JD, Bellaiche L, Hamze B, Naouri JF, Bondeville JM, Tubiana JM. Current status of musculoskeletal interventional radiology. Radiol Clin North Am. 1994;32:377–98.

55. Michel SC, Pfirrmann CW, Boos N, Hodler J. CT-guided core biopsy of subchondral bone and intervertebral space in suspected spondylodiskitis. AJR Am J Roentgenol. 2006;186: 977–80.

56. Tehranzadeh J, Tao C, Browning CA. Percutaneous needle biopsy of the spine. Acta Radiol. 2007;48:860–8.

57. Fyfe IS, Henry AP, Mulholland RC. Closed vertebral biopsy. J Bone Joint Surg Br. 1983;65:140–3.

58. Leffler SG, Chew FS. CT-guided percutaneous biopsy of sclerotic bone lesions: diagnostic yield and accuracy. AJR Am J Roentgenol. 1999;172:1389–92.

59. Kattapuram SV, Khurana JS, Rosenthal DI. Percutaneous needle biopsy of the spine. Spine (Phila Pa 1976). 1992;17:561–4.

60. Logan PM, Connell DG, O'Connell JX, Munk PL, Janzen DL. Image-guided percutaneous biopsy of musculoskeletal tumors: an algorithm for selection of specific biopsy techniques. AJR Am J Roentgenol. 1996;166:137–41.

Anatomic Guidelines and Approaches for Biopsy of the Long Bones

23

Sendasaperumal Navakoti Sendos and Sanjay Gupta

Introduction

Image-guided needle biopsy is generally required for establishing a definite pathologic diagnosis prior to definitive medical or surgical treatment in patients who present with potentially malignant musculoskeletal lesions involving the upper and lower extremities [1–4]. Because needle biopsy intrinsically violates anatomical planes and spaces and malignant seeding of the biopsy tract is possible, standard definitive surgical therapy involves tandem resection of the biopsy tract, particularly if sarcoma is confirmed [1, 5, 6]. Performing safe musculoskeletal biopsy requires a thorough review of available imaging data, a detailed knowledge of the compartmental and neurovascular anatomy, and consultation with the treating orthopedic surgeon. In this chapter, we will review the cross-sectional compartmental anatomy of the upper and lower extremities and some common approaches to needle biopsy of extremity tumors.

Compartmental Anatomy

Musculoskeletal compartments are anatomic spaces bounded by tissues such as joint synovium, articular cartilage, bone cortex, periosteum, fascial planes, and tendinous origins and insertions. These tissues can prevent a tumor spreading from one compartment to another. Regions such as the axilla, antecubital fossa, wrist, groin, popliteal fossa, ankle, and dorsum of the hand or foot are considered extracompartmental [7, 8]. Skin and subcutaneous tissues, bones, parosseous spaces, joints, and muscles are distinct compartments, and lesions confined to these locations are considered intracompartmental.

Upper Extremity Compartments

The cross-sectional anatomy of the upper extremity at different levels is shown in Fig. 23.1. The dorsal periscapular musculature comprises the infraspinatus, teres minor, and rhomboids. The supraspinatus resides in another compartment of this region.

The anterior and posterior compartments of the arm are separated by the medial and lateral intermuscular septa [7, 9]. The anterior compartment contains the biceps, brachialis, brachioradialis, and coracobrachialis muscles, and the posterior compartment contains the triceps muscle. The brachial artery and vein and the median nerve are extracompartmental in the upper arm; however, these neurovascular structures enter the anterior compartment in the distal arm. Likewise, the radial nerve is located in the posterior compartment in the upper arm but crosses over into the anterior compartment in the distal arm. The ulnar nerve remains in an extracompartmental location throughout the arm.

The anatomy of the forearm has been sorted into multiple compartmental classifications [7, 9, 10]. In a commonly used classification, the forearm is divided into three compartments. The dorsal compartment contains the extensor muscles: the supinator, anconeus, extensor digitorum, extensor digiti minimi, extensor carpi ulnaris, extensor pollicis longus, and abductor pollicis longus. The lateral compartment (also known as the "mobile wad of Henry") contains the brachioradialis and two wrist extensors (i.e., the extensor carpi radialis longus and extensor carpi radialis brevis). The volar compartment contains the flexor muscles: the pronator teres, flexor carpi radialis, palmaris longus, flexor digitorum superficialis, flexor carpi ulnaris, flexor pollicis longus, flexor

S.N. Sendos, MD
Department of Radiology, Memorial Hermann Hospital,
7600 Beechnut Street, Houston, TX 77074, USA
e-mail: snsendos@gmail.com

S. Gupta, MD, DNB (✉)
Department of Interventional Radiology,
Department of Diagnostic Radiology,
The University of Texas MD Anderson Cancer Center,
1515 Holcombe Blvd., Unit 1471, Houston TX 77030, USA
e-mail: sgupta@mdanderson.org

K. Ahrar, S. Gupta (eds.), *Percutaneous Image-Guided Biopsy*,
DOI 10.1007/978-1-4614-8217-8_23, © Springer Science+Business Media New York 2014

digitorum profundus, and pronator quadratus. The radius, ulna, and interosseous membrane separate the volar and dorsal compartments, which can be subcategorized as superficial or deep. In the proximal forearm, the radial nerve is located between the lateral and volar compartments. The radial and ulnar arteries and median and ulnar nerves are located in the volar compartment. The anterior and posterior interosseous nerves and vessels are located in the volar and dorsal compartments, respectively.

Lower Extremity Compartments

The cross-sectional anatomy of the lower extremity at different levels is shown in Fig. 23.2. The thigh is divided into anterior, posterior, and medial compartments [7, 8, 11]. The anterior compartment contains the iliotibial tract, tensor fascia lata, quadriceps (i.e., the rectus femoris, vastus lateralis, vastus intermedius, and vastus medialis), and sartorius muscles. The posterior compartment contains the hamstring muscles

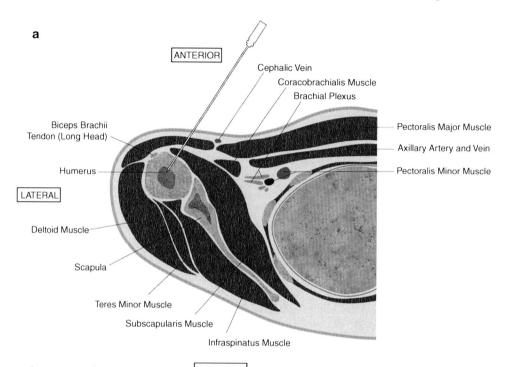

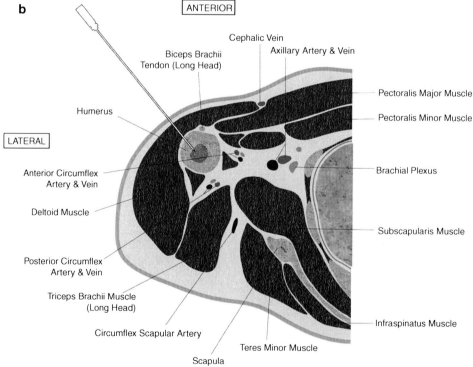

Fig. 23.1 Schematic diagrams of the cross-sectional anatomy, compartments, and recommended needle paths at various levels in the upper extremity. (**a**) Humeral head and proximal metaphysis. (**b**) Proximal humeral diaphysis. (**c**) Mid-humeral diaphysis. (**d**) Distal humeral metaphysis. (**e**) Distal humeral epiphysis and elbow joint. (**f**) Proximal radius and ulna. (**g**) Mid-radial and ulnar diaphyses. (**h**) Distal radial and ulnar diaphyses. (**i**) Distal radial and ulnar metaphyses and epiphyses

Fig. 23.1 (continued)

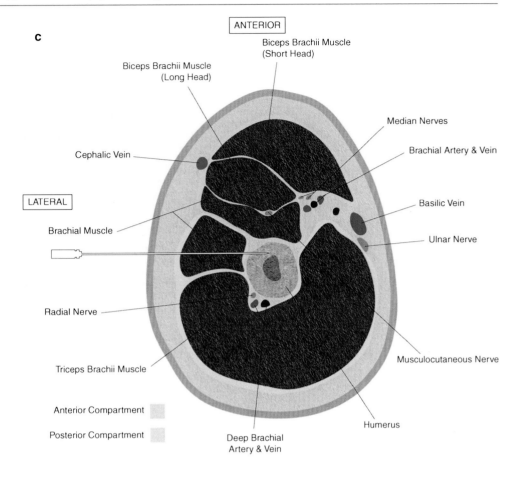

c

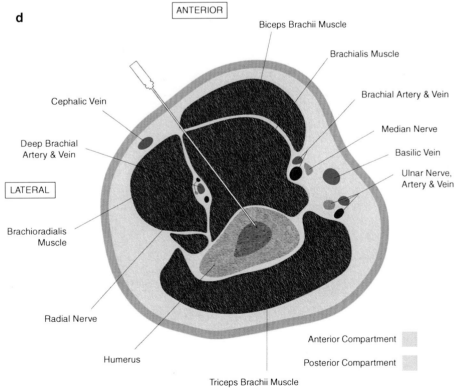

d

Fig. 23.1 (continued)

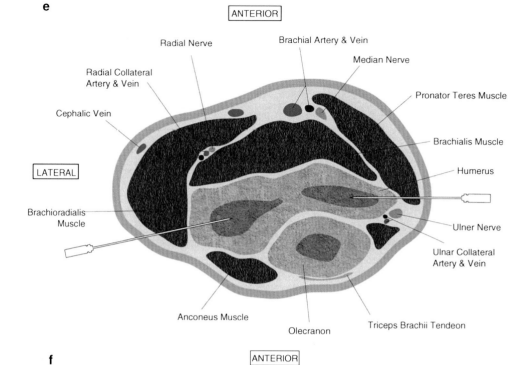

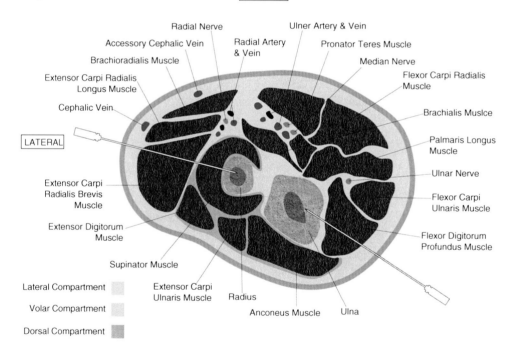

Fig. 23.1   (continued)

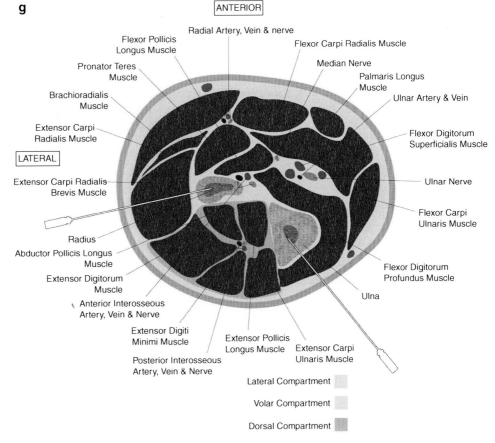

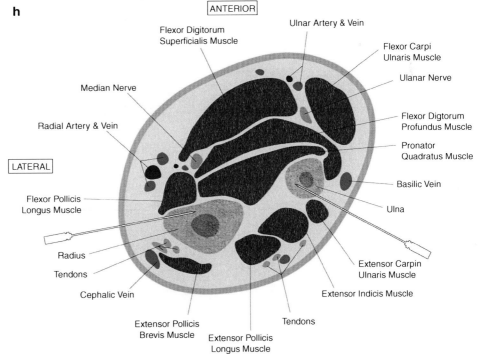

Fig. 23.1 (continued)

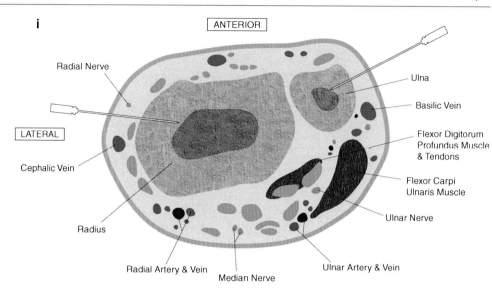

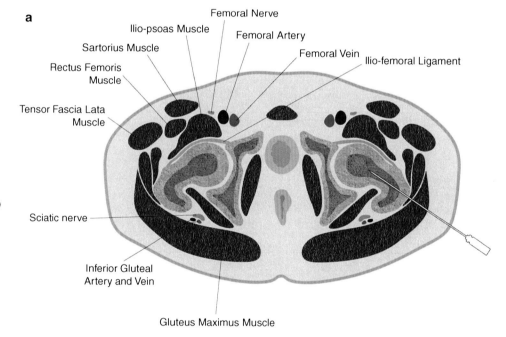

Fig. 23.2 Schematic diagrams of the cross-sectional anatomy, compartments, and recommended needle paths at various levels in the lower extremity. (**a**) Femoral head and neck. (**b**) Proximal femoral diaphysis. (**c**) Mid-femoral diaphysis. (**d**) Distal femoral diaphysis. (**e**) Distal femoral metaphysis. (**f**) Distal femoral epiphysis and knee joint. (**g**) Proximal tibial and fibular epiphyses and metaphyses. (**h**) Proximal tibial and fibular diaphyses. (**i**) Mid-tibial and fibular diaphyses. (**j**). Distal tibial and fibular diaphyses. (**k**) Distal tibial and fibular epiphyses

Fig. 23.2 (continued)

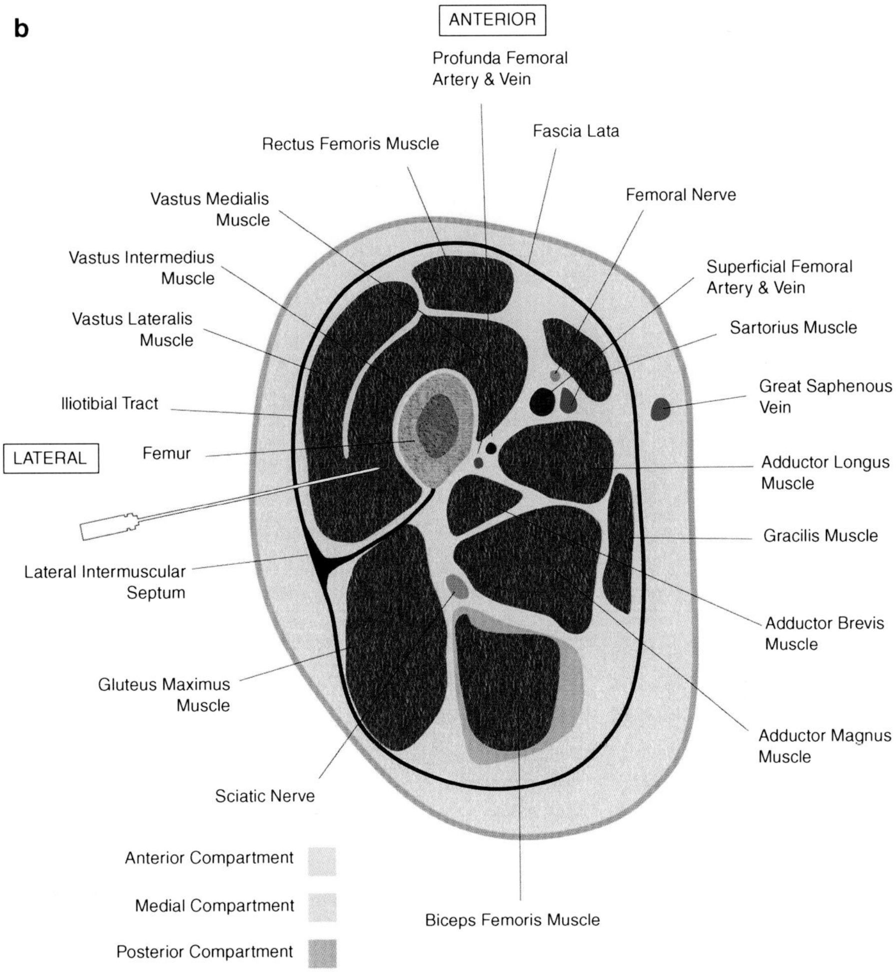

b

ANTERIOR

Profunda Femoral
Artery & Vein

Rectus Femoris Muscle

Fascia Lata

Vastus Medialis
Muscle

Femoral Nerve

Vastus Intermedius
Muscle

Superficial Femoral
Artery & Vein

Vastus Lateralis
Muscle

Sartorius Muscle

Great Saphenous
Vein

Iliotibial Tract

LATERAL   Femur

Adductor Longus
Muscle

Gracilis Muscle

Lateral Intermuscular
Septum

Adductor Brevis
Muscle

Gluteus Maximus
Muscle

Adductor Magnus
Muscle

Sciatic Nerve

Anterior Compartment

Medial Compartment

Posterior Compartment

Biceps Femoris Muscle

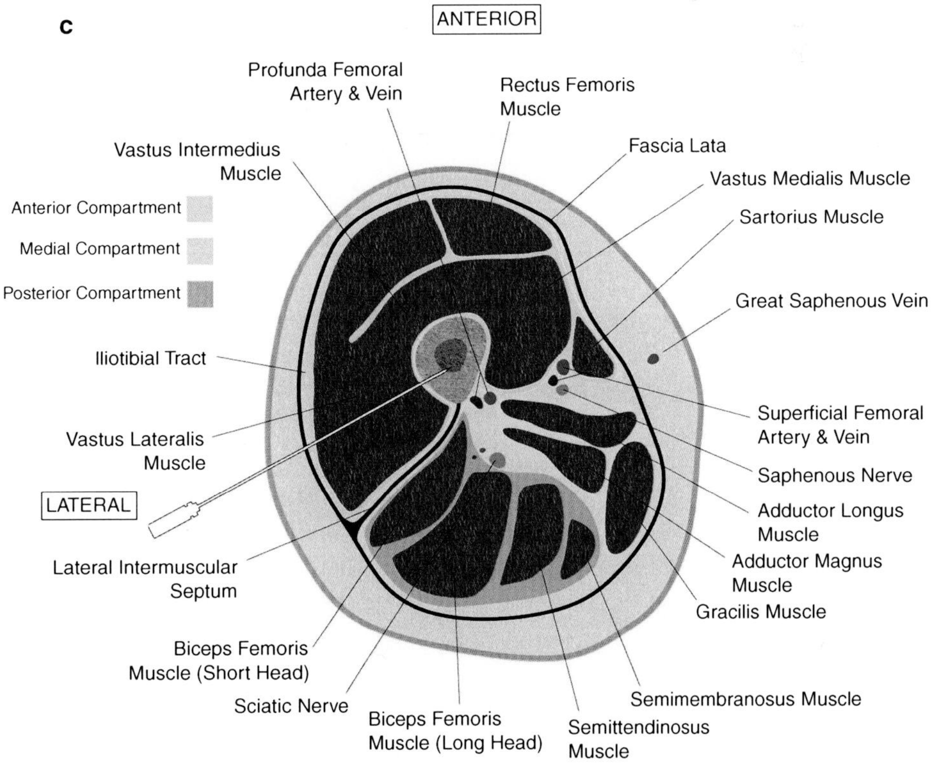

c

ANTERIOR

Profunda Femoral
Artery & Vein

Rectus Femoris
Muscle

Fascia Lata

Vastus Intermedius
Muscle

Anterior Compartment

Vastus Medialis Muscle

Medial Compartment

Sartorius Muscle

Posterior Compartment

Great Saphenous Vein

Iliotibial Tract

Superficial Femoral
Artery & Vein

Vastus Lateralis
Muscle

Saphenous Nerve

LATERAL

Adductor Longus
Muscle

Lateral Intermuscular
Septum

Adductor Magnus
Muscle

Gracilis Muscle

Biceps Femoris
Muscle (Short Head)

Sciatic Nerve

Semimembranosus Muscle

Biceps Femoris
Muscle (Long Head)

Semittendinosus
Muscle

Fig. 23.2 (continued)

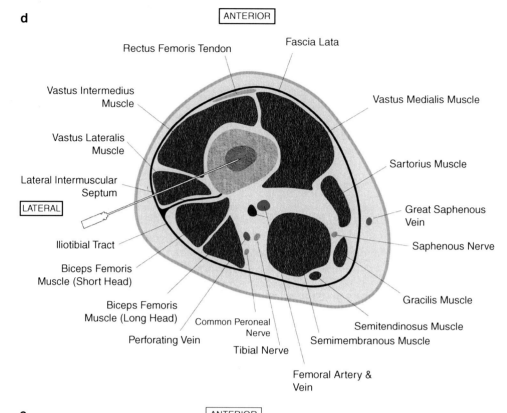

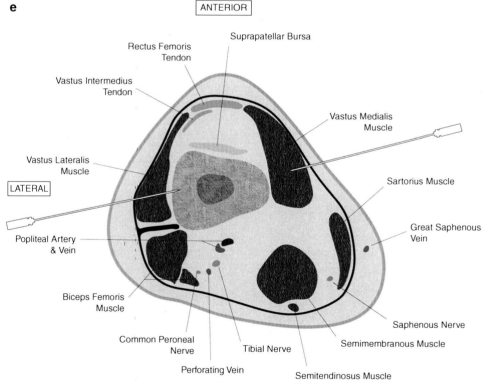

Fig. 23.2 (continued)

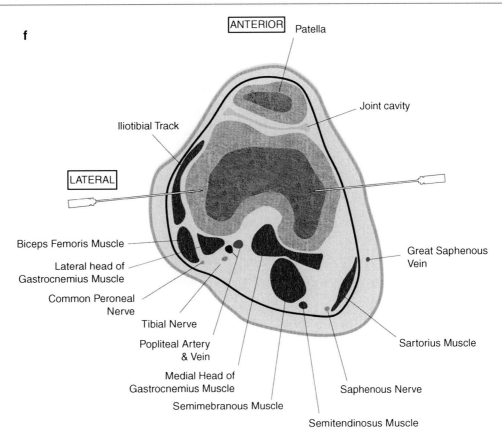

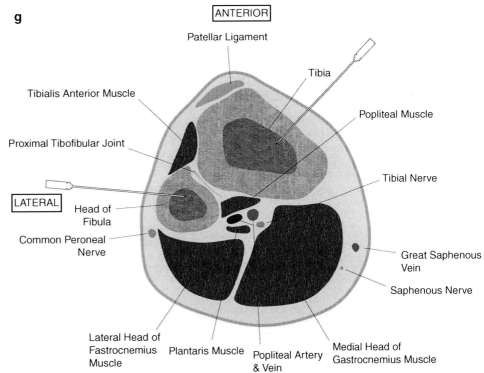

Fig. 23.2 (continued)

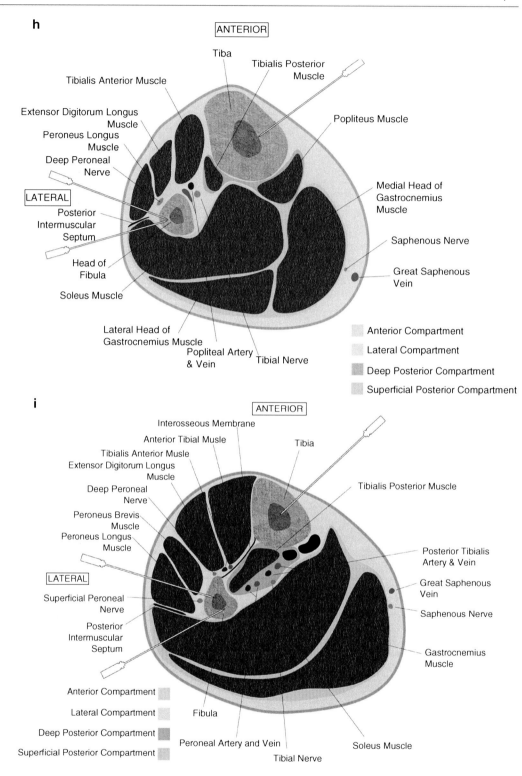

Fig. 23.2 (continued)

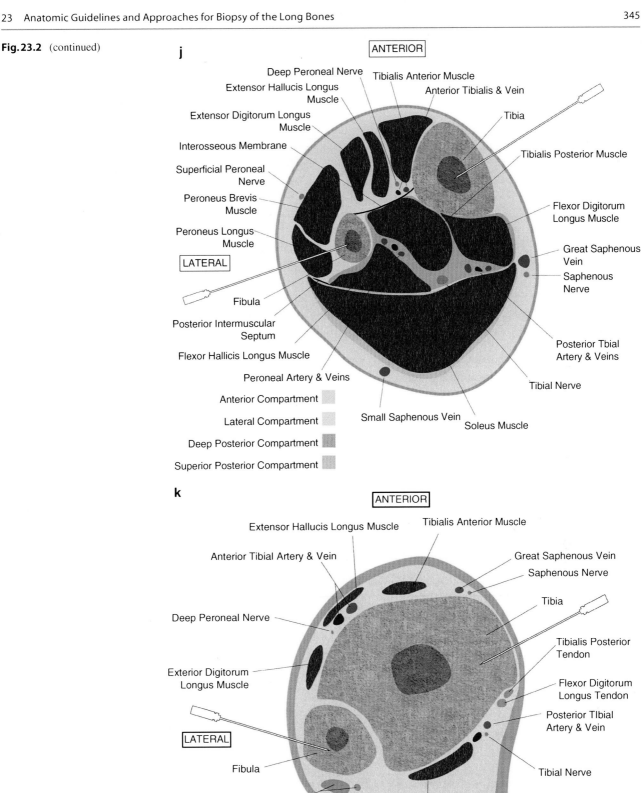

j

ANTERIOR

Deep Peroneal Nerve
Extensor Hallucis Longus Muscle
Extensor Digitorum Longus Muscle
Interosseous Membrane
Superficial Peroneal Nerve
Peroneus Brevis Muscle
Peroneus Longus Muscle
LATERAL
Fibula
Posterior Intermuscular Septum
Flexor Hallicis Longus Muscle
Peroneal Artery & Veins

Tibialis Anterior Muscle
Anterior Tibialis & Vein
Tibia
Tibialis Posterior Muscle
Flexor Digitorum Longus Muscle
Great Saphenous Vein
Saphenous Nerve
Posterior Tbial Artery & Veins
Tibial Nerve
Small Saphenous Vein
Soleus Muscle

Anterior Compartment
Lateral Compartment
Deep Posterior Compartment
Superior Posterior Compartment

k

ANTERIOR

Extensor Hallucis Longus Muscle
Anterior Tibial Artery & Vein
Deep Peroneal Nerve
Exterior Digitorum Longus Muscle
LATERAL
Fibula
Peroneus Longus & Brevis Tendons
Sural Nerve
Small Saphenous Vein

Tibialis Anterior Muscle
Great Saphenous Vein
Saphenous Nerve
Tibia
Tibialis Posterior Tendon
Flexor Digitorum Longus Tendon
Posterior TIbial Artery & Vein
Tibial Nerve
Flexor Hallucis Longus Muscle
Achilles Tendon

(i.e., the biceps femoris, semitendinosus, and semimembranosus), popliteal artery, and sciatic nerve. The femoral artery and vein enter the thigh medially, are contained within the femoral sheath, and are considered extracompartmental, as they are located between the anterior and medial compartments. Distal to the adductor canal, the superficial femoral artery becomes the popliteal artery, which is located in the posterior thigh. A portion of the gluteus maximus resides in the posterior proximal thigh but is not technically within the posterior compartment. The medial compartment contains the gracilis and the adductor muscles. The sciatic nerve is located in the posterior thigh, between the adductor magnus and gluteus maximus in the upper thigh and between the adductor magnus and the biceps femoris in the lower thigh. The fascia lata forms the superficial boundary of all three compartments. The medial and lateral intermuscular septa, which attach to the femur, separate the anterior compartment from the medial and posterior compartments. A thin fascial plane separates the medial and posterior compartments.

The leg has four compartments: anterior, deep posterior, superficial posterior, and lateral [7, 8, 11]. The anterior compartment contains the extensor muscles (i.e., the tibialis anterior, extensor digitorum longus, and extensor hallucis longus), the deep peroneal nerve, and the anterior tibial artery and vein. The deep posterior compartment contains the tibialis posterior, popliteus, flexor digitorum longus, and flexor hallucis longus muscles; the peroneal artery and vein in the lateral part of the compartment; and the posterior tibial artery and vein and the tibial nerve in the medial part of the compartment. The superficial posterior compartment contains the soleus, gastrocnemius, and plantaris muscles and the sural nerve. The lateral compartment contains the peroneus longus and peroneus brevis muscles and the common peroneal nerve, which becomes the superficial peroneal nerve after giving off the deep peroneal nerve. All four compartments are encased superficially by the deep crural fascia. The anterior, posterior, and transverse intermuscular septa and the interosseous membrane form the borders between the various compartments.

Biopsy Approach

The main considerations in planning the biopsy needle path are positioning the tract along the intended surgical incision site and avoiding disease-free compartments, structures that are needed for maintaining function or for reconstructive surgery, and major neurovascular structures. Some general guidelines should be followed [1, 6–8, 12, 13]. For example, the shortest distance possible from the skin surface to the tumor should be selected. It is important to discuss the anticipated needle path with the surgeon who will be performing the definitive surgery.

The key point to consider when selecting a biopsy path is the risk of tumor seeding along the needle tract, specifically when primary musculoskeletal sarcoma is suspected [1, 5, 6]. For this reason, the biopsy tract is resected en bloc during definitive surgery [1, 5, 6]. The needle path must be close to the intended surgical incision site so that the needle path will be amenable to resection during definitive surgery.

Uninvolved compartments should not be traversed by the needle biopsy tract, because potentially consequent tumor seeding to disease-free compartments has significant operative and postoperative implications [14–17]. Mankin and colleagues reviewed 597 percutaneous image-guided biopsies and open biopsies of primary musculoskeletal sarcomas and found that suboptimally planned biopsies resulted in the need for more complex surgical resection or additional chemoradiotherapy in 19 % of patients [16]. Roughly 5–8 % of patients underwent amputation because of improper biopsy planning [16].

The purpose of limb-sparing surgery is total tumor excision with the removal of the least amount of tissue possible to maintain optimal postoperative limb function. Reconstructive surgery is a viable adjunct as needed. Muscles required for optimal postoperative function or reconstruction should not be in the planned biopsy needle path. For example, the rectus femoris should be avoided to preserve the function of knee extensors. The sartorius, gastrocnemius, and gluteus muscles are commonly used for reconstructive flaps and should therefore be avoided if possible. However, transgression of uninvolved structures may not always be avoidable. In these situations, the needle should pass through a small peripheral portion of the muscle.

All attempts should be made to visualize and avoid the crucial neurovascular structures during percutaneous biopsy. Direct needle injury to the nerves or vessels can potentially lead to neural deficits or significant bleeding. More importantly, needle-tract tumor seeding along the neurovascular planes can preclude limb-salvage surgical options, necessitate more extensive surgery, or potentially render the patient inoperable.

Upper Extremity Biopsy Approach

Arm

Approaches to biopsy of the arm vary according to tumor location. When the tumor is in the proximal humerus, the arm is best positioned in external rotation [12]. The needle path should be lateral to the cephalic vein, which should be avoided. The biceps long head tendon, radial nerve, and axillary neurovascular bundle should also be avoided [7–9, 12]. Biopsy of a tumor near the level of the humeral neck should be performed with the tract traversing the anterior third of the deltoid muscle (Fig. 23.1a). The axillary nerve innervation of the deltoid muscle is posterior to anterior. If the posterior aspect of the deltoid is transversed, surgical resection must include this portion of the muscle, resulting in the denervation of the remaining anterior muscle tissue and unnecessarily low postoperative function [7–9, 12]. Similarly, a biopsy tract that transverses the deltopectoral groove is not preferred, as it may contaminate the neurovascular bundle and may preclude the use of the pectoral muscle for reconstruction.

For biopsy of a tumor at the mid-humerus level, the arm may be positioned in internal rotation. The needle path should be posterior to the cephalic vein and biceps (Fig. 23.1b), and the cephalic vein, radial nerve, and radial collateral artery should be avoided [7–9, 12]. At the distal humeral level, the optimal needle path is anterolateral through the brachialis muscle or directly into the medial or lateral epicondyle (Fig. 23.1c, d). The radial nerve and recurrent radial artery should be avoided.

Forearm

When targeting a mass in the proximal radius, specifically the radial head and neck, a direct posterolateral tract should be planned (Fig. 23.1). The radius should be approached from its lateral aspect, whereas a posteromedial or medial trajectory is appropriate for ulnar lesions (Fig. 23.1). The superficial radial nerve, radial artery, and median nerve should be avoided [7–9, 12]. A mass in the olecranon of the ulna should be directly approached posteriorly.

Lower Extremity Biopsy Approach

Pelvis

In general, a mass in the pelvis is intracompartmental if it is confined to an individual muscle or bone. Hence, if feasible, the biopsy needle should not traverse through muscles or bones not involved by the tumor.

Thigh

The femoral head and neck should be accessed laterally, with the needle angled superiorly and medially through the femoral neck (Fig. 23.2a). The femoral neurovascular bundle and the greater trochanteric bursa should be avoided [7, 8, 11, 12]. The femoral shaft should be approached posterolaterally through a small portion of the vastus lateralis muscle, with the patient in the prone or prone-oblique position (Fig. 23.2). The quadriceps tendon should be avoided, along with the sciatic nerve and deep femoral artery. A lateral approach is generally preferred for biopsy of a lesion in the distal femur, with the needle traversing through the vastus lateralis muscle immediately anterior to the lateral intermuscular septum (Fig. 23.2). If a medial approach is needed secondary to the eccentricity of the bone mass or if the lesion is a soft-tissue mass located in the medial compartment, a posteromedial needle trajectory via the vastus medialis should be chosen.

Care should be taken to avoid the superficial femoral artery and nerve, quadriceps tendon, knee joint space, and medial and lateral superior genicular arteries [7, 8, 11, 12].

Leg

The tibia is subcutaneous anteromedially, and biopsy via this trajectory is preferred, as it avoids contamination of the muscular compartments (Fig. 23.2). The tibial tubercle and the peroneus brevis and peroneus longus tendons should not be traversed. The anterior and posterior tibial and peroneal neurovascular bundles should also be avoided [7, 8, 11, 12]. A proximal or distal fibular mass can be approached directly because of the subcutaneous location of the bone. The fibular shaft can be accessed via a lateral approach, immediately anterior or posterior to the posterior intermuscular septum (Fig. 23.2).

Summary

Knowledge of the extremity compartmental anatomy, fascial boundaries, and associated neurovascular elements is critical for interventional radiologists who perform musculoskeletal biopsies. In general, prior to performing the biopsy, the radiologist should confer with the orthopedic surgeon who will perform definitive surgical resection. The surgeon can notify the interventional radiologist of the intended operative path and potential mode of reconstructive surgery, thereby allowing for the selection of a safe needle path.

References

1. Bickels J, Jelinek JS, Shmookler BM, Neff RS, Malawer MM. Biopsy of musculoskeletal tumors. Current concepts. Clin Orthop Relat Res. 1999;368:212–19.
2. Jelinek JS, Murphey MD, Welker JA, et al. Diagnosis of primary bone tumors with image-guided percutaneous biopsy: experience with 110 tumors. Radiology. 2002;223:731–7.
3. Roberts CC, Liu PT, Wenger DE. Musculoskeletal tumor imaging, biopsy, and therapies: self-assessment module. AJR Am J Roentgenol. 2009;193(6 Suppl):S74–8.
4. Yao L, Nelson SD, Seeger LL, Eckardt JJ, Eilber FR. Primary musculoskeletal neoplasms: effectiveness of core-needle biopsy. Radiology. 1999;212:682–6.
5. Davies NM, Livesley PJ, Cannon SR. Recurrence of an osteosarcoma in a needle biopsy track. J Bone Joint Surg Br. 1993;75:977–8.
6. DiCaprio MR, Friedlaender GE. Malignant bone tumors: limb sparing versus amputation. J Am Acad Orthop Surg. 2003;11:25–37.
7. Anderson MW, Temple HT, Dussault RG, Kaplan PA. Compartmental anatomy: relevance to staging and biopsy of musculoskeletal tumors. AJR Am J Roentgenol. 1999;173:1663–71.
8. Bancroft LW, Peterson JJ, Kransdorf MJ, Berquist TH, O'Connor MI. Compartmental anatomy relevant to biopsy planning. Semin Musculoskelet Radiol. 2007;11:16–27.
9. Toomayan GA, Robertson F, Major NM, Brigman BE. Upper extremity compartmental anatomy: clinical relevance to radiologists. Skeletal Radiol. 2006;35:195–201.

10. Boles CA, Kannam S, Cardwell AB. The forearm: anatomy of muscle compartments and nerves. AJR Am J Roentgenol. 2000;174: 151–9.

11. Toomayan GA, Robertson F, Major NM. Lower extremity compartmental anatomy: clinical relevance to radiologists. Skeletal Radiol. 2005;34:307–13.

12. Liu PT, Valadez SD, Chivers FS, Roberts CC, Beauchamp CP. Anatomically based guidelines for core needle biopsy of bone tumors: implications for limb-sparing surgery. Radiographics. 2007;27:189–205; discussion 6.

13. Welker JA, Henshaw RM, Jelinek J, Shmookler BM, Malawer MM. The percutaneous needle biopsy is safe and recommended in the diagnosis of musculoskeletal masses. Cancer. 2000;89:2677–86.

14. Mankin HJ, Lange TA, Spanier SS. The hazards of biopsy in patients with malignant primary bone and soft-tissue tumors. J Bone Joint Surg Am. 1982;64:1121–7.

15. Mankin HJ, Lange TA, Spanier SS. THE CLASSIC: The hazards of biopsy in patients with malignant primary bone and soft-tissue tumors. The Journal of Bone and Joint Surgery, 1982;64:1121–1127. Clin Orthop Relat Res. 2006;450:4–10.

16. Mankin HJ, Mankin CJ, Simon MA. The hazards of the biopsy, revisited. Members of the Musculoskeletal Tumor Society. J Bone Joint Surg Am. 1996;78:656–63.

17. Picci P, Sangiorgi L, Bahamonde L, et al. Risk factors for local recurrences after limb-salvage surgery for high-grade osteosarcoma of the extremities. Ann Oncol. 1997;8:899–903.

Musculoskeletal Biopsies: Extremities

24

David R. Marker and John A. Carrino

Background

The use of percutaneous musculoskeletal needle biopsy (PNB) was reported in the literature as early as 1930 [1]. The initial procedures utilized a stereotactic approach. Through subsequent decades, innovations in imaging technology have resulted in more accurate and effective percutaneous approaches, and musculoskeletal biopsies are now often performed with imaging assistance. Besides enhanced imaging technology, there have been improvements in needle design, histopathologic diagnostic tools, understanding of appropriate indications, and interventional techniques. These advancements have resulted in a large increase in the use of percutaneous biopsies. It was reported that over a recent 7- to 8-year period, the numbers of percutaneous muscle and bone biopsies performed by radiologists increased by 71 % (2,788–4,761) and 60 % (9,259–14,830), respectively [2]. Similarly, reported surgeon utilization of needle biopsy has been estimated to have increased from approximately 10 % in the early 1980s to 40 % in 1999 [3]. Although these increases are substantial, these numbers still suggest underutilization, which is likely associated with the continued perception that needle biopsy does not provide adequate tissue sampling for some pathologic conditions that have traditionally been difficult to diagnose.

The primary role of tissue sampling via musculoskeletal biopsy is to provide histologic analysis for distinguishing among infectious, neoplastic, and tumor-like musculoskeletal lesions (Fig. 24.1). In addition to distinguishing benign from malignant, the biopsy must provide adequate tissue to determine the histologic grade of the lesion. Historically, open surgical biopsy was the accepted standard for this purpose because of its ability to readily obtain sufficient samples representative of the musculoskeletal lesion. However, there are a number of drawbacks or contraindications to this approach. Open surgical biopsy has been reported to be associated with complications in as many as 16 % of cases [4], most often the surgical risks of hemorrhage, infection, and physical and mental discomfort to the patient. Furthermore, surgical biopsy is contraindicated if there is danger of local or general dissemination of the disease or if disruption of tissue may prevent subsequent surgical intervention. Percutaneous image-guided biopsy has emerged as a minimally invasive alternative that is more cost effective [5, 6] and reduces or eliminates many of these drawbacks and risks of open surgical biopsy [3, 7, 8]. For example, needle biopsy has been associated with an approximately twofold decrease in the number of cases for which the initial, preferred treatment had to be abandoned because of the consequences of the biopsy (21 % for open versus 9 % for needle biopsy) [4].

A practical approach to PNB of the musculoskeletal system is to differentiate between biopsy of the appendicular skeleton and biopsy of the axial skeleton. Important differences in anatomy between the two lead to distinct complications and recommendations for imaging and interventional techniques. By virtue of anatomic location, PNB of the appendicular skeleton does not have the inherent risk of damage to vital organs that can occur in procedures for the axial skeleton. For example, complications such as pneumothorax or more serious iatrogenic pathologies such as nerve root injury are specific to the axial skeleton [9]. This chapter focuses on percutaneous image-guided biopsy of the appendicular skeleton, providing an in-depth

D.R. Marker, MD
The Russell H. Morgan Department of Radiology
and Radiological Science,
The Johns Hopkins Hospital, Baltimore, MD, USA
e-mail: markerdr@gmail.com

J.A. Carrino, MD, MPH (✉)
Radiology and Orthopaedic Surgery,
Musculoskeletal Radiology,
The Russell H. Morgan Department of
Radiology and Radiological Science,
The Johns Hopkins University,
Baltimore, MD, USA
e-mail: jcarrin2@jhmi.edu

K. Ahrar, S. Gupta (eds.), *Percutaneous Image-Guided Biopsy*,
DOI 10.1007/978-1-4614-8217-8_24, © Springer Science+Business Media New York 2014

assessment of the interventional techniques and tools that are utilized for lesions of the extremities. The chapter also discusses recommended practice pearls for avoiding the potential pitfalls and complications that can occur in percutaneous image-guided biopsy of lesions of the appendicular skeleton.

Indications and Patient Selection

The first step for ensuring an accurate and clinically useful PNB of the appendicular skeleton is to utilize appropriate indications and patient selection criteria. The decision whether to perform a biopsy should be made by the interventionalist together with the surgeon who will be treating the patient.

Indications for Appendicular Musculoskeletal Biopsy

1. Evaluation of a solitary bone or soft-tissue lesion with nonspecific imaging findings in order to establish its benign or malignant nature.
2. Confirm imaging and staging for cases of suspected metastasis.
3. Confirm diagnosis of suspected infection and identify the organism.
4. Re-biopsy for initially negative or inconclusive findings.
5. Re-biopsy for evaluation of suspected residual/recurrent disease.
6. Determine the nature and extent of systemic diseases.

The question in the case of a suspected primary neoplasm of the appendicular skeleton is whether the musculoskeletal

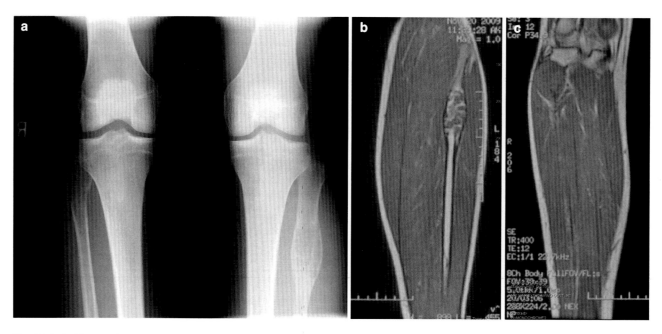

Fig. 24.1 A 23-year-old man presented with a 6-month history of increasing discomfort in his right proximal lateral calf. The patient brought outside images of both fibulas on plain film as well as an MRI scan of each side. Plain radiograph (**a**) showed a lesion of the left fibula with thin internal septations and without evidence of periosteal reaction or cortical break. An expansile destructive lesion was noted within the right fibular head, featuring thinning of the cortex and minimal periosteal reaction. Neoplasm was suspected and MRI was recommended. Sagittal MRI (**b**) demonstrated an expansile lesion within the proximal left fibular diaphysis. There was no evidence of bone marrow edema in the surrounding bone and no evidence of periosteal reaction. On the postcontrast images, there appeared to be central enhancement of this lesion. Coronal MRI (**c**) showed an expansile lesion in the head and proximal metaphysis of the right fibula. A soft-tissue component has extended into the proximal medullary canal. There was edema within the fascial planes surrounding the mass and within the extensor digitorum longus, fibularis longus, and lateral soleus muscles. The periphery of this lesion showed irregular enhancement. The tibial artery and vein ran along the medial border of the lesion and the fat plane was

effaced, but there was no encasement of the artery or vein. The common peroneal nerve was obscured, but the lesion followed the expected course of the nerve. Axial CT image (**d**) showed an expansile lytic lesion of the proximal left fibular shaft with mild internal bony septation. A Bonopty access cannula (outer diameter 2.1 mm) was advanced into this lesion. Appropriate positioning within the targeted lesion was ensured by intermittent CT fluoroscopic observation. A total of four passes were made using 22-gauge needles for fine-needle aspiration. A Bonopty core biopsy device (inner diameter 1.3 mm) also was used for sampling. Two marrow aspirates were also collected. There was no evidence of malignancy on cytopathologic examination. Axial CT image of the right leg (**e**) showed a heterogeneous expansile lesion replacing the right fibular head with areas of cortical disruption. Using intermittent CT fluoroscopic observation to ensure appropriate needle positioning within this lesion, a total of four passes were made using 25-gauge needles for fine-needle aspiration. An additional nine passes were made with a 16-gauge Monopty core biopsy device. The cytopathologic findings were interpreted as a giant cell tumor with aneurysmal bone cyst features

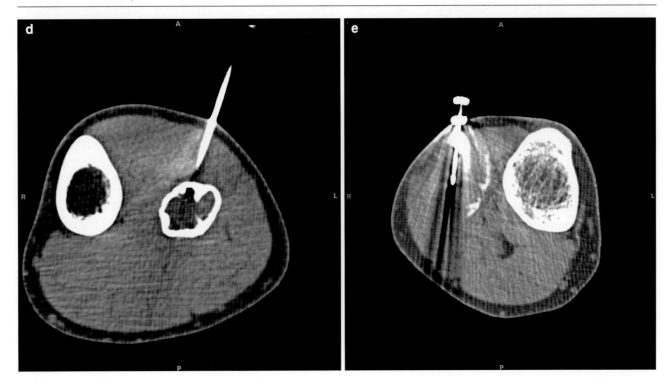

Fig. 24.1 (continued)

lesion is benign or malignant. Previously, there was debate concerning the utility of PNB for primary musculoskeletal neoplasms such as bone sarcomas. However, because of its low complication rates and improvements in its diagnostic accuracy, PNB is now recommended generally for most lytic and blastic lesions in the appendicular skeleton [10]. Some cases of primary lesions still require special considerations, however, including (1) cartilaginous lesions, (2) liposarcomas, and (3) pathologic fractures. For some cartilaginous lesions, differentiation between benign and malignant may be difficult. Cases have been reported in which a chondrosarcoma was erroneously diagnosed as an enchondroma, possibly because of difficulty obtaining adequate tissue from noncalcified areas, which are more representative of the malignancy than calcified areas [11]. If the initial histopathologic analysis of the PNB is read as an enchondroma, the patient should be monitored to confirm this diagnosis. Conversely, some benign lesions such as synovial chondromatosis or chondromyxoid fibromas may show cytologic atypia leading to a misdiagnosis of chondrosarcoma. Ultimately, differentiating benign cartilage lesions from malignant tumors requires evaluation of clinical presentation, imaging, and histopathologic interpretation as well as assessment of changes in the lesion over time [12].

Other lesions that may be difficult to diagnose are soft-tissue tumors that are highly heterogenous [13, 14]. For example, PNB is not recommended for differentiating low-grade liposarcomas from lipomas [15]. Another special

circumstance for biopsy is a pathologic fracture. In some of these cases, imaging may be inconclusive as to whether there is an underlying lesion that led to the fracture. If a malignancy cannot be ruled out on the basis of imaging alone, PNB is recommended.

Percutaneous needle biopsy is utilized to confirm that a suspected metastatic lesion is a metastasis rather than a new primary tumor and to confirm staging of the disease. Biopsy confirmation is especially important when there is uncertainty about diagnosis, as in cases where the lesion appears atypical for the type or stage of the primary tumor or if the lesion is suggestive of metastatic disease but there is no known primary tumor. For cases with no known primary lesion, a number of common sites of neoplastic origin should be considered, such as the lungs, prostate, breasts, kidneys, and thyroid. Successful biopsy of metastatic disease should be considered the final step in staging prior to the referring physician discussing appropriate management options with the patient. Because the biopsy induces subsequent real and artificial radiologic changes that may inhibit future imaging interpretation, the biopsy should be conducted only after completion of imaging studies for staging the disease by assessing any local and/or metastatic spread.

Percutaneous needle biopsy is also utilized in patients who have suspected infection. These patients typically have an initial assessment and laboratory values that are highly suggestive of infection, and the referring physician requests a biopsy to identify the organism and subsequently the appropriate treatment protocol. Suspicion of septic arthritis, either pyogenic or granulomatous, is an important indication for PNB. For patients who have suspected osteomyelitis, the bone biopsy specimens should undergo both microbiologic and histologic evaluation [16]. Percutaneous biopsy may also be requested to distinguish between infection and possible malignant disease.

The case of a negative result or an indeterminate tumor diagnosis presents a difficult decision. As previously noted, some of these may be "negative" in the sense that the lesion is identified as benign rather than the suspected malignant disease. Re-biopsy is typically not recommended unless there is change in the lesion to suggest malignancy. Initially inconclusive cases also are considered for re-biopsy. For example, a cystic or necrotic lesion such as a telangiectatic osteosarcoma may yield only fibrin, blood, or serous fluid that does not allow differentiation from a simple cyst, and re-biopsy is required if there is sufficient clinical suspicion or aggressive imaging appearance. Other reports of normal, inconclusive, or nonspecific biopsies may arise from poor technique, missed lesions, inappropriate handling of specimens, or sampling nonrepresentative portions of the lesion. Either open biopsy or repeat percutaneous biopsy can be utilized for these difficult cases.

Another situation that may warrant re-biopsy is when patients present with a lesion in the appendicular skeleton after they have already undergone therapy with curettage, resection, chemotherapy, and/or radiotherapy. Patients may present with a lesion at the primary site of treatment that is suggestive of local recurrence or a lesion at a new site (often several years later) that is suggestive of metastatic disease. The cases that are suggestive of metastatic disease are especially important for diagnostic biopsy to determine whether the patient has recurrence of primary disease or a new neoplasm that has not yet been identified.

The final reason for biopsy is to determine the nature and extent of systemic diseases. For example, the treatment for connective tissue diseases may be customized on the basis of the findings on biopsy of the synovial membrane [17, 18]. While synovial samples can be obtained via open or arthroscopic surgery, PNB is advantageous because it allows removal of specimens from several regions of the joint with minimal trauma. These biopsies are not always definitive, but rather contribute to the diagnosis when combined with several other criteria.

Contraindications

Although there are a number of relative contraindications for PNB of the appendicular skeleton, the only absolute contraindication is for lesions that can be diagnosed accurately on the basis of clinical and imaging studies alone. The presence of a bone or soft-tissue lesion does not necessarily merit a biopsy, and in cases in which the medical history, physical examination, laboratory results, and appropriate imaging studies allow accurate diagnosis of a musculoskeletal lesion, confirmatory biopsy should not be performed. For example, benign lesions such as intraosseous ganglia, subchondral sclerosis and cystic changes associated with advanced osteoarthritis, and enchondroma bone islands may appear as suspect lucent or sclerotic foci in patients with a known malignancy, but they can be differentiated by utilizing imaging findings and reviewing previous studies. Apophyseal avulsions in young patients are also sometimes mistaken as a malignancy. However, location of the lesion and clinical history are key differentiating points for these cases.

Relative Contraindications for Appendicular Musculoskeletal Biopsy

1. Bleeding diathesis (severe coagulopathy or thrombocytopenia)
2. Lack of safe biopsy tract.
3. Compromised cardiopulmonary function or hemodynamic instability
4. Uncooperative patient or inability to be positioned for the procedure
5. Inadequate institutional infrastructure for the procedure

A simple medical history is typically sufficient to assess for coagulopathy in patients prior to biopsy of an extremity because there is a relatively low risk for vascular complications. For patients with a medical history suggestive of or a known existing bleeding diathesis, laboratory measurements of the patient's prothrombin time, activated partial thromboplastin time, and international normalized ratio are recommended, and abnormalities should be corrected before the biopsy. For patients who require urgent biopsy, fresh frozen plasma can be administered shortly before the procedure to temporarily correct values. When the biopsy site is in close proximity to large vessels, the potential increased risk for bleeding may suggest consideration of alternative approaches. A hematology consultation may be required to deal with coagulopathies that the radiologist does not have experience in correcting. Special attention should be given to patients with a coagulopathy who are taking nonsteroidal anti-inflammatory drugs that can prolong the bleeding time [19]. There have been reports of significant bleeding weeks after discontinuing aspirin, despite normal platelet counts [20].

When determining the planned biopsy tract, the presence of infected soft tissue must be addressed. If the infection is along the planned tract and the target lesion is not considered likely to be infection on the basis of initial clinical and radiographic assessments, another tract should be selected or the patient should be treated for the infection before proceeding with the biopsy. Although there are no sites in the appendicular skeleton that are contraindicated solely because of inaccessible anatomic location, extensive soft-tissue infection may in effect make the targeted biopsy site inaccessible. In contrast, there are sites in the axial skeleton, such as the odontoid process and anterior arch of the first cervical vertebra, that are considered contraindications for PNB because of anatomic features that make the sites inaccessible [21].

Caution should be used in patients who have compromised cardiopulmonary function or hemodynamic instability. Patients who have a history of myocardial infarction, chronic heart failure, or other high-risk chronic medical condition should have a thorough pre-biopsy medical evaluation and clearance by their primary care physician. Because of the low risk for complications of appendicular biopsies, these patients should be considered appropriate candidates for biopsy once their medical condition is optimized.

Uncooperative patients, especially children, may require general anesthesia. As with any surgical case requiring general anesthesia, the risks and benefits of the procedure must be assessed. Patients who are overly concerned about the procedure but are considered high risk for general anesthesia may tolerate a benzodiazepine or other sedating medication that will allow them to undergo the procedure with only local anesthesia.

The last relative contraindication is a function of the treatment center rather than the patient. If the institution is not equipped to perform PNB on a regular basis, the accuracy of the diagnostic studies may be questionable. Definitive diagnosis with appropriate treatment is best performed at an institution that has a team consisting of an orthopedic surgeon, radiologist, and pathologist who coordinate their efforts in selecting appropriate patients, performing the biopsy, providing histopathologic analysis, and subsequently managing the continued care of the patient [4, 22, 23].

Rates of treatment complications have been reported to be two to ten times greater when the biopsy is performed at a center other than where the patient will ultimately receive definitive treatment [24–26].

Technique

The importance of technique in performing a biopsy has been magnified by the change in treatment options. Historically, most malignant tumors of the extremities were treated with amputation. The biopsies that were conducted prior to the amputation were generally performed by an open surgical approach where contamination of the surrounding tissue was inconsequential. However, there has been a significant shift over the last several decades away from amputation and toward limb-sparing surgery. Today, as many as 95 % of patients are able to undergo limb-sparing procedures

without compromising the oncologic outcome [27–29]. Therefore, biopsy must be preceded by careful clinical evaluation and analysis of the imaging studies. The diagnostic accuracy may be greatly influenced by the biopsy method and equipment utilized as well as the location of sampling. Furthermore, a poorly planned or performed biopsy may result in the patient requiring a more radical dissection or amputation with a significant negative impact on long-term survival [4, 30, 31]. The three most critical factors that need be considered for an optimal outcome are (1) preprocedure and intraprocedure imaging, (2) the interventional devices utilized, and (3) the approach and relevant anatomy.

Imaging

Imaging plays an important role in pre-biopsy planning as well as in facilitating localization of the lesion at the time of biopsy. Prior to biopsy, radiographs in two projections as well as CT or MRI scan of the lesion should be obtained for all patients. If more than one site of metastasis is suspected on the basis of initial imaging studies, the most accessible site that will provide adequate tissue should be selected for biopsy. Bone scintigraphy may be useful in patients with metastatic disease to identify additional lesions that are more accessible than initially detected disease sites [32]. In cases where there are multiple lesions with different imaging characteristics, more than one biopsy is needed [33].

The biopsy can be guided by fluoroscopy [10, 11, 34], ultrasound [23, 35], CT [14, 31, 36, 37], or MRI [38, 39]. Each of these imaging modalities has pros and cons in terms of costs, radiation exposure, time required to complete the biopsy, and efficacy in locating the lesion and determining its relevant characteristics. In rare cases, imaging choice is dependent on available imaging modalities and patient positioning.

Fluoroscopy is recommended for lesions of the extremity that do not require careful negotiation of neurovascular structures. Low soft-tissue contrast makes fluoroscopy less ideal for lesions with large cystic or necrotic areas. Biplane fluoroscopy is recommended over conventional fluoroscopy for deeper lesions because of its ability to accurately determine the needle depth. The advantages of fluoroscopy compared to CT and MRI are that it is easy to use; allows fast, multidirectional, near real-time visualization; and costs substantially less.

Ultrasound can be utilized for biopsy of superficial soft-tissue lesions, lesions that have some degree of subperiosteal or extraosseous extension, or bone lesions that demonstrate cortical disruption with an adequate acoustic window for passage of the biopsy needle [40–42]. Lesions that were traditionally targeted with palpation alone are now often visualized with ultrasound to avoid complications such as

Fig. 24.2 An 83-year-old woman was referred for evaluation of a right anterior thigh mass. The patient described a 6-week history of right anterior thigh fullness near the knee. Ultrasound evaluation of the right anterior distal thigh showed a heterogeneously echogenic solid mass (**a**). With ultrasound guidance (**b**), 22-gauge needles were advanced into the mass at four different sites, and eight samples were obtained by the capillary technique. Three core biopsy samples of the lesion were obtained with an 18-gauge Monopty biopsy device. The biopsy revealed a pleomorphic high-grade sarcoma of the right thigh

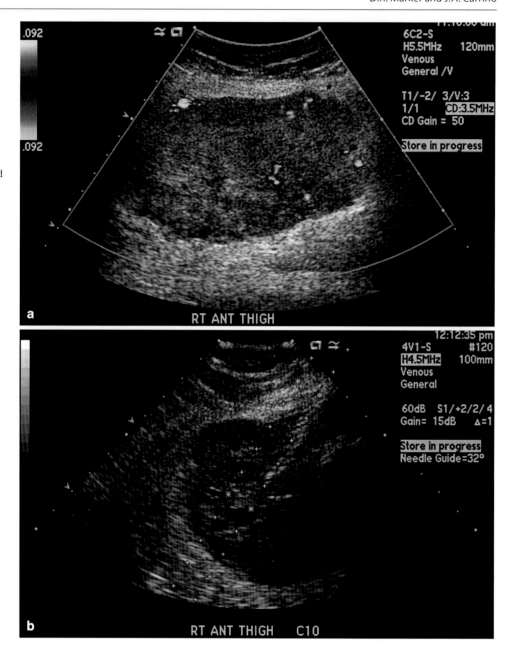

disruption of vascular structures and to ensure intralesional sampling (Fig. 24.2). Ultrasound is inadequate for visualizing deep medullary bone lesions and deep soft-tissue lesions because of poor sound penetration. The advantages of ultrasound are that it provides real-time visualization, color Doppler imaging for regions of variable tissue and adjacent vascular structures, and no radiation to the patient or the interventionalist. Ultrasound is also relatively inexpensive and requires minimal patient and preprocedure preparation, and the procedure can be performed more quickly than a CT-guided biopsy [23].

While CT is frequently required for lesions of the upper thoracic and cervical spine, skull base, and facial bones [21], there are fewer concrete indications for the use of CT in the appendicular skeleton, and some cases are based on operator preference. Deep lesions or lesions adjacent to neurovascular bundles may require a high-resolution "road map" of the compartmental anatomy that is best provided by CT. In comparison to fluoroscopy, CT has an additional element of safety because it can provide better soft-tissue visualization, which allows more precise needle placement within three dimensions [20, 43, 44]. One of the arguments against the use of conventional CT is that it can be time consuming during positioning. However, CT fluoroscopy can address this limitation by providing real-time visualization that allows instantaneous cross-sectional anatomic imaging.

Magnetic resonance imaging is often used for lesions that are not identified on other imaging modalities (Fig. 24.3) and for targeting a focal marrow abnormality or specific portion of a heterogenous lesion that is targeted for biopsy.

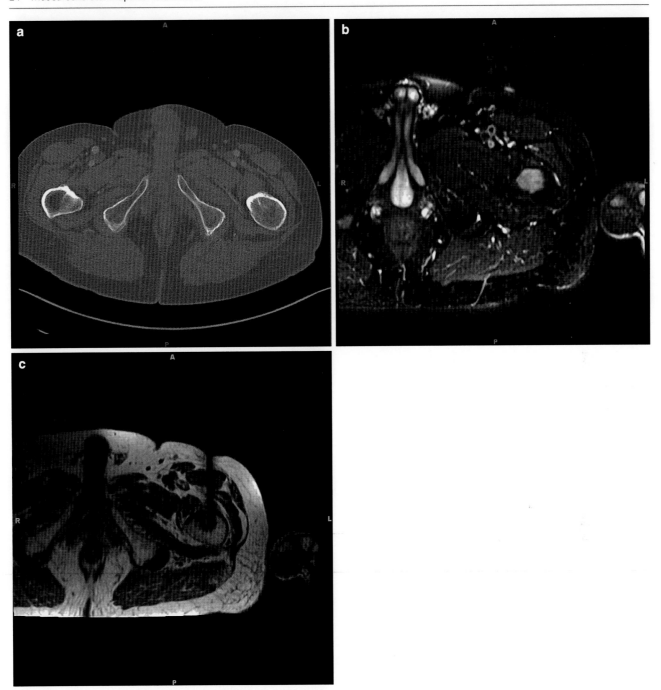

Fig. 24.3 A 78-year-old man with 3 to 4 months of left hip and thigh pain had an MRI at an outside institution which reported a suspicious lesion in the left proximal thigh. With a broad differential inlcuding metastasis of an unknown primary, lyphoma, and myeloma, the patient underwent a screening chest and abdomen CT and presented to our institution for possible biopsy of the lesion. The CT (**a**) showed diffusely osteopenic bones but no definite evidence of discrete lesion that could be target for biopsy. The patient subsequently agreed to undergo MRI-guided biopsy. Pre-biopsy T2, turbo spin echo, fat saturated imaging (**b**) redemonstrated the T2-hyperintense lesion in the proximal femur which was noted on the prior outside MRI study. Under real-time MRI guidance (**c**), a 4 mm MRI compatible coaxial bone biopsy needle system was utilized. A total of 3 core needle biopsies were obtained from the lateral, central and medial portions of the lesion. Pathology reported findings consistent with diffuse large B-cell lymphoma which included bone and marrow space diffusely and extensively involved by an atypical lymphocytic infiltrate composed of large cells that were CD20, CD10, and Bcl-6 positive and had abundant cytoplasm, vesicular chromatin, and conspicuous nucleoli

Intra-articular locations represent a unique group for which lesion conspicuity and real-time guidance are both important issues that are best addressed by MRI. Like CT, MRI is ideal for creating high-resolution reconstructions of the associated compartmental anatomy for deep lesions. Finally, there are some indications for MRI that are more case specific. For example, if a patient has orthopedic hardware near a lesion, use of CT may be limited by streak artifacts.

The advantages of MRI are that there is no radiation, it is a cross-sectional technique with an easily adjustable imaging plane, and it provides superior tissue contrast. Some of the disadvantages are the cost of deploying and maintaining a specialized magnet or modifying an existing magnet and suite for interventional use and the currently higher cost of MR-compatible biopsy equipment. There are also specific contraindications to the use of MR, such as the presence of a pacemaker, certain cerebral aneurysm clips, cochlear implants, or other strongly ferromagnetic material near critical locations.

Devices

Proper needle selection is equally as important as appropriate imaging modality in providing accurate biopsy diagnosis. Core-needle biopsy (CNB) is generally considered more accurate than fine-needle aspiration (FNA) because of the larger yield of specimen available for diagnosis [10, 33]. However, FNA can provide rapid, onsite cytopathologic assessment of the adequacy and character of the tissue specimens to guide additional sampling, whereas CNB results are usually not available for several days. These advantages and disadvantages of CNB and FNA are largely complementary, and multiple studies have reported that CNB and FNA have greater clinical utility when used together than when used alone [45–47].

The choice of needle for CNB depends on the nature, location, and sometimes size of the lesion. Soft-tissue masses, osteolytic lesions that have penetrated the cortex, or medullary lesions (after cortical penetration by drill or bone-cutting needle) can be biopsied with soft-tissue cutting needles or devices such as automated core biopsy guns and vacuum-assisted needles [48]. An outer introducer sheath is affixed in the lesion to minimize repeated imaging and localization. Typically, 14- to 22-gauge needles are utilized for these types of CNB. When choosing large-gauge needles, the advantage of obtaining more tissue sample than smaller gauge needles must be balanced with the risks of increasing crush artifact, obscuring of the CT images, and macerating the soft-tissue mass [4, 9].

Core-needle biopsy of bone lesions that have an intact overlying cortex requires a bone-cutting needle. The bone-cutting needles commonly have a trochar for penetration (10–15 gauge) and a trephine for cutting (12–17 gauge). They can be single pass or coaxial. Because obtaining an adequate sample of sclerotic lesions can be difficult, the use of a needle with a larger inner diameter is recommended. The cutting cannulas have relatively large handles to facilitate trephine needle rotation and application of pressure to the needle tip. A mallet may be employed to force the needle through cortical bone. The cylindrical surface of long bones may cause the needle to slide on the bone. The needle should be positioned perpendicular to the bone, and a mallet can facilitate the anchoring of the bevel or tip of the needle in the cortex before turning the needle into the marrow cavity. Care should be exercised because there is a tendency for weaker needles to bend if tapped too strongly against thick cortex.

Fine-needle aspiration is ideal for providing specimens for culture or cytology. Aspiration needles are commonly 18–25 gauge. The number of passes for FNA varies and is often determined by the operator at the time of the biopsy; between two and six samples is typical. FNA of bone, extra-articular soft-tissue, and intra-articular soft-tissue sites is typically accomplished coaxially by means of an introducer. If soft-tissue lesions are superficial and maintaining the introducer position is difficult, the sampling needle can be placed directly.

Magnetic resonance imaging-assisted biopsies require an MR-compatible needle. These are generally composed of high nickel content steel or titanium alloys. The imaging is then conducted with frequency encoding parallel to the needle path to reduce susceptibility artifact. The studies on MRI-assisted biopsy are limited, but the general recommendations for MR needles are similar to those for other PNB protocols. Employing both CNB and FNA together is recommended whenever possible.

Approach and Relevant Anatomy

Planning of the optimal biopsy tract must be preceded by determination of whether the lesion is benign or if there is widespread disease. In the case of benign lesions that can be diagnosed on the basis of imaging alone with a high level of specificity, such as fibrous dysplasia or osteochondroma, biopsy is not required. Conversely, if there is evidence of widespread malignancy in a limb and evidence that salvage is not possible, CNB would be performed, but there would be no restrictions as to the planned biopsy tract. For all other lesions, which are on the spectrum between being clearly benign and being clearly widespread malignancy and the limb not salvageable, the pertinent anatomic structures and the relationship of the biopsy tract to neurovascular structures, tissue planes, and potential future surgery must be thoroughly considered prior to biopsy.

The initial anatomic consideration in biopsy planning is the lesion's compartment of origin and whether the lesion has spread to other compartments. Compartmental anatomy greatly influences needle approach and is critical for preventing unnecessary surgery, loss of limb function, or even otherwise preventable amputation. A lesion is defined as intracompartmental or extracompartmental on the basis of whether it is confined to or traverses natural barriers such as bone, articular cartilage, fibrous septa, and origins and insertions of muscles. If a lesion remains limited to its original compartment, the barriers of this compartment should not be compromised by the biopsy tract if possible. Although recurrence of the tumor along the needle tract for CNB is rare, it has been shown to result in poor outcome [49, 50], and all compartments transversed by the tract must be resected en bloc. While there is evidence that FNA biopsy tracts are not at risk for tumor seeding [13], precautions similar to those for CNB should be taken, especially considering the recommendation that FNA should be performed together with CNB.

The second anatomic consideration for determining an appropriate biopsy tract is the location of neurovascular bundles. For bone tumors, the biopsy tract should mirror the standard surgical approaches for a given anatomic region. A study by Liu et al. comprehensively assessed these approaches and the vital structures that must be considered in each of the anatomic regions of the extremities [51]. For soft-tissue tumors, the shortest path to the most biologically active area is commonly selected. Exceptions to this approach include if the path compromises the previously discussed compartment considerations, if there are intervening structures, or if biopsy along the long axis of the bone would provide a safer and more optimal sampling approach. Similar to bone tumors, the planned biopsy tract should typically reflect the incision plane that the surgeon would use for future resection. Consultation with the surgeon is recommended, especially if the likely surgical approach is not intuitively obvious.

Finally, functional anatomy must be considered. The study by Liu et al. also comprehensively assessed the functions that would be compromised on the basis of the compartments resected [51]. Again, because of the risk of tumor seeding along the biopsy tract, the functional components transversed by the biopsy needle will likely require surgical resection.

If it is determined prior to biopsy that the patient may require subsequent surgical management, the skin and biopsy tract are often marked to aid the surgeon at the time of resection. The biopsy tract can be marked with methylene blue or sterile India ink, and the skin puncture site can be tattooed with India ink [52]. In all cases, the biopsy route is planned in coordination with the surgeon to avoid tumor contamination of uninvolved tissue compartments, especially tissues that are functionally important.

Potential Complications

Percutaneous needle biopsies of the appendicular skeleton have a relatively low risk for complications. To the authors' knowledge, there are no reports of mortality directly linked to percutaneous biopsy of an extremity.

Overall, the incidence of complications following percutaneous biopsies for studies reporting both axial and extremity data has been between 0.2 and 1.1 % [10, 53]. When only biopsies of the extremities are considered, this rate has been reported to be 0 % in some cohorts and is probably less than 0.2 % at institutions that have dedicated teams of radiologists, pathologists, and surgeons [23, 38, 45, 54]. However, centers that do not perform biopsies routinely may have worse outcomes. As many as 5–8 % of patients have been reported to undergo unnecessary amputation, either for recurrence of disease or as a preventive measure following improper biopsy technique [4]. There is also a risk for nonrepresentative tissue or diagnostic error that leads to mismanagement of the case both in terms of inadequate therapy for malignant disease and contraindicated surgery for a benign lesion.

Some of the more benign risks associated with percutaneous biopsy of the appendicular skeleton include the potential for bleeding, vascular or neural compromise, pain, and infection. Hemorrhage may result from vascular injury or biopsy of a vascular lesion. Neurologic damage is rare in the extremity, but can be devastating to the patient's function if it occurs. There are reports of major motor nerves being anesthetized at the time of biopsy, leading to paresis and paralysis. These complications are transient and should not alarm the interventionalist or the patient [20]. The greatest risk for neurologic damage is when the tumor involves the nerve or originates from the nerve itself. For example, neuropathic-type pain may occur during soft-tissue biopsy of peripheral nerve sheath tumors. Regardless of the tumor type, the percutaneous biopsy needle may cause pain at the site of skin insertion. A biopsy requiring needle penetration of the periosteum or medullar cavity may be unusually painful. Needle entrance into the medullar cavity is especially painful in cases of osteomyelitis and when there is associated negative pressure or needle manipulation within the canal.

Management of Complications

Major complications associated with incorrect diagnosis or potentially preventable amputation may require admission to the hospital for therapy, an unplanned increase in the level of care, or prolonged hospitalization. However, most complications following biopsy are minor and require minimal change in management. Most patients tolerate the biopsy procedure well if adequate local anesthesia (typically 0.5–2 % lidocaine) is provided, but occasional cases require general anesthesia. Post-biopsy pain due to neurological injury can be managed conservatively with pain medication and amitriptyline hydrochloride [38]. This pain may persist for weeks before gradually resolving. In the rare cases of bleeding following biopsy of an extremity, hemostasis can typically be achieved by pressure alone. If an infection occurs at the skin insertion site or along the needle tract, standard antibiotic care and infection control is recommended.

Outcomes and Results

The reported accuracy of needle biopsy in the diagnosis of musculoskeletal lesions has been variable, ranging from 23 % to as high as 97 % in various recent cohorts [4, 36, 47, 55, 56]. This variability is a reflection of the studies' differences in patient and lesion types [31], training and structure of the team associated with the care of the patient [12], whether FNA or CNB was utilized [57], and the imaging modality indicated [38]. There are conflicting reports as to whether the accuracy of percutaneous biopsies is a function of the anatomic site. For example, a recent study reported that the accuracies for the appendicular skeleton and spine/sacrum were similar at 92 % and 84 %, respectively [54]. Similarly, a separate study reported that the effective diagnostic utility was not statistically significantly different for appendicular and axial biopsies (36 % for appendicular versus 52 % for axial lesions) [58]. However, in contradistinction to these studies, another recent study of 359 patients reported that anatomic site was an important factor in biopsy accuracy, spine biopsies having the lowest accuracy rate (61 %) [31]. Another study reported a large variation by anatomic site, with accuracy rates as low as 33 % for abdominal wall lesions and as high as 100 % for sites in the extremities such as the forearm and foot [36]. The difference by anatomic location reported in some studies is likely due the technical difficulty of accessing some sites, such as the spine. Recent studies suggesting that axial and extremity biopsies have similar accuracies may be a reflection of improvements in imaging guidance that help overcome these technical difficulties.

A number of studies have demonstrated that lesion type is one of the most important factors in determining biopsy accuracy. The general rule is that diagnostic yield from highest to lowest is metastatic, primary malignant neoplasm, primary benign tumor, and nonneoplastic lesions [54]. In addition, biopsies of bone lesions with soft-tissue components have a higher diagnostic accuracy (approximately 90 %) than those of lytic lesions (less than 85 %) [52, 53]. Primary bone tumors that are sclerotic are particularly difficult to diagnose accurately because of their low cellularity, and some studies have reported accuracies less than 70 % [52]. Other lesions that are difficult to diagnose are those with hemorrhage or fluid levels, chondroid lesions, and fibrous tumors [53]. Low rates of positive culture in cases of infectious lesions may be due to antibiotic treatment prior to biopsy.

As previously noted, institutions that do not have a dedicated team of surgeons, interventionalists, and pathologists may have less than optimal accuracy for their diagnostic biopsy studies. The integration of treatment and diagnostic teams allows for discussion and planning for difficult cases, especially if the biopsy results are disputable. Ultimately, this coordination of teams allows a seamless process of selecting appropriate patients, performing the biopsy, providing histopathologic analysis, and subsequently managing the continued care of the patient [4, 22, 23]. In institutions that do not have these teams and protocols, the risk for complications may be as much as two to ten times greater [24–26].

In general, the reported accuracies of CNB have been well over 50 %, approaching 100 % in some studies [20]. The reported accuracy of FNA has been more variable, ranging from as low as 23 % to over 97 %. It has been suggested that the lower accuracy for FNA does not necessarily translate into suboptimal clinical outcomes because, for the inconclusive cases, approximately 75 % are sampled from lesions suspected to be benign [47]. As previously noted, FNA and CNB are considered complementary, and many institutions are now using both needle types to sample the same lesion. A recent study by Schweitzer et al. reported that for a cohort of 138 consecutive patients who had both CNB and FNA, the diagnosis was made by CNB only in 17 and by FNA only in 11 [47]. They concluded that having both a cytopathologic and a histopathologic specimen often increases diagnostic accuracy and that both should be performed routinely. Similarly, Ogilvie et al. reported that the clinical utility of CNB and FNA were 67 and 68 %, respectively, when used alone, but 81 % when used together [46].

Optimizing quality of biopsy guidance is a function of using proper indications for choosing the imaging modality. The guidelines for imaging continue to change as the technologies and techniques for the modalities improve. Recently, MRI has been introduced as another potential imaging modality for biopsy guidance. MRI has not been more widely adopted in part because the high-field, closed-bore MRI systems afford only limited access to the patient. Open MRI systems, such as the C-arm or double-doughnut configurations, allow interventionalists to manipulate needles with real-time feedback [59] but offer lower field strength and homogeneity and poorer image quality. Recent technical studies suggest that optical tracking or augmented reality systems have the potential to break down the barriers between patient access and high quality in MRI-guided procedures by allowing imaging data to be first collected in the bore of a conventional superconducting magnet and then projected onto the patient once they are outside the bore (Fig. 24.4) [60–65]. Although no clinical studies have reported the applicability and accuracy of these approaches,

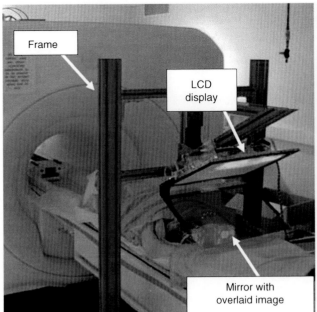

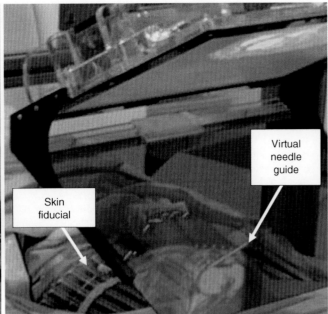

Fig. 24.4 These images show the setup of an augmented reality MRI system currently being tested using phantom models. After an initial scan, the phantom or patient is removed from the scanner bore and an overlay image is projected such that it appears that an axial cut was made through the phantom. This design will allow the MR image, needle, and insertion plan all to be rendered in a single view and will give the operators visual guidance during the procedure without turning attention away from the operative field

biopsy of tumors in the extremities is well suited for this approach because the limb can be immobilized to ensure the projected image accurately represents the true underlying anatomy.

Summary

- Percutaneous image-guided biopsy of the appendicular skeleton is a safe, effective, and accurate tool utilized in histologic analysis for distinguishing among infectious, neoplastic, and tumor-like musculoskeletal lesions.
- There are relatively few contraindications for percutaneous biopsy of the extremities, but caution should be used in patients who have severe coagulopathy or thrombocytopenia, lack a safe biopsy tract, or have compromised cardiopulmonary function or hemodynamic instability.
- Depending on lesion characteristics and patient considerations, appendicular skeleton biopsy can be guided by fluoroscopy, ultrasound, CT, or MR imaging.
- FNA and CNB are considered complementary, and both needle types are frequently utilized to sample the same lesion.
- The relationship of the biopsy tract to neurovascular structures, tissue planes, and future surgery approaches must be thoroughly considered prior to biopsy.
- The reported accuracy of biopsies of the extremities is over 90 % from some institutions that have dedicated teams of surgeons, radiologists, and pathologists.

References

1. Martin HE, Ellis EB. Biopsy by needle puncture and aspiration. Ann Surg. 1930;92:169–81.
2. Kavanagh EC, Roberts CC, Frangos A, et al. Musculoskeletal biopsy: utilization and provider distribution in the United States Medicare population. Acad Radiol. 2007;14:371–5.
3. Welker JA, Henshaw RM, Jelinek J, Shmookler BM, Malawer MM. The percutaneous needle biopsy is safe and recommended in the diagnosis of musculoskeletal masses. Cancer. 2000;89:2677–86.
4. Mankin HJ, Mankin CJ, Simon MA. The hazards of the biopsy, revisited. Members of the Musculoskeletal Tumor Society. J Bone Joint Surg Am. 1996;78:656–63.
5. Fraser-Hill MA, Renfrew DL, Hilsenrath PE. Percutaneous needle biopsy of musculoskeletal lesions. 2. Cost-effectiveness. AJR Am J Roentgenol. 1992;158:813–18.
6. Skrzynski MC, Biermann JS, Montag A, Simon MA. Diagnostic accuracy and charge-savings of outpatient core needle biopsy compared with open biopsy of musculoskeletal tumors. J Bone Joint Surg Am. 1996;78:644–9.
7. Murphy WA. Radiologically guided percutaneous musculoskeletal biopsy. Orthop Clin North Am. 1983;14:233–41.
8. Simon MA. Biopsy of musculoskeletal tumors. J Bone Joint Surg Am. 1982;64:1253–7.
9. Nourbakhsh A, Grady JJ, Garges KJ. Percutaneous spine biopsy: a meta-analysis. J Bone Joint Surg Am. 2008;90:1722–5.
10. Bellaiche L, Hamze B, Parlier-Cuau C, Laredo JD. Percutaneous biopsy of musculoskeletal lesions. Semin Musculoskelet Radiol. 1997;1:177–88.
11. Ghelman B. Biopsies of the musculoskeletal system. Radiol Clin North Am. 1998;36:567–80.
12. McCarthy EF. CT-guided needle biopsies of bone and soft tissue tumors: a pathologist's perspective. Skeletal Radiol. 2007;36:181–2.

13. Kilpatrick SE, Cappellari JO, Bos GD, Gold SH, Ward WG. Is fine-needle aspiration biopsy a practical alternative to open biopsy for the primary diagnosis of sarcoma? Experience with 140 patients. Am J Clin Pathol. 2001;115:59–68.

14. Issakov J, Flusser G, Kollender Y, Merimsky O, Lifschitz-Mercer B, Meller I. Computed tomography-guided core needle biopsy for bone and soft tissue tumors. Isr Med Assoc J. 2003;5:28–30.

15. Mitsuyoshi G, Naito N, Kawai A, et al. Accurate diagnosis of musculoskeletal lesions by core needle biopsy. J Surg Oncol. 2006; 94:21–7.

16. White LM, Schweitzer ME, Deely DM, Gannon F. Study of osteomyelitis: utility of combined histologic and microbiologic evaluation of percutaneous biopsy samples. Radiology. 1995;197:840–2.

17. Beaule V, Laredo JD, Cywiner C, Bard M, Tubiana JM. Synovial membrane: percutaneous biopsy. Radiology. 1990;177:581–5.

18. Parlier-Cuau C, Hamze B, Champsaur P, Nizard R, Laredo JD. Percutaneous biopsy of the synovial membrane. Semin Musculoskelet Radiol. 1997;1:189–96.

19. Lind SE. Prolonged bleeding time. Am J Med. 1984;77:305–12.

20. Kattapuram SV, Rosenthal DI. Percutaneous biopsy of skeletal lesions. AJR Am J Roentgenol. 1991;157:935–42.

21. Long BW. Image-guided percutaneous needle biopsy: an overview. Radiol Technol. 2000;71:335–59.

22. Ward WG Sr, Kilpatrick S. Fine needle aspiration biopsy of primary bone tumors. Clin Orthop Relat Res. 2000;373:80–87.

23. Torriani M, Etchebehere M, Amstalden E. Sonographically guided core needle biopsy of bone and soft tissue tumors. J Ultrasound Med. 2002;21:275–81.

24. Mankin HJ, Lange TA, Spanier SS. THE CLASSIC: The hazards of biopsy in patients with malignant primary bone and soft-tissue tumors. The Journal of Bone and Joint Surgery, 1982;64: 1121–1127. Clin Orthop Relat Res. 2006;450:4–10.

25. Simon MA, Finn HA. Diagnostic strategy for bone and soft-tissue tumors. J Bone Joint Surg Am. 1993;75:622–31.

26. Simon MA, Finn HA. Diagnostic strategy for bone and soft-tissue tumors. Instr Course Lect. 1994;43:527–36.

27. Bacci G, Ferrari S, Bertoni F, et al. Long-term outcome for patients with nonmetastatic osteosarcoma of the extremity treated at the Istituto Ortopedico Rizzoli according to the Istituto Ortopedico Rizzoli/osteosarcoma-2 protocol: an updated report. J Clin Oncol. 2000;18:4016–27.

28. Ferrari S, Smeland S, Mercuri M, et al. Neoadjuvant chemotherapy with high-dose Ifosfamide, high-dose methotrexate, cisplatin, and doxorubicin for patients with localized osteosarcoma of the extremity: a joint study by the Italian and Scandinavian Sarcoma Groups. J Clin Oncol. 2005;23:8845–52.

29. Grimer RJ. Surgical options for children with osteosarcoma. Lancet Oncol. 2005;6:85–92.

30. Clark CR, Morgan C, Sonstegard DA, Matthews LS. The effect of biopsy-hole shape and size on bone strength. J Bone Joint Surg Am. 1977;59:213–17.

31. Hau A, Kim I, Kattapuram S, et al. Accuracy of CT-guided biopsies in 359 patients with musculoskeletal lesions. Skeletal Radiol. 2002;31:349–53.

32. Telfer N. Nuclear medicine in the management of musculoskeletal tumors. Orthop Clin North Am. 1977;8:1011–21.

33. Murphy WA, Destouet JM, Gilula LA. Percutaneous skeletal biopsy 1981: a procedure for radiologists–results, review, and recommendations. Radiology. 1981;139:545–9.

34. Choi JJ, Davis KW, Blankenbaker DG. Percutaneous musculoskeletal biopsy. Semin Roentgenol. 2004;39:114–28.

35. Ahrar K, Himmerich JU, Herzog CE, et al. Percutaneous ultrasound-guided biopsy in the definitive diagnosis of osteosarcoma. J Vasc Interv Radiol. 2004;15:1329–33.

36. Altuntas AO, Slavin J, Smith PJ, et al. Accuracy of computed tomography guided core needle biopsy of musculoskeletal tumours. ANZ J Surg. 2005;75:187–91.

37. Krause ND, Haddad ZK, Winalski CS, Ready JE, Nawfel RD, Carrino JA. Musculoskeletal biopsies using computed tomography fluoroscopy. J Comput Assist Tomogr. 2008;32:458–62.

38. Carrino JA, Khurana B, Ready JE, Silverman SG, Winalski CS. Magnetic resonance imaging-guided percutaneous biopsy of musculoskeletal lesions. J Bone Joint Surg Am. 2007;89:2179–87.

39. Neuerburg JM, Adam G, Hunter D. New trends in musculoskeletal interventional radiology: percutaneous, MR-guided skeletal biopsy. Semin Musculoskelet Radiol. 1997;1:339–48.

40. Carrasco CH, Wallace S, Richli WR. Percutaneous skeletal biopsy. Cardiovasc Intervent Radiol. 1991;14:69–72.

41. Civardi G, Livraghi T, Colombo P, Fornari F, Cavanna L, Buscarini L. Lytic bone lesions suspected for metastasis: ultrasonically guided fine-needle aspiration biopsy. J Clin Ultrasound. 1994; 22:307–11.

42. Yeow KM, Tan CF, Chen JS, Hsueh C. Diagnostic sensitivity of ultrasound-guided needle biopsy in soft tissue masses about superficial bone lesions. J Ultrasound Med. 2000;19:849–55.

43. Haaga JR. New techniques for CT-guided biopsies. AJR Am J Roentgenol. 1979;133:633–41.

44. Hardy DC, Murphy WA, Gilula LA. Computed tomography in planning percutaneous bone biopsy. Radiology. 1980;134:447–50.

45. Hodge JC. Percutaneous biopsy of the musculoskeletal system: a review of 77 cases. Can Assoc Radiol J. 1999;50:121–5.

46. Ogilvie CM, Torbert JT, Finstein JL, Fox EJ, Lackman RD. Clinical utility of percutaneous biopsies of musculoskeletal tumors. Clin Orthop Relat Res. 2006;450:95–100.

47. Schweitzer ME, Gannon FH, Deely DM, O'Hara BJ, Juneja V. Percutaneous skeletal aspiration and core biopsy: complementary techniques. AJR Am J Roentgenol. 1996;166:415–18.

48. White LM, Schweitzer ME, Deely DM. Coaxial percutaneous needle biopsy of osteolytic lesions with intact cortical bone. AJR Am J Roentgenol. 1996;166:143–4.

49. Davies NM, Livesley PJ, Cannon SR. Recurrence of an osteosarcoma in a needle biopsy track. J Bone Joint Surg Br. 1993;75: 977–8.

50. Schwartz HS, Spengler DM. Needle tract recurrences after closed biopsy for sarcoma: three cases and review of the literature. Ann Surg Oncol. 1997;4:228–36.

51. Liu PT, Valadez SD, Chivers FS, Roberts CC, Beauchamp CP. Anatomically based guidelines for core needle biopsy of bone tumors: implications for limb-sparing surgery. Radiographics. 2007;27:189–205; discussion 206.

52. Logan PM, Connell DG, O'Connell JX, Munk PL, Janzen DL. Image-guided percutaneous biopsy of musculoskeletal tumors: an algorithm for selection of specific biopsy techniques. AJR Am J Roentgenol. 1996;166:137–41.

53. Jelinek J, Buick M, Shmookler B. Image-guided percutaneous biopsies of musculoskeletal lesions. AJR Am J Roentgenol. 1996;167:532–3.

54. Tsukushi S, Katagiri H, Nakashima H, Shido Y, Arai E. Application and utility of computed tomography-guided needle biopsy with musculoskeletal lesions. J Orthop Sci. 2004;9:122–5.

55. Ayala AG, Zornosa J. Primary bone tumors: percutaneous needle biopsy. Radiologic-pathologic study of 222 biopsies. Radiology. 1983;149:675–9.

56. Puri A, Shingade VU, Agarwal MG, et al. CT-guided percutaneous core needle biopsy in deep seated musculoskeletal lesions: a prospective study of 128 cases. Skeletal Radiol. 2006; 35:138–43.

57. Barth Jr RJ, Merino MJ, Solomon D, Yang JC, Baker AR. A prospective study of the value of core needle biopsy and fine needle aspiration in the diagnosis of soft tissue masses. Surgery. 1992;112:536–43.

58. Fraser-Hill MA, Renfrew DL. Percutaneous needle biopsy of musculoskeletal lesions. 1. Effective accuracy and diagnostic utility. AJR Am J Roentgenol. 1992;158:809–12.

59. Lewin JS, Petersilge CA, Hatem SF, et al. Interactive MR imaging-guided biopsy and aspiration with a modified clinical C-arm system. AJR Am J Roentgenol. 1998;170:1593–601.

60. Fischer GS, Deguet A, Csoma C, et al. MRI image overlay: application to arthrography needle insertion. Comput Aided Surg. 2007;12:2–14.

61. Fischer GS, Deguet A, Schlattman D, et al. MRI image overlay: applications to arthrography needle insertion. Stud Health Technol Inform. 2006;119:150–5.

62. Fischer GS, Dyer E, Csoma C, Deguet A, Fichtinger G. Validation system of MR image overlay and other needle insertion techniques. Stud Health Technol Inform. 2007; 125:130–5.

63. Fischer GS, Taylor RH. Electromagnetic tracker measurement error simulation and tool design. Med Image Comput Comput Assist Interv. 2005;8:73–80.

64. George S, Kesavadas T. Low cost augmented reality for training of MRI-guided needle biopsy of the spine. Stud Health Technol Inform. 2008;132:138–40.

65. Ojala R, Sequeiros RB, Klemola R, Vahala E, Jyrkinen L, Tervonen O. MR-guided bone biopsy: preliminary report of a new guiding method. J Magn Reson Imaging. 2002;15:82–6.

Index

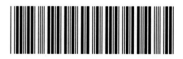